MENOPAUSE PRACTICE

A CLINICIAN'S GUIDE

5th EDITION

MENOPAUSE PRACTICE

A CLINICIAN'S GUIDE

5th EDITION

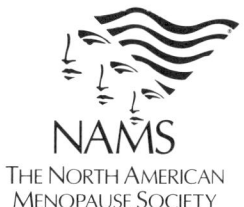

The North American Menopause Society

Mayfield Heights, Ohio

© 2014 North American Menopause Society

The North American Menopause Society
5900 Landerbook Drive, Suite 390
Mayfield Heights, OH 44124, USA
Tel: 440-442-7550
Fax: 440-442-2660
E-mail: info@menopause.org
Web: www.menopause.org

All rights reserved. No part of this publication may be reproduced in any form or by any means, electronic or mechanical, including photocopy, recording, or any information storage and retrieval system, without written permission from the publisher.

Although every effort has been made to ensure that all owners of copyrighted material have been acknowledged in this publication, we would be glad to acknowledge in subsequent reprints or editions any omissions brought to our attention.

The information presented in this clinician's guide is provided as a compilation of the existing state of knowledge on the subject matter. It is not meant to substitute for a provider's experience and judgment brought to each clinical situation.

The field of menopause management is constantly changing. As with all reference resources, this guide reflects the best understanding of the science of menopause management at the time of publication, but it should be used with the clear understanding that continuing research and clinical experience may result in new knowledge.

Cover design by Brent Stowe
ISBN 978-0-692-26135-4
Printed in the United States of America

CONTENTS

Contributors and Acknowledgments vii

Continuing Medical Education (CME) Information and Disclosures xv

Preface xvii

1 Menopause 1
Overview of menopause 1
    Demographics 1
    Quality of life 1
    Menopause terminology 2
Ovarian aging and hormone production 3
    Stages of reproductive aging 3
    Menopause transition overview 6
Hypothalamic-pituitary-ovarian axis 9
Adrenal physiology and menopause 10
Receptor activity 11
    Estrogen receptors 11
    Progesterone receptors 12
    Androgen receptors 12
Premature menopause and primary ovarian insufficiency 12

2 Midlife Body Changes 21
Vulvovaginal changes 21
Body weight 22
Skin 27
Hair 31
Eyes 34
Ears 37
Teeth and oral cavity 37

3 Clinical Issues 45
Decline in fertility 45
Uterine bleeding 47
Vasomotor symptoms 55
Genitourinary syndrome of menopause 60
Other vulvar and vaginal clinical issues 63
Other urinary tract clinical issues 68
Sexual function 73
Sleep disturbances 79
Headache 82
Cognition 85
Psychological symptoms 87
Sexually transmitted infections 92

4 Disease Risk 107
Cardiovascular health 107
Diabetes mellitus 116
Osteoporosis 121
Gallbladder disease 132
Arthritis and arthralgia 133
Thyroid disease 136
Epilepsy 139
Asthma 140
Cancer 141
    Breast cancer 141
    Endometrial cancer 148
    Cervical cancer 153
    Ovarian cancer 154
    Lung cancer 158
    Colorectal cancer 158
    Pancreatic cancer 161
    Skin cancer 162

5 Clinical Evaluation and Counseling 181
History gathering 181
Physical examination 183
Identification of modifiable health-risk factors 186
Diagnostic and screening tests 188
Counseling issues 193
Quality-of-life assessment tools 201

6 Complementary and Alternative Medicine 207
Integrative medicine 207
Whole medical systems 208
- Naturopathy and homeopathy 208
- Chinese medicine 209
- Ayurveda 211
- Yoga 211

Biologically based practices 212
- Isoflavones 212
- Herbal therapies 216

Safety 221

7 Nonprescription Options 227
Government regulation of dietary supplements 227
Vitamins and minerals 229
- Vitamins 230
- Minerals 237

Other supplements 243
Over-the-counter hormones 246

8 Prescription Therapies 255
Contraceptives 255
Estrogen therapy and estrogen-progestogen therapy 263
Selective estrogen-receptor modulators 280
Selective serotonin-reuptake inhibitors and serotonin norepinephrine-reuptake inhibitors 282
Androgens 282

Appendix: How to Evaluate Scientific Literature 289

Index 293

Continuing Medical Education (CME) Activity 305
Self-assessment examination 305
Answer sheet 309

CONTRIBUTORS AND ACKNOWLEDGMENTS

NAMS greatly appreciates the efforts of all contributors to the content of this *Clinician's Guide*.

Sherihan H Allam, MD, MSc
Research Fellow, Dermatology Department
Cleveland Clinic
Cleveland, OH
Assistant Lecturer, Dermatology Department
Mansoura University, Egypt

Rebecca H Allen, MD, MPH
Assistant Professor of Obstetrics and Gynecology
Warren Alpert Medical School of Brown University
Women and Infants Hospital
Providence, RI

Gloria A Bachmann, MD
Interim Chair, Department of Obstetrics, Gynecology, and Reproductive Sciences
Associate Dean for Women's Health
Rutgers Robert Wood Johnson Medical School
New Brunswick, NJ

C Noel Bairey Merz, MD, FACC, FAHA
Women's Guild Endowed Chair in Women's Health
Director, Barbra Streisand Women's Heart Center
Director, Linda Joy Pollin Women's Heart Health Program
Director, Preventive Cardiac Center
Professor of Medicine
Cedars-Sinai Medical Center
Los Angeles, CA

Wilma F Bergfeld, MD, FAAD
Senior Dermatologist and Co-Director, Dermatopathology
Departments of Dermatology and Pathology
Cleveland Clinic
Cleveland, OH

Diana L Bitner, MD, NCMP, FACOG
Director, Midlife and Menopause Health Services
Spectrum Health Medical Group
Assistant Professor, Department of Obstetrics and Gynecology
Michigan State University, School of Human Medicine
Grand Rapids, MI

Joel A Block, MD
Willard L Wood, MD, Professor
Director, Division of Rheumatology
Rush Medical College
Rush University Medical Center
Chicago, IL

Frank Bonura, MD, FACOG, CCD, NCMP
Director, Obstetrics and Gynecology
Director, Osteoporosis Program
St Catherine of Siena Medical Center
Clinical Associate Professor, Obstetrics and Gynecology
State University of New York at Stony Brook
Stony Brook, NY

Mindy S Christianson, MD
Assistant Professor, Division of Reproductive Endocrinology and Infertility
Department of Gynecology and Obstetrics
Johns Hopkins University School of Medicine
Lutherville, MD

Thomas B Clarkson, DVM
Professor of Comparative Medicine
Wake Forest University School of Medicine
Winston-Salem, NC

Janine Austin Clayton, MD
Director, Office of Research on Women's Health
Associate Director for Research on Women's Health
National Institutes of Health
Bethesda, MD

Carolyn J Crandall, MD, MS, NCMP
Professor of Medicine
David Geffen School of Medicine at the University of California
Los Angeles, CA

Carrie Cwiak, MD, MPH
Director, Family Planning Division
Associate Professor of Gynecology and Obstetrics
Emory University School of Medicine
Atlanta, GA

Susan R Davis, MBBS, FRACP, PhD
Professor of Women's Health and NHMRC Principal
  Research Fellow
Director, the Women's Health Research Program
Department of Epidemiology and Preventive Medicine
School of Public Health and Preventive Medicine
Monash University
Melbourne, Vic, Australia

Dima L Diab, MD
Assistant Professor of Clinical Medicine and Associate
  Program Director
Director, University of Cincinnati Bone Health
  and Osteoporosis Center
Division of Endocrinology, Diabetes, and Metabolism
University of Cincinnati College of Medicine
Cincinnati, OH

Julia Schlam Edelman, MD, FACOG, NCMP
Consultant, Massachusetts General Hospital, Boston
Clinical Instructor, Harvard Medical School
Adjunct Clinical Instructor, Brown Medical School
Providence, RI
Private Practice
Middleboro, MA

Bernard A Eskin MS, MD
Professor of Obstetrics and Gynecology
Drexel University College of Medicine
Philadelphia, PA

Robert R Freedman, PhD
Professor, Departments of Psychiatry and Obstetrics
  and Gynecology
Director, Behavioral Medicine
Wayne State University School of Medicine
Detroit, MI

Ruth Freeman, MD
Professor of Medicine and Obstetrics and Gynecology
Montefiore Medical Center
Albert Einstein College of Medicine of Yeshiva University
Bronx, NY

Steven R Goldstein, MD, FACOG, CCD, NCMP
Professor of Obstetrics and Gynecology
New York University School of Medicine
New York, NY

Susan Goldstein, MD, CCFP, FCFP, NCMP
Course Director, Family Medicine Longitudinal Experience
Assistant Professor
Department of Family and Community Medicine
University of Toronto
Toronto, Ontario, Canada

George I Gorodeski, MD, MSc, PhD, NCMP
Professor Emeritus
Case Western Reserve University
Cleveland, OH

Jeffrey M Gould, LAc
Johns Hopkins Integrative Medicine and Digestive Center
Lutherville, MD

George Helmrich, MD, CCD, NCMP
Clinical Assistant Professor
University of South Carolina School
  of Medicine-Greenville
Department of Obstetrics and Gynecology,
  Greenville Health System
Greenville, SC
Chief Medical Officer
Baptist Easley Hospital
Easley, SC

Victor W Henderson, MD, MS, NCMP
Professor of Health Research and Policy (Epidemiology)
  and Neurology and Neurological Sciences
Chief, Division of Epidemiology
Stanford University
Stanford, CA

Catherine A Henry, MD, FACP
Head and Neck Institute
Cleveland Clinic
Cleveland, OH

Andrew G Herzog, MD, MSc
Professor of Neurology, Harvard Medical School
Director, Neuroendocrine Unit
Beth Israel Deaconess Medical Center
Boston, MA

David A Hutchins, MD, NCMP
Clinical Associate Professor, General Obstetrics
  and Gynecology
Co-Director, Center for Vulvar Disorders
University of Arkansas for Medical Sciences
Little Rock, AR

Michelle Inkster, MD, PhD, FACG
Staff Gastroenterologist
Department of Gastroenterology and Hepatology
Cleveland Clinic
Cleveland, OH

Nancy Roberson Jasper, MD, FACOG, NCMP
Assistant Clinical Professor
Department of Obstetrics and Gynecology
Columbia University Medical Center
New York, NY

Xuezhi (Daniel) Jiang, MD, FACOG, NCMP
Assistant Professor of Obstetrics and Gynecology
Jefferson Medical College of Thomas Jefferson University
Faculty Associate and Clerkship Director,
  Department of Obstetrics and Gynecology
Reading Health System
West Reading, PA

Hadine Joffe, MD, MSc
Associate Professor, Harvard Medical School
Director, Women's Hormone and Aging Research Program
Director of Research Development, Department
  of Psychiatry
Brigham and Women's Hospital
Director, Psycho-Oncology Research
Department of Psychosocial Oncology and Palliative Care
Dana Farber Cancer Institute
Boston, MA

Risa Kagan, MD, FACOG, CCD, NCMP
Clinical Professor
Department of Obstetrics, Gynecology,
  and Reproductive Sciences
University of California San Francisco
Sutter East Bay Physicians Medical Foundation
Berkeley, CA

Andrew M Kaunitz, MD, NCMP
Professor and Associate Chair, Department of Obstetrics
  and Gynecology
Associate Program Director, Residency Program
  in Obstetrics and Gynecology
University of Florida College of Medicine
Jacksonville, FL

Fredi Kronenberg, PhD
Consulting Professor, Department of Anesthesia
Stanford University School of Medicine
Stanford, CA

Michael L Krychman, MD
Executive Director
Southern California Center for Sexual Health
  and Survivorship Medicine
Newport Beach, CA

Shelagh B Larson, MS, RNC, WHNP, NCMP
Faculty, Department of Obstetrics and Gynecology
University of North Texas Health Science Center
Fort Worth, TX

James H Liu, MD
Arthur H Bill Professor and Chair
Department of Obstetrics and Gynecology
University Hospitals Case Medical Center
MacDonald Women's Hospital
Department of Reproductive Biology
Case Western Reserve University School of Medicine
Cleveland, OH

Tieraona Low Dog, MD
Fellowship Director, Arizona Center for Integrative
  Medicine
Clinical Associate Professor, Department of Medicine
University of Arizona Health Sciences
Tucson, AZ

Kathryn Macaulay, MD
Clinical Professor
Director, University of California San Diego
  Menopause Health Program
Department of Reproductive Medicine
University of California San Diego Medical Center
San Diego, CA

JoAnn E Manson, MD, DrPH, NCMP
Professor of Medicine and the Michael and Lee Bell
  Professor of Women's Health
Harvard Medical School
Chief of Preventive Medicine
Co-Director, Connors Center for Women's Health
  and Gender Biology
Brigham and Women's Hospital
Boston, MA

Mark G Martens, MD, NCMP
Chair, Department of Obstetrics and Gynecology
Director, Division of OB-GYN Infectious Diseases
Jersey Shore University Medical Center
Vice-Chair and Clinical Professor
Rutgers Robert Wood Johnson Medical School
Neptune, NJ

Susan C Modesitt, MD, FACOG, FACS
Director, Gynecologic Oncology Division
Co-Director, High Risk Breast/Ovarian Cancer Clinic
Richard N and Louise R Crockett Professor of Obstetrics
  and Gynecology
University of Virginia Health System
Charlottesville, VA

Anne Moore, DNP, APN, WHNP/ANP-BC, FAANP
Nurse Practitioner
Department of Family Health and Wellness
Tennessee Department of Health
Nashville, TN

Jeri W Nieves, PhD
Associate Professor of Clinical Epidemiology
Columbia University
Director, Bone Density Testing
Clinical Research Center
Helen Hayes Hospital
West Haverstraw, NY

Joan Otomo-Corgel, DDS, MPH, FACD
Clinical Associate Professor
University of California Los Angeles School of Dentistry
Department of Periodontics
Faculty, Greater Los Angeles VA Health Care Center
Los Angeles, CA

Diane T Pace, PhD, FNP-BC, NCMP, FAANP
Clinical Associate Professor
University of Memphis/Loewenberg School of Nursing
Memphis, TN

Bruce Patsner, MD, JD
Global Safety Officer
Pharmacovigilance and Epidemiology
Genzyme
Cambridge, MA
Affiliate Scholar, Chicago-Kent School of Law
Chicago, IL

Rebecca B Perkins, MD, MSc
Assistant Professor of Obstetrics and Gynecology
Boston University School of Medicine/Boston Medical Center
Boston, MA

Nancy A Phillips, MD
Clinical Assistant Professor, Department of Obstetrics, Gynecology, and Reproductive Science
Rutgers Robert Wood Johnson Medical School
New Brunswick, NJ

JoAnn V Pinkerton, MD, NCMP
Professor of Obstetrics and Gynecology
Director, Midlife Health
University of Virginia Health Sciences Center
Charlottesville, VA

Brenda Powell, MD, ABIHM
Clinical Faculty, Family Medicine University of Washington
Associate Medical Director, Integrative Medicine
University of Washington Neighborhood Clinics
Consultant, Cleveland Clinic Wellness Institute
Cleveland, OH

Beth A Prairie, MD, MPH
Assistant Professor of Obstetrics and Gynecology
Temple University School of Medicine
The Western Pennsylvania Hospital
Pittsburgh, PA

Dana L Redick, MD
Associate Professor
Department of Obstetrics and Gynecology— Generalist Division
University of Virginia
Charlottesville, VA

Laurel Rice, MD
Ben Miller Peckham, MD, PhD, Distinguished Professor and Chair
Department of Obstetrics and Gynecology
University of Wisconsin School of Medicine and Public Health
Madison, WI

Sheila M Rice Dane, MD, FACP, NCMP
Staff Physician, Department of Community Internal Medicine
Medicine Institute, Cleveland Clinic Foundation
Associate Professor of Medicine
Cleveland Clinic Lerner College of Medicine of Case Western Reserve University
Cleveland, OH

Gloria Richard-Davis, MD, FACOG
Professor and Division Director
Reproductive Endocrinology and Infertility
Department of Obstetrics and Gynecology
University of Arkansas Medical Sciences
Little Rock, AR

Marcie K Richardson, MD, NCMP
Director, Harvard Vanguard Menopause Consultation Service
Assistant Professor, Obstetrics, Gynecology, and Reproductive Medicine
Harvard Medical School
Boston, MA

Michelle Rindos, MD
Assistant Professor
Department of Obstetrics and Gynecology—
 Midlife Division
University of Virginia Health System
Charlottesville, VA

David E. Rogers, MD, MBA
Assistant Professor, Department of Obstetrics
 and Gynecology
University of Texas Southwestern Medical Center
Dallas, TX

Nanette Santoro, MD
Professor and E Stewart Taylor Chair of Obstetrics
 and Gynecology
University of Colorado School of Medicine
Aurora, CO

Kristi M Saunders, MD, MS, FACOG, NCMP
Hospice Medical Director
Lake Sunapee Region VNA and Hospice
Attending, Good Neighbors Neighborhood Clinic
New London, NH

Wen Shen, MD, MPH
Assistant Professor of Gynecology and Obstetrics
Johns Hopkins Medicine
Johns Hopkins Integrative Medicine Center
Baltimore, MD

Jan L Shifren, MD, NCMP
Associate Professor of Obstetrics, Gynecology,
 and Reproductive Biology
Harvard Medical School
Director, Massachusetts General Midlife Women's
 Health Center
Massachusetts General Hospital
Boston, MA

Chrisandra Shufelt, MD, MS, FACP, NCMP
Associate Director, Barbra Streisand Women's Heart
 Center and Preventive and Rehabilitative Cardiac Center
Director, Women's Hormone and Menopause Program
Assistant Professor, Cedars-Sinai Medical Center
Los Angeles, CA

Andrea Sikon, MD, FACP, NCMP
Chair, Department of Internal Medicine, Medicine Institute
Center for Specialized Women's Health, Women's
 Health Institute
Director, Staff Mentorship Program
Associate Professor of Medicine, Cleveland Clinic Lerner
 COM of Case Western Reserve University
Cleveland, OH

Barbara A Soltes, MD, NCMP
Associate Professor, Department of Obstetrics
 and Gynecology
Division of Reproductive Endocrinology
Rush Presbyterian St Luke's Medical Center
Chicago, IL

Carrie Sopata, MD
Assistant Professor
Department of Obstetrics and Gynecology—
 Generalist Division
University of Virginia
Charlottesville, VA

Sahar M Stephens, MD
Clinical Fellow, Reproductive Endocrinology
 and Infertility
University of Colorado School of Medicine
Aurora, CO

Cynthia A Stuenkel, MD, NCMP
Clinical Professor of Medicine, Endocrinology,
 and Metabolism
University of California, San Diego
La Jolla, CA

Eliza L Sutton, MD, FACP
Associate Professor, General Internal Medicine
Medical Director, Women's Health Care Center
University of Washington
Seattle, WA

Holly L Thacker, MD, FACP, CCD, NCMP
Professor and Director, Center for Specialized
 Women's Health
OB-GYN and Women's Health Institute
Cleveland Clinic Lerner College of Medicine of CWRU
Executive Director, Speaking of Women's Health
Cleveland, OH

Wulf H Utian, MD, PhD, DSc(Med)
Professor Emeritus
Case Western Reserve University School of Medicine
Cleveland, OH

Victor G Vogel, MD, MHS
Director, Breast Medical Oncology/Research
Geisinger Health System
Danville, PA

L Elaine Waetjen, MD
Professor, Department of Obstetrics and Gynecology
University of California Davis Medical Center
Sacramento, CA

Nelson Watts, MD
Director, Mercy Health Osteoporosis and Bone
 Health Services
Cincinnati, OH

Melissa Wellons, MD, MHS
Assistant Professor, Medicine-Division of Diabetes,
 Endocrinology, and Metabolism
Vanderbilt University Medical Center
Nashville, TN

Robert A Wild, MD, PhD, MPH, NCMP
Professor of Obstetrics and Gynecology, Clinical
 Epidemiology and Biostatistics
Oklahoma University Health Sciences Center
Chief of Gynecology, VA Medical Center
Oklahoma City, OK

Barbara B Wilson, MD
Edward P Cawley Professor and Chair of Dermatology
University of Virginia Health System
Charlottesville, VA

Nancy Fugate Woods, PhD, RN, FAAN
Department of Biobehavioral Nursing
University of Washington School of Nursing
Seattle, WA

Tonita E Wroolie, PhD
Clinical Assistant Professor
Department of Psychiatry and Behavioral Science
Stanford School of Medicine
Stanford, CA

Manisha Yadav, MD, NCMP, CCD
Department of Internal Medicine
Palo Alto Medical Foundation
Sutter Health
Santa Clara, CA

Jeanne Young, MD
Department of Dermatology
University of Virginia Health System
Charlottesville, VA

Nese Yuksel, BScPharm, PharmD, FCSHP, NCMP
Associate Professor, Faculty of Pharmacy
 and Pharmaceutical Sciences
University of Alberta
Edmonton, Alberta, Canada

Acknowledgments

NAMS extends great appreciation for the review and approval of the voting members of the 2013-2014 NAMS Board of Trustees.

Jan L Shifren, MD, NCMP, *President*
Associate Professor of Obstetrics, Gynecology,
 and Reproductive Biology
Harvard Medical School
Director, Massachusetts General Midlife Women's
 Health Center
Massachusetts General Hospital
Boston, MA

Pauline M Maki, PhD, *President-Elect*
Professor of Psychiatry and Psychology
Director, Women's Mental Health Research
Research Director, UIC Center for Research in Women
 and Gender
University of Illinois at Chicago
Chicago, IL

Diane T Pace, PhD, FNP-BC, FAANP, NCMP
Immediate Past President
Clinical Associate Professor
University of Memphis/Loewenberg School of Nursing
Memphis, TN

Andrew M Kaunitz, MD, *Secretary*
Professor and Associate Chair
Department of Obstetrics and Gynecology
Associate Program Director, Residency Program
 in Obstetrics and Gynecology
University of Florida College of Medicine
Jacksonville, FL

Peter F Schnatz, DO, FACOG, FACP, NCMP
Treasurer
Associate Chair and Residency Program Director
Department of Obstetrics and Gynecology
The Reading Hospital
Reading, PA

Margery L.S. Gass, MD, NCMP
Executive Director
Consultant, Cleveland Clinic Center for Specialized
 Women's Health
Clinical Professor, Case Western Reserve University
 School of Medicine
Cleveland, OH

Howard N Hodis, MD
Harry J Bauer and Dorothy Bauer Rawlins Professor
  of Cardiology
Professor of Medicine and Preventive Medicine
Professor of Molecular Pharmacology and Toxicology
Director, Atherosclerosis Research Unit
Division of Cardiovascular Medicine
Keck School of Medicine
University of Southern California
Los Angeles, CA

Sheryl A Kingsberg, PhD
Chief, Division of Behavioral Medicine
University Hospitals Case Medical Center
MacDonald Women's Hospital
Professor, Departments of Reproductive Biology
  and Psychiatry
Case Western Reserve University School of Medicine
Cleveland, OH

James H Liu, MD
Arthur H Bill Professor and Chair
Department of Obstetrics and Gynecology
University Hospitals Case Medical Center
MacDonald Women's Hospital
Department of Reproductive Biology
Case Western Reserve University School of Medicine
Cleveland, OH

JoAnn E Manson, MD, DrPH, NCMP
Professor of Medicine and the Michael and Lee Bell
  Professor of Women's Health
Harvard Medical School
Chief of Preventive Medicine
Co-Director, Connors Center for Women's Health
  and General Biology
Brigham and Women's Hospital
Boston, MA

Gloria Richard-Davis, MD, FACOG
Professor and Division Director
Reproductive Endocrinology and Infertility
Department of Obstetrics and Gynecology
University of Arkansas Medical Sciences
Little Rock, AR

Marla Shapiro, MDCM, CCFP, MHSc,
  FRCP(C), FCFP, NCMP
Associate Professor
Department of Family and Community Medicine
University of Toronto
Toronto, Ontario, Canada

Lynnette Leidy Sievert, BSN, PhD
Professor, Department of Anthropology
University of Massachusetts, Amherst
Amherst, MA

Isaac Schiff, MD, *Ex Officio*
Joe Vincent Meigs Professor of Gynecology
Harvard Medical School
Chief, Vincent Obstetrics and Gynecology Service
Massachusetts General Hospital
Boston, MA

Wulf H Utian, MD, PhD, DSc(Med), *Ex Officio*
Professor Emeritus
Case Western Reserve University School of Medicine
Beachwood, OH

NAMS would also like to acknowledge the editorial contributions of Marjorie L. S. Gass, MD, NCMP, and NAMS Executive Director, and Kathy Method, MA, NAMS Project Manager, and the Continuing Medical Education contributions of Penny Allen, NAMS Education Manager.

NAMS is grateful to Noven Women's Health for the unrestricted educational grant that helps in part to defray development costs for this textbook. This company did not exercise any control over its content.

CONTINUING MEDICAL EDUCATION (CME) INFORMATION

This essential guide to menopause management for all healthcare professionals who treat or counsel women at midlife and beyond is certified as a continuing medical education (CME) activity.

Release date: October 15, 2014

Expiration date: October 15, 2017

The North American Menopause Society (NAMS) is accredited by the Accreditation Council for Continuing Medical Education (ACCME) to provide continuing medical education for physicians.

NAMS designates this activity for a maximum of 26.0 *AMA PRA Category 1 Credits™*.

On successful completion of the examination at the end of the text, physicians will receive CME credits, and other learners will receive a certificate of participation. Other learners should consult their professional licensing boards for information on the applicability and acceptance of continuing education credit for this activity

Learning objectives

At the conclusion of this activity, participants should be able to

- Initiate discussion with patients on menopause and healthy aging, including its effect on quality of life and sexuality
- Perform appropriate clinical assessments to diagnose conditions of menopause and aging, assess health risks, and identify any contraindications to medications
- Discuss a full range of management options with patients on the basis of their health risks, goals, and preferences
- Collaborate with other healthcare professionals to offer effective, individualized therapy for menopausal symptoms and conditions
- Instruct and encourage patients to achieve a healthy lifestyle

Grant support

This CME activity is supported in part by an unrestricted grant from Noven Women's Health.

Claiming CME credit

To claim CME credit, please read and study the entire *Clinician's Guide*, complete the examination and evaluation, and submit them to NAMS by the expiration date of October 15, 2017. Certificates will be issued to those who achieve a passing grade of 70%. The examination and evaluation with instructions on submission begin on page **305**.

Other learners will be issued a certificate of participation. The activity includes 11.5 hours of pharmacotherapeutics education, which will be noted on the certificate of participation. These learners should consult their professional licensing boards for information on the applicability and acceptance of continuing education credit for this activity.

Disclosures of Financial Interests

To maintain the independence of its CME activities and in accordance with the policies of ACCME, NAMS requires all persons in control of content of this activity (contributors, reviewers, and program staff) to disclose any financial relationships that they or their spouses or partners have had with any relevant commercial interests within the past 12 months. Any conflicts of interest were resolved before this activity was released with review of content by reviewers who had no conflicts of interest.

For the contributors

Dr. Bachman reports: Consultant/Advisory Board: TEVA; Royalties/Patents and Authorship: UpToDate. Dr. Bairey Merz reports: Consultant/Advisory Board: Gilead, Japanese Circulation Society; Grant/Research Support: Cardiac Research Institute, University of New Mexico, National Institutes of Health Special Emphasis Panel; Lectures, Mayo Foundation, Bryn Mawr Hospital, Practice Point Communications, Allegheny General Hospital, Duke University, Vox Media, Emory University, Preventive Cardiovascular Nurses Association, Kaiser Permanente, Garden State American Heart Association; Honorarium, University of California, San Francisco. Dr. Block reports: Royalties/Patents: GlaxoSmithKline, Daichii-Sankyo, Agios; Chair: Data and Safety Monitoring Board; Royalties (use of unique human chondrocyte cell lines): PLx Pharma. Dr. Christianson reports: Grant/Research Support: Ferring. Dr. Cwiak reports: Faculty Trainer: Merck; Grant/Research Support: Medicines 360; Royalties/Patents: Springer. Dr. Davis reports: Consultant/Advisory Board: Trimel; Grant/Research Support: Lawley. Dr. Susan Goldstein reports: Consultant/Advisory Board: Pfizer, AstraZeneca; Moderator Fee: Warner Chilcott, Merck. Dr. Joffe reports: Grant/Research Support: Cephalon, Noven, Sunovion. Dr. Kagan reports: Consultant/Advisory Board: Depomed, Merck, Noven, Novo Nordisk, Pfizer, Shionogi; Grant/Research Support: Therapeutics MD; Speakers Bureau: Noven, Novo Nordisk, Pfizer, Shionogi; Legal Consulting: Actavis, Merck. Dr. Kaunitz reports: Consultant/Advisory Board: Actavis, Bayer, Merck, Teva (contraception only); Grant/Research Support: Bayer, Endoceutics, Medical Diagnostic Laboratories, Noven, Teva, Trimel; Royalties/Patents: UpToDate. Dr. Krychman reports: Consultant/

Advisory Board: Bayer, Sprout, Pfizer, Palatin Technologies, Shionogi, Noven; Speakers Bureau: Bayer, Sprout, Pfizer, Palatin Technologies, Shionogi, Noven. Dr. Liu reports: Consultant/Advisory Board: Noven, Shionogi, Ferring, Pfizer. Dr. Low Dog reports: Consultant/Advisory Board: Pharmaca, Weil Lifestyle. Dr. Pace reports: Consultant/Advisory Board: Hologic, Pfizer. Dr. Pinkerton reports: Consultant/Advisory Board: Pfizer, Shionogi, Noven, Novo Nordisk; Grant/Research Support: Therapeutics, Endoceutics. Dr. Santoro reports Grant/Research Support: Bayer; Stock/Ownership: Menogenix. Dr. Shifren reports: Consultant/Advisory Board: New England Research Institutes; Royalties/Patents: UpToDate. Dr. Thacker reports: Consultant/Advisory Board: Noven, Pfizer, Myriad; Speakers Bureau: Novo Nordisk, Amgen, Shionogi, Novartis. Dr. Utian reports: Consultant/Advisory Board: Metagenics, Pharmavite, Primus Pharmaceuticals, SenoSENSE. Dr. Watts reports: Consultant/Advisory Board: AbbVie, Amarin, Amgen, Bristol-Meyers Squibb, Corcept, Endo, Imagepace, Janssen, Lilly, Merck, Novartis, Noven, Pfizer/Wyeth, Radius, Sanofi-Aventis; Grant/Research Support: Merck, NPS; Stock/Ownership/Royalties: OsteoDynamics; Honoraria: Amgen, Merck.

Dr. Allam, Dr. Allen, Dr. Bergfeld, Dr. Bitner, Dr. Bonura, Dr. Clarkson, Dr. Clayton, Dr. Crandall, Dr. Diab, Dr. Edelman, Dr. Eskin, Dr. Freedman, Dr. Freeman, Dr. Steven Goldstein, Dr. Gorodeski, Mr. Gould, Dr. Helmrich, Dr. Henderson, Dr. Henry, Dr. Herzog, Dr. Hutchins, Dr. Inkster, Dr. Jasper, Dr. Jiang, Dr. Kronenberg, Ms. Larson, Dr. Macaulay, Dr. Manson, Dr. Martens, Dr. Modesitt, Ms. Moore, Dr. Nieves, Dr. Otomo-Corgel, Dr. Patsner, Dr. Perkins, Dr. Phillips, Dr. Powell, Dr. Prairie, Dr. Redick, Dr. Rice, Dr. Rice Dane, Dr. Richardson, Dr. Rindos, Dr. Rogers, Dr. Saunders, Dr. Shen, Dr. Shufelt, Dr. Sikon, Dr. Soltes, Dr. Sopata, Dr. Stephens, Dr. Stuenkel, Dr. Sutton, Dr. Vogel, Dr. Waetjen, Dr. Wellons, Dr. Wild, Dr. Wilson, Dr. Woods, Dr. Wroolie, Dr. Yadav, Dr. Young, and Dr. Yuksel each reports: No relevant financial relationships.

For the 2013-2014 Board of Trustees who were not contributors

Dr. Maki reports: Consultant: Pfizer; Speaking Honorarium: Abbott. Dr. Schnatz reports: Board of Directors/Trustees: FaithCare. Dr. Kingsberg reports: Consultant/Advisory Board: Apricus, Emotional Brain, Novo Nordisk, Palatin, Pfizer, Shionogi, Sprout, SST, Teva, Trimel Biopharm, Viveve. Dr. Richard-Davis reports: Consultant/Advisory Board: Pfizer. Dr. Shapiro reports: Board of Directors/Trustees: Women's College Hospital, Research Canada, Dairy Farmers of Canada, Canadian Foundation for Women and Health; Employment: Consultant, CTV Canada AM, CTV National News, CTV NewsChannel, Parents Canada; Consultant/Advisory Board: Amgen, AstraZeneca, Merck, Novartis, Pfizer, Actavis; Speaker's Bureau: Amgen, Merck, Novartis, Novo Nordisk, Pfizer; Website Writer: CTV.ca, healthandbone.ca. Dr. Hodis, Dr. Sievert, and Dr. Schiff each reports: No relevant financial relationships.

For additional contributors

Dr. Gass, Ms. Method, and Ms. Allen report: No relevant financial relationships.

PREFACE

Welcome to the 5th edition of *Menopause Practice: A Clinician's Guide*. This edition brings you the most current information that clinicians need in order to provide excellent care for perimenopausal and postmenopausal women. It is available in print and digital formats.

Entirely new with this edition is the companion piece, *The North American Menopause Society Recommendations for Clinical Care of Midlife Women*, a set of key points and recommendations published separately in the October 2014 issue of our journal, *Menopause*. Thank you to Dr. Jan Shifren who served as Editor-in-Chief and spearheaded the publication of these recommendations.

This edition also serves as one of our leading educational initiatives, offering 26.0 hours of continuing medical education as well as 11.5 pharmacotherapeutics hours.

Many dedicated professionals have contributed to this edition. I want to thank the authors who gave generously of their time and expertise, the members of the Professional Education Committee who reviewed the chapters, and the Board of Trustees who reviewed and approved the final edition. A special word of gratitude goes to Ms. Kathy Method, medical writer and project manager.

Margery Gass, MD, NCMP
Executive Director
The North American Menopause Society

CHAPTER 1

Menopause

Overview of menopause

Menopause represents the permanent cessation of menses resulting from loss of ovarian follicular function, usually because of aging. Menopause is a normal, physiological event, defined as a woman's final menstrual period (FMP). Menopause can occur naturally (spontaneously)—on average around age 52—or be induced through a medical intervention (surgery, chemotherapy, or pelvic radiation therapy). Women have experienced menopause for thousands of years. The difference today is that most women live far beyond their menopause, not as in the past.

Aging is the natural progression of changes in structure and function that occur with the passage of time in the absence of known disease. Aging of the female reproductive system begins in utero at 20 weeks' gestation with regard to follicle atresia and proceeds as a continuum.[1] It consists of a steady loss of oocytes from atresia or ovulation and does not necessarily occur at a constant rate. Because of the relatively wide age range (40-58 y) for natural menopause, chronologic age is a poor indicator of the beginning or the end of the menopause transition.[2]

During the transition from the reproductive years through menopause and beyond, a woman experiences many physical changes, most of which are normal consequences of menopause and aging. Some of the physical changes observed around the time of menopause may be signs of illness that develop during midlife, such as diabetes mellitus (DM). Sometimes, health problems arise when changing hormone levels and the physical effects of aging are coupled with a person's genetic makeup, certain unhealthy lifestyles, and other stresses of midlife.

Accurate information about physiologic changes, management of menopause symptoms, and reducing disease risk is essential at midlife. Although menopause is perhaps the most obvious physical event, general knowledge about the aging process is also needed. Additionally, psychological support may be required for the many psychosocial issues women encounter in midlife.

Demographics

Menopause affects every woman, if she is fortunate enough to survive to middle adulthood. As the large baby-boom generation reaches midlife and beyond, an unprecedented number of women are postmenopausal. An estimated 6,000 US women reach menopause every day (more than 2 million per year). In addition, more women are living beyond age 65. Exact figures on the number of postmenopausal women and the number reaching menopause each year are difficult to obtain. There were an estimated 50 million postmenopausal women in the United States in 2010.[3] About 45 million of them were aged older than 52 years, the average age of natural menopause in the Western world. By the year 2020, the number of US women aged older than 51 years is expected to be more than 50 million.

Canadian statistics also demonstrate an increase in life expectancy for midlife women.[4] In 1922, a 50-year-old woman lived to be 75 years old, on average. Today, a woman the same age can expect to live until her mid-80s. By 2026, it is estimated that almost one-quarter (22%) of the Canadian population will be composed of women older than age 50. A woman's life expectancy in the Western world is estimated at 80.8 years, so women can expect to spend approximately a third of their lives beyond menopause.[5]

Quality of life

Survey research does not verify the concept of a "midlife crisis" as universal or even widely present in the general population. However, women in midlife may fear aging for a variety of reasons, some of which are universal, some peculiar to their culture, and the rest reflecting their personal and family circumstances. Women at midlife may be reacting to a multitude of financial, relationship, and care-giving changes that are common at this time of life and that can elicit fear and anxiety.

All women experience menopause, but each one does so in a unique way. How a woman responds to the physical changes of menopause may be similar to the way her mother responded, although the evidence to support this notion is limited.

Chapter 1

Lifestyle, demographic factors, and attitudes all influence a woman's perception of menopause.[6] The menopause experience is often perceived as merely the cessation of menses. A woman may view the end of fertility as liberation from the possibility of pregnancy, or she may grieve for the children she never had. For women who have had an unexpected early menopause, either natural or induced, their experience may be more negative. The level of menopause-related symptoms will also have an influence. Some women will have troublesome symptoms, whereas others may navigate the transition with few or even no symptoms at all.[7,8] Diverse social and cultural differences also can affect a woman's experience of menopause and her view of menopause treatments, as well as her overall health and well-being.[7,9]

Risk factors, patterns of disease and mortality, access to healthcare, economic status, existing medical therapies, and societal norms related to femininity and aging all differ across groups of women. There is very little research on how these differences affect the experience of menopause. To date, menopause research has focused mostly on middle-class white women. Although different populations are being studied, considerable information is needed before many aspects of menopause are better understood.[10]

In one study, 80% of women experiencing menopause reported no decrease in quality of life (QOL); 75% of the women denied experiencing any loss in their attractiveness.[11] Most (62%) women reported positive attitudes toward menopause itself. Another study showed that most women viewed menopause as inconsequential and suggested that other events of midlife were more important or stressful.[12] A cohort of well-educated, midlife women described the menopause transition as a normal developmental event.[13] Only about 10% of perimenopausal and postmenopausal women participating in community-based studies reported feelings of despair, irritability, or fatigue during the menopause transition.

The QOL and health status of a generally low-income and poorly educated population of menopause-aged women were examined in a cross-sectional study.[8] Women who were employed and had attained higher levels of education or income reported better overall health and fewer menopause symptoms. There were no significant differences between ethnic groups with respect to either menopause QOL or health status. Hysterectomy with bilateral oophorectomy did not seem to be a factor in decreasing QOL. Compared with women with an intact uterus, women who underwent hysterectomy expressed more improvement, especially in the areas of sexual relationships, spouse or partner relationships, personal fulfillment, and physical health. This improvement did not seem to be related to the use of menopausal hormone therapy (HT).

Most (51%) US postmenopausal women surveyed in a Gallup Poll reported being happiest and most fulfilled when aged between 50 and 65 years compared with when they were in their 20s (10%), 30s (17%), or 40s (16%).[14] Many women reported improvement in various aspects of their lives since menopause. They reported a sense of personal fulfillment, an ability to focus on hobbies or other interests, and improved relationships with their spouses or partners and with friends. Most (51%) said that their sexual relationships had remained unchanged. Lifestyle changes were often initiated during this midlife period.

Fortunately, menopause is better understood and more openly discussed than ever before. Menopause can be viewed as a sentinel event that presents a unique opportunity for women, working with healthcare professionals, to evaluate personal health and improve health practices. Collaboration between a woman and her healthcare professional, characterized by mutual respect and trust, is the goal of menopause counseling. Menopause counseling can facilitate informed decision-making and validate a woman's confidence in her decisions and in her ability to carry them out or modify them over time.[15] Individualized screening and management approaches are essential components of this collaboration.[16,17]

By considering a woman's preferences, values, and concerns, the menopause practitioner will enhance the woman's sense of well-being, not only around the time of menopause but for the rest of her life. Please see Chapter 5 for more on clinical evaluation and counseling.

Menopause terminology

Clinicians and researchers have long recognized the need for universally accepted menopause terminology.

Menopause. *Menopause* is the FMP resulting from the physiologic permanent decline in gonadal hormone levels confirmed by 12 months of amenorrhea in women with a uterus. For some women, menstrual bleeding criteria cannot be used to define menopause, and the diagnosis can be supported with criteria including history of bilateral oophorectomy and/or symptoms and/or serial measurement of endocrine markers.

Premenopause/Premenopausal. The terms *premenopause* and *premenopausal* refer to the phase of life that precedes menopause.

Postmenopause/Postmenopausal. The terms *postmenopause* and *postmenopausal* refer to the phase of life after menopause. Among women aged 40 to 45 years, an estimated 5% have experienced natural menopause, based primarily on data from the Study of Women Across the Nation (SWAN).[18] For naturally postmenopausal women in the next oldest category (45-55 y), a rough estimate is 25%.

Menopause transition. According to the Stages of Reproductive Workshop (STRAW), the term *menopause transition* refers to the span of time that begins with the onset of intermenstrual cycle irregularities (± 7 days) and/or other menopause-related symptoms and extends through menopause (the FMP).[19]

Perimenopause. The term *perimenopause* literally means "around menopause." It begins with the onset of intermenstrual cycle irregularities (± 7 days) and/or other menopause-related symptoms and extends beyond menopause (the FMP) to include the 12 months after menopause, thus lasting 1 year longer than the menopause transition. Perimenopause is a clinically useful term because it encompasses the highly symptomatic years.

Early menopause and late menopause. *Early menopause* and *late menopause* are vague terms that can be used to describe menopause that occurs earlier or later in the normal range of menopause.

Premature menopause. *Premature menopause* refers to menopause that occurs before age 40. Several studies, including SWAN, indicate that the percentage of US women experiencing premature natural menopause is approximately 1%.[18] Applying this 1% estimate to the projected number of US women who will be aged 15 to 44 years in 2015 (approximately 49 million), approximately 490,000 US women will experience premature natural menopause.[3]

Premature ovarian failure. It has been recommended by the North American Menopause Society and the American Congress of Obstetricians and Gynecologists that the term *premature ovarian failure* no longer be used.

Primary ovarian insufficiency. *Primary ovarian insufficiency* is a condition characterized by hypergonadotrophic hypogonadism in women aged younger than 40 years (also known as premature ovarian failure).

Induced menopause. *Induced menopause* is defined as the cessation of menstruation that follows either surgical removal of both ovaries (bilateral oophorectomy, with or without hysterectomy) or iatrogenic ablation of ovarian function (eg, by chemotherapy or pelvic radiation therapy). Bilateral oophorectomy is the most common cause of induced menopause.

Climacteric. The term *climacteric* has been defined as the period of endocrinal, somatic, and transitory psychologic changes occurring at the time of menopause. It is sometimes used interchangeably with perimenopause.

As women move from the reproductive phase through the menopause transition into postmenopause, physical and psychological changes occur. Women and their healthcare professionals may be challenged to distinguish menopause-related changes from those attributable to normal aging. A number of endocrine systems manifest age-related changes that may or may not have their onset during the menopause transition. Furthermore, concurrent medical disorders such as obesity, DM, dyslipidemia, thyroid disease, and hypertension often develop during midlife and may influence reproductive aging.

Ovarian aging and hormone production

Menopause is an obvious marker of ovarian aging. The ovary contains the maximal number of oocytes during fetal development. Follicular loss begins in utero; women are born with 1 to 2 million follicles. By the menopause transition, a few hundred to a few thousand remain. Most follicular loss results from atresia versus ovulation (<500 follicles ovulated over a lifetime). The number of follicles falls at a constantly increasing rate; thus, the number of follicles declines more rapidly with increasing age.[20] The parallel decline in oocyte quality (as well as quantity) contributes to the associated decline in fertility.[21]

Stages of reproductive aging

Chronologic age is a poor predictor of reproductive age, and women vary widely in timing of the menopause transition. To provide nomenclature and encourage consistency in research and reporting, a standardized definition of reproductive aging based on menstrual cycle bleeding criteria and follicle-stimulating hormone (FSH) levels was initially proposed in 2001 by STRAW and was subsequently validated.[19,22,23] In 2011, a multidisciplinary, multinational, STRAW+10 workshop was convened with the goal of reevaluating the criteria for the staging system to incorporate new data related to FSH, antral follicle count (AFC), antimüllerian hormone (AMH), and inhibin B, as well as added evidence regarding postmenopausal changes in FSH and estradiol.[24] The STRAW+10 writing group acknowledged the challenges of applying the STRAW criteria to women based on variations in body size, lifestyle characteristics, and health status.

The reproductive-aging continuum created by STRAW is divided into 7 stages: 5 precede and 2 follow the FMP. Not all healthy women will follow this pattern, and some will seesaw between stages or skip a stage altogether.

STRAW+10 staging system for reproductive aging in women

As in the original STRAW paradigm, the primary stages of reproductive aging include the reproductive stage, the menopause transition, and the postmenopause (Figure 1).[24] These 3 major categories are further subdivided into several additional stages, each with specific clinical criteria, endocrine parameters, and characteristic markers of reproductive aging.

Reproductive stages (STRAW stages −5, −4, and −3b and −3a). The reproductive phase includes 3 stages (Figure 1)[24]: early (stage −5), peak (stage −4), and late (stages −3b and −3a). Hormonal changes reflecting ovarian aging are best appreciated from the perspective of an understanding of the normal menstrual cycle (characteristic of stages −5, −4, and −3b).[21,25,26]

The normal menstrual cycle involves 3 phases (Figure 2): follicular (proliferative), periovulatory, and luteal (secretory).

Chapter 1

By convention, the first day of menses marks the onset of the menstrual cycle as well as the beginning of the *follicular phase*. Circulating levels of estrogen and progesterone are low, signaling the hypothalamus and pituitary through a negative feedback loop to increase FSH. Follicle-stimulating hormone initiates the process of follicular maturation, and the follicle (the fluid-filled sac containing an ovum, or egg) increases estrogen production, which stimulates new endometrial growth. At the end of the follicular phase, the endometrium thickens 3-fold, and a primordial follicle matures in preparation for ovulation, the release of an ovum.

During the *periovulatory phase*, increased estrogen from the mature follicle, through a positive feedback mechanism, triggers a sharp increase in luteinizing hormone (LH)—the LH surge—leading to ovulation (release of the ovum). Pituitary LH continues to stimulate the residual ovarian follicle, transforming it into the corpus luteum.

The *luteal phase* is marked by secretion of estrogen and progesterone from the corpus luteum. Increasing serum progesterone concentration supports and enriches the thickened endometrium in preparation for embryo implantation and pregnancy. If fertilization of the ovum does not occur, the corpus luteum regresses, estrogen and progesterone levels fall, and menses (shedding of the endometrial lining and uterine bleeding) ensues.

The cyclical release of FSH and LH from the pituitary gland is tightly regulated and easily perturbed. If the pituitary gland does not release appropriate quantities of FSH and LH in characteristic pulsatile fashion, ovulation may not occur, potentially disrupting the normal menstrual cycle.

Estradiol is the primary estrogen produced by the ovaries. In the normal menstrual cycle, circulating serum estradiol levels fluctuate between 10 pg/mL and 100 pg/mL (37-370 pmol/L) in the early follicular phase, 200 pg/mL and 800 pg/mL (730-2,930 pmol/L) at midcycle,

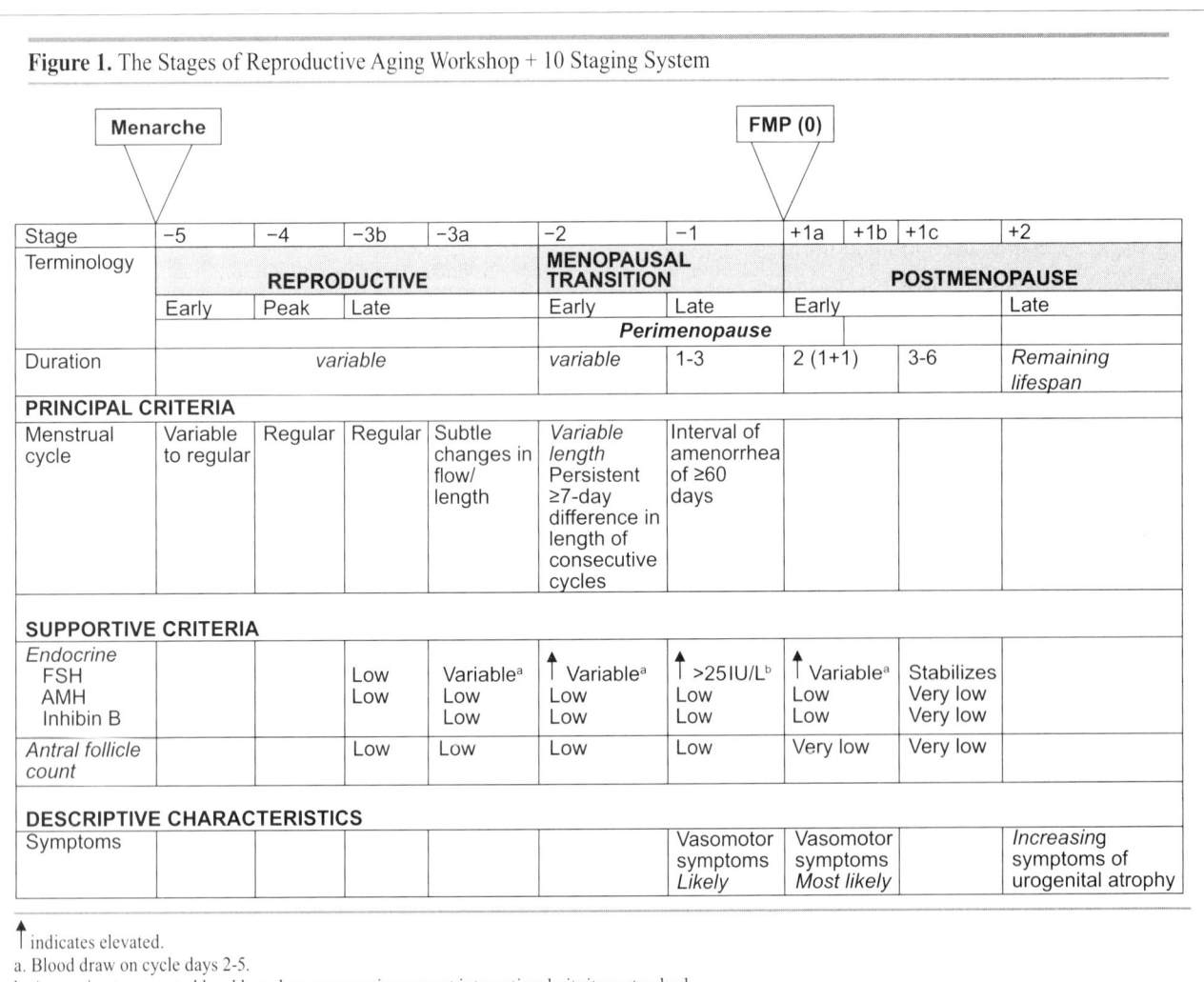

Figure 1. The Stages of Reproductive Aging Workshop + 10 Staging System

↑ indicates elevated.
a. Blood draw on cycle days 2-5.
b. Approximate expected level based on assays using current international pituitary standard.
Abbreviations: AMH, antimüllerian hormone; FMP, final menstrual period; FSH, follicle-stimulating hormone.
Adapted from Harlow SD, et al.[24] © North American Menopause Society.

and 200 pg/mL and 340 pg/mL (730-1,250 pmol/L) during the luteal phase.

During the menstrual cycle, ovarian production of estradiol ranges from 36 μg per day in the follicular phase to 250 μg per day in the luteal phase. More than 95% of the circulatory estradiol comes from the dominant follicle and corpus luteum; the remainder is derived from peripheral conversion of estrone.

Estrone is the second most abundant estrogen in women. Estrone is derived primarily from the metabolism of estradiol and from peripheral aromatization of androstenedione to estrone in adipose tissue and muscle. Ovarian and adrenal secretion supplies a small portion. During the menstrual cycle, serum estrone levels vary from 30 pg/mL to 180 pg/mL (110-660 pmol/L). In premenopausal women, estradiol is the predominant circulating estrogen; the ratio of circulating estradiol to estrone is greater than 1.0.

Progesterone secretion is predominantly confined to the luteal phase of the menstrual cycle, with serum concentrations ranging from 2 ng/mL to 20 ng/mL (310-660 pmol/L). The production rate is 25 mg per day in the midluteal phase.

In reproductive-aged women, circulating *androgens* are produced by the ovaries, the adrenal glands, and through peripheral conversion of circulating androstenedione and dehydroepiandrosterone (DHEA) to testosterone. Five androgens are clinically important: testosterone, dihydrotestosterone (DHT), androstenedione, DHEA, and dehydroepiandrosterone sulfate (DHEAS). Some androgens circulate in blood bound to proteins; others circulate in an unbound state. Dehydroepiandrosterone sulfate binds strongly to albumin, resulting in a very low metabolic clearance rate. Dehydroepiandrosterone and androstenedione bind weakly to albumin; their metabolic clearance rates are higher. One-quarter of circulating testosterone originates in the ovaries, one-quarter in the adrenals, and one-half from peripheral conversion of androstenedione. Testosterone levels range from 0.2 ng/mL to 0.81 ng/mL (0.7-2.8 nmol/L). During the menstrual cycle, there is a slight but significant preovulatory rise in serum testosterone concentration.

The major ovarian peptides involved in pituitary feedback are inhibin A and inhibin B.[26] During the menstrual cycle, inhibin A levels are low for most of the follicular phase, then rise in midcycle, subsequently falling and then rising again to reach the highest levels during the luteal phase. Inhibin A is secreted in parallel with estradiol and progesterone. Inhibin B levels rise and fall in the first half of the follicular phase, exhibit a midcycle peak, and then subsequently fall to their lowest concentrations during the luteal phase. Inhibin B and FSH form a closed-loop negative feedback system during the first half of the cycle, with the levels of

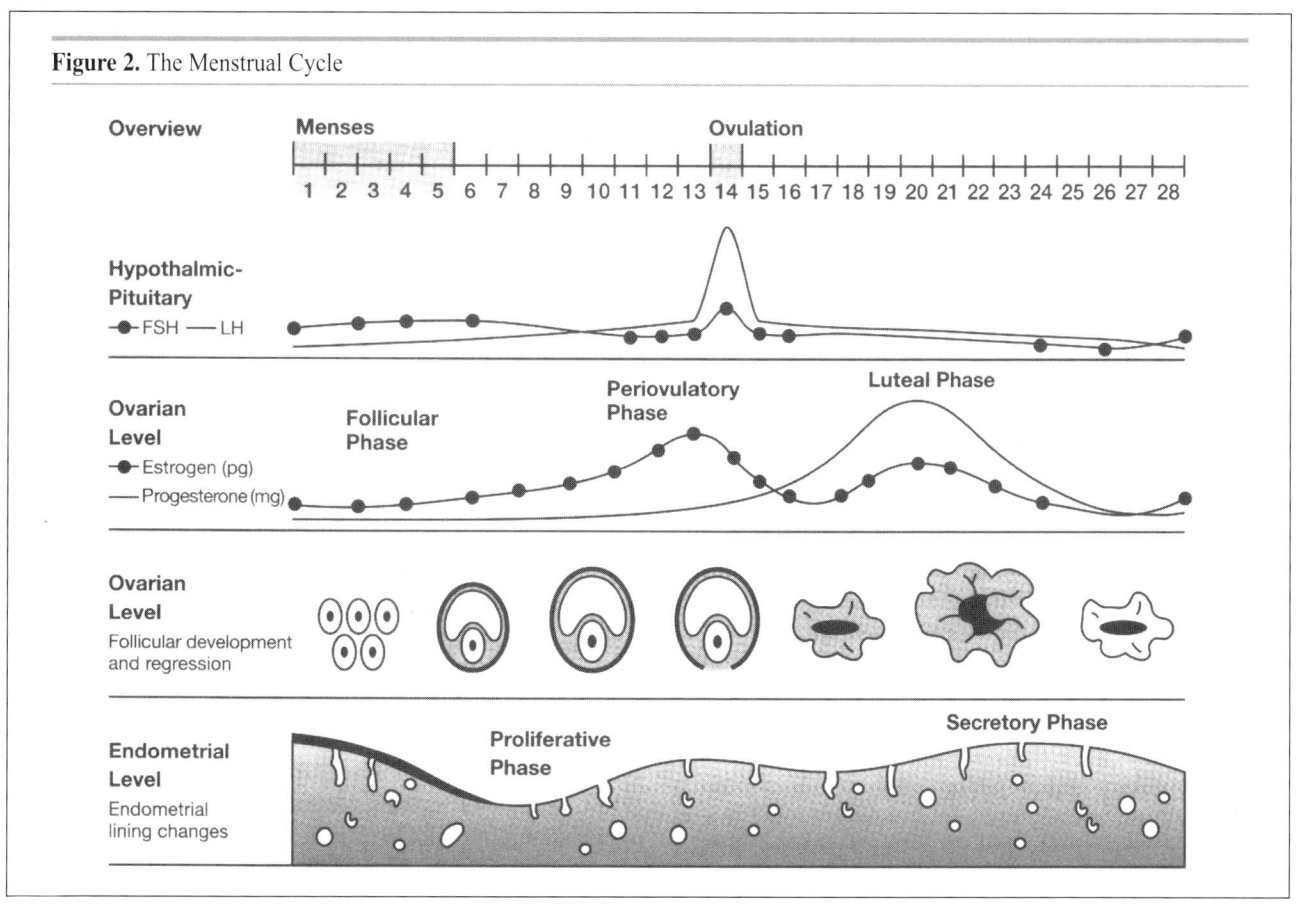

Figure 2. The Menstrual Cycle

inhibin B fine-tuning pituitary FSH regulation. Thus, both ovarian estradiol and the inhibins contribute to pituitary gonadotropin feedback.

Antimüllerian hormone (AMH) is produced exclusively by the granulosa cells of preantral and small ovarian follicles and reflects the transition of resting primordial follicles to growing follicles.[22] Antimüllerian hormone inhibits FSH-dependent follicle growth and may play a role in follicle recruitment and selection. Although AMH had been thought not to vary across the menstrual cycle, variation of AMH in the early follicular phase may occur in younger women.[27]

Antimüllerian hormone has been identified as a marker of ovarian reserve. In one study, AMH fell more than 10-fold in women aged 29 to 37 years compared with younger women, although there was minimal change in FSH.[22] In another study, AMH levels declined 20-fold in women aged between 31 and 35 years and 45 and 50 years.[28] The FSH-inhibin B ratio has been reported to be inversely correlated with AMH and might be useful in conjunction with AMH to characterize menopause status.

Antimüllerian hormone levels have been used primarily to assess ovarian reserve in women seeking fertility assessment. In 17,120 women aged 24 to 50 years who presented to fertility centers in the United States, serum AMH levels ranged from 4.1 ng/mL to 3.2 ng/mL for women aged 24 to 30 years, with a continual age-related gradual decline such that by age 41, AMH levels were on average 1.0 ng/mL, further dropping to zero by age 50.[29]

Additional longitudinal studies demonstrate this age-related decline, with AMH falling to undetectable levels approximately 5 years before menopause.[30] Serial measurements of AMH have been proposed in a number of reports as a means of predicting age of menopause. In the largest study to date, in 1,015 women (aged 20-50 y) with regular and predictable menstrual cycles at baseline, a model based on age and AMH predicted age at menopause within 6 months.[31] Lack of standardized assays and adequate data from non-infertile populations, however, remain important limitations to incorporating AMH into the clinic of menopause practitioners.[24,32]

Antral follicle count, as determined by ultrasound evaluation of the ovary, has also been included in the STRAW+10 staging paradigm, although as with AMH, qualitative criteria rather than specific cut-offs have been provided. Although AFC has been used primarily as a factor in fertility counseling, the role in predicting reproductive aging related to time of menopause continues to be explored.[33-35] Identification of genetic associations linking follicle number and menopausal age support this association.[36]

Late reproductive stage (STRAW stage −3). This phase marks the time when fecundability begins to decline and during which a woman may begin to notice changes in her menstrual cycles.[24] To acknowledge that critical endocrine changes occur before changes in the menstrual cycle and that these endocrine changes are important when assessing potential fertility, in the STRAW+10 update, the late reproductive stage has been divided into 2 phases: −3b and −3a. In −3b, the earlier phase, menstrual cycles and early follicular FSH remain normal; however, AMH levels and AFC are low. The later stage, −3a, is characterized by subtle menstrual cycle changes in flow and length (shorter cycles) and variable FSH levels.

As the number of ovarian follicles declines in stage −3a, inhibin B levels also fall. With a reduction in negative feedback from inhibin B, FSH levels rise. Early follicular-phase FSH elevation is the first commonly measured clinical sign of reproductive aging.[22] The increase in FSH could contribute to the advancement of follicles leaving the resting phase. Follicular phase shortening by approximately 2 to 4 days manifests as shorter menstrual cycles (luteal phase length remains unchanged).

Menopause transition overview (STRAW stages −2 and −1)

The menopause transition is characterized by menstrual cycle irregularity, reflecting an increase in variability of hormone secretion and inconsistent ovulation.[37] The transition culminates with menopause, the complete cessation of menses.[22,26] Changes in central nervous system control of ovarian function and accelerated ovarian follicular atresia both likely contribute to the initiation and progression of the menopause transition. There is no specific endocrine marker of the early or late transition, so although understanding the hormonal milieu of the menopause transition is important, measurements of FSH or estradiol are unreliable when trying to assign reproductive stage to an individual woman.[26]

Early menopause transition (STRAW stage −2). Consistent with the original STRAW classification and the ReSTAGE Collaboration,[19,23,38] the formal onset of the early menopause transition as defined in STRAW+10 is marked by a persistent difference of 7 days or more in the length of consecutive cycles. *Persistence* is defined as recurrence within 10 cycles of the first variable length cycle. Cycles in the early menopause transition are also characterized by elevated but variable early follicular-phase FSH levels and low AMH levels and AFC.[24]

Late menopause transition (STRAW stage −1). According to STRAW+10 (consistent with the original STRAW and ReSTAGE),[19,23] the criteria for the late menopause transition is 60 consecutive days (or longer) of amenorrhea.[24] One such episode is sufficient to stage women aged 45 years and older.[39] For women aged 40 to 44 years, recurrence of an episode of amenorrhea of 60 days or longer within a year improves prediction of entry into the late menopause transition. Menstrual cycles are characterized by increased variability in cycle length, extreme fluctuations in hormone levels, and increased prevalence of anovulation.[24] Follicle-stimulating hormone levels fluctuate between postmenopausal levels and those consistent with the reproductive stages. Serum FSH levels of 25 IU/L or higher in a random blood draw have been incorporated into the STRAW+10 classification criteria as an independent marker for the late menopause transition. This stage is estimated to last, on average, 1 to 3 years.

Clinical implications of endocrine characteristics of the menopause transition

An explanation for the elevated serum estradiol levels during some cycles in the menopause transition reflects a physiologic phenomenon termed *luteal out-of-phase* (LOOP) *event* (Figure 3).[40,41] In a LOOP cycle, which occurs in about 1 in 4 cycles in women studied during the early menopause transition (and approximately one-third of women in the late menopause transition), elevated FSH levels are adequate to recruit a second follicle during the luteal phase of an ongoing cycle. Recruitment of a second follicle results in a follicular phase-like rise in estradiol secretion superimposed on the mid- to late-luteal phase of the ongoing ovulatory cycle. Follicle-stimulating hormone levels drop to midreproductive levels during the menstrual and follicular phases of the subsequent cycle; estradiol levels peak during the subsequent menstrual phase. Concurrent with persistent estradiol elevations are marked falls in luteal progesterone.[40]

About half the time, an LH surge and ovulation follow within the first 5 days of the cycle.[40] As a result, the final length of the second cycle is unusually short (<21 d). If ovulation does not occur, estradiol levels drop until the onset of a new follicular phase; the resulting cycle is then longer than average (>36 d).

Overproduction of estradiol by an enlarged cohort of recruited follicles or a LOOP cycle may result in mastalgia, migraine, menorrhagia, growth of uterine fibroids, or endometrial hyperplasia. Conversion of androgen to estrogen through aromatization increases with age and body weight, another mechanism resulting in elevated estradiol levels during the menopause transition.[42] Women with a longer menopause transition might experience increased exposure to unopposed estrogen, an important risk for reproductive cancers.[43]

Despite the reduction in fertility with reproductive aging, women should be aware that pregnancy can occur until

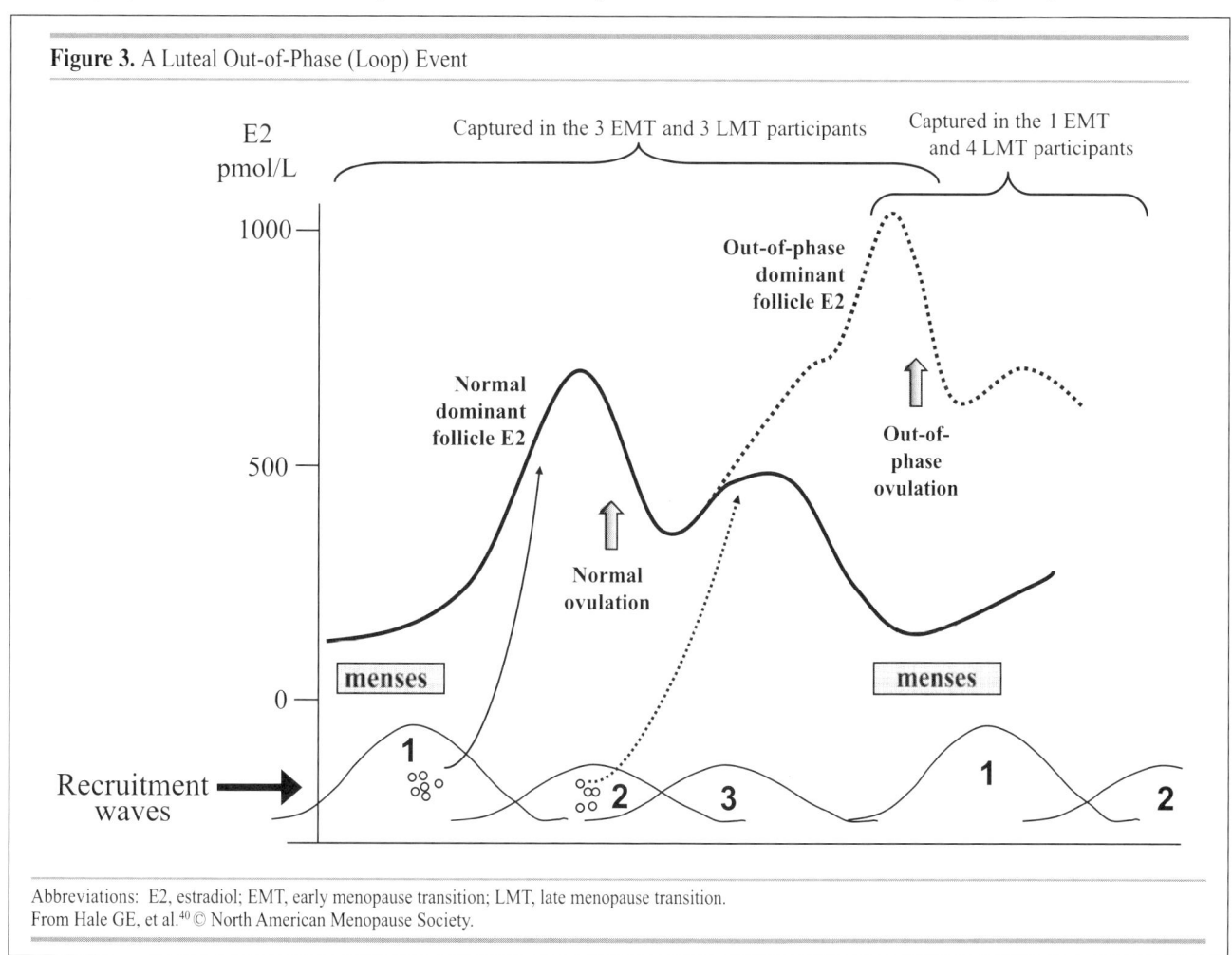

Figure 3. A Luteal Out-of-Phase (Loop) Event

Abbreviations: E2, estradiol; EMT, early menopause transition; LMT, late menopause transition.
From Hale GE, et al.[40] © North American Menopause Society.

menopause. In one study of the menopause transition, fully 25% of all cycles longer than 60 days were ovulatory; the average day of ovulation occurred on day 27 of the cycle.[44] In other studies, approximately 40% to 60% of cycles are anovulatory,[37,44] whereas several follicles may be released during other cycles, perhaps accounting for the increased incidence of twins born to midlife women.

In SWAN, 3 patterns of anovulatory cycles were initially described.[45] One group of women had a normal increase in estradiol and midcycle LH surge but very low progesterone production, consistent with compromised corpus luteal function; a second group had a normal increase in estradiol but the LH surge was absent, implying an inadequate hypothalamic-pituitary response; and a third group had a hormonal pattern characterized by elevated levels of LH and FSH and low levels of both estradiol and progesterone, similar to the hormonal pattern in postmenopausal women.

As women progress through the menopause transition, the number of anovulatory cycles increases and the proportion of anovulatory cycles associated with bleeding progressively decreases.[46] As anticipated, progesterone levels are low during anovulatory cycles. Measures of overall progesterone secretion show a linear decline from STRAW stages −3 to −1 and +1.[44,46] In other studies, progesterone levels are reduced late in the menopause transition or not reduced at all in ovulatory cycles.[22,37]

In SWAN, estradiol levels varied; in anovulatory cycles that ended in bleeding, estradiol levels were comparable with those of women who had ovulated. In cycles without bleeding, estradiol levels were low, approximately one-third the level characteristic of ovulatory cycles. Women who were obese were more likely to have anovulatory cycles characterized by high estradiol levels.[44,46] Women who were obese also were more likely to have lower premenopausal yet higher postmenopausal estradiol levels compared with women of normal weight.[48,49]

In SWAN, women of different races and ethnic groups demonstrated similar patterns of hormonal changes with the menopause transition, but the concentration of hormones differed.[50] Chinese and Japanese women had lower estradiol levels than white, black, and Hispanic women. Follicle-stimulating hormone concentrations were higher in black women than in women of other races. Testosterone levels did not change in the longitudinal Melbourne Women's Midlife Health Study, which followed women during the menopause transition (from 4 y before menopause to 2 y after the FMP).[51]

Other studies that evaluated testosterone concentrations during the menopause transition present conflicting data. In one small study, the midcycle rise in testosterone and androstenedione, characteristic of younger (19-37 y), regularly cycling women, was found to be consistently and significantly absent in older (43-47 y) regularly cycling women.[52]

Total testosterone levels did not differ significantly in any cycle stage between older and younger women. Data from the Rancho Bernardo Study suggest that reductions in testosterone levels at menopause may be transient and followed by normalization of testosterone levels in older women.[53] In a large cross-sectional Australian study, serum androgen levels were shown to decline with age from the early reproductive years without changing at the menopause transition.[54] As in the Rancho Bernardo study, testosterone levels increased slightly during the seventh decade.

In the Melbourne Women's Midlife Health Study, the menopause transition was associated with a drop in the levels of *sex hormone-binding globulin* (SHBG).[51] During the 4 years before menopause to 2 years after menopause, SHBG levels decreased by approximately 40%. The greatest change occurred 2 years before menopause, concurrent with a dramatic decline in serum estradiol. Reduced SHBG levels alter the free androgen index, calculated as the ratio of testosterone to SHBG. The free androgen index rises by nearly 80% during the menopause transition, with the maximal change occurring 2 years before the FMP.

Postmenopause (STRAW stages +1a, +1b, +1c, and +2)
The hallmark for initiation of the postmenopause is the FMP. There is no single specific endocrine marker of the postmenopause, which may primarily be considered an endometrial event.[26]

Early postmenopause (STRAW stages +1a, +1b, and +1c). STRAW stage +1a is defined as the 12 months after the FMP, which also is defined as the end of the perimenopause. Stage +1b encompasses the second postmenopausal year and ends at the time point at which FSH and estradiol levels begin to stabilize. Vasomotor symptoms (VMS) are most likely to occur during stages +1a and +1b, which in general lasts 2 years.[24] During the 3- to 6-year period defined as stage +1c, high FSH levels and low estradiol levels stabilize.

Late postmenopause (STRAW stage +2). Stage +2 begins 6 years after the FMP and continues for the remaining lifespan. Further changes in reproductive endocrine function are limited, and somatic aging predominates.[24] This phase is marked by increasing genitourinary symptoms.

Endocrine findings during the postmenopause include elevated FSH and LH levels (increased 10- to 15-fold), with FSH greater than LH and marked reductions in estradiol and estrone. Characteristically high gonadotropin levels after menopause progressively diminish with age. Postmenopausal estradiol levels are 10% or less of concentrations attained during reproductive life and range from less than 10 pg/mL to 20 pg/mL (37-135 pmol/L). Estrone levels range from 6 pg/mL to 63 pg/mL (22-233 pmol/L). The ratio of estradiol to estrone reverses, and estrone becomes the predominant circulating estrogen. Estrone is derived primarily from peripheral conversion (ie, aromatization) of androstenedione. Consequently, estrogen levels may be increased in women who are obese as aromatization increases in proportion to adipose tissue volume.

Transient elevations of estradiol in postmenopausal women may reflect activity in a residual follicle, but such activity does not usually result in ovulation. At least 1 such case, however, has been formally reported,[55] and many clinicians can attest to at least 1 patient who has described a "normal" menstrual cycle accompanied by premenstrual molimina and normal pattern of menstrual bleeding after menopause. These episodes, nevertheless, constitute unscheduled postmenopausal bleeding and as such must be formally evaluated.

The postmenopausal ovary continues to produce androstenedione and testosterone. Higher levels of androgens in some postmenopausal women might reflect ovarian stromal hyperplasia and luteinization.[56] In the Rancho Bernardo Study, women aged 50 to 89 years with intact ovaries had total testosterone levels that increased with age, reaching premenopausal levels by age 70, with relatively stable levels thereafter.[53] In a report from the Cardiovascular Health Study, total testosterone levels declined with age until age 80, whereas free testosterone levels did not vary by age.[57] White race, higher education level, lower body mass index (BMI), current use of estrogens, and oral corticosteroid use were each associated with lower total and free testosterone levels in women aged older than 65 years.[58]

Surgical menopause results in lower testosterone levels. In the Rancho Bernardo study, women who had undergone bilateral oophorectomy with hysterectomy had testosterone levels that did not vary with age and were 40% to 50% lower than levels in women with intact uterus and ovaries.[53]

Hypothalamic-pituitary-ovarian axis

The normal menstrual cycle is controlled via a complex interplay of multiple components of the hypothalamic-pituitary-ovarian (HPO) axis. Although ovarian aging is thought to be the predominant event leading to menopause, alterations of the central hypothalamic-pituitary axis with aging may contribute.

Pulsatile hypothalamic release of gonadotropin-releasing hormone (GnRH) stimulates the pituitary gland to secrete FSH and LH. The gonadotropins then stimulate the ovary to secrete estrogen and progesterone. The pattern of pulsatile release of GnRH, pituitary hormones, and subsequent ovarian hormone secretion varies throughout the normal menstrual cycle (Figure 2).

As reproductive aging ensues, the HPO axis changes in several ways.[59] An early measurable sign is an increase in serum FSH levels. Ovarian inhibin production declines, resulting in a loss in negative feedback or *disinhibition* of pituitary FSH secretion. A rise in serum FSH can be detected as early as the STRAW+10 late reproductive stage.

Postmenopausal FSH levels increase and then plateau. Although FSH levels eventually decline in the years after menopause, they remain elevated above premenopausal concentrations, even in older postmenopausal women.

Concurrent with or possibly preceding the decline in ovarian inhibin production and the resultant increase in FSH secretion, the neuroendocrine control of GnRH secretion also is altered. There is speculation based on animal and some human studies that GnRH neurons change in their capacity to synthesize and release GnRH and to respond to neural inputs and steroid hormone sensitivity.[59-63] Alterations of the GnRH pulse generator and regulatory (both excitatory and inhibitory) neuropeptides might contribute to the compromise or complete absence of the midcycle LH surge in perimenopausal women, also consistent with a reduction in the sensitivity of the hypothalamus and pituitary to positive feedback by estrogen.[45,60] Estrogen exerts a direct inhibitory effect (negative feedback) on pituitary responsiveness to GnRH, which contributes to the differential regulation of FSH and LH secretion.[64]

During the menopause transition, LH levels usually remain in the normal range or increase slightly. After menopause, basal LH levels continue to rise and then plateau in about 1 year. The loss of gonadal steroid feedback after menopause alters the forms of LH and FSH secreted, resulting in slower clearance and prolonged half-life.[59]

After menopause, the steady age-related decline in serum levels of LH and FSH provides clear evidence for additional hypothalamic-pituitary changes independent of those caused by loss of ovarian hormonal feedback. The capacity of the hypothalamus to secrete GnRH is not diminished with age, although the dynamics of its control are altered. The amount of GnRH secreted with each GnRH pulse is increased in postmenopausal women, although accompanied by a decrease in GnRH pulse frequency. The decline of LH and FSH in the presence of increased GnRH secretion results from an age-related diminution in pituitary responsiveness to GnRH.[65] Studies also demonstrate a differential effect of aging on ovarian steroid negative and positive feedback as required to generate an LH surge. The magnitude of the positive-feedback LH response to ovarian steroids is attenuated with aging in women, whereas the magnitude of estrogen negative feedback is unaffected.[66]

Gonadotropin secretion in postmenopausal women does not follow a circadian rhythm, although circadian rhythmicity of the pituitary hormones adrenocorticotropic hormone (ACTH) and thyroid-stimulating hormone (TSH) remains intact.[67,68]

Low-level pituitary production of human chorionic gonadotropin (hCG) seems to be normal in postmenopausal women (levels <32 mIU/mL [IU/L]). Pituitary hCG in postmenopausal women is the pregnancy-type hCG, and production parallels the increasing postmenopausal production of LH. Pituitary origin of hCG in a postmenopausal woman can be confirmed by suppression of hCG to less than 2 mIU/mL (IU/L) after 2 weeks of menopausal HT.

Adrenal physiology and menopause

The adrenal gland consists of 2 main regions—the outer cortex and the inner medulla. The adrenal medulla secretes epinephrine, norepinephrine, and dopamine in response to neural signals. The adrenal cortex is made up of 3 distinct zones, each of which primarily secretes 1 class of steroid hormone: mineralocorticoids, glucocorticoids, and androgens.

The *zona glomerulosa* (the outermost layer of the adrenal cortex) secretes mineralocorticoids, predominantly aldosterone. Secretion is primarily regulated by the renin-angiotensin system. Other regulators include sodium and potassium concentrations, ACTH, and neural components of the adrenergic and dopaminergic systems. Mineralocorticoid feedback at the level of the hippocampus might have important implications for regulation of glucocorticoid and adrenal androgen secretion, particularly with aging.[70]

The *zona fasciculata* (the middle layer of the adrenal cortex) secretes glucocorticoids, primarily cortisol, under control of the pituitary hormones ACTH and arginine vasopressin, as well as neural elements of the stress response. Adrenocorticotropic hormone is regulated by hypothalamic corticotropin-releasing hormone (CRH) and by other central influences. Glucocorticoids provide feedback inhibition to ACTH and CRH.

Adrenal glucocorticoid secretion follows a circadian pattern of secretion, with peak values in the morning and a nadir in the late afternoon. Cortisol and ACTH levels rise with increasing age, and serum concentrations at all ages are higher in women than in men.[71] Blunting of the cortisol circadian rhythm is characteristic of aging in both sexes. Feedback inhibition of ACTH secretion by cortisol may be impaired in older persons, leading to prolonged glucocorticoid exposure.[72]

In the Seattle Midlife Women's Health Study, during the 7 to 12 months after the onset of the late menopause transition stage (defined as skipped menstrual periods), cortisol levels were reported to rise significantly, coinciding with an increase in DHEAS, urinary metabolites of estrogen, and FSH.[73,74] Women with an increase in cortisol were found to have significantly more severe hot flashes. Cortisol levels stabilized around the time of the FMP. In a separate study of postmenopausal women, serum LH correlated significantly with 24-hour urinary free cortisol, suggesting that LH may act directly by binding to adrenal LH receptors.[75] Because of a previous study suggesting a lack of association between LH and cortisol if the LH was greater than 41 mIU/mL, analysis was restricted to women with an LH of less than 41 mIU/mL.[76]

Serum cortisol circulates bound to cortisol-binding globulin (CBG). In a cross-sectional study comparing postmenopausal women receiving oral estrogen therapy (ET), transdermal ET, or placebo, total serum cortisol concentrations were 67% higher in those receiving oral ET than in controls or in women receiving transdermal ET.[77] The increase in total serum cortisol was associated with a higher level of CBG in women taking oral ET. Salivary cortisol concentration, a measure of free cortisol, was similar in all 3 groups.

In a separate study, transdermal ET administration for 3 months did not alter adrenal steroid levels or adrenal response to ACTH.[78] Estrogen effects on the hypothalamic-pituitary-adrenal axis may differ on the basis of a woman's weight and weight distribution. Transdermal ET induced a significant reduction in ACTH response to CRH stimulation in women who had a high waist-to-hip ratio, whereas adrenal sensitivity was improved in women with a low waist-to-hip ratio.

In a study of 11 postmenopausal women, 1 year of raloxifene therapy reduced circulating levels of adrenal steroids, adrenal sensitivity to ACTH, and estrogen levels, all hypothesized to be of benefit by reducing exposure to endogenous glucocorticoids and reducing breast exposure to endogenous estrogens.[79]

The *zona reticularis* (the innermost layer of the adrenal cortex) secretes the adrenal androgens DHEA and androstenedione and is also regulated by pituitary ACTH. Serum concentrations of adrenal androgens, particularly DHEA and its sulfated conjugate, DHEAS, fall progressively with age and are lower in women than in men.[71] In older postmenopausal women, the inverse relationship between DHEAS (decreased) and cortisol secretion (increased) is thought to be related to a defect in adrenal production of DHEAS.[80] The capacity of the adrenal gland to produce androstenedione does not seem compromised, and the age-related decrease in androstenedione likely reflects reduced production by the ovary.[81] Smoking is associated with increased adrenal androgens; in the Rancho Bernardo study, the levels of DHEA and androstenedione increased concomitantly with cigarette smoking.[82]

Reports of changes in DHEAS during the menopause transition have been inconsistent. In the Melbourne Women's Midlife Health Project, DHEAS levels were reportedly unchanged during the menopause transition.[83] When 10 years of annual data from the SWAN study were analyzed by participant ovarian status, a transient rise in DHEAS level during the late menopause transition was sustained through the early postmenopause stage; analysis by chronologic age, however, was consistent with the anticipated age-related decline in DHEAS.[84,85] Further analysis demonstrated that the transient rise in DHEAS during the menopause transition is also accompanied by increases in mean circulating testosterone, androstenedione, and androstenediol.[86] The strongest correlation was between DHEAS and androstenediol, which achieved a 5-fold increase during the menopause transition. Research suggests that the inherent estrogenic activity of androstenediol might modulate differences in menopausal symptoms when estradiol levels fall and possibly affect eventual health outcomes.[87] The rise in DHEAS also has been reported in women who underwent bilateral oophorectomy during the menopause transition, providing additional support for an adrenal source.[88]

Evidence that LH controls the increase in adrenal androgen secretion during the menopause transition is supported by studies in nonhuman primates, which demonstrate a positive adrenal androgen response to LH-chorionic gonadotropin administration, consistent with the presence of LH receptors in the adrenal cortex.[89]

Receptor activity

Steroid hormones are released from the cells in which they are synthesized and are then transported in the bloodstream throughout the body to target cells in different tissues in which they trigger a response. Ovarian steroid hormones (estrogen, progesterone, testosterone) diffuse freely into cells, but activity within a tissue or individual cell usually depends on the presence and density of specific hormone receptors, binding proteins, coactivators, and corepressors.

Estrogen receptors

Estrogen is the dominant hormone in women. Two distinct estrogen receptors (ERs) have been identified: ER-α and ER-β.[90] The concentration of the 2 receptors varies in different tissues with states of health and possibly with age.[91] Estrogen receptors-α are primarily expressed in organs of the reproductive system (eg, uterus, ovary, and breast) but also are found in liver, bone, adipose tissue, and brain. Estrogen receptors-β are more prevalent in other tissues (eg, colon, vascular endothelium, lung, bladder, and brain). Both ER-α and ER-β are present in the ovary, the central nervous system, and cardiovascular tissues.[92] A high ER-α to ER-β ratio correlates with high levels of cellular proliferation, whereas dominance of ER-β correlates with repression of proliferation.[93]

A number of ER-gene polymorphisms have been identified that may contribute to individual differences in menopause symptoms and development of osteoporosis, cardiovascular disease (CVD), cognitive dysfunction, DM, depression, and possibly breast cancer.[92,94] More research is required to determine how best to apply knowledge about ER polymorphisms to clinical practice.

The ER is receptive to a variety of substances known as *ligands*. Different ligands (eg, estradiol, estrone, phytoestrogens, selective estrogen-receptor modulators [SERMs]) have different affinities for ER-α and ER-β. For example, 17β-estradiol binds to both ER-α and ER-β, whereas phytoestrogens seem to have a higher affinity for ER-β.[95,96] Ligand binding to the ER initiates receptor activation. Depending on the specific ligand, the shape, or conformation, of the ER is altered in a unique ligand-specific manner. This conformational change of the ligand-receptor complex affects subsequent DNA binding and cofactor interactions. Four distinct estrogen and ER-signaling pathways have been described.[91]

Pathway 1: Estrogen receptor-dependent, nuclear-initiated estrogen signaling. In the classical pathway of hormone action, estrogen enters the cytoplasm of the cell and binds to an ER.[97] Dimerization of the ligand-receptor complex (homodimers, ER-α/ER-α and ER-β/ER-β, and heterodimers, ER-α/ER-β) is followed by translocation to the cell nucleus. Depending on the tissue in which the particular ligand-receptor complex resides, specific cofactors interact with both the receptor-ligand complex and specific locations on the target gene known as estrogen response elements (EREs).[98,99] The DNA receptor-ligand complex will either turn on (activate) or turn off (repress) gene transcription, depending on the ligand, the receptor, the tissue, and which of the more than 300-plus identified cofactors (coactivators or corepressors) are involved. The process of ligand-receptor binding culminating in gene transcription transpires over hours or days. After transcription, the ER or coactivator can be degraded by the 26S proteasome. Thus, a cycle of assembly, activation, and destruction occurs.[93]

In addition to the classical pathway, ligand-activated nuclear ERs can regulate transcription through ER-DNA indirect association by interacting with other transcription factors: stimulating protein-1, activator protein 1, nuclear factor κB, and c-jun.[91] Approximately one-third of estradiol-responsive gene transcription occurs in this manner.

Pathway 2: Estrogen receptor-dependent, membrane-initiated estrogen signaling. Alternatively, rapidly acting ERs are located in proximity to plasma membranes.[100,101] This pathway effects acute, rapid estrogen actions in the nervous system, skeleton, liver, and other tissues that occur much faster than transcriptional processes.[91] Membrane-initiated estrogen signaling involves modifying growth factors, neurotransmitter receptors, tyrosine kinase receptors, and insulin-like growth hormone receptors.

In addition, the G-protein-coupled receptor GPR30 has been identified as an estrogen-binding protein involved in rapid nongenomic cell signaling, although controversy exists regarding this receptor.[102,103] GPR30 is located in the plasma membrane, Golgi apparatus, and endoplasmic reticulum. Another receptor, ER-X, is a membrane-associated ER prominent in the brain, uterus, and lungs.[91]

Pathway 3: The estrogen receptor-independent pathway. Studies have demonstrated that estrogens can exert antioxidant effects and suppress oxidative stress in an ER-independent pathway.[91] This pathway might be prominent in neurons. There is also some evidence that estradiol can promote breast cancer in mice with deleted endogenous

ER-α and ER-β. Vascular effects are also thought to be mediated via non-sex hormone nuclear receptors.

Pathway 4: Ligand-independent activation of estrogen receptors. Estrogen receptors can be activated by a variety of factors, including neurotransmitters such as dopamine, growth factors such as epidermal growth factor and insulin-like growth factor, and activators of intracellular signaling pathways such as protein kinase.[91] These lead to phosphorylation and activation of nuclear ERs at EREs.

Estrogen-related receptors (-α, -β, -γ) are orphan nuclear receptors that do not seem to require a classic ligand to facilitate interactions with coactivators and hormone response elements within target genes to stimulate transcription. Study of these estrogen-related receptors indicates an emerging role in modulating estrogen responsiveness, substituting for ER activities, and serving as prognosticators in breast, ovarian, and colorectal cancers.[104]

Clinical implications of estrogen-receptor modulation

The evolving understanding of ER action has broad clinical implications for the health of postmenopausal women, strategies for disease prevention, and refinement of therapies for breast cancer and menopause symptoms.

Awareness that ER action closely reflects characteristics of the ligand to which it bound has led to a better understanding of SERMs (also known as estrogen agonist/antagonists), agents that act as ER agonists in some tissues and antagonist action in others.[93,97] Tamoxifen for breast cancer treatment and prevention, raloxifene for osteoporosis prevention and treatment and breast cancer prevention, and ospemifene for treatment of dyspareunia from vaginal symptoms associated with menopause are familiar examples. The pharmacology of each individual SERM is influenced by binding affinity for the ER, the density of ER in a given tissue, characteristics of coregulators, the role of signaling pathways, and specifics of the ERE within the target gene.[97]

Antiestrogens such as fulvestrant and the SERM bazedoxifene have been shown in cellular models of breast cancer to enhance ER corepressor functions and thereby contribute to a proteasome-mediated degradation in cellular ER-α. These agents, referred to as *selective estrogen-receptor downregulators*, may have potential for treating tamoxifen- and aromatase inhibitor-resistant breast cancers, an area of active investigation.[98,105]

One challenge has been to understand the mechanism of *tissue-selective estrogen complexes* (TSEC), combination therapies in which a SERM and an ER agonist are combined to yield distinct clinical actions, for example, bazedoxifene with conjugated estrogens (CE).[106] Genes have been identified that are regulated by various TSEC combinations but not by the estrogen or SERM alone. Receptor studies demonstrate an ER heteroligand dimer complex that consists of 1 subunit of the receptor dimer bound to agonist with the other bound to antagonist.[107]

Progesterone receptors

Two progesterone receptors (PRs), PR-α and PR-β, are coexpressed in most tissues, with PR-α predominating in the uterus and ovary and PR-β in the breast. Pure progesterone antagonists (eg, mifepristone, RU-486) bind to progesterone receptors and recruit corepressors to prevent progesterone action. *Selective progesterone-receptor modulators*, such as ulipristal acetate, have mixed agonist/antagonist activity, depending on the structure of the ligand and the tissue where binding occurs.[108] Clinical applications of progesterone antagonists and selective progesterone-receptor modulators include emergency contraception and pregnancy termination.[109] Potential uses under investigation include treatment of endometriosis and uterine leiomyoma and long-term estrogen-free contraception.[109,110]

Androgen receptors

Less well studied in women, yet of increasing interest in several important clinical spheres, the androgen receptor (AR) mediates the biologic effects of testosterone and other androgens.[111] Similar to ER action, the AR is a ligand-dependent transcriptional factor that modulates gene expression through interaction with coregulator complexes and target genes. In women, ARs have been detected in the mucosa and stroma of the vagina.[112] In vaginal mucosa, the density of ARs decreases with age and does not respond to androgen therapy. In the stromal tissue, AR density score does not change with age, yet it increases significantly after administration of testosterone. In a systematic review of women with early breast cancer, tumor expression of AR was associated with better overall survival and disease-free survival, regardless of ER status.[113] Evaluation of the role of AR in ovarian cancer, polycystic ovary syndrome (PCOS), and anxiety disorders is under way.

Premature menopause and primary ovarian insufficiency

Premature menopause is a general term used to describe menopause that occurs before age 40. *Primary ovarian insufficiency* (POI) is a condition characterized by hypergonadotrophic hypogonadism in women aged younger than 40 years (also known as *premature ovarian failure* [POF]).

Premature menopause is thought to affect approximately 1% of US women by age 40.[114] Premature menopause is either *induced* as a result of medical intervention or is *spontaneous*. The diagnosis also can be applied with certainty to women who have had their ovaries removed before age 40. It is less clear how to distinguish spontaneous premature menopause from POI.

Induced menopause occurs as a result of bilateral oophorectomy or secondary to chemotherapy or radiation therapy, with subsequent ovarian damage. In some cases, chemotherapy and radiation therapy will result in a transient state of ovarian insufficiency that only can be diagnosed retrospectively once menses resume. With induced menopause, levels of ovarian hormones (including estrogens, progesterone, and androgens) often drop rapidly. Similar changes occur with the use of GnRH for treatment of endometriosis or fibroids. Cancer treatments, especially surgery and radiation therapy, can damage the vaginal epithelium, the vascular supply, and the anatomy of the vaginal canal. Some treated women experience a narrowed or shortened vagina. These changes can produce pain with pelvic examinations, dyspareunia, and an increased risk of vaginal infections.[115] Menopause that is surgically induced is referred to as *surgical menopause*.

The term *primary ovarian insufficiency* is preferred to the older term *premature ovarian failure* because the condition is neither always complete ovarian failure nor is it always permanent.[116] Although POI may be transient or even wax and wane, permanent loss of ovarian function resulting in premature menopause is the eventual outcome.[117]

There are no accurate figures of the prevalence of POI. Most estimates are derived from the percentage of women with infertility, oligomenorrhea (infrequent menstrual flow), or amenorrhea presenting for evaluation. Estimates are subject to referral bias and range from 2% to 10% of women presenting with secondary amenorrhea.[118,119] Conceptually, POI can arise from 2 different causes: ovarian follicular dysfunction or ovarian follicular depletion.[120,121]

Premature menopause can also be an inadvertent sequela of hysterectomy or uterine artery embolization, hypothesized to be because of compromised ovarian blood flow from the uterus.[122,123] In the experience of one institution, the mean age of ovarian failure in a group of women who had undergone hysterectomy was 45.4 ± 4.0 years—significantly younger than the mean age of 49.5 ± 4.04 years in women who had not had this surgery.[124] Women undergoing hysterectomy or uterine artery embolization should be informed about the possible risk for decreased ovarian function earlier than expected.

Despite episodes of amenorrhea and elevated FSH levels, ovulation in women with POI may occur intermittently and unpredictably for several years. It is estimated that between 5% and 25% of women with POI will experience at least 1 spontaneous return of ovarian function. Among women with POI who have a normal karyotype, one-half may still have ovarian follicles capable of functioning intermittently. Perhaps 5% to 10% conceive spontaneously.[125] Primordial follicles in the ovaries of some women with POI do not adequately respond to gonadotropin stimulation. These follicles, however, may still function sufficiently to produce estradiol. In other women, the ovaries demonstrate complete depletion of follicles, stemming from an inadequate initial pool of follicles, accelerated follicular atresia, or follicular destruction through immune, infectious, or toxic insults.

Etiology
Primary ovarian insufficiency has multiple etiologies including genetic (X chromosome-related and autosomal), environmental insults, metabolic dysfunction, and immune disturbances (Table 1).[116,117,120,126-133] It seems to be sporadic and idiopathic in 74% to 90% of cases; it can also be familial (4%-33%).[69,126]

Familial clusters of POI exist. Approximately 10% to 15% of women with POI have a family history of the disorder.[126] In a large Italian study, early ovarian failure had a recognizable heritable association in nearly one-third of the women evaluated.[134] The most consistent predictable factor for early menopause is maternal age at menopause.[135] Although genetic or familial factors may influence ovarian aging, the prevalence of these factors, the relative expression, and the proportion of early ovarian failure attributed to genetic or familial causes are not well studied. Two percent of cases of POI appear to be caused by fragile X mental retardation 1 (FMR1) mutations with associated mental retardation in those with the highest number of CGG repeats.[136,137] Sporadic and familial forms of fragile X syndrome associated with premature and POI menopause have been widely recognized.

Autoimmune causes of POI are common and may be associated with other immune disorders such as adrenal insufficiency, hypothyroidism, or hyperthyroidism and as part of the multiple autoimmune endocrine abnormalities.[138,139] This form is often caused by follicular dysfunction rather than absence of follicles.

A gene locus on the X chromosome is related to ovarian failure.[140] Women with a single X chromosome, such as those with Turner syndrome, develop normal ovaries with a normal complement of primordial follicles. They experience accelerated atresia, which leads to ovarian failure, often before birth and usually before the age of menarche. Women with a mosaic karyotype (eg, 45XO, 46XX) may experience normal reproductive function and pregnancy before presenting with POI. The X chromosome mutations POF1, POF2, and fragile X are associated with point mutations on the X chromosome.

Most women with galactosemia (an autosomal-recessive condition) eventually develop POI, along with hepatocellular damage, renal cellular damage, development of cataracts, and mental retardation.[141]

Mumps has been the classic but rare example of an infectious disease associated with oophoritis and potentially POI. Data are scarce. When a postpubertal female develops mumps parotiditis, oophoritis should be suspected when lower abdominal tenderness or ovarian pain occurs.[142]

Evaluation of primary ovarian insufficiency and nonsurgical premature menopause
The standard diagnostic criterion for menopause (12 months with no menses) as applied to women aged 40 years and older does not apply to younger women. Women with POI typically present with 1) disordered uterine bleeding (abnormal uterine bleeding [AUB], oligomenorrhea, or amenorrhea), 2) elevated FSH levels, 3) low or undetectable

Chapter 1

Table 1. Known Causes of Premature Menopause and Primary Ovarian Insufficiency

Genetic disorders
- X chromosome disorders (monosomy, trisomy, or translocations, deletions), reduced gene dosage, nonspecific impairment of meiosis, and accelerated atresia
- Specific genetic disorders on the long arm of the X chromosome (POF1, POF2, and FMR1 genes)
- Autosomal genes such as FOXL2 that codes for the forkhead transcription factor that plays a major role in development of the ovary
- Mutations involving enzymes important for reproduction
  - Galactosemia
  - 17α-hydroxylase deficiency (CYP17A1)
  - Aromatase deficiency
- Mutations involving reproductive hormones, their receptors, and actions
  - FSH receptor mutations
  - Mutations involving postreceptor steps in FSH actions
  - LH-receptor mutations

Associated autoimmune disorders
- Autoimmune polyendocrine syndromes
  - Hypothyroidism
  - Adrenal insufficiency
  - Hypoparathyroidism
  - Type 1 DM
- Dry eye syndrome
- Myasthenia gravis
- Rheumatoid arthritis
- Systemic lupus erythematosus
- Congenital thymic aplasia

Miscellaneous disorders
- Metabolic syndromes
- Infections (mumps, HIV)
- Idiopathic

Iatrogenic causes
- Pelvic radiation
- Chemotherapy (alkylating agents)

Surgical menopause
- Oophorectomy
- Ovarian cystectomy
- Consequence of hysterectomy or uterine artery embolization

Abbreviations: DM, diabetes mellitus; FMR1, fragile X retardation 1; FOXL2, forkhead box L2; FSH, follicle-stimulating hormone; HIV, human immunodeficiency virus; POF1, premature ovarian failure 1; POF2, premature ovarian failure 2.
Nelson LM[116]; Progetto Menopausa Italia Study Group[117]; Aittomäki K, et al[120]; Van Kasteren YM, et al[126]; Vegetti W, et al[127]; Luborsky JL, et al[128]; Rebar RW[129]; Vearncombe KL, et al[130]; Vujovic S[131]; Harris SE, et al[132]; Latronico AC, et al[133].

AMH levels,[143] and 4) low ovarian AFC. At least 4 months of disordered bleeding in conjunction with more than 1 elevated FSH level are needed to consider the diagnosis.

Unfortunately, there is no characteristic menstrual history preceding either POI or premature menopause. The presentation of POI may begin as a shortened intercycle menstrual interval, oligomenorrhea, AUB, or an abrupt cessation of menses. Primary ovarian insufficiency can occur immediately postpartum or after cessation of oral contraceptives. During the transition from normal to abnormal ovarian function, estrogen levels and FSH levels fluctuate.[144] Some women have typical menopause symptoms, at least intermittently, whereas others do not, at least not that they recognize as such.

Severe menopause symptoms often occur in women who experience induced menopause by oophorectomy, chemotherapy or radiotherapy. Symptoms include hot flashes, mood changes, a lack of energy, depression, and insomnia. These symptoms and their severity are similar to those in younger women who experience shutdown of their menstrual cycles with GnRH agonists for treatment of endometriosis or uterine myomas and reflect the abrupt reduction of estrogen production.

Studies have not determined which women with signs and symptoms of POI are likely to progress to premature menopause. This makes individual patient counseling regarding fertility and contraception challenging. It is important to outline the trajectory or timeframe when expected changes may occur. Because early estrogen deficiency has a negative effect on bone density and possibly on cognitive function and sexual function, a timely diagnosis is warranted.[145-148]

A careful history and physical examination are needed to rule out other causes of menstrual dysfunction, particularly secondary amenorrhea (Table 2).[116] The medical history should identify prior ovarian surgery, chemotherapy, or pelvic radiation, as well as a personal or family history of POI or other autoimmune disorders (hypothyroidism, Hashimoto thyroiditis, Addison disease, diabetes mellitus, Graves disease, vitiligo, systemic lupus erythematosus, rheumatoid arthritis, Sjögren syndrome, inflammatory bowel disease, or celiac disease).

Family history of fragile X syndrome, intellectual disability, dementia, tremor or ataxia, or symptoms similar to Parkinson disease might suggest a premutation in the FMR1 gene.[116]

Questions about vaginal dryness are relevant as is evidence of vaginal atrophy on examination. The pelvic examination should evaluate for conditions associated with AUB such as uterine fibroids, ovarian cysts, endometriosis, or pelvic inflammatory disease.

Initial laboratory evaluation after a negative pregnancy test includes serum prolactin, FSH, estradiol, and thyroid-stimulating hormone and is warranted for any woman aged younger than 40 years who misses 3 or more consecutive menstrual cycles.[129] If the FSH level is elevated, repeat in

1 month along with a serum estradiol level done on day 2 or 3 of the cycle if she is still menstruating. Estradiol and FSH levels should always be evaluated together in assessing ovarian reserve because testing may have been performed at the time of midcycle gonadotropin surge if FSH and estradiol are elevated. In addition, a low FSH value in the setting of a high estradiol level does not provide reassurance of adequate ovarian reserve because of the negative feedback effect of estradiol on FSH. Additional laboratory tests should be performed to exclude a variety of other causes (Table 3).

Measuring circulating FSH, LH, and estradiol concentrations at intervals may determine whether functional follicles are present. An estradiol concentration greater than 50 pg/mL (183 pmol/L) suggests the presence of functional follicles. A low AMH level has been shown to correlate with decreased ovarian reserve and low ovarian AFC.[149] Intermittent uterine bleeding also suggests the presence of remaining follicles with sporadic estrogen production, although other sources of uterine pathology associated with bleeding should be ruled out. Because of sporadic estrogen production, the progesterone withdrawal test can be misleading in the setting of POI and is not routinely recommended.

Transvaginal ultrasound imaging is useful to provide information regarding the ovarian volume and AFC. A karyotype is also recommended particularly in those who are amenorrheic with premature menopause. This may be important in counseling; if a Y chromosome fragment is present, the gonads have increased malignant potential and should be removed. The karyotype might also be helpful in diagnosing familial syndromes that include POI and identifying a Turner mosaic condition. Testing for fragile X syndrome may have important implications for her family.

Women with POI may not achieve peak bone mass if the condition presents at a very young age, and they may lose bone mass because of their low estrogen state. If HT is part of the management plan, bone mineral density (BMD) testing is not necessary in the absence of fractures. If BMD testing is performed, it should be noted that the diagnostic criteria were developed for women who experienced natural menopause at the typical age. Extrapolation to younger women is problematic. In younger patients, attention should be given to the Z-score for their own age and ethnic group rather than the T-score. Bisphosphonate therapy should be avoided in young women, because most of them are not losing bone but fail to have sufficient bone formation to achieve peak bone mass, and in those who might conceive.

It may be of value to assess ovarian reserve in women at risk for POI (previous ovarian surgery, pelvic radiation, exposure to cytotoxic drugs, autoimmune diseases, and smokers). Tests to identify decreased ovarian reserve include cycle day 2 or 3 determination of FSH and circulating estradiol. Clinicians should be aware that assays for such testing often use different reference standards, and normal cutoff values may vary. In centers with extensive experience using assays with appropriate validity and reproducibility, FSH levels greater than 10 mIU/mL (IU/L) portend diminished ovarian reserve.[129] Other testing options for ovarian reserve include vaginal ultrasound examination to determine mean ovarian volume and number of antral follicles, as well as AMH and inhibin B measurements.[143,150]

Table 2. Differential Diagnosis of S Amenorrhea (Short List)

Low FSH conditions
- Pregnancy
- Hypothalamic amenorrhea
  - Secondary to constitutional disorder
    - Uncontrolled DM
    - Celiac disease
  - Extremes of lifestyle
    - Exercise
    - Caloric restriction
    - Perceived stress
  - Lesions of the hypothalamus/pituitary
  - GnRH agonist/antagonist therapy
- Hyperprolactinemia
- Hypothyroidism and hyperthyroidism
- PCOS

Elevated FSH condition
- POI

Abbreviations: DM, diabetes mellitus; FSH, follicle-stimulating hormone; GnRH, gonadotropin-releasing hormone; PCOS, polycystic ovary syndrome; POI, primary ovarian insufficiency.
Nelson LM.[116]

Management

Although research to guide clinical management of POI and premature menopause is lacking, there are several management approaches to physical and emotional health issues. Management differs significantly between those who already have amenorrhea with very high FSH and deficient estradiol levels versus those who have irregular or occasional menses.

Hormone treatment. For those who have lost all ovarian function, HT, if not contraindicated, is advised to treat acute menopause-related symptoms as well as maintain bone and other tissues. Because these women are younger than typical menopause patients, many experts recommend treating with the equivalent of the 100-μg transdermal estradiol patch or 1.25 CE orally. If the uterus is present, a cyclical progestogen

Table 3. Clinical Evaluation in Women With Suspected Primary Ovarian Insufficiency

- Complete history and physical examination
- Family history of early menopause
- LH, FSH, estradiol, and prolactin levels
- If FSH initially elevated, repeat FSH and estradiol levels on at least 2 occasions, usually 1 month apart
- Karyotype (consider molecular cytogenetic studies of the X chromosome)
- FMR1 gene premutation testing
- Adrenal antibodies (evaluate adrenal reserve with ACTH testing if positive)
- TSH and thyroid peroxidase antibodies
- Fasting blood glucose
- Serum calcium and phosphorus concentrations
- Pelvic ultrasound

Not indicated

- Progesterone withdrawal test
- Ovarian antibodies
- Ovarian biopsy

Abbreviations: ACTH, adrenocorticotropic hormone; FMR1, fragile X mental retardation 1; FSH, follicle-stimulating hormone; LH, luteinizing hormone; TSH, thyroid-stimulating hormone.

should be added for 14 days of the month. Although clinical trial data are lacking regarding the optimal length of HT for women with premature menopause, most healthcare professionals recommend continuing until at least age 50 years (the median age of menopause), provided no adverse effects are observed.[16] If the woman does not want to risk becoming pregnant, hormonal contraceptives can be used to provide estrogen.

Therapy can continue for an individual woman as long as the benefits outweigh the risks. It is important to realize that the findings of most clinical trials regarding the benefits and risks of HT pertain to women aged 50 years and older. For women experiencing an early menopause, especially before age 45, the benefits of using HT until the average age of natural menopause will likely outweigh the risks. Not only is treatment of vasomotor symptoms and vaginal atrophy and maintenance of BMD important for younger women, premature menopause or POI appear to be associated with an increased risk of cardiovascular disease and cognitive impairment with aging, especially for women experiencing menopause before age 45 who do not receive HT.[146,151,152] It is also possible that cardiovascular and cognitive impairment are related to the genetic condition associated with early menopause.

Psychological support. Women experiencing premature menopause or POI may experience significant psychological consequences.[147] For some women, particularly those who are younger, infertility can precipitate a range of emotions. Offer psychological support for concerns about early loss of fertility, self-image, and sexual function.

Childbearing options. If possible, provide counseling regarding childbearing options before chemotherapy, radiation, or surgery that may induce premature menopause. Consider referral to a fertility specialist in all situations in which early loss of fertility is possible. Options for preserving fertility include ovarian hyperstimulation with oocyte retrieval followed by oocyte or embryo cryopreservation, ovarian tissue cryopreservation, ovarian suppression with hormones, ovarian transposition, and conservative gynecologic surgery (eg, trachelectomy for cervical cancer). However, diminished ovarian reserve correlates with poor pregnancy rates with all options listed above and not all options are available for all women, and some techniques such as ovarian tissue cryopreservation are still experimental.

For women with premature menopause or POI, discuss their concerns about childbearing and their options. Pregnancy through in vitro fertilization with oocytes from a known or anonymous donor is commonly recommended and performed with high success rates. Embryo donation is available, and adoption is another alternative. Whether a woman chooses these options depends on age, general health, financial status, and the cause of premature menopause.

Because of the possibility of spontaneous and unexpected pregnancy, women with POI should be counseled early in their course regarding their desire to conceive. If pregnancy is not desired, oral contraceptives, barrier methods, or an intrauterine device are suggested to prevent the unlikely occurrence of an unintentional pregnancy. Oral contraceptives provide additional benefits, including relief of vasomotor symptoms and vaginal dryness and maintenance of BMD. A discussion of contraception is especially important for women with FMR1 who carry a higher risk for a child with mental retardation.

Sexual concerns. Because premature menopause and POI occur at an age when women usually engage in more frequent sexual activity, they may be more adversely affected by any sexual function change than older women experiencing natural menopause. Most women experiencing premature menopause and POI are able to maintain their sex life. Clinicians can provide information regarding what to expect during this time of change to make coping easier.

The causes of sexual concerns in women with premature menopause are multifactorial and often related to their diagnosis or to the medical problem that precipitated menopause. Etiologies include depression, anxiety, relationship conflict, stress, fatigue, medications, or physical problems that make sexual activity uncomfortable. A thorough evaluation should be performed before considering treatment options. Counseling and sex therapy help patients and couples overcome a wide variety of sexual problems. Vaginal dryness and dyspareunia can be treated the same as they are in natural menopause

Special concerns for women undergoing cancer therapy. Because the effect of pelvic radiation and chemotherapy on ovarian function is sometimes not readily apparent, sexually active, reproductive-aged women facing these interventions should discuss fertility preservation or the need for birth control with their healthcare clinician. Fertility can often be preserved in women undergoing either chemotherapy or radiation treatment for cancer.[153] The effect of cancer treatment on fertility and POI depends on the type of chemotherapy, size of the radiation field and dose intensity, the disease, the patient's age, and the patient's pretreatment fertility.

After chemotherapy, the ovaries of younger women (<30 years) are more likely to recover. Some women may experience temporary ovarian insufficiency, with subsequent resumption of menstruation and fertility. Women aged 40 years or older are more likely to have induced menopause. Certain chemotherapeutic agents, such as alkylating agents, are more toxic. In a randomized trial, the use of a GnRH agonist to shut down the menstrual cycle appeared to reduce the cytotoxic damage from chemotherapy.[154]

Pelvic radiation is more likely to cause induced menopause if the ovaries receive high doses of radiation (such as during the treatment for cervical cancer). Estrogen levels often decline quickly. If lower doses of pelvic radiation are used (such as for Hodgkin lymphoma), the ovaries may recover. In these circumstances, surgical transposition of the ovaries away from the radiation field may be an option.

Premature menopause and POI have many different causes. Evaluation for these disorders is complex but needs to start with the finding of elevated FSH and reduced estradiol (intermittent or constant), together with reduced AMH and inhibin B, as well as reduced numbers or function of follicles. Management depends on the patient's wishes, her age, and previous fertility, as well as on the probable cause of the disorder. Further research is necessary as to the causes and proper type and length of treatment.

References

1. Wallace WH, Kelsey TW. Human ovarian reserve from conception to the menopause. *PLoS One*. 2010;5(1):e8772.
2. Miro F, Parker SW, Aspinall LJ, Coley J, Perry PW, Ellis JE. Sequential classification of endocrine stages during reproductive aging in women: the FREEDOM study. *Menopause*. 2005;12(3):281-290.
3. US Census Bureau. Population Division. *Projections of the Population by Selected Age Groups and Sex for the United States: 2015 to 2060*. US Census Bureau Web site. Published December 2012. www.census.gov/population/projections/data/national/2012/summarytables.html. Accessed June 2, 2014.
4. Statistics Canada. Demography Division. *Population Projections for Canada, Provinces and Territories: 2009 to 2036*. Ottawa, Ontario, Canada: Ministry of Industry; 2010. www.statcan.gc.ca/pub/91-520-x/91-520-x2010001-eng.pdf. Accessed June 2, 2014.
5. Murphy SL, Xu J, Kockanek KD. *Deaths: Final Data for 2010*. Hyattsville, MD: National Center for Health Statistics; 2013. National Vital Statistics Reports, vol. 61, no. 4.
6. Gold EB, Sternfeld B, Kelsey JL, et al. Relation of demographic and lifestyle factors to symptoms in a multi-racial/ethnic population of women 40-55 years of age. *Am J Epidemiol*. 2000;152(5):463-473.
7. Avis NE, Stellato R, Crawford S, et al. Is there a menopausal syndrome? Menopausal status and symptoms across racial/ethnic groups. *Soc Sci Med*. 2001;52(3):345-356.
8. Brzyski RG, Medrano MA, Hyatt-Santos JM, Ross JS. Quality of life in low-income menopausal women attending primary care clinics. *Fertil Steril*. 2001;76(1):44-50.
9. Lock M, Kaufert P. Menopause, local biologies, and cultures of aging. *Am J Hum Biol*. 2001;13(4):494-504.
10. Palmer JR, Rosenberg L, Wise LA, Horton NJ, Adams-Campbell LL. Onset of natural menopause in African American women. *Am J Public Health*. 2003;93(2):299-306.
11. Sommer B, Avis N, Meyer P, et al. Attitudes toward menopause and aging across ethnic/racial groups. *Psychosom Med*. 1999;61(6):868-875. Erratum in: *Psychosom Med*. 2000;62(1):96.
12. Winterich JA, Umberson D. How women experience menopause: the importance of social context. *J Women Aging*. 1999;11(4):57-73.
13. Woods NF, Mitchell ES. Anticipating menopause: observations from the Seattle Midlife Women's Health Study. *Menopause*. 1999;6(2):167-173.
14. Utian WH, Boggs PP. The North American Menopause Society 1998 Menopause Survey. Part I: Postmenopausal women's perceptions about menopause and midlife. *Menopause*. 1999;6(2):122-128.
15. Martin KA, Manson JE. Approach to the patient with menopausal symptoms. *J Clin Endocrinol Metab*. 2008;93(12):4567-4575.
16. North American Menopause Society. The 2012 hormone therapy position statement of: The North American Menopause Society. *Menopause*. 2012;19(3):257-271.
17. Jacobs Institute of Women's Health Expert Panel on Menopause Counseling. *Guidelines for Counseling Women on the Management of Menopause*. Washington, DC: Jacobs Institute of Women's Health; 2000.
18. Johnston JM, Colvin A, Johnson BD, et al. Comparison of SWAN and WISE menopausal status classification algorithms. *J Womens Health (Larchmt)*. 2006;15(10):1184-1194.
19. Soules MR, Sherman S, Parrott E, et al. Executive summary: Stages of Reproductive Aging Workshop (STRAW) Park City, Utah, July, 2001. *Menopause*. 2001;8(6):402-407.
20. Hansen KR, Knowlton NS, Thyer AC, Charleston JS, Soules MR, Klein NA. A new model of reproductive aging: the decline in ovarian non-growing follicle number from birth to menopause. *Hum Reprod*. 2008;23(3):699-708.
21. Broekmans FJ, Soules MR, Fauser BC. Ovarian aging: mechanisms and clinical consequences. *Endocr Rev*. 2009;30(5):465-493.
22. Harlow SD, Cain K, Crawford S, et al. Evaluation of four proposed bleeding criteria for the onset of late menopausal transition. *J Clin Endocrinol Metab*. 2006;91(9):3432-3438.
23. Harlow SD, Crawford S, Dennerstein L, Burger HG, Mitchell ES, Sowers MF; ReSTAGE Collaboration. Recommendations from a multi-study evaluation of proposed criteria for staging reproductive aging. *Climacteric*. 2007;10(2):112-119.
24. Harlow SD, Gass M, Hall JE, et al; STRAW 10 Collaborative Group. Executive summary of the Stages of Reproductive Aging Workshop + 10: addressing the unfinished agenda of staging reproductive aging. *Menopause*. 2012;19(4):387-395.
25. Hale GE, Burger HG. Hormonal changes and biomarkers in late reproductive age, menopausal transition and menopause. *Best Pract Res Clin Obstet Gynaecol*. 2009;23(1):7-23.
26. Burger HG, Hale GE, Dennerstein L, Robertson DM. Cycle and hormone changes during perimenopause: the key role of ovarian function. *Menopause*. 2008;15(4 pt 1):603-612.

27. Sowers M, McConnell D, Gast K, et al. Anti-Müllerian hormone and inhibin B variability during normal menstrual cycles. *Fertil Steril.* 2010;94(4):1482-1486.
28. Robertson DM, Hale GE, Fraser IS, Hughes CL, Burger HG. A proposed classification system for menstrual cycles in the menopause transition based on changes in serum hormone profiles. *Menopause.* 2008;15(6):1139-1144.
29. Seifer DB, Baker VL, Leader B. Age-specific serum anti-Müllerian hormone values for 17,120 women presenting to fertility centers within the United States. *Fertil Steril.* 2011;95(2):747-750.
30. Sowers MR, Eyvazzadeh AD, McConnell D, et al. Anti-mullerian hormone and inhibin B in the definition of ovarian aging and the menopause transition. *J Clin Endocrinol Metab.* 2008;93(9):3478-3483.
31. Tehrani FR, Solaymani-Dodaran M, Tohidi M, Gohari MR, Azizi F. Modeling age at menopause using serum concentration of anti-mullerian hormone. *J Clin Endocrinol Metab.* 2013;98(2):729-735. Erratum in: *J Clin Endocrinol Metab.* 2013;98(4):1766.
32. Dewailly D, Andersen CY, Balen A, et al. The physiology and clinical utility of anti-Mullerian hormone in women. *Hum Reprod Update.* 2014;20(3): 370-385.
33. Bentzen JC, Forman JL, Larsen EC, et al. Maternal menopause as a predictor of anti-Mullerian hormone level and antral follicle count in daughters during reproductive age. *Hum Reprod.* 2013;28(1):247-255.
34. Bentzen JG, Forman JL, Johannsen TH, Pinborg A, Larsen EC, Andersen AN. Ovarian antral follicle subclasses and anti-mullerian hormone during normal reproductive aging. *J Clin Endocrinol Metab.* 2013;98(4):1602-1611.
35. Wellons MF, Bates GW, Schreiner PJ, Siscovick DS, Sternfeld B, Lewis CE. Antral follicle count predicts natural menopause in a population-based sample: the Coronary Artery Risk Development in Young Adults Women's Study. *Menopause.* 2013;20(8):825-830.
36. Schuh-Huerta SM, Johnson NA, Rosen MP, Sternfeld B, Cedars MI, Reijo Pera RA. Genetic markers of ovarian follicle number and menopause in women of multiple ethnicities. *Hum Genet.* 2012;131(11):1709-1724.
37. Hale GE, Zhao X, Hughes CL, Burger HG, Robertson DM, Fraser IS. Endocrine features of menstrual cycles in middle and late reproductive age and the menopausal transition classified according to the Staging of Reproductive Aging Workshop (STRAW) staging system. *J Clin Endocrinol Metab.* 2007;92(8):3060-3067.
38. Harlow SD, Mitchell ES, Crawford S, Nan B, Little R, Taffe J; ReSTAGE Collaboration. The ReSTAGE Collaboration: defining optimal bleeding criteria for onset of early menopausal transition. *Fertil Steril.* 2008;89(1): 129-140.
39. Taffe JR, Cain KC, Mitchell ES, Woods NF, Crawford SL, Harlow SD. "Persistence" improves the 60-day amenorrhea marker of entry to late-stage menopausal transition for women aged 40 to 44 years. *Menopause.* 2010; 17(1):191-193.
40. Hale GE, Hughes CL, Burger HG, Robertson DM, Fraser IS. Atypical estradiol secretion and ovulation patterns caused by luteal out-of-phase (LOOP) events underlying irregular ovulatory menstrual cycles in the menopausal transition. *Menopause.* 2009;16(1):50-59.
41. Hale GE, Robertson DM, Burger HG. The perimenopausal woman: endocrinology and management. *J Steroid Biochem Mol Biol.* 2014; 142C:121-131..
42. Welt CK, Jimenez Y, Sluss PM, Smith PC, Hall JE. Control of estradiol secretion in reproductive ageing. *Hum Reprod.* 2006;21(8):2189-2193.
43. O'Connor KA, Ferrell RJ, Brindle E, et al. Total and unopposed estrogen exposure across stages of the transition to menopause. *Cancer Epidemiol Biomarkers Prev.* 2009;18(3):828-836.
44. O'Connor KA, Ferrell R, Brindle E, et al. Progesterone and ovulation across stages of the transition to menopause. *Menopause.* 2009;16(6):1178-1187.
45. Weiss G, Skurnick JH, Goldsmith LT, Santoro NF, Park SJ. Menopause and hypothalamic-pituitary sensitivity to estrogen. *JAMA.* 2004;292(24): 2991-2996. Erratum in: *JAMA.* 2005;293(2):163; *JAMA.* 2007;298(3):288.
46. Santoro N, Crawford SL, Lasley WL, et al. Factors related to declining luteal function in women during the menopausal transition. *J Clin Endocrinol Metab.* 2008;93(5):1711-1721.
47. Santoro N, Lasley B, McConnell D, et al. Body size and ethnicity are associated with menstrual cycle alterations in women in the early menopausal transition: the Study of Women's Health across the Nation (SWAN) Daily Hormone Study. *J Clin Endocrinol Metab.* 2004;89(6):2622-2631.
48. Freeman EW, Sammel MD, Lin H, Gracia CR. Obesity and reproductive hormone levels in the transition to menopause. *Menopause.* 2010;17(4): 718-726.
49. Randolph JF Jr, Zheng H, Sowers MR, et al. Change in follicle-stimulating hormone and estradiol across the menopausal transition: effect of age at the final menstrual period. *J Clin Endocrinol Metab.* 2011;96(3):746-754.
50. Randolph JF Jr, Sowers M, Bondarenko IV, Harlow SD, Luborsky JL, Little RJ. Change in estradiol and follicle-stimulating hormone across the early menopausal transition: effects of ethnicity and age. *J Clin Endocrinol Metab.* 2004;89(4):1555-1561.
51. Burger HG, Dudley EC, Cui J, Dennerstein L, Hopper JL. A prospective longitudinal study of serum testosterone, dehydroepiandrosterone sulfate, and sex hormone-binding globulin levels through the menopause transition. *J Clin Endocrinol Metab.* 2000;85(8):2832-2838.
52. Mushayandebvu T, Castracane VD, Gimpel T, Adel T, Santoro N. Evidence for diminished midcycle ovarian androgen production in older reproductive aged women. *Fertil Steril.* 1996;65(4):721-723.
53. Laughlin GA, Barrett-Connor E, Kritz-Silverstein D, von Mühlen D. Hysterectomy, oophorectomy, and endogenous sex hormone levels in older women: the Rancho Bernardo Study. *J Clin Endocrinol Metab.* 2000;85(2):645-651.
54. Davison SL, Bell R, Donath S, Montalto JG, Davis SR. Androgen levels in adult females: changes with age, menopause, and oophorectomy. *J Clin Endocrinol Metab.* 2005;90(7):3847-3853.
55. Seungdamrong A, Weiss G. Ovulation in a postmenopausal woman. *Fertil Steril.* 2007;88(5):1438.e1-e2.
56. Rinaudo P, Strauss JF 3rd. Endocrine function of the postmenopausal ovary. *Endocrinol Metab Clin North Am.* 2004;33(4):661-674.
57. Cappola AR, Ratcliffe SJ, Bhasin S, et al. Determinants of serum total and free testosterone levels in women over the age of 65 years. *J Clin Endocrinol Metab.* 2007;92(2):509-516.
58. Spencer JB, Klein M, Kumar A, Azziz R. The age-associated decline of androgens in reproductive age and menopausal black and white women. *J Clin Endocrinol Metab.* 2007;92(12):4730-4733.
59. Hall JE. Neuroendocrine changes with reproductive aging in women. *Semin Reprod Med.* 2007;25(5):344-351.
60. Downs JL, Wise PM. The role of the brain in female reproductive aging. *Mol Cell Endocrinol.* 2009;299(1):32-38.
61. Yin W, Wu D, Noel ML, Gore AC. Gonadotropin-releasing hormone neuroterminals and their microenvironment in the median eminence: effects of aging and estradiol treatment. *Endocrinology.* 2009;150(12):5498-5508.
62. Yin W, Gore AC. Neuroendocrine control of reproductive aging: roles of GnRH neurons. *Reproduction.* 2006;131(3):403-413.
63. Kermath BA, Gore AC. Neuroendocrine control of the transition to reproductive senescence: lessons learned from the female rodent model. *Neuroendocrinology.* 2012;96(1):1-12.
64. Shaw ND, Histed SN, Srouji SS, Yang J, Lee H, Hall JE. Estrogen negative feedback on gonadotropin secretion: evidence for a direct pituitary effect in women. *J Clin Endocrinol Metab.* 2010;95(4):1955-1961.
65. Shaw ND, Srouji SS, Histed SN, McCurnin KE, Hall JE. Aging attenuates the pituitary response to gonadotropin-releasing hormone. *J Clin Endocrinol Metab.* 2009;94(9):3259-3264.
66. Shaw ND, Srouji SS, Histed SN, Hall JE. Differential effects of aging on estrogen negative and positive feedback. *Am J Physiol Endocrinol Metab.* 2011;301(2):E351-E355.
67. Lavoie HB, Marsh EE, Hall JE. Absence of apparent circadian rhythms of gonadotropins and free alpha-subunit in postmenopausal women: evidence for distinct regulation relative to other hormonal rhythms. *J Biol Rhythms.* 2006;21(1):58-67.
68. Klingman KM, Marsh EE, Klerman EB, Anderson EJ, Hall JE. Absence of circadian rhythms of gonadotropin secretion in women. *J Clin Endocrinol Metab.* 2011;96(5):1456-1461.
69. Cole LA, Sasaki Y, Muller CY. Normal production of human chorionic gonadotropin in menopause. *N Engl J Med.* 2007;356(11):1184-1186.
70. Giordano R, Bo M, Pellegrino M, et al. Hypothalamus-pituitary-adrenal hyperactivity in human aging is partially refractory to stimulation by mineralocorticoid receptor blockade. *J Clin Endocrinol Metab.* 2005; 90(10):5656-5662.
71. Laughlin GA, Barrett-Connor E. Sexual dimorphism in the influence of advanced aging on adrenal hormone levels: the Rancho Bernardo Study. *J Clin Endocrinol Metab.* 2000;85(10):3561-3568.
72. Wilkinson CW, Petrie EC, Murray SR, Colasurdo EA, Raskind MA, Peskind ER. Human glucocorticoid feedback inhibition is reduced in older individuals: evening study. *J Clin Endocrinol Metab.* 2001;86(2):545-550.
73. Woods NF, Carr MC, Tao EY, Taylor HJ, Mitchell ES. Increased urinary cortisol levels during the menopausal transition. *Menopause.* 2006;13(2):212-221.

74. Woods NF, Mitchell ES, Smith-Dijulio K. Cortisol levels during the menopausal transition and early postmenopause: observations from the Seattle Midlife Women's Health Study. *Menopause.* 2009;16(4):708-718.
75. Saxena AR, Seely EW. Luteinizing hormone correlates with adrenal function in postmenopausal women. *Menopause.* 2012;19(11):1280-1283.
76. Alevizaki M, Saltiki K, Mantzou E, Anastasiou E, Huhtaniemi I. The adrenal gland may be a target of LH action in postmenopausal women. *Eur J Endocrinol.* 2006;154(6):875-881.
77. Qureshi AC, Bahri A, Breen LA, et al. The influence of the route of oestrogen administration on serum levels of cortisol-binding globulin and total cholesterol. *Clin Endocrinol (Oxf).* 2007;66(5):632-635.
78. Cucinelli F, Soranna L, Barini A, et al. Estrogen treatment and body fat distribution are involved in corticotropin and cortisol response to corticotropin-releasing hormone in postmenopausal women. *Metabolism.* 2002;51(2):137-143.
79. Genazzani AR, Lombardi I, Borgioli G, et al. Adrenal function under long-term raloxifene administration. *Gynecol Endocrinol.* 2003;17(2):159-168.
80. Liu CH, Laughlin GA, Fischer UG, Yen SS. Marked attenuation of ultradian and circadian rhythms of dehydroepiandrosterone in postmenopausal women: evidence for a reduced 17,20-desmolase enzymatic activity. *J Clin Endocrinol Metab.* 1990;71(4):900-906.
81. Parker CR Jr, Slayden SM, Azziz R, et al. Effects of aging on adrenal function in the human: responsiveness and sensitivity of adrenal androgens and cortisol to adrenocorticotropin in premenopausal and postmenopausal women. *J Clin Endocrinol Metab.* 2000;85(1):48-54.
82. Khaw KT, Tazuke S, Barrett-Connor E. Cigarette smoking and levels of adrenal androgens in postmenopausal women. *N Engl J Med.* 1988;318(26):1705-1709.
83. Guthrie JR, Dennerstein L, Taffe JR, Lehert P, Burger HG. The menopausal transition: a 9-year prospective population-based study. The Melbourne Women's Midlife Health Project. *Climacteric.* 2004;7(4):375-389.
84. Lasley BL, Santoro N, Randolf JF, et al. The relationship of circulating dehydroepiandrosterone, testosterone, and estradiol to stages of the menopausal transition and ethnicity. *J Clin Endocrinol Metab.* 2002;87(8):3760-3767.
85. Crawford S, Santoro N, Laughlin GA, et al. Circulating dehydroepiandrosterone sulfate concentrations during the menopausal transition. *J Clin Endocrinol Metab.* 2009;94(8):2945-2951.
86. McConnell DS, Stanczyk FZ, Sowers MR, Randolph JF Jr, Lasley BL. Menopausal transition stage-specific changes in circulating adrenal androgens. *Menopause.* 2012;19(6):658-663.
87. Lasley BL, Chen J, Stanczyk FZ, et al. Androstenediol complements estrogenic bioactivity during the menopausal transition. *Menopause.* 2012;19(6):650-657.
88. Lasley BL, Crawford SL, Laughlin GA, et al. Circulating dehydroepiandrosterone sulfate levels in women who underwent bilateral salpingo-oophorectomy during the menopause transition. *Menopause.* 2011;18(5):494-498.
89. Moran FM, Chen J, Gee NA, Lohstroh PN, Lasley BL. Dehydroepiandrosterone sulfate levels reflect endogenous luteinizing hormone production and response to human chorionic gonadotropin challenge in older female macaque (Macaca fascicularis). *Menopause.* 2013;20(3):329-335.
90. Jensen EV, Jordan VC. The estrogen receptor: a model for molecular medicine. *Clin Cancer Res.* 2003;9(6):1980-1989.
91. Cui J, Shen Y, Li R. Estrogen synthesis and signaling pathways during aging: from periphery to brain. *Trends Mol Med.* 2013;19(3):197-209.
92. Deroo BJ, Korach KS. Estrogen receptors and human disease. *J Clin Invest.* 2006;116(3):561-570.
93. Maximov PY, Lee TM, Jordan VC. The discovery and development of selective estrogen receptor molulators (SERMs) for clinical practice. *Curr Clin Pharmacol.* 2013;8(2):135-155.
94. Kjaergaard AD, Ellervik C, Tybjaerg-Hansen A, et al. Estrogen receptor alpha polymorphism and risk of cardiovascular disease, cancer, and hip fracture: cross-sectional, cohort, and case-control studies and a meta-analysis. *Circulation.* 2007;115(7):861-871.
95. Chang EC, Charn TH, Park SH, et al. Estrogen receptors alpha and beta as determinants of gene expression: influence of ligand, dose, and chromatin binding. *Mol Endocrinol.* 2008;22(5):1032-1043.
96. Minutolo F, Macchia M, Katzenellenbogen BS, Katzenellenbogen JA. Estrogen receptor β ligands: recent advances and biomedical applications. *Med Res Rev.* 2011;31(3):364-442.
97. Nelson ER, Wardell SE, McDonnell DP. The molecular mechanisms underlying the pharmacological actions of estrogens, SERMs and oxysterols: implications for the treatment and prevention of osteoporosis. *Bone.* 2013;53(1):42-50.
98. McDonnell DP. The molecular determinants of estrogen receptor pharmacology. *Maturitas.* 2004;48(suppl 1):S7-S12.
99. Hall JM, McDonnell DP. Coregulators in nuclear estrogen receptor action: from concept to therapeutic targeting. *Mol Interv.* 2005;5(6):343-357.
100. Levin ER. Plasma membrane estrogen receptors. *Trends Endocrinol Metab.* 2009;20(10):477-482.
101. Moriarty K, Kim KH, Bender JR. Minireview: estrogen receptor-mediated rapid signaling. *Endocrinology.* 2006;147(12):5557-5563.
102. Maggiolini M, Picard D. The unfolding stories of GPR30, a new membrane-bound estrogen receptor. *J Endocrinol.* 2010;204(2):105-114.
103. Langer G, Bader B, Meoli L, et al. A critical review of fundamental controversies in the field of GPR30 research. *Steroids.* 2009;75(8-9):603-610.
104. Ariazi EA, Jordan VC. Estrogen-related receptors as emerging targets in cancer and metabolic disorders. *Curr Top Med Chem.* 2006;6(3):203-215.
105. Wardell SE, Nelson ER, Chao CA, McDonnell DP. Bazedoxifene exhibits antiestrogenic activity in animal models of tamoxifen-resistant breast cancer: implications for treatment of advanced disease. *Clin Cancer Res.* 2013;19(9):2420-2431.
106. Wardell SE, Kazmin D, McDonnell DP. Research resource: transcriptional profiling in a cellular model of breast cancer reveals functional and mechanistic differences between clinically relevant SERM and between SERM/estrogen complexes. *Mol Endocrinol.* 2012;26(7):1235-1248.
107. Liu S, Han SJ, Smith CL. Cooperative activation of gene expression by agonists and antagonists mediated by estrogen receptor heteroligand dimer complexes. *Mol Pharmacol.* 2013;83(5):1066-1077.
108. Chabbert-Buffet N, Meduri G, Bouchard P, Spitz IM. Selective progesterone receptor modulators and progesterone antagonists: mechanisms of action and clinical applications. *Hum Reprod Update.* 2005;11(3):293-307.
109. Bouchard P, Chabbert-Buffet N, Fauser BC. Selective progesterone receptor modulators in reproductive medicine: pharmacology, clinical efficacy and safety. *Fertil Steril.* 2011;96(5):1175-1189.
110. Chabbert-Buffet N, Pintiaux A, Bouchard P. The imminent dawn of SPRMs in obstetrics and gynecology. *Mol Cell Endocrinol.* 2012;358(2):232-243.
111. Matsumoto T, Sakari M, Okada M, et al. The androgen receptor in health and disease. *Annu Rev Physiol.* 2013;75:201-204.
112. Baldassarre M, Perrone AM, Giannone FA, et al. Androgen receptor expression in the human vagina under different physiological and treatment conditions. *Int J Impot Res.* 2013;25(1):7-11.
113. Vera-Badillo FE, Templeton AJ, de Gouveia P, et al. Androgen receptor expression and outcomes in early breast cancer: a systematic review and meta-analysis. *J Natl Cancer Inst.* 2014;106(1):djt319.
114. Coulam CB, Bustillo M, Schulman JD. Empty follicle syndrome. *Fertil Steril.* 1986;46(6):1153-1155.
115. Kirchheiner K, Fidarova E, Nout RA, et al. Radiation-induced morphological changes in the vagina. *Strahlenther Onkol.* 2012;188(11):1010-1017.
116. Nelson LM. Clinical practice. Primary ovarian insufficiency. *N Engl J Med.* 2009;360(6):606-614.
117. Progetto Menopausa Italia Study Group. Premature ovarian failure: frequency and risk factors among women attending a network of menopause clinics in Italy. *BJOG.* 2003;110(1):59-63.
118. de Moraes-Ruehsen M, Jones GS. Premature ovarian failure. *Fertil Steril.* 1967;18(4):440-461.
119. Alper MM, Garner PR, Seibel MM. Premature ovarian failure. Current concepts. *J Reprod Med.* 1986;31(8):699-708.
120. Aittomäki K, Lucena JL, Pakarinem P, et al. Mutations in the follicle-stimulating hormone receptor gene causes hereditary hypergonadotropic ovarian failure. *Cell.* 1995;82(6):959-968.
121. Bakalov VK, Anasti JN, Calis KA, et al. Autoimmune oophoritis as a mechanism of follicular dysfunction in women with 46,XX spontaneous premature ovarian failure. *Fertil Steril.* 2005;84(4):958-965.
122. Farquhar CM, Sadler L, Harvey SA, Stewart AW. The association of hysterectomy and menopause: a prospective cohort study. *BJOG.* 2005;112(7):956-962.
123. Tulandi T, Salamah K. Fertility and uterine artery embolization. *Obstet Gynecol.* 2010;115(4):857-860.
124. Siddle N, Sarrel P, Whitehead M. The effect of hysterectomy on the age of ovarian failure: identification of a subgroup of women with premature loss of ovarian function and literature review. *Fertil Steril.* 1987;47(1):94-100.

Chapter 1

125. Rebar RW, Connolly HV. Clinical features of young women with hypergonadotropic amenorrhea. *Fertil Steril*. 1990;53(5):804-810.
126. van Kasteren YM, Hundscheid RD, Smits AP, Cremers FP, van Zonneveld P, Braat DD. Familial idiopathic premature ovarian failure: an overrated and underestimated genetic disease? *Hum Reprod*. 1999;14(10):2455-2459.
127. Vegetti W, Marozzi A, Manfredini E, et al. Premature ovarian failure. *Mol Cell Endocrinol*. 2000;161(1-2):53-57.
128. Luborsky JL, Meyer P, Sowers MF, Gold EB, Santoro N. Premature menopause in a multi-ethnic population study of the menopause transition. *Hum Reprod*. 2003;18(1):199-206.
129. Rebar RW. Premature ovarian failure. *Obstet Gynecol*. 2009;113(6):1355-1363.
130. Vearncombe KJ, Pachana NA. Is cognitive functioning detrimentally affected after early, induced menopause? *Menopause*. 2009;16(1):188-198.
131. Vujovic S. Aetiology of premature ovarian failure. *Menopause Int*. 2009;15(2):72-75.
132. Harris SE, Chand AL, Winship IM, Gersak K, Aittomäki K, Shelling AN. Identification of novel mutations in FOXL2 associated with premature ovarian failure. *Mol Hum Reprod*. 2002;8(8):729-733.
133. Latronico AC, Chai Y, Arnhold IJ, Liu X, Mendonca BB, Segaloff DL. A homozygous microdeletion in helix 7 of the luteinizing hormone receptor associated with familial testicular and ovarian resistance is due to both decreased cell surface expression and impaired effector activation by the cell surface receptor. *Mol Endocrinol*. 1998;12(3):442-450.
134. Vegetti W, Grazia Tibiletti M, Testa G, et al. Inheritance in idiopathic premature ovarian failure: analysis of 71 cases. *Hum Reprod*. 1998;13(7):1796-1800.
135. Mishra G, Hardy R, Kuh D. Are the effects of risk factors for timing of menopause modified by age? Results from a British birth cohort study. *Menopause*. 2007;14(4):717-724.
136. Murray A, Schoemaker MJ, Bennett CE, et al. Population-based estimates of the prevalence of FMR1 expansion mutations in women with early menopause and primary ovarian insufficiency. *Genet Med*. 2014;16(1):19-24.
137. Wittenberger MD, Hagerman RJ, Sherman SL, et al. The FMR1 premutation and reproduction. *Fertil Steril*. 2007;87(3):456-465.
138. Hoek A, Schoemaker J, Drexhage HA. Premature ovarian failure and ovarian autoimmunity. *Endocr Rev*. 1997;18(1):107-134.
139. Alper MM, Garner PR. Premature ovarian failure: its relationship to autoimmune disease. *Obstet Gynecol*. 1985;66(1):27-30.
140. Zinn AR. The X chromosome and the ovary. *J Soc Gynecol Investig*. 2001;8(1 suppl proceedings):S34-S36.
141. Spencer JB, Badik JR, Ryan EL, et al. Modifiers of ovarian function in girls and women with classic galactosemia. *J Clin Endocrinol Metab*. 2013;98(7):E1257-E1265.
142. Morrison JC, Given JR, Wiser WL, Fish SA. Mumps oophoritis: a cause of premature menopause. *Fertil Steril*. 1975;26(7):655-659.
143. Méduri G, Massin N, Guibourdenche J, et al. Serum anti-Müllerian hormone expression in women with premature ovarian failure. *Hum Reprod*. 2007;22(1):117-123.
144. Chalmers C, Lindsay M, Usher D, Warner P, Evans D, Ferguson M. Hysterectomy and ovarian function: levels of follicle stimulating hormone and incidence of menopausal symptoms are not affected by hysterectomy in women under age 45 years. *Climacteric*. 2002;5(4):366-373.
145. Gallagher JC. Effects of early menopause on bone mineral density and fractures. *Menopause*. 2007;14(3 pt 2):567-571.
146. Rocca WA, Bower JC, Maraganote DM, et al. Increased risk of cognitive impairment or dementia in women who underwent oophorectomy before menopause. *Neurology*. 2007;69(11):1074-1083.
147. van der Stege JG, Groen H, van Zadelhoff SJ, et al. Decreased androgen concentrations and diminished general and sexual well-being in women with premature ovarian failure. *Menopause*. 2008;15(1):23-31.
148. Kalantaridou SN, Vanderhoof VH, Calis KA, Corrigan EC, Troendle JF, Nelson LM. Sexual function in young women with spontaneous 46,XX primary ovarian insufficiency. *Fertil Steril*. 2008;90(5):1805-1811.
149. Knauff EA, Eijkemans MJ, Lambalk CB, et al; Dutch Premature Ovarian Failure Consortium. Anti-mullerian hormone, inhibin B, and antral follicle count in young women with ovarian failure. *J Clin Endocrinol Metab*. 2009;94(3):786-792. Erratum in: *J Clin Endocrinol Metab*. 2010;95(1):465.
150. Su HI, Sammel MD, Green J, et al. Antimullerian hormone and inhibin B are hormone measures of ovarian function in late reproductive-aged breast cancer survivors. *Cancer*. 2010;116(3):592-599.
151. Parker WH, Broder MS, Chang E, et al. Ovarian conservation at the time of hysterectomy and long-term health outcomes in the Nurses' Health Study. *Obstet Gynecol*. 2009;113(5):1027-1037.
152. Rivera CM, Grossardt BR, Rhodes DJ, et al. Increased cardiovascular mortality after early bilateral oophorectomy. *Menopause*. 2009;16(1):15-23.
153. Loren AW, Mangu PB, Beck LN, et al; American Society of Clinical Oncology. Fertility preservation for patients with cancer: American Society of Clinical Oncology clinical practice guideline update. *J Clin Oncol*. 2013;31(10):2500-2510.
154. Del Mastro L, Boni L, Michelotti A, et al. Effect of the gonadotropin-releasing hormone analogue triptorelin on the occurrence of chemotherapy-induced early menopause in premenopausal women with breast cancer: a randomized trial. *JAMA*. 2011;306(3):269-276.

CHAPTER 2

Midlife Body Changes

Perimenopausal and postmenopausal women often report body changes that may or may not be attributed to the menopause transition. These include weight changes and changes to the vagina, skin, hair, eyes, ears, teeth, and oral cavity, to name a few.

Vulvovaginal changes

In premenopausal women, the vagina is lined with glycogen-rich squamous epithelium, which is nonkeratinized in the vagina, vestibule, and introitus and keratinized in the labia and vulva. Vaginal fluid is composed of transudate from the surrounding blood vessels, mixed with vulvar and cervical secretions, exfoliated epithelial cells, and endometrial and tubal fluids. Normal vaginal fluid may appear clear or white, sometimes flocculent, but it is odorless and does not cause vulvovaginal pruritus, odor, or irritation.

The vaginal vault is populated by complex communities of microorganisms and protective bacteria. In reproductive-aged women, the vaginal flora is dominated by lactobacilli that convert epithelial glycogen into lactic acid, with a resultant pH between 3.5 and 4.5. Lactobacilli also produce hydrogen peroxide, which helps suppress colonization of pathologic organisms.

Vaginal squamous epithelium is composed of 3 layers: immature parabasal cells, intermediate cells, and mature superficial cells. Estrogen stimulation thickens the epithelial layer primarily because of an increase in mature superficial cells.

The vaginal maturation index (VMI) is a clinical laboratory means of evaluating vaginal estrogen status. A vaginal smear is evaluated for percentage of each cell type. Wright's staining aids in identification of each cell. A premenopausal vagina will have a higher proportion of superficial cells, whereas a postmenopausal or estrogen-deprived vagina will have a higher proportion of parabasal cells.

At menopause, the decrease in estrogen along with concomitant changes in the vaginal microbiome increases the vaginal pH from an acidic environment to an alkaline one. Lactobacilli are replaced by other flora that may include organisms commonly found in bacterial vaginosis. Previously, microbiome changes were considered unhealthy, but current research has found that some beneficial microbial communities are associated with a higher pH.[1] This research changes the underlying premise that the menopausal vagina's flora is abnormal and not healthy.

Even though the makeup of the microbial communities is different, a healthy production of lactic acid continues.[2] The menopausal vagina appears to be able to adapt to the tremendous changes at this time by transitioning to previously uncultivated *Lactobacillus* species and other lactic acid-producing bacteria such as *Atopobium*.

The term *vaginal atrophy* describes vaginal walls that are thin, smooth, pale, dry, and sometimes inflamed (*atrophic vaginitis*). (Strictly speaking, atrophic vaginitis reflects either inflammation or infection of the vagina.) Vaginal walls can exhibit small petechiae (pinpoint, nonraised, round, purple-red spots caused by intradermal or submucous hemorrhage) and may be friable to touch. These changes increase the likelihood of trauma from activities such as intercourse, douching, and speculum insertion during a pelvic examination. Vaginal bleeding or spotting, tearing of fragile vaginal tissue, dyspareunia, or pain during any vaginal penetration is often the presenting and most bothersome complaint. Although not all women develop troublesome symptoms after menopause, for some women, the condition can be progressive and severe, resulting in significant vaginal stenosis that prevents sexual intercourse.

Although assessment of the VMI and vaginal pH are routinely part of clinical trials, they are not essential to make diagnoses in clinical practice if examination findings are characteristic of vaginal atrophy.

Atrophy and phimosis of the prepuce of the clitoris may result in dyspareunia that leads to decreased interest in and avoidance of sexual activity. Dyspareunia has been shown to be strongly associated with female sexual dysfunction in postmenopausal women.[3]

Vulvovaginal atrophy may occur in hypoestrogenic states other than natural menopause.[4] Examples include surgical menopause (bilateral oophorectomy, with or without hysterectomy); use of gonadotropin-releasing hormone agonists to manage conditions such as endometriosis and uterine leiomyomata; hypothalamic amenorrhea caused by excessive exercise, disordered eating, or the postpartum state; and by cancer treatments, such as surgery, pelvic radiation therapy, chemotherapy, or endocrine therapy, that remove ovaries or render them inactive, either temporarily or permanently.

Body weight

Many women gain weight during the menopause transition. Although neither menopause nor hormone therapy (HT) is responsible for the added pounds, one study found that postmenopausal women are less likely to lose visceral adipose tissue than premenopausal women during a weight reduction program.[5] Consequently, postmenopausal women may find it more difficult to overcome the increased risk of certain serious diseases such as cardiovascular disease (CVD) that are linked to obesity.

In the United States, 66% of women aged 40 to 59 years and more than 73% of women aged 60 years or older are overweight, defined as a body mass index (BMI) greater than 25 kg/m^2. Approximately 40% of those age groups are obese, defined as a BMI at or above 30 kg/m^2. The prevalence of obesity has been increasing over time, although it appears to have stabilized over the past 10 years at approximately 35% for adult women.[6]

During the menopause transition, many women gain weight, averaging approximately 5 lb (2.27 kg).[7] This increase is sometimes attributed to menopause or to treatment for menopause-related conditions, including the use of HT. However, the notion that menopause or HT is responsible for weight gain is not supported by scientific evidence.[8,9] Weight gain during the menopause transition seems to be related mostly to aging and lifestyle. Several pieces of evidence support this conclusion. Body fat accumulates throughout adult life, and thus any fat accumulated during perimenopause will add to the existing fat deposits. Also, lean body mass decreases with age, which is compounded by the more sedentary lifestyle of older women.[10] Burning fewer calories through less physical activity also increases fat mass and weight gain.[11]

Sleep deprivation also has been associated with weight gain. The mechanisms are unclear, but women with sleep deprivation may experience daytime fatigue and reduced activity. In addition, studies show that sleep deprivation can cause changes in serum leptin and ghrelin levels, subsequently increasing hunger and appetite. A 2006 study reported an association between reduced sleep and increased weight gain in more than 68,000 women followed in the Nurses' Health Study (median follow-up, 12 y).[12] Investigators found that women who slept 5 hours or less gained 2.5 lb (1.14 kg) more than those sleeping 7 hours. Women sleeping 6 hours gained 1.6 lb (0.71 kg) more than those sleeping 7 hours.

Although research suggests that age, rather than menopause, is associated with weight gain, there is some evidence that menopause may be related to changes in body composition and fat distribution. Several studies have shown that menopause is associated with increased fat in the abdominal region as well as decreased lean body mass, independent of age.[13] The change in distribution of fat from subcutaneous stores to visceral abdominal fat may have detrimental metabolic effects. Increased trunk-mass-to-leg-fat-mass ratio has been associated with increases in blood pressure (BP), fasting glucose, and abnormal lipoprotein profiles.[14] Women who are obese with increased visceral adipose tissue stores compared to subcutaneous abdominal adipose tissue are more likely to have DM, metabolic syndrome, hepatic steatosis, and aortic plaque.[15]

The effects of HT on weight are conflicting, with some evidence supporting a slight benefit.[16,17] In the Postmenopausal Estrogen/Progestin Interventions trial (N=847 aged 45 to 64 y), women using estrogen with or without progestogen weighed, on average, 2.2 lb (1 kg) less than placebo recipients at the end of the 3-year trial.[18] No difference in weight was noted between the groups using estrogen therapy (ET) or estrogen-progestogen therapy (EPT). In the Women's Health Initiative (WHI) trial of 10,739 postmenopausal women aged 50 to 79 years randomized to conjugated estrogens (CE) 0.625 mg daily or placebo, BMI had increased 0.5 kg/m^2 in both groups by the 6-year follow-up.[19] Waist circumference increased 1.4 cm in the CE group and 1.9 cm in the placebo group, a difference that was not statistically significant.

Regardless of sex, higher levels of body weight and body fat are associated with increased risk for numerous adverse health consequences such as CVD, type 2 diabetes mellitus (DM), hypertension, some cancers, osteoarthritis, and premature mortality.[20,21] Postmenopausal women who are obese also have a higher rate of breast cancer than nonobese postmenopausal women.[22-24] One study found that gaining 15 lb to 20 lb (6.8-9.0 kg) after age 18 increases the risk of myocardial infarction later in life. Conversely, overweight women who lose just 10% of their body weight can reap many health benefits, including a significant lowering of BP.[25,26]

The metabolic syndrome is a combination of medical disorders that increases a patient's risk for CVD and type 2 DM. According to the National Cholesterol Education Program Adult Treatment Panel (ATP III), the definition includes the presence of any 3 of these 5 traits[27]:

- Central obesity (waist circumference ≥35 in [88 cm] in women)
- Elevated triglycerides (≥150 mg/dL; 1.70 mmol/L) or drug treatment for elevated triglycerides
- Reduced high-density lipoprotein cholesterol (HDL-C; <50 mg/dL in women; 1.3 mmol/L) or drug treatment for low HDL-C

- Elevated blood pressure (BP; ≥130/85 mm Hg) or use of antihypertensive medication
- Elevated fasting glucose levels (≥110 mg/dL; 6.1 mmol/L) or use of medication for hyperglycemia

Diagnosing women with this syndrome is crucial because it helps identify those who need aggressive lifestyle modification, focusing on weight reduction, increased physical activity, and medication, if necessary.[28]

Elevated BMI has been associated with more frequent or severe hot flashes, and increases in body fat have been associated with greater hot flash reporting during the menopause transition.[29] Conversely, weight loss in women who are overweight and obese has been shown to improve the occurrence of bothersome hot flashes.[30] In the WHI Dietary Modification trial, a reduced fat diet with increased intake of fruit, vegetables, and whole grains was associated with a reduction in vasomotor symptoms (VMS), although the effect was more pronounced in women with concomitant weight loss.[31]

Moderating factors—including age, sex, family history, body fat distribution, diet, and physical activity—can affect a person's risk of becoming overweight.

Being underweight can also be unhealthy. Very thin women are at increased risk for osteoporosis. Premenopausal women who overdiet or overexercise can become so underweight that their menstrual cycles stop temporarily, placing them at higher risk for osteoporosis later in life.[32]

Optimization of body weight

Efforts to manage weight in perimenopausal and postmenopausal women are essential. The advice to eat a healthy diet, increase physical activity, and avoid further weight gain is appropriate for almost all women at or above a healthy weight.[33] For those who are overweight or obese, weight loss is indicated. Underweight persons need counseling on achieving a healthy body weight.

Physical activity and controlled caloric intake are necessary to achieve or maintain a healthy body weight. In the Women's Healthy Lifestyle Project, women prevented weight gain (and minimized low-density lipoprotein cholesterol [LDL-C] elevations) during the menopause transition by increasing physical activity and consuming a low-fat diet with moderate caloric restrictions.[34,35]

Several different types of diets have become popular for weight loss, including low-fat, low-calorie diets; moderate-fat, low-calorie diets; low-carbohydrate diets; and high-protein diets. No single diet or eating regimen is right for all women. Women seeking to lose weight should be encouraged to set realistic goals achieved through long-term lifestyle change. Emphasis should be placed on changing eating habits rather than relying on diets, especially fad diets. Support can be obtained from family members, coworkers, and friends. Various organization and support groups (Weight Watchers, Overeaters Anonymous) offer help with dieting, but no single program has been proven superior.[36] A randomized trial compared adherence rates and effectiveness of 4 popular diets: Atkins (carbohydrate restriction), Zone (macronutrient balance), Weight Watchers (calorie restriction), and Ornish (fat restriction).[37] Results showed that all 4 diets modestly decreased body weight and significantly decreased the LDL-C:HDL-C ratio, although overall adherence rates were low. Discontinuation rates were slightly higher in the more extreme diet groups (Atkins and Ornish), although this was not statistically significant. All 4 diets showed greater weight loss and reductions in cardiac risk factors in patients with increased adherence.

Weight loss management tools such as calorie-counting apps or online communities can be effective. The National Weight Control Registry (www.nwcr.ws) is an online resource that describes the behaviors of a large cohort of people who have sustained at least a 30-lb weight loss over time. These resources can provide patients with a "toolbox" approach to weight loss in which they sample a variety of behaviors and adaptations and incorporate the ones that are most helpful to achieve their weight loss goals. Early evidence indicates that online and telephone resources are at least as effective as in-person counseling.[38]

The WHI Dietary Modification Trial examined the long-term benefits and risks of a low-fat diet as well as increasing vegetable, fruit, and grain intake. The intervention group included group and individual sessions to promote decreased fat intake and increased vegetable, fruit, and grain consumption without weight-loss or calorie-restriction goals. In comparison, the control group received diet-related educational materials. Results showed that women in the intervention group lost weight in the first year and maintained a lower weight than the control group during an average 7.5-year follow-up period. These findings refuted claims that low-fat eating results in weight gain in postmenopausal women.[39]

A meta-analysis evaluating the benefit of an increased protein-carbohydrate ratio in a low-fat diet suggest that a high-protein, low-fat diet results in greater reduction in weight, fat mass, and triglyceride levels.[40] A high-protein diet was also shown to improve weight loss as well as total body fat reduction compared with a high-fiber diet in women who were overweight and obese.[41]

No one diet has proven superior for sustained long-term weight loss. However, one review of the literature found maintenance of weight loss to be most closely associated with a daily caloric deficit of 400 to 600 calories, regular physical activity, low fat intake, consumption of fruits and vegetables, self-monitoring, and ongoing behavior support.[42] The benefits of eating at regular intervals (every 4-5 h) and engaging in a regular exercise program—perhaps the most important element—must be emphasized. Regular exercise seems to have the most beneficial effect on minimizing weight gain in midlife women around menopause. Although aerobic and resistance exercises will consume calories and eventually decrease weight, evidence suggests that perimenopausal and postmenopausal women striving for a lower body-fat ratio will benefit more from resistance-type exercise.[43] This type of exercise builds more lean body muscle tissue and may help to create a more slender phenotype. Because lean muscle mass is more metabolically active, muscle building allows women to lose weight without excessively decreasing food consumption. In a randomized study of 107 nonobese postmenopausal women, resistance exercise plus calorie restriction resulted in greater losses in fat mass parameters than did calorie restriction alone.[44] No differences were noted in fasting lipids and insulin resistance, although both groups showed improvement. Increased activity alone will not necessarily result in weight loss. Calories must be restricted in excess of those expended by the exercise.

Recommendations from the US Preventive Services Task Force (USPSTF) are to screen all adults for obesity and offer or refer for intensive, multicomponent behavioral intervention.[45] Intensive, multicomponent behavioral interventions include behavioral management activities, improving diet and increasing physical activity, addressing barriers to change, self-monitoring and strategizing how to maintain lifestyle changes. The level of intervention required depends on the woman's BMI and the presence of comorbidities (Table 1).[46] The benefits and risks of obesity treatment must be assessed on an individual basis.

For overweight women, the initial goal should be to reduce body weight by approximately 10% over 6 to 12 months. This can be accomplished through a management program that includes a controlled diet with a deficit of 500 to 1,000 calories per day, reducing dietary fat intake to less than 30% of total energy intake, and participating in regular physical activity.

Nonpharmacologic interventions

Various herbal remedies and nutritional supplements are advertised to promote weight loss by boosting the metabolic rate; however, controlled clinical studies have not been conducted. Chromium picolinate is touted to help burn fat and build muscle. Studies are conflicting regarding chromium's effect on weight, although at least 1 study found that when combined with a diet and exercise program chromium produced favorable changes in body composition (more lean tissue and less fat). Improvements in metabolic parameters such as insulin resistance, C-reactive protein, and serum lipids have not been demonstrated.[47] A meta-analysis of 11 randomized, controlled trials (RCTs) showed a decrease in weight with chromium supplementation; however, the mean difference was only 0.5 kg, making the clinical significance questionable.[48] Toxic effects are not well known. Remedies containing ephedra should be avoided. This plant contains the stimulant ephedrine, which can cause adverse events (AEs) on the central nervous system, heart rate, and BP.

Many excellent print and Web-based tools are available to supplement the information given by the healthcare professional.[49,50] In conjunction with the Department of Agriculture, the US Department of Health and Human Services publishes the *Dietary Guide for Americans* every 5 years.[51] Controlling portions can be achieved by using a smaller or premeasured portion-control plate. Women with special considerations or medical conditions are best referred to a dietitian for specific dietary advice.

Of special significance to the population of perimenopausal and postmenopausal women are strategies to prevent CVD, which is the leading cause of death for North American women. General diet and lifestyle recommendations from the American Heart Association (AHA), if rigorously applied with other lifestyle recommendations, will significantly decrease the risk for CVD and noncardiac disease as well.[52,53] For persons who are at high risk of CVD, the recommendations may have to be intensified.[28,54]

- *Maintain a healthy body weight.* To avoid weight gain, adults must achieve energy balance (caloric intake= energy expenditure). Knowledge about the caloric content of foods and beverages per portion consumed may increase control of portion size and calorie intake. The macronutrient composition of a diet (the amount of fat, carbohydrate, and protein) has little effect on energy balance unless manipulation of those macronutrients influences total energy intake.

- *Exercise to achieve and maintain a healthy body weight.* Regular aerobic and resistance training exercises help to build and maintain lean muscle mass and strength. Both are needed to maintain not only weight but also short- and long-term health, including memory, attention, and cognitive functioning. The American College of Sports Medicine and the AHA have drafted a set of recommendations on physical activity for older adults (Table 2).[55]

- *Consume a diet rich in vegetables and fruit.* Increasing intake of vegetables and fruits meets micronutrient, macronutrient, and fiber requirements without adding substantially to overall energy consumption. Deeply colored vegetables and fruits (spinach, carrots, peaches, berries) tend to be higher in micronutrients than others (potatoes, corn). Whole fruit is preferred over fruit juice because it contains more fiber.

- *Choose whole-grain, high-fiber foods.* These products have been associated with better diet quality and decreased risk of CVD and some cancers. At least half of grain intake needs to come from whole grains, which include wild rice, barley, quinoa, millet, and wheat berries.[56]

- *Consume fish, especially oily fish, at least twice a week.* Eating 2 servings (approximately 8 oz) per week of fish high in omega-3 polyunsaturated fatty acids (eg, salmon) is associated with a decreased risk of sudden death and

Table 1. Intervention by Body Mass Index Category

BMI (kg/m²)	Intervention options
<18.5	Lifestyle changes[a]
18.5-24.9	No treatment needed
25-26.9	Lifestyle changes if comorbidity present[b]
27-29.9	Lifestyle changes plus drug therapy, if comorbidity present
30-34.9	Lifestyle changes plus drug therapy
35-39.9	Lifestyle changes plus drug therapy; surgery if comorbidity present
>40	Lifestyle changes, drug therapy, and surgery

Abbreviation: BMI, body mass index.
a. Lifestyle changes are diet, exercise, and behavior therapy.
b. Comorbidities include hypertension, type 2 diabetes mellitus, and hyperlipidemia.
National Institutes of Health, National Heart, Lung, and Blood Institute, North American Association for the Study of Obesity.[46]

death from coronary artery disease in adults. Contamination of some fish (especially large, predatory fish such as shark, swordfish, king mackerel, or tilefish) with mercury and other organic compounds is of concern, especially in children and pregnant women. For middle-aged and older men and postmenopausal women, the benefits of fish consumption far outweigh the potential risks when the amounts eaten are within the recommendations established by the US Food and Drug Administration (FDA) and Environmental Protection Agency. Potential exposure to some contaminants can be reduced by removing the skin and surface fat from fish before cooking and by eating smaller fish.

- *Limit intake of saturated and trans fat and cholesterol.* The AHA recommends intakes of less than 7% of energy as saturated fat, less than 1% as trans fat, and less than 300 mg of cholesterol per day.[57] Strategies to reduce saturated fat and cholesterol usually involve replacement of animal fats with unsaturated (polyunsaturated and monounsaturated) fats and selection of lower-fat versions of foods, such as replacing full-fat dairy products with nonfat or low-fat versions. Replacing meats with vegetable alternatives and/or fish is another option. Reduction of trans-fatty acids usually requires substitution of partially hydrogenated fats with liquid vegetable oils, except for tropical oils. Some margarines or butter products contain plant sterols useful in lowering cholesterol.

- *Minimize intake of beverages and foods with added sugars and caffeine.* The primary reasons for this recommendation are to lower total caloric intake and promote nutrient adequacy. Evidence suggests that calories consumed as liquids have less satiety than those from solid foods. This may, in turn, negatively affect attempts to maintain a healthy body weight.

Caffeine-containing drinks (coffee, tea, colas, soft drinks) can have a negative effect on health (trigger hot flashes, contribute to insomnia, increase dehydration). Because women are often unaware of the effects of caffeine or its sources, discuss their intake.

- *Choose and prepare foods with little or no salt.* Reduced sodium intake can prevent hypertension, act as an adjunct to antihypertensive medication, and facilitate hypertension control. Because of the currently high-sodium food supply and high levels of sodium consumption, an interim recommendation for sodium intake has been set at 2.3 g per day (100 mmol/d). An optimal sodium intake is 1.5 g per day (65 mmol/d), which may not be easily achievable at present.

- *Consume alcohol in moderation.* Alcohol can be addictive, and high intake has been associated with serious health and social consequences. The AHA recommends that alcohol consumption be limited to no more than 2 drinks per day for men and 1 drink per day for women, ideally consumed with meals.[58]

- *Follow the AHA diet and lifestyle recommendations when eating food prepared outside the home.*[59] Foods prepared outside the home or "take-away" foods tend to come in large portions and have high-energy density. They are often also high in saturated fat, trans fat, cholesterol, added sugars, and sodium and low in fiber and micronutrients. There is an association between increased consumption of fast food, total energy intake, weight gain, and insulin resistance. People must be vigilant and make wise choices when eating food prepared outside of the home.

Pharmacologic interventions

Pharmacologic therapy can be offered to patients who are obese who have failed to achieve their weight loss goals through an adequate trial of diet, exercise, and lifestyle changes. It should be included as part of a comprehensive program including diet and physical activity in women with

Chapter 2

Table 2. Physical Activity in Older Adults: Recommendations From the American College of Sports Medicine and the American Heart Association

Aerobic activity
- Minimum of 30 min/day, 5 d/wk, of moderate-intensity activity or 20 min/d, 3 d/wk, of vigorous-intensity activity
- On a 10-point scale, in which sitting is 0, moderate-intensity activity is a 5 or 6; vigorous intensity is a 7 or 8
- These activities are in addition to routine activities of daily living

Muscle-strengthening activity
- Resistance exercise involving major muscle groups for a minimum of 2 nonconsecutive d/wk
- 10-15 repetitions of 8-10 exercises
- On a 10-point scale, in which no movement is 0 and maximal effort of a muscle group is a 10, moderate-intensity effort is a 5 or 6; vigorous intensity is a 7 or 8

Flexibility activity
- Exercises that maintain or increase flexibility and improve joint range of motion on at least 2 d/wk for at least 10 min each day

Balance exercise
- In community-dwelling adults with substantial risk of falls (frequent falls or mobility problems), exercises that maintain or improve balance are recommended

Nelson ME, et al.[55]

a BMI greater than 30 kg/m^2 or those with a BMI greater than 27 kg/m^2 with comorbidities.[60] The amount of weight loss that can be attributed to medications is modest (approximately 5 kg/y), but this may be enough to halt progression of some comorbid conditions. For example, medication may prevent or slow the progression of impaired glucose tolerance to type 2 DM, improve lipid profiles, and decrease BP levels. Long-term safety profiles for many of these medications are lacking. Patients often return to their original weight after cessation of therapy.[61]

Several medications that had been approved for the treatment of obesity have been removed from the market or have had length of use restricted for various health concerns. The off-label combination of fenfluramine and dexfenfluramine was removed from the market for concerns regarding valvular heart disease. Rimonabant, an appetite suppressant, was associated with depression and suicidal behaviors and also was removed, and sibutramine has been removed because of an increased risk of adverse cardiovascular events.[62]

Prescription drug therapies often used for the treatment of obesity include phentermine HCl, diethylpropion, and orlistat. Half-strength orlistat has been FDA approved for sale without a prescription to be used in combination with a reduced-calorie, low-fat diet. More recent FDA-approved medications for the treatment of obesity are lorcaserin and phentermine/topiramate extended release. Some of these medications may not be available for use in Canada.

Phentermine and diethylpropion are sympathomimetic drugs that work as appetite suppressants. Because of the abuse potential associated with these medications, they are approved only for short-term use (widely interpreted as 12 wk).

Orlistat works by inhibiting pancreatic lipases, preventing absorption of dietary fat (30% with 120 mg orlistat and 25% with 60 mg orlistat). A 16-week RCT of 60 mg orlistat 3 times a day with meals in overweight (not obese) patients (average BMI, 26.8 kg/m^2) on a reduced-calorie, low-fat diet found that patients taking the drug lost 2.5 lb (1.15 kg) more than those taking placebo.[63] Orlistat causes flatulence with oily spotting, loose stools, and fecal urgency in 2% to 40% of patients on a low-fat diet. Adverse events would presumably increase with higher doses or higher fat intake. Fat-soluble vitamins and beta-carotene absorption are often decreased, and supplementation may be necessary. The drug possibly interferes with the absorption of other drugs and may increase the anticoagulant effect of warfarin.

Lorcaserin is a selective serotonin receptor 2C (5-HTC2C) agonist that promotes satiety. The recommended dose is 10 mg orally twice a day. If patients have not lost 5% of their body weight by 12 weeks of use, they are unlikely to have significant weight loss with continued use, and discontinuation should be considered. People with diabetes should be monitored for hypoglycemia; care should be taken in those with renal or hepatic impairment, although mild disease does not require dose adjustment.[62] Serotonin syndrome is a serious potential complication, and caution should be exercised when considering lorcaserin initiation in those already on other serotinergic agents. Lorcaserin is generally well tolerated, with headache being the most commonly reported AE.[64]

Phentermine/Topiramate extended release works as an appetite suppressant and is available in multiple dosing formulations. It is recommended to start with 3.75 mg phentermine/23 mg topiramate extended release daily for 14 days, then increase to 7.5 mg/46 mg, respectively, daily. If 5% weight loss is not achieved by 12 weeks of use, the dose may be increased to the maximum dose of 15 mg/

92 mg, respectively, daily, or discontinuation may be considered. Dosage should be tapered before complete discontinuation because seizures have been seen with abrupt discontinuation.[64] Phentermine has been associated with increases in heart rate; care should be taken in those with CVD. Patients should be monitored for changes in mood because topiramate has been associated with depression and suicidal ideation. Other potential complications include acute angle closure glaucoma and hypoglycemia in patients with DM.[62]

A combination drug of naltrexone sustained release (SR) and bupropion SR has shown promising results in phase 3 studies, with a loss of 9.3% of initial body weight compared with 5.1% in the placebo group after 56 weeks.[65] The CONTRAVE Obesity Research-II study showed naltrexone SR-bupropion SR use resulted in more participants reaching at least 5% weight loss at week 28 and at week 56 of treatment compared with placebo. Patients on naltrexone SR-bupropion SR also had improvement in cardiometabolic risk factors and patient-reported QOL.[66] Naltrexone SR-bupropion SR is currently being evaluated in patients with cardiovascular risk factors for the occurrence of adverse cardiac events.[67]

In clinical trials, liraglutide, a once-daily human glucagon-like peptide-a analog currently approved for treatment of type 2 DM, induced meaningful weight loss in a phase 2 study in patients who were obese without DM.[68] In a phase 3 trial, with diet and exercise, liraglutide 3 mg per day also maintained weight loss achieved through calorie restriction and induced further weight loss over 56 weeks. Liraglutide produces small but significant improvements in several cardiometabolic risk factors compared with placebo.

Two prescription drugs used off label for obesity treatment include fluoxetine and bupropion. Fluoxetine and bupropion are approved for the treatment of depression but also may facilitate weight loss. Bupropion is approved to prevent weight gain during smoking cessation.

Surgery

The National Institutes of Health has created an obesity management and referral algorithm that incorporates treatment approaches and interventions in the quest for nonsurgical interventions to treat obesity (Figure).[46] Ultimately, however, referral to a bariatric surgeon may be the only option left for patients with a BMI of 40 kg/m² or higher who have failed an adequate trial of diet, exercise, and lifestyle modification or with a BMI of 35 kg/m² or higher who suffer from a comorbid condition such as hypertension, impaired glucose tolerance, type 2 DM, hyperlipidemia, or obstructive sleep apnea. The goal of surgery is to reduce the morbidity and mortality associated with obesity.

Bariatric surgery refers to surgical procedures used to promote weight loss and can be divided into 3 groups: restrictive, malabsorptive, or mixed procedures. Restrictive procedures reduce the size of the stomach, thereby limiting the amount of food that can be consumed. They include vertical banded gastroplasty ("stomach stapling"), laparoscopic gastric banding, and sleeve gastrectomy. These restrictive procedures promote more gradual weight loss than the malabsorptive procedures and are often simpler to perform.

Malabsorptive surgery, such as the biliopancreatic diversion with or without duodenal switch, decreases the effective length of the small intestine, reducing absorption and inducing weight loss. These malabsorptive procedures can result in profound weight loss; however, significant metabolic complications such as protein calorie malnutrition and various micronutrient deficiencies can occur.

Mixed procedures combine both restrictive and malabsorptive components and include gastric bypass. Literature has shown that patients experience better surgical outcomes when referred to high-volume centers with experienced surgeons.

Two meta-analyses have summarized data on the effectiveness of bariatric surgery. One group reviewed 136 studies in which patients underwent a variety of bariatric procedures.[69] The mean overall percentage of excess weight loss was 61%, with the most weight loss occurring after malabsorptive surgery (70.1%) and the least after gastric banding (47.5%). The 30-day mortality was 0.1% for restrictive procedures, 1.1% for malabsorptive procedures, and 0.5% for mixed procedures. Comorbidity resolution and improvement rates were excellent in these surgical patients.

Another meta-analysis included 147 studies and found the largest benefit of bariatric surgery in patients with a BMI greater than 40 kg/m², whereas benefits in patients with BMIs of 35 kg/m² to 39 kg/m² were less clear.[70] Greater weight loss was observed with gastric bypass than with gastroplasty. Adverse events occurred in approximately 20% of patients, and overall mortality was less than 1%. Data have shown a reduction in all-cause mortality of 40% among bariatric surgery patients with a history of major cardiovascular events compared with obese surgical controls and a near 50% reduction in cardiovascular death.[71,72]

Skin

The skin is composed of 3 layers: the epidermis, dermis, and subcutis. The top layer is the epidermis. The stratum corneum, the outermost part of the epidermis, consists of dead keratinocytes (squamous cells) that are continually shed. Below the stratum corneum are layers of living keratinocytes that produce keratin, sulfur-containing fibrous proteins that form the chemical basis of horny epidermal tissues such as hair and nails. At the lowest part of the epidermis are basal cells that continually divide to produce new keratinocytes. Also present in the epidermis are melanocytes, cells that produce melanin, the protective brown pigment that makes skin tan or brown. Melanin is formed to protect the deeper layers of the skin from the harmful effects of the sun.

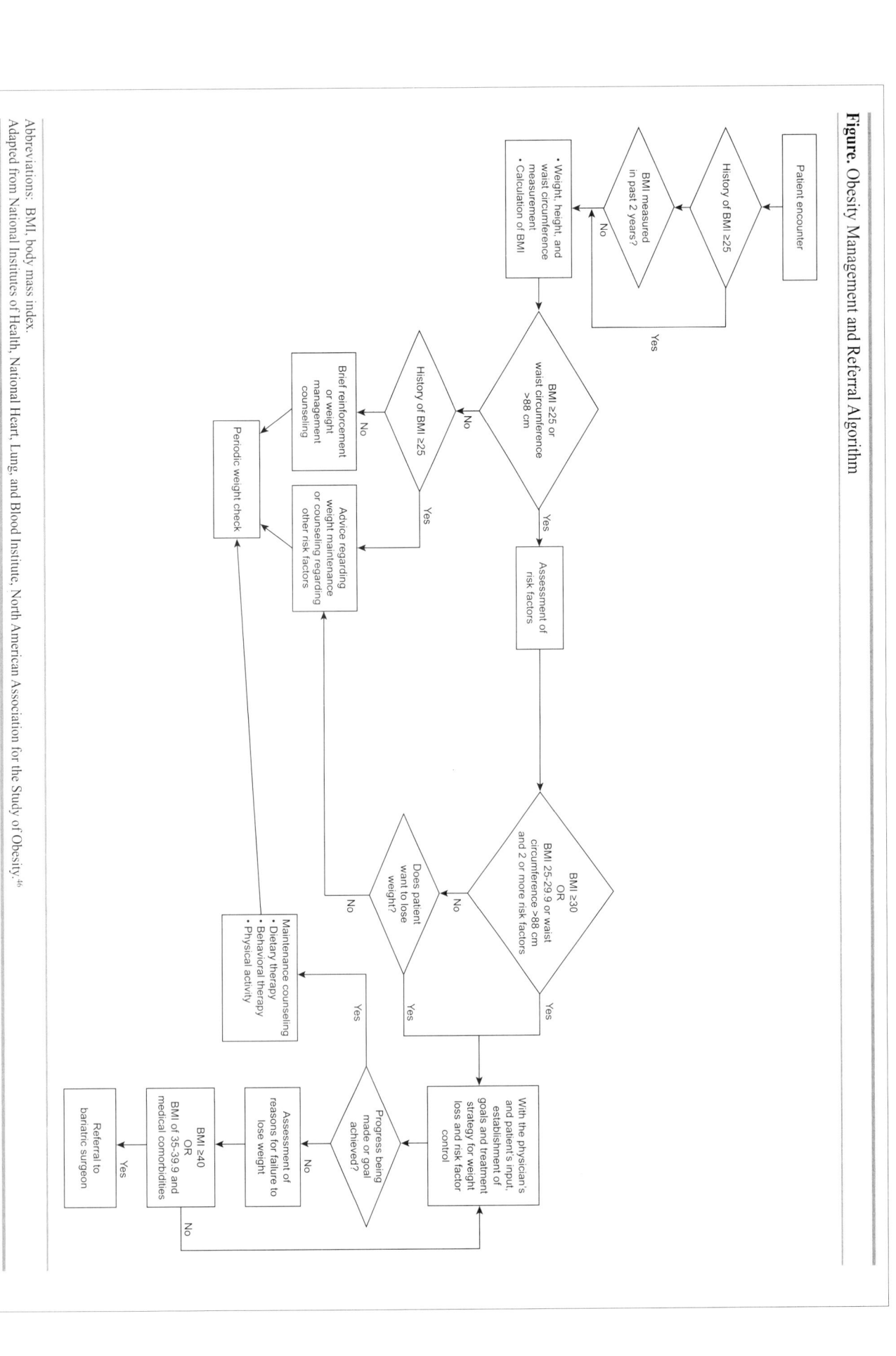

Figure. Obesity Management and Referral Algorithm

Abbreviations: BMI, body mass index.
Adapted from National Institutes of Health, National Heart, Lung, and Blood Institute, North American Association for the Study of Obesity.[46]

The dermis forms the main bulk of the skin. Fibroblasts are the dominant cell in the dermis and are specialized in producing dermal proteins. The fibers present in the dermis consist primarily of 2 types of fibrous protein: collagen and elastin. Collagen fibers make up about 70% to 75% of the proteins in the dermis and are responsible for its mass and resilience. Skin ages relatively well. It is only with exposure to extrinsic factors, primarily sunlight, that a more marked aging of the skin occurs. In sun-damaged locations in the dermis, elastin becomes fragmented as a direct consequence of ultraviolet (UV) light absorption. Dark clumps of elastin proteins can be seen in stained specimens of sun-damaged skin, giving it an appearance that clearly differs from that of the fine elastin fibers seen in young skin. Skin changes are also influenced by subcutaneous fat, which is diminished or redistributed with age. This change adds to increases in skin laxity. Weight fluctuations can also increase laxity because as skin elasticity is reduced with aging, the skin does not retract after loss of body fat, leaving excess skin. Loss of underlying muscle mass contributes to sagging skin because muscle acts as a skin filler, especially on the face.

Role of hormones

Hormones play an important role in skin physiology.[73,74] The androgen hormones modulate sebum (oil) production. Acne can result from androgen-induced excessive sebum production. The effects of androgens on acne are more evident in adult women than in adolescents. Levels of circulating androgens, although typically in the normal range, are often higher in women with acne than in women without acne.

Estrogen has a number of functions in the skin, in which ERs are present in significant numbers. Cross-sectional data have shown a highly significant correlation between the declines in skin collagen and skin thickness and the years since menopause. No such correlation has been found between these parameters and actual chronologic age, however, supporting the role of hormone effects on these skin changes. The decline in skin collagen after menopause occurs at a much more rapid rate in the early postmenopause years. Some 30% of skin collagen is lost during the first 5 years after menopause, followed by an average decline of 2% per postmenopause year over 20 years. These statistics are similar to those for bone loss after menopause. Increases in skin laxity and wrinkling, as well as decreases in skin elasticity, also occur after menopause.

Photoaging

Exposure to the sun induces clinical and histologic changes to the skin, commonly called photoaging. Clinically, photoaging can be manifested as wrinkles, skin roughness and dryness, irregular pigmentation, sallowness, and solar lentigines (brown spots). Benign conditions of vascular proliferation, including linear telangiectasia, cherry angiomas, and spider angiomas, often occur with aging and cutaneous photodamage. Other common age-related skin changes include seborrheic keratoses (tan, brown, or black raised spots with a waxy texture or rough surface), actinic keratoses (premalignant, sun-induced growths that are sometimes burning and tender. These are usually dry and scaly in consistency, and "frown lines," which result from facial muscles interacting with less elastic, sun-damaged skin.

Risk factors of photoaging and skin cancer include fair skin, difficulty tanning, ease of sunburning, sunburns before the age of 20 years, tanning-bed use, and advancing age. Smoking is an independent risk factor for wrinkling, telangiectasia, and squamous cell cancer.[75] Women with substantial photoaging should be examined periodically for actinic keratoses and skin cancers.[76]

Most changes that occur as a result of photoaging have similar causes and risk factors, but the extent and consequences of these changes vary among women. The decision about whether to recommend treatment depends on the nature of the changes, their severity, the degree to which they bother the woman, and the patient's willingness to accept the risks and costs of treatment, which most insurance plans do not cover.[75]

Although skin collagen content and skin thickness decline significantly with age, it is only with exposure to extrinsic factors such as sunlight and tobacco smoke that aging of the skin occurs in a more marked fashion.[75] Although this problem is often medically insignificant, it is of profound cosmetic concern and will detract from the QOL for many women at midlife and beyond.

Management of photoaging. At any age, protection from the sun reduces the risk of actinic keratoses and squamous cell cancer and the progression of photoaging. (Reducing the risk of basal cell cancer depends primarily on reducing sun exposure during childhood.)

- *Sunscreen*. Ample use of a moisturizing sunscreen will have the greatest effect in protecting and improving the appearance of aging skin. Data support the importance of preventing UVA and UVB radiation. For optimal skin protection, women should use a broad-spectrum, water-resistant sunscreen with a minimal sun protection factor (SPF) of 30 throughout the year. Tanning should be discouraged.

  It has long been believed that UVB radiation (wavelengths from 290-320 nm) is mainly responsible for cutaneous photocarcinogenesis and that the longer wavelength UVA radiation is primarily to blame for the deeper dermal changes of photoaging. This implicated UVA radiation in the pathogenesis of melanoma. Subsequent data do not support an increased risk of melanoma associated with sunscreen use.[77] However, the association of tanning bed use, which uses primarily UVA radiation, with melanoma also points the finger at UVA radiation as a carcinogen. Newer research supports a role for UVA and UVB in cutaneous carcinogenesis and photoaging.[78]

FDA announced new labeling requirements for sunscreen in June 2011. These new guidelines better standardize labels and avoid ambiguous previously unregulated claims made by sunscreen manufacturers. As a result, only sunscreen with an SPF of 15 or higher can claim to reduce skin cancer risk. Water-resistant claims must be accompanied by a time specification, and terms such as *water-proof* or *sweat-proof* cannot be used. All sunscreens must include standard "drug facts" on the label. Current guidelines in sunscreen use recommend broad-spectrum, water-resistant formulations with an SPF of 30 or higher, which provide protection against both UVA and UVB.[79]

Sunscreens that provide protection against UVB radiation decrease the synthesis of vitamin D. However, people generally do not apply a sufficient amount of sunscreen, do not cover all sun-exposed skin, or do not reapply often enough to prevent sufficient synthesis of vitamin D.[80] Ultraviolet B radiation from natural and artificial sources carries significant risk of photoaging and skin cancer and cannot be recommended as a main source of vitamin D. Women using sunscreen coverage should obtain vitamin D through diet and nutritional supplementation to reach the recommended daily allowance.[81]

- *Other treatments.* Antioxidants, α-hydroxy acids, and topical retinoids (vitamin A derivatives) have been used to repair photoaged skin. Only topical retinoids have demonstrated a well-documented ability to repair skin at the clinical, histologic, and molecular level.[82] Two topical retinoid products (tretinoin and tazarotene) have been government approved for the palliation of fine wrinkles and irregular pigmentation of photoaging. There is limited evidence to support the efficacy of other vitamin A derivatives often found in over-the-counter preparations, including retinol and retinaldehyde. Of the literature that exists, retinaldehyde has been shown to have the most beneficial effect on aging skin.[83]

  Many products and procedures are advocated for facial rejuvenation. For example, injections of collagen or botulinum toxin type A are popular wrinkle treatments. Data collected over the past 2 decades show an impressive safety and efficacy record with the use of botulinum toxin when used appropriately and by trained professionals. Adverse events, including unintended muscle paralysis (eyelid ptosis), headache, local injection reaction, and infection, are most often transient and mild.[84]

- *Hormone therapy.* Clinical trial evidence indicates that systemic HT has some beneficial effects on skin.[85,86] Systemic HT has been shown to limit the loss of skin collagen, maintain skin thickness, improve skin elasticity and firmness, increase skin moisture, and decrease wrinkle depth and pore size.[87] Systemic HT also seems to limit skin extensibility during perimenopause, exerting a preventive effect on skin slackness, although no effect on skin viscoelasticity has been noted. Although the data are not convincing enough to initiate HT for skin benefits alone, the potential facial skin benefits may appeal to some women. Hormone therapy is not government approved for any skin benefit.

  Hormone therapy neither alters the effects of genetic aging or damage caused by sun exposure or tobacco use nor does it affect the risk of skin cancer. Some women taking high doses of estrogen may experience increased pigmentation (melasma or chloasma) that may not be reversible.

  Studies suggest that HT has a positive effect on facial skin elasticity parameters and other aging properties.[88-90] However, the evidence is mixed and controversial, especially in light of the known risks associated with HT.[91] Compared with HT, estrogen agonist/antagonist raloxifene has yielded similar results related to skin elasticity.[89] Other estrogen agonists/antagonists are being studied to identify their potential role in modifying skin aging.[92,93] However, in a trial that assessed global appearance ratings by dermatologists and postmenopausal participants, low-dose systemic HT did not alter moderate age-related facial skin changes.[94]

  Studies of topical estradiol therapy for skin aging have yielded mixed results from small studies. There is some evidence that facial epithelial and dermal thickness is enhanced by topical therapy, whereas other evidence suggests that topical therapy is ineffective in stimulating collagen development in photoaged skin.[95-97] The application of topical isoflavones has been shown to be less effective than topical estradiol but may be a promising alternative.[74,95] There is also some evidence that facial application of 2% progesterone cream improves skin elasticity parameters.[98]

  Systemic HT cannot be recommended for treatment of aging skin, and the minimal safe concentration of topical estrogen has not been established.[74]

Dry skin

Xerosis (dry skin), the most common condition of aging skin, is a consequence of decreased water and lipid content in the skin as well as reduced oil production and sweating. By age 70 years, nearly all adults are affected.[99] Xerosis is usually more pronounced on the back and the ankles and can cause significant itching and discomfort. It tends to be more marked in dry climates and during winter months.

Management of dry skin. The key to managing xerosis in the aging patient is to first hydrate the skin and then seal in the hydration with topical emollients. Women should be advised to use a bath oil or heavy lotion on wet skin immediately after showering or bathing. Products that have an oily feel, such as petroleum jelly and baby oil, are most effective, inasmuch as common hand lotions often contain alcohol and little oil. Skin will become more resistant to physical and chemical insults if it is kept lubricated. Hot water and harsh soaps that strip the skin of natural lipids can further aggravate xerosis and should be avoided. Severely dry skin can occasionally lead to an inflammatory eczematous dermatitis that can be treated with topical steroids.

It is important to keep skin hydrated by drinking adequate amounts of water. Most women consume far too little water. (Liquids such as coffee, tea, and caffeinated soft drinks may quench thirst, but their diuretic action decreases hydration.) Avoidance of excessive alcohol consumption also will contribute to skin health. Other skin-healthy habits include getting adequate exercise and sleep and avoiding stress and smoking. Because underlying muscle mass acts as a skin filler to reduce sagging, especially on the face, there is merit to exercising the facial muscles for bulk.

Acne

Some women will develop acne around menopause, usually because of an increase in the ratio of androgen to estrogen. Circulating androgens are typically in the normal range, but levels have been shown to be significantly higher in women with acne than in women without. The effects of androgens on acne are most evident in adult women. Women who had acne during their teen years will almost always have acne in midlife. Clinically, the adult variety of acne occurs mostly on the lower face, particularly along the chin, jaw line, and neck. Lesions are predominantly papulonodular and are often tender.

Management of acne. The net effect of systemic hormonal treatment for acne is a reduction of sebum production from the sebaceous gland. Neither topical acne preparations nor oral antibiotics influence sebum production. The first US government-approved estrogen-containing contraceptive for the treatment of acne was norgestimate plus ethinyl estradiol. Efficacy has been demonstrated in 2 multicenter trials. At least 2 other estrogen-progestin contraceptives—norethindrone acetate plus ethinyl estradiol, and drospirenone plus ethinyl estradiol—also have been approved for acne treatment. Cyproterone acetate plus ethinyl estradiol is approved in Canada for the treatment of severe acne in women who have associated symptoms of androgenization, including seborrhea and mild hirsutism. It also provides reliable contraception.[100] Spironolactone, a mild diuretic with antiandrogen effects, is also commonly used in the treatment of hormonally induced acne.

Formication

Women presenting with formication (tactile sensation of insects crawling on the skin) may respond to treatment with HT or with psychopharmacologic therapies or both. However, no clinical studies have addressed this problem, and no therapy has been identified as effective.

When to refer

A referral to a dermatologist is recommended for treating any skin condition with which the menopause practitioner is not experienced. Effective procedures to treat benign conditions are available from the dermatologist, including those using lasers, cryosurgery, electrosurgery, and microdermabrasion. Any serious skin disease, including suspicion of precancerous lesions and skin carcinoma, should be referred to a dermatologist.

Hair

Some women experience thinning of hair on the scalp or unwanted growth of hair on the face (hirsutism) in midlife and associate these hair changes with menopause. The phenomenon has been called *androgenetic alopecia* (AGA), perhaps inappropriately because the actual cause is unknown but seems to be caused by multiple factors including genetic predisposition, local androgen metabolism, growth factors (especially cytokines), hormones, and stress. It has been postulated that the increase in the ratio of androgen to estrogen during the midlife transition may influence hair changes in some women. This is evidenced by the increase in hair density that can be attained with antiandrogen treatments. The cause of the variable physiologic responses of hair follicles in different sites (crown vs occipital scalp) from identical hormone signals remains unknown. Hair growth aberrations can have significant psychological consequences that affect body image, self-esteem, and QOL, underscoring the importance of effective medical management.

Hair loss

The onset of hair loss during the menopause transition and in postmenopausal women may be caused by a variety of conditions. Female pattern hair loss (FPHL) and telogen effluvium are the most common causes. Female pattern hair loss is more common after menopause: the altered estrogen-to-androgen ratio may play a role in pathogenesis. A sudden onset of hair shedding usually indicates a disruption of the hair cycle (telogen effluvium), whereas gradual hair thinning typically occurs in FPHL.[101]

In FPHL, the hair thins mainly on the crown of the scalp. It usually starts with a widening through the center hair part. The front hairline remains intact, and the hair loss rarely progresses to total or near total baldness as it may in male pattern hair loss (MPHL). Male pattern hair loss can also occur in women, involving vertex balding and bitemporal recession. Another form of hair loss, frontal fibrosing alopecia—a lichen planopilaris variant—occurs predominantly in postmenopausal women and is associated with symmetrical regression of the frontal and temporal hairline, with partial or total loss of the eyebrows.[102,103] Other causes of hair loss, including thyroid disease, cicatricial alopecias, trichotillomania, alopecia neoplastica, tinea capitis, and alopecia areata, are less common and should be excluded.

Hormones influence hair growth.[85] Estrogen and androgen receptors have been found on hair follicles.[104,105] The exact mechanism of action of estrogen on hair follicles is unknown; however, estrogen is believed to protect against hair loss, with the ER pathway involved with telogen-anagen follicle cycling.[85,106] This is illustrated by women's increased hair density during pregnancy from prolongation of anagen and the postpartum telogen effluvium (gravidarum) that accompanies the decline in maternal estrogen levels.

Androgens, importantly DHT, which is converted from testosterone by 5α-reductase at the level of the hair follicle, act via the androgen receptor.[105] Androgens have differential effects on hair follicles, depending on the body site, and cause progressive miniaturization of susceptible hair follicles and shortening of anagen on the scalp.[105,107,108] This androgen effect occurs in genetically susceptible people and causes hair loss, although in FPHL the role of androgens is less clear than in MPHL.[109]

During postmenopause, estrogen levels are low, and testosterone levels are usually normal or only slightly decreased, leading to a hypoestrogenic and relative hyperandrogenic state, causing an increase in the androgen-to-estrogen ratio that may lead to patterned hair loss (PHL) in susceptible women.[74,110] In a study of a group of premenopausal women with FPHL, the ratio of estrogen to androgen was found to be significantly lower than in the control group and was suggested as the hair loss trigger.[111] Other factors, such as alterations in the activity of the aromatase enzyme, the androgen receptor, or androgen and estrogen metabolism in the hair follicle, may be involved in FPHL.

In the menopause transition, FPHL is the most likely diagnosis for alopecia. History, examination, and laboratory investigations should confirm the diagnosis and exclude other disorders.

Clinical history and examination. A thorough clinical history, including the onset, duration, pattern, and percentage of hair loss, is required. A detailed female history is needed, including menstrual history, number of pregnancies, age at menopause, menopause symptoms, HT use, and associated symptoms of androgen excess such as acne, seborrhea, and hirsutism. A family history is needed, focusing on PHL, autoimmune conditions, thyroid disorders, and malignancies. Further hair loss triggers, including medication history, severe illness, surgery, or weight loss, should be sought.

A detailed dietary and hair care history should be obtained. A medical history and systems review should also be performed. Clinical examination should confirm the distinctive pattern of loss over the crown, with the widening of the central part and retention of the frontal hairline seen in FPHL, and exclude other types of hair loss, including a cicatricial alopecia such as frontal fibrosing alopecia with loss of visible follicular openings.[109] Women can also show a male-type pattern of alopecia with vertex balding and bitemporal recession. Other signs of hyperandrogenism should be screened for, including acne, seborrhea, obesity, clitoromegaly, increased muscle mass, deepened voice, and hirsutism. Hair pull test results may be positive early in FPHL.

Laboratory investigations. In any woman presenting with hair loss, additional causes should be excluded. A complete blood count, comprehensive metabolic panel, thyroid function tests (TSH, thyroxine levels), iron, ferritin, and zinc level will exclude systemic disease, thyroid disease, and nutritional deficiency. In women with FPHL or other signs of androgen excess (or both), an androgen screen is required to exclude an androgen-secreting tumor or other endocrinopathy.[109] A total or free testosterone level (or both) and levels of SHBG and DHEAS can identify high androgen levels. Further investigation such as autoimmune screening and referral to an endocrinologist may be required.

A small study has suggested that some postmenopausal women with FPHL do not have statistically significant differences in their levels of testosterone, estradiol, or SHBG compared with matched controls without FPHL.[112] Levels of testosterone and DHEAS greater than 200 ng/dL (6.9 nmol/L) and 700 μg/dL (19 μmol/L), respectively, are suggestive of an ovarian or adrenal tumor.[113] Estradiol and FSH levels can demonstrate postmenopausal hormone levels.[110] Histology, if needed, can confirm the diagnosis of FPHL, with miniaturization of terminal hair follicles into vellus hairs, leading to a diagnostic ratio of terminal to vellus hairs of less than 4:1.[114] The diagnostic yield for finding a laboratory abnormality in random patients with FPHL is low; generally, women with a more advanced presentation of FPHL or with clinical signs and symptoms of virilization or endocrinopathy show an abnormality.

General treatment of hair loss. A healthy diet consisting of less red meat, low calories, and a high content of zinc, iron, and vitamin D is recommended. Nutritional deficiencies should be corrected, and biotin and multivitamin supplements can be given to support hair regrowth.[115] Topical minoxidil 2% or 5% is beneficial for hair regrowth but is a nonspecific hair promoter.[109,116] Although it has been used for more than 30 years, there is limited understanding about its mechanism of action: possibly prolongation of anagen, increase of follicle size, promotion of perifollicular blood flow, or stimulatory effects on hair growth because of the opening of potassium channels.[73] For FPHL, only the 2% solution is approved by the US government, but the 5% solution is more effective by patient subjective rating.[116] Facial hypertrichosis, contact dermatitis, and irritation are possible AEs for the 5% solution.[109,116] Several products that include minoxidil, sometimes combined with other active ingredients such as tretinoin, are available from different manufacturers in the United States.[117] No RCTs using the combination of minoxidil and an antiandrogen for treatment of FPHL exist; however, this therapeutic combination is commonly used in patients with FPHL. Where appropriate, creative hair styles, hairpieces, or hair transplant can be helpful as adjunctive treatments.[109]

Two types of hormonal treatments have been studied for hair loss: antiandrogens and menopausal ET. The hypothesis that FPHL is a relatively high androgen state has led to the use of antiandrogens or androgen suppressors. However, the use of these agents and their efficacy are questionable. All the agents discussed for the treatment of FPHL are off-label treatments. Also of concern is that studies of these treatments were small and not double blinded or placebo controlled. Patients with hair loss who have testosterone measurements sometimes have very low levels, and using antiandrogens in this clinical scenario is questionable. The use of these agents in patients without overt hyperandrogenism has not been shown to be effective.

- *Antiandrogens* compete with circulating androgens for the high-affinity androgen receptor.[109,118] The aim of treatment is to prevent progression of the hair loss rather than promote hair regrowth. Although none of the agents are government approved for treatment of FPHL, they can be helpful in some women. In particular, these agents may be useful in those women with other indirect evidence of hyperandrogenism, such as hirsutism, acne, and MPHL.[109,119] It is still unclear, however, whether women with FPHL and measurable levels of androgen excess respond differently to antiandrogen therapy compared with women with FPHL and normal androgen levels. There have been no large randomized trials investigating antiandrogens in perimenopausal or postmenopausal women with FPHL.

Spironolactone competitively blocks the AR and suppresses ovarian androgen synthesis.[118] It has been used in doses of 50 mg to 200 mg daily as an antiandrogen for FPHL.[109,118,120,121] Hyperkalemia is a risk; baseline and continued monitoring of serum potassium is needed.[122] Other AEs include fatigue, postural hypotension, and liver abnormalities.[109,118,122] Spironolactone was found to be tumorigenic and teratogenic in animal studies, although the significance to humans is unknown.[122] Therapies such as antiandrogens that alter the hormonal milieu should be avoided in women with a personal or family history of estrogen-dependent cancers such as breast, uterine, or ovarian. Because of the potential teratogenic and tumorigenic potential, women prescribed spironolactone should be counseled to use birth control. Topical compounded spironolactone 5% solution exists and has been used in combination with minoxidil with variable success.[123]

The antiandrogen cyproterone acetate is also used for the treatment of FPHL in postmenopausal women (not available in the United States). Cyproterone acetate competitively inhibits the AR and inhibits LH release.[109,120,124] It can be used continuously in postmenopausal women at 50 mg daily, alone or in combination with menopausal ET.[109,118] Adverse effects include nausea, weight gain, depression, breast tenderness, and decreased libido.[118]

Finasteride, a type II 5α-reductase inhibitor, prevents conversion of testosterone to the more potent DHT.[125] Finasteride is government approved and effective for treatment of MPHL. It is not government approved for any indication in women. In postmenopausal women with FPHL, finasteride is ineffective at doses of 1 mg daily. Higher doses of 2.5 mg to 5.0 mg daily of finasteride may be effective in some women with FPHL.[126] Finasteride has also been tried without success in postmenopausal women with frontal fibrosing alopecia.[127]

Dutasteride is a 5α-reductase inhibitor that inhibits both type I and type II 5α-reductase enzymes and is effective, but not government approved, for MPHL.[128] Some cases are reported of oral dutasteride treatment for FPHL in postmenopausal women.[129] There is currently no effective treatment of frontal fibrosing alopecia, the most effective being oral finasteride or oral dutasteride, drugs that possibly affect the accompanying AGA.[130]

Flutamide is a potent antiandrogen but is associated with significant risk of hepatotoxicity. It is not used for treatment of FPHL and has no government-approved indications for use in women.[120] Topical estrogen preparations are not available for FPHL treatment in the United States.

Fluridil is a topical antiandrogen. In an open clinical study, fluridil 2% solution prevented progression of hair loss and increased hair diameter in women with FPHL.[131] Fluridil is used in Europe but is still awaiting approval in the United States.[123]

- *Menopausal estrogen therapy*. In some women, cessation of menopausal ET can precipitate hair shedding and unmask FPHL. Menopausal ET, if appropriate to continue prescribing, can support hair growth as it supports other skin structures. The decision to continue menopausal ET should be directed by the patient's primary care provider and depends on the woman's individual risk factors, menopausal symptoms, and other indications for use.

- *Adjunctive therapies*. Bimatoprost is a prostaglandin analog/prodrug used to control the progression of glaucoma and in the management of ocular hypertension. In December 2008, the indication to lengthen eyelashes was approved by FDA.[132] Latanoprost, another glaucoma treatment, has been investigated for its potential to promote scalp hair growth. Latanoprost significantly increased hair density and may also promote pigmentation compared with baseline and placebo.[133]

Ketoconazole shampoo 2% can be used as an antiandrogen and has been suggested to reduce shedding and promote hair growth in AGA through androgen-dependent pathways.[134,135] A study of antidandruff shampoos containing 1% zinc pyrithione was also suggestive of potential hair growth.[136] Hair count results showed a sustained improvement in hair growth with daily use.

Another treatment option includes the low-energy laser-light products that are available for treatment of alopecia.[137] They are designed as a hairbrush or comb that shines red light directly on the scalp. One such handheld, noninvasive device was cleared by FDA for men in 2007 and for women with FPHL in 2011.

Camouflaging topical sprays, powders, or keratin fibers may be alternatives to achieve an adequate cosmetic result for women with FPHL.[123]

- *Cell-mediated treatments for androgenetic alopecia.* There are 2 main approaches to cell-mediated treatments for AGA: the direct injection of cultured cells or the use of cell-secreted factors as a hair growth-promoting product. Preclinical studies have shown that cells from the hair follicle mesenchyme cells can be cultured and used to induce new hair follicle formation.[138] The injected cells can also increase the size of the resident hair follicles. Alternatively, cells are cultured, and the culture supernatant is processed to produce a compound rich in hair growth-promoting factors for use in treatment. These cell-mediated treatment approaches may be available in a few years. Also, platelet-rich plasma isolated from whole blood associated with multiple growth factors is currently gaining popularity in the marketplace.[139]

Analogous to their male counterparts, one study found that women with early onset FPHL have a higher prevalence of hypertension and hyperaldosteronemia than do age-matched controls.[140] Although specific studies in menopausal women are lacking, BP screening in all women presenting with PHL loss may be worthwhile for earlier diagnosis and treatment of unsuspected hypertension.

Hirsutism

Coarse facial hairs in females typically arise in areas of the body where the hair follicles are the most androgen-sensitive, including the chin, upper lip, and cheeks. Hirsutism affects between 5% and 15% of women. Except for rare cases of virilizing tumors or adrenal hyperplasia caused by enzymatic defects, hirsutism is caused mainly by ovarian androgen overproduction (eg, polycystic ovary syndrome) or by peripheral hypersensitivity to normal levels of circulating androgen (idiopathic hirsutism). The role of androgens in women with hirsutism is further evidenced by the reduction in hair density that can be attained with antiandrogen treatments, including hormonal contraceptives with low androgenicity.[100]

Most women with hirsutism have an exaggerated local production of potent androgens as a result of enhanced local 5α-reductase activity. Other clinical disorders that have been observed with acute or transient androgen excess include FPHL, seborrhea (oily face and scalp, frequently with associated seborrheic dermatitis), and acne. If chronic androgen excess exists, polycystic ovary syndrome is the most common cause (70%-80% of cases); androgen-secreting tumors, androgenic drug intake, and endocrinopathies are less frequent causes. Polycystic ovary syndrome is associated with insulin resistance, which must be screened for in suspected cases.

Menopausal facial hair. Another hair-growth phenomenon of concern to many women is the appearance of fine hairs ("peach fuzz") on the face, most commonly on the upper lip and chin but sometimes generalized in appearance. Rapidly growing, large "rogue hairs" can sometimes be found on the chin. The growth of unwanted hair is common, and sometimes occurs long before menopause.

Management of hirsutism. The diagnostic evaluation of women with hirsutism first focuses on confirming the condition and whether excess levels of androgen are present. Other associated abnormalities and conditions, including ovulatory dysfunction, adrenal hyperplasia, DM, and thyroid hormone abnormalities, need to be ruled out.

Treatment for hirsutism focuses on a combination of therapies including hormonal drugs, peripheral androgen blockage, and mechanical depilation. A woman can remove hair by plucking, waxing, or shaving. Shaving is less traumatic than the other methods, but it may lead to folliculitis and ingrown hairs. Bleaching is also useful, particularly for mild conditions. Chemical depilatory agents may irritate the skin, especially facial skin. Electrolysis can usually destroy terminal hairs after 6 months of treatment. Electrolysis can be complicated by folliculitis and postinflammatory dyspigmentation.[141]

Laser treatment is effective for large areas.[140] Dyspigmentation, hypertrophic scars, and thermal burns (blistering, ulceration) can occur as AEs of laser treatment.[142,143] Other uncommon AEs may include premature graying of hair and tunneling of hair under the skin.[144] Also, paradoxical hypertrichosis is a rare AE seen in patients treated with intense pulsed light devices, diode lasers, and alexandrite lasers.[145]

Eflornithine hydrochloride cream is a prescription topical enzyme inhibitor of hair growth (not available in Canada). It is indicated for reducing unwanted facial hair in women. The cream is applied twice daily.

Menopausal ET may delay the progression of hirsutism, but it will not change coarse terminal hairs into softer and less noticeable vellus hairs. Off-label treatment options include estrogen-containing contraceptives and antiandrogens (eg, spironolactone) as well as 5α-reductase inhibitors (eg, finasteride).

To avoid progression of hirsutism symptoms, treatment of androgen excess should begin as soon as the diagnosis is established. Response to therapy may require 6 to 8 months. Hormonal suppression may need to be continued indefinitely. Androgen levels should be measured at regular intervals.

Eyes

Various ocular changes may occur during the menstrual cycle, during pregnancy, and at menopause.[146] Ocular complaints reported by postmenopausal women include dry eye syndrome, blurred vision, increased lacrimation, tired eyes, and swollen and reddened eyelids. Presbyopia often starts just before menopause, and many women require reading glasses.

Visual performance may be altered by increased corneal, lid, and conjunctival edema during certain phases of the menstrual cycle and during perimenopause. These effects may reduce contact lens tolerance. In addition, hormonal and menopausal status may adversely affect clinical outcomes after refractive surgery, which is now recognized to cause dry eye (keratoconjunctivitis sicca) in some men and women.

Dry eye syndrome

One of the most common ocular complaints associated with menopause is dry eye syndrome. It is characterized by symptoms of ocular irritation such as dryness, pressure, foreign-body sensation, scratchiness, and burning as well as photophobia (light intolerance). The signs of ocular surface damage include redness, aberrant mucus production, and even corneal scarring. Any event that contributes to abnormalities of tear stability or flow can induce or exacerbate dry eye, such as environmental triggers (eg, low humidity or wind) and autoimmune diseases (eg, Sjögren syndrome or rheumatoid arthritis). Drugs such as diuretics, antihistamines, or psychotropics may also be a factor.

Management of dry eye. Women presenting with symptoms of dry eye can be advised to use ocular lubricants such as drops, gels, and ointments. This treatment is palliative at best, resulting in temporary reduction of ocular surface-to-eyelid shear forces and transient symptomatic relief. Small studies show oral fish oil intake may improve health and normal functioning.[147] Plugging of the lacrimal punctae, the openings through which tears drain from the surface of the eye into the nose, can increase the volume of tears on the ocular surface despite a decreased rate of tear production. This can be accomplished with temporary collagen plugs or with silicone plugs or cauterization; however, it may not relieve symptoms in all women.

Although there are many causes of dry eye, an underlying cytokine receptor-mediated inflammatory process is common to many ocular surface diseases. By treating this process, it may be possible to normalize the ocular surface lacrimal neural reflex and facilitate ocular surface healing. Anti-inflammatory medications are now recognized as an appropriate therapeutic strategy for dry eye to address the underlying pathophysiology. In women with moderate to severe dry eye, topical cyclosporine A has been shown to significantly increase tear production and significantly decrease ocular surface damage. Histopathologic evidence indicates that cyclosporine A treatment significantly reduces the numbers of activated T lymphocytes within the conjunctiva.[148]

Similarly, there have been reports of symptomatic relief and reduction of signs of dry eye with the use of topical corticosteroids. Corticosteroids may have significant AEs, such as cataract formation and increased intraocular pressure, making them unsuitable for chronic use. Oral pilocarpine, a parasympathomimetic, and cevimeline HCl, a selective muscarinic cholinergic agonist, are indicated to treat dry mouth in Sjögren syndrome. These drugs may also have beneficial effects in treating severe dry eye. A clinical trial studying the effect of topical cyclosporine A in the treatment of moderate to severe dry eye in patients with Sjögren syndrome and in postmenopausal women found that cyclosporine A significantly reduced the numbers of activated lymphocytes within the conjunctiva.[149]

Role of hormones. Sex hormone receptors have been identified in many ocular tissues, including the meibomian glands, the lacrimal gland, the lens, the cornea, and the conjunctiva, suggesting involvement of sex hormones in the maintenance of ocular surface homeostasis.[150,151]

Studies in animal models have revealed that lacrimal gland function is significantly influenced by sex hormones.[152] Androgens specifically have been shown to exert essential and specific effects on maintaining normal glandular functions and suppressing inflammation.[153] Researchers found that topical androgen treatment (19-nortestosterone) improved signs of dry eye when administered to dogs.

It has been proposed that the pathology of dry eye may be initiated when systemic androgen levels fall below the threshold necessary to support secretory function and maintain an anti-inflammatory environment. The decrease in systemic androgen levels that comes with aging may have a direct effect on dry eye syndrome. A possible effect of changes in androgens or estrogens affecting dry eye is supported clinically by studies in humans comparing tear production in perimenopausal and postmenopausal women in which both quality and amount of tear production were reduced in the postmenopausal group. Further, women report worse dry eye symptoms and more severe effects on daily life than do men.[154]

The results of topical application of estrogens or androgens in humans, however, have not been consistent. A few studies have reported improvement in dry eye signs and symptoms with ET, but these have involved relatively few patients. A review of data on 25,665 women from the Women's Health Study suggested that ET is actually associated with an increased risk of either clinically diagnosed dry eye or severe symptoms of both ocular dryness and irritation.[155] Treatment with EPT was associated with an intermediate risk. Women who had never used estrogen had the lowest risk. Although several smaller studies have confirmed the finding that unopposed estrogen use may worsen dry eye, a separate small study showed that treatment with combined esterified estrogens and methyltestosterone resulted in improvement in dry eye symptoms.[156] Phytoestrogen supplementation has been shown to improve signs and symptoms of dry eye by increasing tears and tear quality.[157]

Cataracts

The prevalence of cataract (lens opacity) is higher in postmenopausal women than in men of the same age. The reason for this sex difference is unclear. Population-based studies have reported a greater incidence of cortical and nuclear cataracts in women compared with men. Long-term follow-up (10-15 y) data from 2 large cross-sectional studies with postmenopausal women showed a significantly higher incidence of cataract in women than in men, although the specific type of cataract differed.[158-160]

Inconsistent results have been reported related to the association between cataracts and reproductive factors such as exogenous hormone administration and age at menopause. Although administration of estrogen is protective against cataract formation in several animal models, there have been mixed reports regarding the effect of menopausal HT on cataract incidence or extraction.[161,162] Cross-sectional studies have reported associations between HT and cataract, whereas several US prospective studies showed an inverse relationship between ET and nuclear cataract. No longitudinal evaluations have found significant associations between HT and cataract; for instance, a study with a 10-year follow-up failed to identify any significant association between HT, age at menarche, duration of exposure to exogenous estrogen, parity, or type of menopause with cataract or cataract extraction.[160] Similarly, a long-term population-based US study showed no association between age at menarche, age at menopause, and years of contraceptive use with cataract incidence.[158,159] This was substantiated in the Singapore Malay Eye Study, a population-based, cross-sectional epidemiologic study that examined the associations between reproductive factors and eye disease in 3,280 persons. Glaucoma was the only disease found to have any association.[163]

The Salisbury Eye Evaluation Project showed a protective association between the use of HT and nuclear and posterior subcapsular cataract.[164] In the Framingham Heart Study, 10 or more years of ET use was inversely associated with nuclear cataract.[165] Women who have undergone surgical menopause are more likely to develop posterior subcapsular cataract than women who reach menopause spontaneously. Women with breast cancer treated with tamoxifen have an increased risk of cataract, which may be consistent with a protective role for estrogen in lens opacification.[166]

Glaucoma

Glaucoma is another ocular condition for which age is an independent risk factor, regardless of sex. Some studies have demonstrated a hormonal effect on intraocular pressure. Increased intraocular pressure is itself a risk factor for development of glaucoma.[167] The mean intraocular pressure of postmenopausal women is greater than that of women of the same age who have not yet reached menopause. The Nurses' Health Study included 66,417 women aged 40 years or older who were followed from 1980 to 2002.[168] Postmenopausal women who reached menopause before age 45 years or at or after age 54 years did not have a higher incidence of primary open-angle glaucoma than women reaching menopause aged between 50 and 54 years.

Another large population-based study among postmenopausal women reported an association between early menopause and a higher risk of glaucoma.[169] Other large studies have reported results such as an increased risk of primary open-angle glaucoma with increasing parity. A retrospective, longitudinal cohort study of a managed-care population of 150,000 women aged older than 50 years reported a smaller fraction of women treated with ET, but not EPT or androgen, developed primary open-angle glaucoma than nonusers.[170] The effects of menopausal HT on glaucoma risk are complex and may be dependent on genotype or gene-environment interactions. Further study is needed.

Management of glaucoma. Management of glaucoma includes use of ocular antihypertensive medications such as topical beta-blockers, α-agonists, prostaglandin analogs, and topical or oral carbonic anhydrase inhibitors. A variety of laser and surgical procedures also are available to reduce intraocular pressure.

Retina and vitreous

Several changes in the retina and vitreous have been found to be more prevalent in postmenopausal women than in age-matched men. One study showed a possible increased risk of posterior vitreous detachment in postmenopausal women.[171] Posterior vitreous detachment in itself is not a vision-threatening condition; however, it may cause new floaters and slightly increase the risk of retinal tears or detachment in the acute phase. Posterior vitreous detachment also is a risk factor for macular hole formation, which would help explain the higher incidence of macular hole in postmenopausal women than in age-matched men. Estrogen use has been reported to be inversely related to the prevalence of macular holes. The exact mechanism by which sex hormones influence these retinal and vitreous changes is not yet known.

Age-related macular degeneration is a leading cause of blindness in the United States and Canada, and there is no clear evidence for sex differences in risk; however, the burden of age-related macular degeneration is greater in women because of the longer life expectancy of women compared with men. Some researchers have suggested that HT may help to prevent macular degeneration in postmenopausal women. The WHI Sight Exam Study assessed possible protective effects of EPT against progression of macular degeneration.[23] Although no significant benefit for early or late age-related macular degeneration with ET or EPT was found, EPT and antioxidants such as vitamins C, D, and E, β-carotene, and zinc were associated with a reduced risk of progression to late macular degeneration in a subgroup of patients with high-risk features.

Genetic and environmental risk factors for age-related macular degeneration have been demonstrated, and interactions with the effects of HT warrant further study. For example, one study reported significant inverse associations with HT and oral contraceptive use and age-related macular degeneration risk and significant interactions between a particular gene variant, *ARMS2*, and HT.[172] Treatment modalities for neovascular age-related macular degeneration include laser photocoagulation, photodynamic therapy, and intravitreal antivascular endothelial growth factor medications.[173]

Other ocular changes

The effects of hormone changes at menopause have been studied in ocular tissues other than the lacrimal gland, lens, retina, and vitreous. Sex hormone receptors have been found in conjunctiva, iris, and ciliary body, but the role of these receptors has yet to be determined.

Ears

Hearing loss has been reported to be 5.5-fold higher in men than in women and 70% lower in blacks than in whites.[174] Earlier onset of hearing loss has been associated with smoking, noise exposure, cardiovascular risks, and chemotherapy for breast, endometrial, and ovarian cancer.[174-176]

Hearing impairment increases beyond age 50 with presbycusis (ie, progressive hearing impairment associated with aging, characterized by hearing loss and degeneration of cochlear structures) being the most important contributor to this increase. About 25% of persons aged 51 to 65 years have decreased hearing in at least one ear, and objective hearing loss can be identified in more than 33% of those aged 65 years and older. It is unclear if or how much the menopause transition acts as a trigger for a relatively rapid age-related hearing decline in healthy women, starting in the left ear.[177,178]

There is some evidence of a relationship among menopause, estrogens, and hearing. The question is whether sex steroids, specifically estrogen, preserve hearing during aging. Some researchers have concluded that physiologic levels of estrogen would appear to have a possible protective effect on hearing function.[179] Women with Turner syndrome have earlier presbycusis, and women using HT have slightly better hearing than those who do not.

Hormone therapy has a positive effect on auditory brain stem response in postmenopausal women, an important objective measure of hearing. Hormone therapy use was shown to improve conduction auditory pathways at the brain stem and thalamocortex. Estrogen-only users benefited more, and the addition of progestin to estrogen did not have a negative or potentiating effect.[180] There is a report, however, that progestin as a component of HT resulted in poorer hearing abilities in postmenopausal women, affecting both the peripheral (ear) and central (brain) auditory systems, interfering with the perception of speech in background noise.[181] Tibolone, which has both estrogenic and progestogenic/androgenic effects, has not been shown to have any effect on hearing in postmenopausal women.[182]

The USPSTF confirms that the incidence of hearing impairment, largely presbycusis, rises quickly after age 50.[183] They also report that self-assessment questionnaires to identify hearing impairment probably represent the most rapid and least expensive way to screen for hearing loss in the adult because they are 70% to 80% accurate, depending on the audiometric criteria.[184] Although no controlled study has proven the effectiveness of screening for hearing impairment in the adult population, there is evidence for measured improvement in social, cognitive, emotional, and communication function from hearing aid use.

The Canadian Task Force on the Periodic Health Examination states that "there is fair evidence to include screening for hearing impairment in the periodic health examination in the elderly."[185] The USPSTF has concluded that "current evidence is insufficient to assess the balance of benefits and harms of screening for hearing loss in asymptomatic adults aged 50 years or older."[183]

Teeth and oral cavity

Oral cavity health is multifactorial. Important features include lifetime oral hygiene, socioeconomic status, professional dental care, and treatment of early problems, as well as general health status, with particular emphasis on smoking and DM. Tooth loss also has been associated with osteoporosis through a sequence that begins with atrophy of bony tooth sockets, leading to gum recession and exposure of nonenameled tooth surfaces (roots), periodontal pocket development, bacterial invasion, and clinical periodontitis.[186] Although women appear to have better periodontal health than men, men tend to retain more teeth by a mean of less than one tooth in each age group (Table 3).[187]

The rate of systemic bone loss in postmenopausal women is a predictor of tooth loss.[188] For each 1% per year decrease in whole-body bone mineral density, the risk for tooth loss more than quadruples. A study of women with severe osteoporosis found them to be 3 times more likely than healthy, age-matched controls to have no teeth. In HT users, longitudinal studies have found higher tooth counts, reduced risk of tooth loss, and reduced alveolar bone loss from periodontal disease progression, thereby implying a relationship to menopause or healthy-user effect.[189]

Several studies also suggest a relationship between low bone mineral density and periodontal disease.[190] Most studies that enrolled women with osteoporosis or osteopenia show a higher frequency of alveolar bone height and crestal/subcrestal loss than in normal controls.[191]

Prevention and treatment of osteoporosis are important factors in maintaining postmenopausal dental health. Patients who are using long-term oral bisphosphonate therapy should be cautioned about reported cases of altered bone healing and bone necrosis (although the risk appears low) and should have frequent periodontal/dental maintenance and meticulous home care.[192-195]

CHAPTER 2

Table 3. Number of Teeth by Age and Sex, Mean

Age group, y					
20-40		>40-60		>60	
Women	Men	Women	Men	Women	Men
24.8 ± 4.0	25.0 ± 3.7	18.9 ± 7.4	19.6 ± 7.3	8.5 ± 8.6	8.8 ± 8.7

Excludes third molars.
Adapted from Meisel P, et al.[187]

Although the exact mechanism is unclear, risk factors for bisphosphonate-related osteonecrosis include 1) incident periodontal disease, 2) duration of bisphosphonate use, 3) intravenous (IV) delivery of the bisphosphonate, 4) dental surgery, and 5) underlying malignancy.[196] With current emphasis on prevention in higher-risk patients, dental surgery and extraction should be performed before initiation of therapy. Also, procedures that involve osseous damage and/or dental implants should be avoided in oncology patients exposed to the more potent IV bisphosphonates. Low-risk patients may undergo elective dentoalveolar surgery. In patients with established bisphosphonate-related osteonecrosis, long-term discontinuation of IV bisphosphonates may be beneficial in stabilizing current sites and reduce the risk of new site development. Cessation of oral therapy may be of similar, but lesser, benefit over 6 to 12 months. Discontinuation of therapy needs to be done in consultation with the patient, the treating physician, and the oral maxillofacial surgeon. There is no short-term benefit to discontinuation and no benefit of a drug holiday.

Fluctuations of sex hormones around the time of menopause have been implicated in inflammatory changes in gingiva.[197] Estrogen affects cellular proliferation, differentiation, and keratinization of the gingival epithelium. Periodontal infections can increase the systemic release of inflammatory cytokines, which accelerate systemic bone resorption. Vitamin D deficiency has been associated with a cytokine profile that favors greater inflammation.[198] It is suggested that menopausal women should maintain an adequate vitamin D status to prevent and treat osteoporosis-associated periodontal disease.[199,200]

Thinning of the oral epithelium is reflected in increased gingival recession, enhanced susceptibility to tissue injury, and sensitivity (eg, burning mouth and tongue, root sensitivity, generalized increased tissue sensitivity). Hormone receptors have been identified in basal and spinous layers of the epithelium and connective tissue, implicating gingival and other oral tissues as targets manifesting hormone deficiencies.[201]

A burning sensation in the mouth can be a symptom of another disease such as anemia or type 2 DM or can be a syndrome in its own right. It has been suggested that when no underlying dental or medical causes are identified and no oral signs are found, the term *burning mouth syndrome* should be used to identify the condition.[202] The prominent feature is burning pain that is usually localized to the tongue and/or lips but can involve the entire oral cavity. Prevalence rates in general populations have been reported to vary from 0.7% to 15%. Many of these patients show evidence of anxiety, depression, and personality disorders, which has led to treating burning mouth syndrome as an emotional problem. However, research shows that burning mouth syndrome may be the result of nerve damage. When nerves that carry taste signals are damaged, especially in people with sensitive taste buds, the brain seems to magnify mouth pain. Although a small percentage of women reaching menopause report burning mouth syndrome, it has not been associated with menopause.

Clinicians are urged to stress the importance of regular dental visits. Dental examinations should include full periodontal charting and caries evaluation. Postmenopausal women tend to have drier mouths, thus having an increased susceptibility to dental caries. As with all patients, menopausal women should be encouraged to floss and brush with fluoride-containing toothpaste daily, and use antimicrobial rinses as indicated. Additionally, it is clear that adequate calcium and vitamin D intake across a woman's lifespan are important for both bone and periodontal health.[203,204]

References

1. Ravel J, Gajer P, Abdo Z, et al. Vaginal microbiome of reproductive-age women. *Proc Natl Acad Sci U S A*. 2011;108(suppl 1):4680-4687.
2. Lamont RF, Sobel JD, Akins RA, et al. The vaginal microbiome: new information about genital tract flora using molecular based techniques. *BJOG*. 2011;118(5):533-549.
3. Levine KB, Williams RE, Hartmann KE. Vulvovaginal atrophy is strongly associated with female sexual dysfunction among sexually active postmenopausal women. *Menopause*. 2008;15(4 pt 1):661-666.
4. Management of symptomatic vulvovaginal atrophy: 2013 position statement of The North American Menopause Society. *Menopause*. 2013;20(9):903-904.
5. Park HS, Lee KU. Postmenopausal women lose less visceral adipose tissue during a weight reduction program. *Menopause*. 2003;10(3):222-227.
6. Flegal KM, Carroll MD, Kit BK, Ogden CL. Prevalence of obesity and trends in the distribution of body mass index among US adults, 1999-2010. *JAMA*. 2012;307(5):491-497.
7. Brown WJ, Williams L, Ford JH, Ball K, Dobson AJ. Identifying the energy gap: magnitude and determinants of 5-year weight gain in midage women. *Obes Res*. 2005;13(8):1431-1441. Erratum in: *Obes Res*. 2006;14(2):342.
8. Milewicz A, Tworowska U, Demissie A. Menopausal obesity—myth or fact? *Climacteric*. 2001;4(4):273-283.

9. Crawford SI, Casey VA, Avis NE, McKinlay SM. A longitudinal study of weight and the menopause transition: results from the Massachusetts Women's Health Study. *Menopause.* 2000;7(2):96-104.

10. Douchi T, Yamamoto S, Yoshimitsu N, Andoh T, Matsuo T, Nagata Y. Relative contribution of aging and menopause to changes in lean and fat mass in segmental regions. *Maturitas.* 2002;42(4):301-306.

11. Drewnowski A, Warren-Mears VA. Does aging change nutrition requirements? *J Nutr Health Aging.* 2001;5(2):70-74.

12. Patel SR, Malhotra A, White DP, Gottlieb DJ, Hu FB. Association between reduced sleep and weight gain in women. *Am J Epidemiol.* 2006;164(10):947-954.

13. Franklin RM, Ploutz-Snyder L, Kanaley JA. Longitudinal changes in abdominal fat distribution with menopause. *Metabolism.* 2009;58(3):311-315.

14. Park JK, Lim YH, Kim KS, et al. Body fat distribution after menopause and cardiovascular disease risk factors: Korean National Health and Nutrition Examination Survey 2010. *J Womens Health (Larchmt).* 2013;22(7):587-594.

15. Neeland IJ, Ayers CR, Rohatqi AK, et al. Associations of visceral and abdominal subcutaneous adipose tissue with markers of cardiac and metabolic risk in obese adults. *Obesity (Silver Spring).* 2013;21(9):E439-E447.

16. Thorneycroft IH, Lindsay R, Pickar JH. Body composition during treatment with conjugated estrogens with and without medroxyprogesterone acetate: analysis of the women's Health, Osteoporosis, Progestin, Estrogen (HOPE) trial. *Am J Obstet Gynecol.* 2007;197(2):137.e1-e7.

17. Utian WH, Gass ML, Pickar JH. Body mass index does not influence response to treatment, nor does body weight change with lower doses of conjugated estrogens and medroxyprogesterone acetate in early postmenopausal women. *Menopause.* 2004;11(3):306-314.

18. Barrett-Connor E, Slone S, Greendale G, et al. The Postmenopausal Estrogen/Progestin Interventions Study: primary outcomes in adherent women. *Maturitas.* 1997;27(3):261-274.

19. Bonds DE, Lasser N, Qi L, et al. The effect of conjugated equine oestrogen on diabetes incidence: the Women's Health Initiative randomised trial. *Diabetologia.* 2006;49(3):459-468.

20. Folsom AR, Kushi LH, Anderson KE, et al. Associations of general and abdominal obesity with multiple health outcomes in older women: the Iowa Women's Health Study. *Arch Intern Med.* 2000;160(14):2117-2128.

21. Calle EE, Rodriguez C, Walker-Thurmond K, Thun MJ. Overweight, obesity, and mortality from cancer in a prospectively studied cohort of US adults. *N Engl J Med.* 2003;348(17):1625-1638.

22. Eliassen AH, Colditz GA, Rosner B, Willett WC, Hankinson SE. Adult weight change and risk of postmenopausal breast cancer. *JAMA.* 2006;296(2):193-201.

23. Haan MN, Klein R, Klein BE, et al. Hormone therapy and age-related macular degeneration: the Women's Health Initiative Sight Exam Study. *Arch Ophthalmol.* 2006;124(7):988-992.

24. Velie E, Kulldorff M, Schairer C, Block G, Albanes D, Schatzkin A. Dietary fat, fat subtypes, and breast cancer in postmenopausal women: a prospective cohort study. *J Natl Cancer Inst.* 2000;92(10):833-839.

25. National Task Force on the Prevention and Treatment of Obesity. Overweight, obesity, and health risk. *Arch Intern Med.* 2000;160(7):898-904.

26. Schneider HJ, Glaesner H, Klotsche J, et al; DETECT Study Group. Accuracy of anthropometric indicators of obesity to predict cardiovascular risk. *J Clin Endocrinol Metab.* 2007;92(2):589-594.

27. Grundy SM, Brewer HB Jr, Cleeman JI, Smith SC Jr, Lenfant C; American Heart Association; National Heart, Lung and Blood Institute. Definition of metabolic syndrome: report of the National Heart, Lung, and Blood Institute/American Heart Association conference on scientific issues related to definition. *Circulation.* 2004;109(3):433-438.

28. Grundy SM, Cleeman JI, Daniels SR, et al; American Heart Association/National Heart, Lung, and Blood Institute Scientific Statement. Diagnosis and management of the metabolic syndrome: an American Heart Association/National Heart, Lung, and Blood Institute Scientific Statement. *Circulation.* 2005;112(17):2735-2752. Erratum in: *Circulation.* 2005;112(17):e297; *Circulation.* 2005;112(17).e298.

29. Thurston RC, Sowers MR, Sternfeld B, et al. Gains in body fat and vasomotor symptom reporting over the menopausal transition: the study of women's health across the nation. *Am J Epidemiol.* 2009;170(6):766-774.

30. Huang AJ, Subak LL, Wing R, et al; Program to Reduce Incontinence by Diet and Exercise Investigators. An intensive behavioral weight loss intervention and hot flushes in women. *Arch Intern Med.* 2010;170(13):1161-1167. Erratum in: *Arch Intern Med.* 2010;170(17):1601.

31. Kroenke CH, Caan BJ, Stefanick ML, et al. Effects of dietary intervention and weight change on vasomotor symptoms in the Women's Health Initiative. *Menopause.* 2012;19(9):980-988.

32. Marcus MD, Bromberger JT, Wei HL, Brown C, Kravitz HM. Prevalence and selected correlates of eating disorder symptoms among a multiethnic community sample of midlife women. *Ann Behav Med.* 2007;33(3):269-277.

33. Warren MP, Artacho CA. Role of exercise and nutrition. In: Lobo RA, ed. *Treatment of the Postmenopausal Woman: Basic and Clinical Aspects.* 3rd ed. San Diego, CA: Academic Press; 2007:655-682.

34. Kuller LH, Simkin-Silverman LR, Wing RR, Meilahn EN, Ives DG. Women's Healthy Lifestyle Project: a randomized clinical trial: results at 54 months. *Circulation.* 2001;103(1):32-37.

35. Koffman DM, Bazzarre T, Mosca L, Redberg R, Schmid T, Wattigney WA. An evaluation of Choose to Move 1999: an American Heart Association physical activity program for women. *Arch Intern Med.* 2001;161(18):2193-2199.

36. Dansinger ML, Gleason JA, Griffith JL, Selker HP, Schaefer EJ. Comparison of the Atkins, Ornish, Weight Watchers, and Zone diets for weight loss and heart disease risk reduction. *JAMA.* 2005;293(1):43-53.

37. Gardner CD, Kiazand A, Alhassan S, et al. Comparison of the Atkins, Zone, Ornish, and LEARN diets for change in weight and related risk factors among overweight premenopausal women. The A to Z Weight Loss Study: a randomized trial. *JAMA.* 2007;297(9):969-977. Erratum in: *JAMA.* 2007;298(2):178.

38. Appel LJ, Clark JM, Yeh HC, et al. Comparative effectiveness of weight-loss interventions in clinical practice. *N Engl J Med.* 2011;365(21):1959-1968.

39. Howard BV, Van Horn L, Hsia J, et al. Low-fat dietary pattern and risk of cardiovascular disease: the Women's Health Initiative Randomized Controlled Dietary Modification Trial. *JAMA.* 2006;295(6):655-666.

40. Wycherley TP, Moran LJ, Clifton PM, Noakes M, Brinkworth GD. Effects of energy-restricted high-protein, low-fat compared with standard-protein, low-fat diets: a meta-analysis of randomized controlled trials. *Am J Clin Nutr.* 2012;96(6):1281-1298.

41. Te Morenga LA, Levers MT, Williams SM, Brown RC, Mann J. Comparison of high protein and high fiber weight-loss diets in women with risk factors for the metabolic syndrome: a randomized trial. *Nutr J.* 2011;10:40.

42. Korczak D, Kister C. Overweight and obesity: the efficacy of diets for weight maintenance after weight loss. *GMS Health Technol Assess.* 2013;10(9):1-8.

43. Jakicic JM, Marcus BH, Gallagher KI, Napolitano M, Lang W. Effect of exercise duration and intensity on weight loss in overweight, sedentary women: a randomized trial. *JAMA.* 2003;290(10):1323-1330.

44. Brochu M, Malita MF, Messier V, et al. Resistance training does not contribute to improving the metabolic profile after a 6-month weight loss program in overweight and obese postmenopausal women. *J Clin Endocrinol Metab.* 2009;94(9):3226-3233.

45. Moyer VA; US Preventive Services Task Force. Screening for and management of obesity in adults: US Preventive Services Task Force recommendation statement. *Ann Intern Med.* 2012;157(5):373-378.

46. National Institutes of Health, National Heart, Lung, and Blood Institute, North American Association for the Study of Obesity. *The Practical Guide: Identification, Evaluation, and Treatment of Overweight and Obesity in Adults.* October 2000. www.nhlbi.nih.gov/guidelines/obesity/prctgd_c.pdf. Accessed June 6, 2014.

47. Iqbal N, Cardillo S, Volger S, et al. Chromium picolinate does not improve key features of metabolic syndrome in obese nondiabetic adults. *Metab Syndr Relat Disord.* 2009;7(2):143-150.

48. Onakpoya I, Posadzki P, Ernst E. Chromium supplementation in overweight and obesity: a systematic review and meta-analysis of randomized clinical trials. *Obes Rev.* 2013;14(6):496-507.

49. US Dept of Health and Human Services. *Healthy People 2020.* HealthyPeople.gov Web site. November 2010. www.healthypeople.gov/2020/topicsobjectives2020/pdfs/HP2020_brochure_with_LHI_508.pdf. Accessed June 6, 2014.

50. Health Canada. *Eating Well With Canada's Food Guide.* Health Canada Web site. Revised May 23, 2012. www.hc-sc.gc.ca/fn-an/alt_formats/hpfb-dgpsa/pdf/food-guide-aliment/view_eatwell_vue_bienmang-eng.pdf. Accessed June 6, 2014.

51. US Dept of Health and Human Services. *Dietary Guidelines for Americans, 2015.* DietaryGuidelines.gov Web site. Updated June 6, 2014. www.health.gov/dietaryguidelines/2015.asp. Accessed June 6, 2014.

Chapter 2

52. American Heart Association Nutrition Committee, Lichtenstein AH, Appel LJ, et al. Diet and lifestyle recommendations revision 2006: a scientific statement from the American Heart Association Nutrition Committee. *Circulation.* 2006;114(1):82-96. Erratum in: *Circulation.* 2006;114(1):e27; *Circulation.* 2006;114(23):e629.

53. Appel LJ, Brands MW, Daniels SR, Karanja N, Elmer PJ, Sacks FM; American Heart Association. Dietary approaches to prevent and treat hypertension: a scientific statement from the American Heart Association. *Hypertension.* 2006;47(2):296-308.

54. Kris-Etherton P, Eckel RH, Howard BV, St Jeor S, Bazzarre TL; Nutrition Committee Population Science Committee and Clinical Science Committee of the American Heart Association. AHA science advisory: Lyon Diet Heart Study. Benefits of a Mediterranean-style, National Cholesterol Education Program/American Heart Association Step I dietary pattern on cardiovascular disease. *Circulation.*2001;103(13):1823-1825.

55. Nelson ME, Rejeski WJ, Blair SN, et al; American College of Sports Medicine; American Heart Association. Physical activity and public health in older adults: recommendation from the American College of Sports Medicine and the American Heart Association. *Circulation.* 2007;116(8):1094-1105.

56. Slavin JL, Jacobs D, Marquart L, Wiemer K. The role of whole grains in disease prevention. *J Am Diet Assoc.* 2001;101(7):780-785.

57. American Heart Association. *Know Your Fats.* American Heart Association Web site. Updated May 14, 2014. www.heart.org/HEARTORG/Conditions/Cholesterol/PreventionTreatmentofHighCholesterol/Know-Your-Fats_UCM_305628_Article.jsp. Accessed June 6, 2014.

58. American Heart Association. *Alcohol and Heart Disease.* American Heart Association Web site. Updated March 14, 2014. www.heart.org/HEARTORG/Conditions/More/MyHeartandStrokeNews/Alcohol-and-Heart-Disease_UCM_305173_Article.jsp. Accessed June 6, 2014.

59. American Heart Association. *Dining Out.* American Heart Association Web site. www.heart.org/HEARTORG/GettingHealthy/NutritionCenter/DiningOut/Dining-Out_UCM_304183_SubHomePage.jsp. Accessed June 6, 2014.

60. Snow V, Barry P, Fitterman N, Qaseem A, Weiss K; Clinical Efficacy Assessment Subcommittee of the American College of Physicians. Pharmacologic and surgical management of obesity in primary care: a clinical practice guideline from the American College of Physicians. *Ann Intern Med.* 2005;142(7):525-531.

61. Mann T, Tomiyama AJ, Westling E, Lew AM, Samuels B, Chatman J. Medicare's search for effective obesity treatments: diets are not the answer. *Am Psychol.* 2007;62(3):220-233.

62. Holes-Lewis KA, Malcolm R, O'Neil PM. Pharmacotherapy of obesity: clinical treatments and considerations. *Am J Med Sci.* 2013;345(4):284-288.

63. Anderson JW, Schwartz SM, Hauptman J, et al. Low-dose orlistat effects on body weight of mildly to moderately overweight individuals: a 16 week, double-blind, placebo-controlled trial. *Ann Pharmacother.* 2006;40(10):1717-1723.

64. Boulghassoul-Pietrzykowska N, Franceschelli J, Still C. New medications for obesity management: changing the landscape of obesity treatment. *Curr Opin Endocrinol Diabetes Obes.* 2013;20(5):407-411.

65. Wadden TA, Foreyt JP, Foster GD, et al. Weight loss with naltrexone SR/bupropion SR combination therapy as an adjunct to behavior modification: the COR-BMOD trial. *Obesity (Silver Spring).* 2011;19(1):110-120.

66. Apovian CM, Aronne L, Rubino D, et al; COR-II Study Group. A randomized, phase 3 trial of naltrexone SR/bupropion SR on weight and obesity-related risk factors (COR-II). *Obesity (Silver Spring).* 2013;21(5):935-943.

67. Orexigen Therapeutics. Cardiovascular outcomes study of naltrexone SR/bupropion SR in overweight and obese subjects with cardiovascular risk factors (The Light Study). ClinicalTrials.gov Web site. Updated May 20, 2014. http://clinicaltrials.gov/show/NCT01601704. Accessed June 6, 2014. NLM Identifier: NCT01601704.

68. Wadden TA, Hollander P, Klein S, et al; NN8022-1923 Investigators. Weight maintenance and additional weight loss with liraglutide after low-calorie-diet-induced weight loss; the SCALE Maintenance randomized study. *Int J Obesity (Lond).* 2013;37(11):1443-1451. Erratum in: *Int J Obes (Lond).* 2013;37(11):1514.

69. Buchwald H, Avidor Y, Braunwald E, et al. Bariatric surgery: a systematic review and meta-analysis. *JAMA.* 2004;292(14):1724-1737. *Erratum in: JAMA.* 2005;293(14):1728.

70. Maggard MA, Shugarman LR, Suttorp M, et al. Meta-analysis: surgical treatment of obesity. *Ann Intern Med.* 2005;142(7):547-559.

71. Johnson RJ, Johnson BL, Blackhurst DW, et al. Bariatric surgery is associated with a reduced risk of mortality in morbidly obese patients with a history of major cardiovascular events. *Am Surg.* 2012;78(6):685-692.

72. Sjöström L, Peltonen M, Jacobson P, et al. Bariatric surgery and long-term cardiovascular events. *JAMA.* 2012;307(1):56-65.

73. Mercurio MG, Gogstetter DS. Androgen physiology and the cutaneous pilosebaceous unit. *J Gend Specif Med.* 2000;3(4):59-64.

74. Verdier-Sévrain S, Bonté F, Gilchrest B. Biology of estrogens in skin: implications for skin aging. *Exp Dermatol.* 2006;15(2):83-94.

75. Kennedy C, Bastiaens MT, Bajdik CD, Willemze R, Westendorp RG, Bouwes Bavinck JN; Leiden Skin Cancer Study. Effect of smoking and sun on the aging skin. *J Invest Dermatol.* 2003;120(4):548-554.

76. Foote JA, Harris RB, Giuliano AR, et al. Predictors for cutaneous basal- and squamous-cell carcinoma among actinically damaged adults. *Int J Cancer.* 2001;95(1):7-11.

77. Huncharek M, Kupelnick B. Use of topical sunscreens and the risk of malignant melanoma: a meta-analysis of 9067 patients from 11 case-control studies. *Am J Public Health.* 2002;92(7):1173-1177.

78. Halliday GM, Byrne SN, Damian DL. Ultraviolet A radiation: its role in immunosuppression and carcinogenesis. *Semin Cutan Med Surg.* 2011;30(4):214-221.

79. American Academy of Dermatology. Sunscreen 101: Dermatologists answer burning questions about sunscreens [press release]. American Academy of Dermatology Web site. May 20, 2013. www.aad.org/stories-and-news/news-releases/sunscreen-101-dermatologists-answer-burning-questions-about-sunscreens. Accessed June 6, 2014.

80. National Institutes of Health. *Dietary Supplements Fact Sheet: Vitamin D.* Office of Dietary Supplements Web site. Reviewed June 24, 2011. http://ods.od.nih.gov/pdf/factsheets/VitaminD-HealthProfessional.pdf. Accessed June 6, 2014.

81. Lim HW, Gilchrest BA, Cooper KD, et al. Sunlight, tanning booths, and vitamin D. *J Am Acad Dermatol.* 2005; 52(5):868-876. Erratum in: *J Am Acad Dermatol.* 2005;53(3):496.

82. Seité S, Bredoux C, Compan D, et al. Histological evaluation of a topically applied retinol-vitamin C combination. *Skin Pharmacol Physiol.* 2005;18(2):81-87.

83. Babamiri K, Nassab R. Cosmeceuticals: the evidence behind the retinoids. *Aesthet Surg J.* 2010;30(1):74-77.

84. Carruthers J, Carruthers A. Botulinum toxin in facial rejuvenation: an update. *Dermatol Clin.* 2009;27(4):417-425.

85. Raine-Fenning NJ, Brincat MP, Muscat-Baron Y. Skin aging and menopause: implications for treatment. *Am J Clin Dermatol.* 2003;4(6):371-378.

86. Quatresooz P, Pierard-Franchimont C, Gaspard U, Pierard GE. Skin climacteric aging and hormone replacement therapy. *J Cosmet Dermatol.* 2006;5(1):3-8.

87. Sauerbronn AV, Fonseca AM, Bagnoli VR, Saldiva PH, Pinotti JA. The effects of systemic hormonal replacement therapy on the skin of postmenopausal women. *Int J Gynaecol Obstet.* 2000;68(1):35-41.

88. Sator PG, Sator MO, Schmidt JB, et al. A prospective, randomized, double-blind, placebo-controlled study on the influence of a hormone replacement therapy on skin aging in postmenopausal women. *Climacteric.* 2007;10(4):320-324.

89. Sumino H, Ichikawa S, Kasama S, et al. Effects of raloxifene and hormone replacement therapy on forearm skin elasticity in postmenopausal women. *Maturitas.* 2009;62(1):53-57.

90. Wolff EF, Narayan D, Taylor HS. Long-term effect of hormone therapy on skin rigidity and wrinkles. *Fertil Steril.* 2005;8(2):285-288.

91. Hall G, Phillips TJ. Estrogen and the skin: the effects of estrogen, menopause, and hormone replacement therapy on the skin. *J Am Acad Dermatol.* 2005;53(4):555-568.

92. Stevenson S, Thornton J. Effect of estrogens on skin aging and the potential role of SERMs. *Clin Interven Aging.* 2007;2(3):283-297.

93. Verdier-Sévrain S. Effect of estrogens on skin aging and the potential role of selective estrogen receptor modulators. *Climacteric.* 2007;10(4):289-297.

94. Phillips TJ, Symons J, Menon S; HT Study Group. Does hormone therapy improve age-related skin changes in postmenopausal women? A randomized, double-blind, double-dummy, placebo-controlled multicenter study assessing the effects of norethindrone acetate and ethinyl estradiol in the improvement of mild to moderate age-related skin changes in postmenopausal women. *J Am Acad Dermatol.* 2008;59(3):397-404.

95. Moraes AB, Haidar MA, Soares Júnior JM, Simões MJ, Baracat ED, Patriarca MT. The effect of topical isoflavones on postmenopausal skin: double-blind and randomized clinical trial of efficacy. *Eur J Obstet Gynecol Reprod Biol.* 2009;146(2):188-192.
96. Patriarca MT, Goldman KZ, Dos Santos JM, et al. Effects of topical estradiol on the facial skin collagen of postmenopausal women under oral hormone therapy: a pilot study. *Eur J Obstet Gynecol Reprod Biol.* 2006;130(2):202-205.
97. Rittié L, Kang S, Voorhees JJ, Fisher GJ. Induction of collagen by estradiol: difference between sun-protected and photodamaged human skin in vivo. *Arch Dermatol.* 2008;144(9):1129-1140.
98. Holzer G, Riegler E, Hönigsmann H, Farokhnia S, Shmidt JB. Effects and side-effects of 2% progesterone cream on the skin of peri- and postmenopausal women: results from a double-blind, vehicle-controlled, randomized study. *Br J Dermatol.* 2005;153(3):626-634. Erratum in: *Br J Dermatol.* 2005;153(5):1092.
99. Farage MA, Miller KW, Berardesca E, Maibach HI. Clinical implications of aging skin: cutaneous disorders in the elderly. *Am J Clin Dermatol.* 2009;10(2):73-86.
100. Azziz R. The evaluation and management of hirsutism. *Obstet Gynecol.* 2003;101(5 pt 1):995-1007.
101. Mirmirani P. Managing hair loss in midlife women. *Maturitas.* 2013;74(2):119-122.
102. Tosti A, Paraccini BM, Iorizzo M, Misciali C. Frontal fibrosing alopecia in postmenopausal women. *J Am Acad Dermatol.* 2005;52(1):55-60.
103. Rallis E, Gregoriou S, Christofdou E, Rigopoulis D. Frontal fibrosing alopecia: to treat or not to treat? *J Cutan Med Surg.* 2010;14(4):161-166.
104. Yoo HG, Won CH, Lee SR, et al. Expression of androgen and estrogen receptors in human scalp mesenchymal cells in vitro. *Arch Dermatol Res.* 2007;298(10):505-509.
105. Zouboulis CC, Chen WC, Thornton MJ, Qin K, Rosenfield R. Sexual hormones in human skin. *Horm Metab Res.* 2007;39(2):85-95.
106. Oh HS, Smart RC. An estrogen receptor pathway regulates the telogen-anagen hair follicle transition and influences epidermal cell proliferation. *Proc Natl Acad Sci U S A.* 1996;93(22):12525-12530.
107. Rebora A. Pathogenesis of androgenetic alopecia. *J Am Acad Dermatol.* 2004;50(5):777-779.
108. Deplewski D, Rosenfield RL. Role of hormones in pilosebaceous unit development. *Endocr Rev.* 2000;21(4):363-392.
109. Olsen EA, Messenger AG, Shapiro J, et al. Evaluation and treatment of male and female pattern hair loss. *J Am Acad Dermatol.* 2005;52(2):301-311.
110. Nathan L. Menopause and postmenopause. In: DeCherney AH, Nathan L, Goodwin TM, Laufer N, Roman A, eds. *Current Diagnosis and Treatment: Obstetrics and Gynecology.* 11th ed. New York: McGraw Hill Medical; 2012:948-970.
111. Riedel-Baima B, Riedel A. Female pattern hair loss may be triggered by low oestrogen to androgen ratio. *Endocr Regul.* 2008;42(1):13-16.
112. Georgala S, Gourgiotou K, Kassouli S, Stratigos JD. Hormonal status in postmenopausal androgenetic alopecia. *Int J Dermatol.* 1992;31(12):858-859.
113. Waggoner W, Boots LR, Azziz R. Total testosterone and DHEAS levels as predictors of androgen-secreting neoplasms: a populational study. *Gynecol Endocrinol.* 1999;13(6):394-400.
114. Sellheyer K, Bergfeld WF. Histopathologic evaluation of alopecias. *Am J Dermatopathol.* 2006;28(3):236-259.
115. Rushton DH. Nutritional factors and hair loss. *Clin Exp Dermatol.* 2002;27(5):396-404.
116. Lucky AW, Piacquadio DJ, Ditre CM, et al. A randomized, placebo-controlled trial of 5% and 2% topical minoxidil solutions in the treatment of female pattern hair loss. *J Am Acad Dermatol.* 2004;50(4):541-553.
117. McElwee KJ, Shapiro JS. Promising therapies for treating and/or preventing androgenic alopecia. *Skin Therapy Lett.* 2012;17(6):1-4.
118. Sinclair R, Wewerinke M, Jolley D. Treatment of female pattern hair loss with oral antiandrogens. *Br J Dermatol.* 2005;152(3):466-473.
119. Shapiro J. Clinical practice. Hair loss in women. *N Engl J Med.* 2007;357(16):1620-1630.
120. Scheinfeld N. A review of hormonal therapy for female pattern (androgenic) alopecia. *Dermatol Online J.* 2008;14(3):1.
121. Burke BM, Cunliffe WJ. Oral spironolactone therapy for female patients with acne, hirsutism or androgenetic alopecia. *Br J Dermatol.* 1985;112(1):124-125.
122. Burova EP. Antiandrogens. In: Wakelin SH, Maibach HI, eds. *Handbook of Systemic Drug Treatment in Dermatology.* London: Thieme; 2002:32-40.
123. Atanaskova Mesinkovska N, Bergfeld WF. Hair: what is new in diagnosis and management? Female pattern hair loss update: diagnosis and treatment. *Dermatol Clin.* 2013;31(1):119-127.
124. Dawber RP, Sonnex T, Ralfs I. Oral antiandrogen treatment of common baldness in women. *Br J Dermatol.* 1982;107(suppl):20-21.
125. Price VH, Roberts JL, Hordinsky M, et al. Lack of efficacy of finasteride in postmenopausal women with androgenetic alopecia. *J Am Acad Dermatol.* 2000;43(5 pt 1):768-776.
126. Trueb RM; Swiss Trichology Study Group. Finasteride treatment of patterned hair loss in normoandrogenic postmenopausal women. *Dermatology.* 2004;209(3):202-207.
127. Harries MJ, Sinclair RD, MacDonald-Hulls, Whiting DA, Griffiths CE, Paus R. Management of primary cicatricial alopecias: options for treatment. *Br J Dermatol.* 2008;159(1):1-22.
128. Olsen EA, Hordinsky M, Whiting D, et al; Dutasteride Alopecia Research Team. The importance of dual 5alpha-reductase inhibition in the treatment of male pattern hair loss: results of a randomized placebo-controlled study of dutasteride versus finasteride. *J Am Acad Dermatol.* 2006;55(6):1014-1023.
129. Georgala S, Katoulis AC, Befon A, Danopoulou I, Georgala C. Treatment of postmenopausal frontal fibrosing alopecia with oral dutasteride. *J Am Acad Dermatol.* 2009;61(1):157-158.
130. Rácz E, Gho C, Moorman PW, Noordhoek Hegt V, Neumann HA. Treatment of frontal fibrosing alopecia and lichen planopilaris: a systematic review. *J Eur Acad Dermatol Venereol.* 2013;27(12):1461-1470.
131. Kučerová R, Bienová M, Novotný R, Fiurášková M, Hajdúch M, Sovak M. Current therapies of female androgenetic alopecia and use of fluridil, a novel topical antiandrogen. *Scr Med (Brno).* 2006;79(1):35-48.
132. Banaszek A. Company profits from side effects of glaucoma treatment. *CMAJ.* 2011;183(14):E1058.
133. Blume-Peytavi U, Lönnfors S, Hillmann K, Garcia Bartels N. A randomized double-blind placebo-controlled pilot study to assess the efficacy of a 24-week topical treatment by latanoprost 0.1% on hair growth and pigmentation in healthy volunteers with androgenetic alopecia. *J Am Acad Dermatol.* 2012;66(5):794-800.
134. Hugo Perez BS. Ketocazole as an adjunct to finasteride in the treatment of androgenetic alopecia in men. *Med Hypotheses.* 2004;62(1):112-115.
135. Inui S, Itami S. Reversal of androgenetic alopecia by topical ketoconzole: relevance of anti-androgenic activity. *J Dermatol Sci.* 2007;45(1):66-68.
136. Berger RS, Fu JL, Smiles KA, et al. The effects of minoxidil, 1% pyrithione zinc and a combination of both on hair density: a randomized controlled trial. *Br J Dermatol.* 2003;149(2):354-362.
137. Leavitt M, Charles G, Heyman E, Michaels D. HairMax LaserComb laser phototherapy device in the treatment of male androgenetic alopecia: a randomized, double-blind, sham device-controlled, multicentre trial. *Clin Drug Investig.* 2009;29(5):283-292.
138. McElwee KJ, Kissling S, Wenzel E, Huth A, Hoffmann R. Cultured peribulbar dermal sheath cells can induce hair follicle development and contribute to the dermal sheath and dermal papilla. *J Invest Dermatol.* 2003;121(6):1267-1275.
139. Takikawa M, Nakamura S, Nakamura S, et al. Enhanced effect of platelet-rich plasma containing a new carrier on hair growth. *Dermatol Surg.* 2011;37(12):1721-1729.
140. Arias-Santiago S, Gutierrez-Salmerón MT, Buendía-Eisman A, Girón-Prieto MS, Naranjo-Sintes R. Hypertension and aldosterone levels in women with early-onset androgenetic alopecia. *Br J Dermatol.* 2009;162(4):786-789.
141. Richards RN, Meharg GE. Electrolysis: observations from 13 years and 140,000 hours of experience. *J Am Acad Dermatol.* 1995;33(4):662-666.
142. Moreno-Arias GA, Camps-Fresneda A. Long-lasting hypopigmentation induced by long-pulsed alexandrite laser photo-epilation. *Dermatol Surg.* 2003;29(4):420-422.
143. Alster TS, Khoury RR. Treatment of laser complications. *Facial Plast Surg.* 2009;25(5):316-323.
144. Rasheed AI. Uncommonly reported side effects of hair removal by long pulsed-alexandrite laser. *J Cosmet Dermatol.* 2009;8(4):267-274.
145. Desai S, Mahmoud BH, Bhatia AC, Hamzavi IH. Paradoxical hypertrichosis after laser therapy: a review. *Dermatol Surg.* 2010;36(3):291-298.

Chapter 2

146. Qureshi IA. Intraocular pressure: association with menstrual cycle, pregnancy and menopause in apparently healthy women. *Chin J Physiol.* 1995;38(4):229-234. Erratum in: *Chin J Physiol.* 1996;39(1):63.
147. Kangari H, Eftekhari MH, Sardari S, et al. Short term consumption of oral omega-3 and dry eye syndrome. *Ophthalmology.* 2013;120(11):2191-2196.
148. Sall K, Stevenson OD, Mundorf TK, Reis B. Two multicenter, randomized studies of the efficacy and safety of cyclosporine ophthalmic emulsion in moderate to severe dry eye disease. CsA Phase 3 Study Group. *Ophthalmology.* 2000;107(4):631-639. Erratum in: *Ophthalmology.* 2000;107(7):1220.
149. Kunert KS, Tisdale AS, Stern ME, Smith JA, Gipson IK. Analysis of topical cyclosporine treatment of patients with dry eye syndrome: effect on conjunctival lymphocytes. *Arch Ophthalmol.* 2000;118(11):1489-1496.
150. Toker E, Yenice O, Akpinar I, Aribal E, Kazokoglu H. The influence of sex hormones on ocular blood flow in women. *Acta Ophthalmol Scand.* 2003;81(6):617-624.
151. Smith JA, Vitale S, Reed GF, et al. Dry eye signs and symptoms in women with premature ovarian failure. *Arch Ophthalmol.* 2004;122(2):151-156.
152. Hales AM, Chamberlain CG, Murphy CR, McAvoy JW. Estrogen protects lenses against cataract induced by transforming growth factor-beta (TGFbeta). *J Exp Med.* 1997;185(2):273-280.
153. Sullivan DA, ed. *Lacrimal Gland, Tear Film, and Dry Eye Syndromes: Basic Science and Clinical Relevance.* New York: Springer; 2007.
154. Schaumberg DA, Uchino M, Christen WG, Semba RD, Buring JE, Li JZ. Patient reported differences in dry eye disease between men and women: impact, management, and patient satisfaction. *PLoS One.* 2013;8(9):e76121.
155. Schaumberg DA, Buring JE, Sullivan DA, Dana MR. Hormone replacement therapy and dry eye syndrome. *JAMA.* 2001;286(17):2114-2119.
156. Khurana RN, LaBree LD, Scott G, Smith RE, Yiu SC. Esterified estrogens combined with methyltestosterone raise intraocular pressure in postmenopausal women. *Am J Ophthalmol.* 2006;142(3):494-495.
157. Scuderi G, Contestabile MT, Gagliano C, Iacovello D, Scuderi L, Avitabile T. Effects of phytoestrogen supplementation in postmenopausal women with dry eye syndrome: a randomized clinical trial. *Can J Ophthalmol.* 2012;47(6):489-492.
158. Klein BE, Klein R, Lee KE. Reproductive exposures, incident age-related cataracts, and age-related maculopathy in women: the Beaver Dam Eye Study. *Am J Ophthalmol.* 2000;130(3):322-326.
159. Klein BE, Klein R, Lee KE. Incidence of age-related cataract over a 10-year interval: the Beaver Dam Eye Study. *Ophthalmology.* 2002;109(11):2052-2057.
160. Kanthan GL, Wang JJ, Rochtchina E, et al. Ten-year incidence of age-related cataract and cataract surgery in an older Australian population. The Blue Mountains Eye Study. *Ophthalmology.* 2008;115(5):808-814.e1.
161. Bigsby RM, Cardenas H, Caperell-Grant A, Grubbs CJ. Protective effects of estrogen in a rat model of age-related cataracts. *Proc Natl Acad Sci USA.* 1999;96(16):9328-9332.
162. Deschênes MC, Descovich D, Moreau M, et al. Postmenopausal hormone therapy increases retinal blood flow and protects the retinal nerve fiber layer. *Invest Ophthalmol Vis Sci.* 2009;51(5):2587-2600.
163. Lam JS, Tay WT, Aung T, Saw SM, Wong TY. Female reproductive factors and major eye diseases in Asian women—The Singapore Malay Eye Study. *Ophthalmic Epidem.* 2014;21(2):92-98.
164. Freeman EE, Munoz B, Schein O, West SK. Hormone replacement therapy and lens opacities: the Salisbury Eye Evaluation Project. *Arch Ophthalmol.* 2001;119(11):1687-1692.
165. Worzola K, Hiller R, Sperduto RD, et al. Postmenopausal estrogen use, type of menopause, and lens opacities: the Framingham studies. *Arch Intern Med.* 2001;161(11):1448-1454.
166. Paganini-Hill A, Clark LJ. Eye problems in breast cancer patients treated with tamoxifen. *Breast Cancer Res Treat.* 2000;60(2):167-172.
167. Hulsman CA, Westendorp IC, Ramrattan RS, et al. Is open-angle glaucoma associated with early menopause? The Rotterdam Study. *Am J Epidemiol.* 2001;154(2):138-144.
168. Pasquale LR, Rosner BA, Hankinsons SE, Kang JH. Attributes of female reproductive aging and their relation to primary open-angle glaucoma: a prospective study. *J Glaucoma.* 2007;16(7):598-605.
169. Lee AJ, Mitchell P, Rochtchina E, Healey PR; Blue Mountains Eye Study. Female reproductive factors and open-angle glaucoma: the Blue Mountains Eye Study. *Br J Ophthalmol.* 2003;87(11):1324-1328.
170. Newman-Casey PA, Talwar N, Nan B, Musch DC, Pasquale LR, Stein JD. The potential association between postmenopausal hormone use and primary open-angle glaucoma. *JAMA Ophthalmol.* 132(3):298-303.
171. Chuo JY, Lee TY, Hollands H, et al. Risk factors for posterior vitreous detachment: a case-control study. *Am J Ophthalmol.* 2006;142(6):931-937.
172. Edwards DR, Gallins P, Polk M, et al. Inverse association of female hormone replacement therapy with age-related macular degeneration and interactions with ARMS2 polymorphisms. *Invest Ophthalmol Vis Sci.* 2010;51(4):1873-1879.
173. Yaffe K, Clemons TE, McBee WL, Lendblad AS; Age-Related Eye Disease Study Research Group. Impact of antioxidants, zinc, and copper on cognition in the elderly: a randomized, controlled trial. *Neurology.* 2004;63(9):1705-1707.
174. Agrawal Y, Platz EA, Niparko JK. Prevalence of hearing loss and differences by demographic characteristics among US adults: data from the National Health and Nutrition Examination Survey, 1999-2004. *Arch Intern Med.* 2008;168(14):1522-1530.
175. Travis LB, Fossa SD, Sesso HD, et al; Platinum Study Group. Chemotherapy-induced peripheral neurotoxicity and ototoxicity: new paradigms for translational genomics. *J Natl Cancer Inst.* 2014;106(5):pii: dju044.
176. Jenkins V, Low R, Mitra S. Hearing sensitivity in women following chemotherapy treatment for breast cancer: results from a pilot study. *Breast.* 2009;18(5):279-283.
177. Hederstierna C, Hultcrantz M, Collins A, Rosenhall U. The menopause triggers hearing decline in healthy women. *Hear Res.* 2009;259(1-2):31-35.
178. Oghan F, Coksuer H. Comparative audiometric evaluation of hearing loss between the premenopausal and postmenopausal period in young women. *Am J Otolaryngol.* 2012;33(3):322-325.
179. Hultcrantz M, Simonska R, Sternberg AE. Estrogen and hearing: a summary of recent investigations. *Acta Otolaryngol.* 2006;126(1):10-14.
180. Khaliq F, Tandon OP, Goel N. Differential effects of exogenous estrogen versus estrogen-progesterone combination on auditory evoked potentials in menopausal women. *Indian J Physiol Pharmacol.* 2005;49(3):345-352.
181. Guimaraes P, Frisina ST, Mapes F, Tadros SF, Frisina DR, Frisina RD. Progestin negatively affects hearing in aged women. *Proc Natl Acad Sci U S A.* 2006;103(38):14246-14249.
182. Köşüş N, Köşüş A, Turhan NÖ, Kurtaran H. Hearing levels in menopausal women and the effect of tibolone on audiological functions. *J Obstet Gynaecol.* 2012;32(3):294-297.
183. Moyer V; US Preventive Services Task Force. Screening for hearing loss in older adults: US Preventive Services Task Force recommendation statement. *Ann Intern Med.* 2012;157(9):655-661.
184. Hederstierna C, Hultcrantz M, Collins A, Rosenhall U. Hearing in women at menopause. Prevalence of hearing loss, audiometric configuration and relation to hormone replacement therapy. *Acta Otolaryngol.* 2007;127(2):149-155.
185. Patterson C. Prevention of hearing impairment and disability in the elderly. In: Goldbloom R, ed. *The Canadian Guide to Clinical Preventive Health Care.* Canadian Task Force on the Periodic Health Examination. Ottawa, ON: Canada Communication Group; 1994.
186. Tezal M, Wactawski-Wende J, Grossi SG, Ho AW, Dunford R, Genco RJ. The relationship between bone mineral density and periodontitis in postmenopausal women. *J Periodontol.* 2000;71(9):1492-1498.
187. Meisel P. Reifenberger J, Haase R, Nauck M, Bandt C, Kocher T. Women are periodontally healthier than men, but why don't they have more teeth than men? *Menopause.* 2008;15(2):270-275.
188. Krall EA, Dawson-Hughes B, Papas A, Garcia RI. Tooth loss and skeletal bone density in healthy postmenopausal women. *Osteoporos Int.* 1994;4(2):104-109.
189. Krall EA, Dawson-Hughes B, Hannan MT, Wilson PW, Kiel DP. Postmenopausal estrogen replacement and tooth retention. *Am J Med.* 1997;102(6):536-542.
190. Lerner UH. Inflammation-induced bone remodeling in periodontal disease and the influence of post-menopausal osteoporosis. *J Dent Res.* 2006;85(7):596-607.
191. Wactawski-Wende J. Periodontal diseases and osteoporosis: association and mechanisms. *Ann Periodontol.* 2001;6(1):197-208.
192. Management of osteoporosis in postmenopausal women: 2010 position statement of The North American Menopause Society. *Menopause.* 2010;17(1):23-54; quiz 55-56.
193. Edwards BJ, Hellstein JW, Jacobsen PL, Kaltman S, Mariotti A, Migliorati CA; American Dental Association Council on Scientific Affairs Expert Panel on Bisphosphonate-Associated Osteonecrosis of the Jaw. Updated recommendations for managing the care of patients receiving oral bisphosphonate therapy: an advisory statement from the American Dental Association Council on Scientific Affairs. *J Am Dent Assoc.* 2008;130(12):1674-1677. Erratum in: *J Am Dent Assoc.* 2009;140(5):522.

194. Migliorati CA, Casiglia J, Epstein J, Jacobsen PL, Siegel MA, Woo SB. Managing the care of patients with bisphosphonate-associated osteonecrosis: an American Academy of Oral Medicine position paper. *J Am Dent Assoc.* 2005;136(12):1658-1668. Erratum in: *J Am Dent Assoc.* 2006;137(1):26.
195. Woo SB, Hellstein JW, Kalmar JR. Narrative [corrected] review: bisphosphonates and osteonecrosis of the jaws. *Ann Intern Med.* 2006;144(10):753-761. Erratum in: *Ann Intern Med.* 2006;145(3):235.
196. Ruggiero SL, Dodson TB, Fantasia J, et al; American Association of Oral and Maxillofacial Surgeons. *Position Paper: Medication-Related Osteonecrosis of the Jaw—2014 Update.* www.aaoms.org/docs/position_papers/mronj_position_paper.pdf?pdf=MRONJ-Position-Paper. Accessed June 9, 2014.
197. Yildirim TT, Kaya FA. The effects of menopause on periodontal tissues. *Int Dent Res.* 2011;1(3):81-86.
198. Mascitelli L, Pezzetta F, Goldstein MR. Menopause, vitamin D, and oral health (August 2009). *Cleve Clin J Med.* 2009;76(11):629-630.
199. Anand N, Chandraselearan SC, Rajput NS. Vitamin D and periodontal health: current concepts. *J Indian Soc Periodontal.* 2013;7(3):302-308.
200. Kayce EK. Bone and Oral Health. *J Am Dental Assoc.* 2007;138(5):616-619.
201. Genco RJ, Grossi SG. Is estrogen deficiency a risk factor for periodontal disease? *Compend Contin Educ Dent Suppl.* 1998;(22):S23-S29.
202. Zakrzewska JM, Forssell H. Glenny AM. Interventions for the treatment of burning mouth syndrome. *Cochrane Database Syst Rev.* 2005;(1):CD002779.
203. Gunsolley JC. Clinical effectiveness of antimicrobial mouthrinses. *J Dent.* 2010;38(suppl 1):s6-s10.
204. Stewart S, Hanning R. Building osteoporosis prevention into dental practice. *J Can Dent Assoc.* 2012;78:c29.

Chapter 3

Clinical Issues

Women moving through the menopause transition often experience 1 or more various menopause-related symptoms and other health effects.

Decline in fertility

Social trends have led to delayed or deferred childbearing, which has been associated with an increase in age-related infertility and pregnancy loss.[1] Fertility declines with increasing age, becoming significant in women aged around 35 to 38 years, or 10 to 15 years before menopause. Age-related infertility has been shown in studies of donor insemination and in vitro fertilization (IVF) embryo-transfer programs. In addition, advanced maternal age (≥35 y) is associated with increased risks for spontaneous miscarriage (50% by age 45), chromosomal abnormalities in the fetus, and other pregnancy complications (premature labor, fetal mortality, or need for cesarean delivery).[2,3] The most frequent chromosomal abnormality is autosomal trisomy, which is related in part to changes in the meiotic spindle that predispose to nondisjunction.[4]

Many women in industrialized countries are delaying childbearing and thus may face increased risk of fertility problems. The American Congress of Obstetricians and Gynecologists (ACOG) recommends that women desiring pregnancy after age 35 should receive expedited evaluation and treatment after 6 months of failed attempts at conception or sooner if clinically indicated.[1]

Evaluation for ovarian reserve

Diminished ovarian reserve is associated with decreased oocyte quality, oocyte quantity, and the ability to become pregnant. The functional activity of the ovary changes more with age than does almost any other organ in the human body. There is no single, highly reliable test for assessing ovarian reserve and predicting pregnancy potential; thus, a number of screening tests may be used. Furthermore, hormone test results may differ, depending on the laboratory.[5] For women aged older than 35 years or for whom there is concern about ovarian reserve, a day-3 (day 1 is the first day of full menstrual flow) follicle-stimulating hormone (FSH) level test may be helpful. An estradiol level should be drawn on day 3 as well, because FSH levels are not predictive of ovarian reserve when estradiol levels are high.

With aging, there is a subtle but real increase in FSH and a decrease in antral follicle production of inhibin B.[6] Inhibin B normally inhibits the pituitary's FSH production.[7]

Well-functioning ovaries produce ovarian hormones from small follicles early in the menstrual cycle and maintain FSH at a low level, whereas women with a reduced pool of follicles and oocytes have an insufficient production of ovarian hormones that does not provide normal inhibition of FSH, leading to an early cycle increase (a value <10 mIU/mL is suggestive of adequate ovarian reserve; levels of 10-15 mIU/mL are considered borderline). A reduction in pregnancy rate and live births is seen at higher levels of basal FSH (>10 mIU/mL). High basal FSH is suggestive of diminished ovarian reserve.

Day-3 estradiol less than 80 pg/mL is also suggestive of normal ovarian reserve. Elevated day-3 estradiol levels are seen in women with poor ovarian reserve as a result of premature follicle recruitment. Elevated estradiol can inhibit pituitary FSH production, which can mask one of the signs of decreased ovarian reserve. Measuring FSH and estradiol levels on day 3 helps to avoid falsely reassuring FSH testing.

The clomiphene citrate challenge is another test used for assessing ovarian reserve. It is usually recommended for patients aged 38 years or older, those with unexplained infertility, those with a prior history of ovarian surgery, those with poor responses to fertility medications, and those in whom other symptoms may be suggestive of decreased ovarian reserve (such as shorter menstrual cycles). Oral clomiphene citrate 100 mg is prescribed for cycle days 5 through 9. Follicle-stimulating hormone is measured on days 3 and 10 and estradiol level on day 3.

Referral to a reproductive specialist for consideration of ovulation induction, IVF, or use of donor oocytes is recommended if the day-3 FSH level or clomiphene citrate challenge test is abnormal. Women who have markedly diminished ovarian reserve rarely conceive without the use of donor eggs.

Additional tests include the antral follicle count (AFC) and antimüllerian hormone (AMH) level. The AFC, defined as the number of follicles measuring 2 mm to 10 mm in diameter using ultrasonographic measurement, is another measure of ovarian reserve. On transvaginal ultrasound, a low AFC of 3 to 10 antral follicles between cycle days 2 to 4 suggests diminished ovarian reserve.

Low AFC is associated with poor ovarian reserve and response.[8] Once the oocyte pool decreases to approximately 1,000 follicles, menopause is reached.[9]

Antimüllerian hormone is expressed by the small preantral and early antral follicles. Antimüllerian hormone levels gradually decline as the size of the primordial follicle pool declines with age,[10] but there is no consensus on the appropriate threshold values. In general, levels of serum AMH above 0.5 ng/mL are consistent with good ovarian reserve, whereas lower levels suggest the presence of a depleted ovarian follicle pool. Very low levels (<0.15 ng/mL) suggest poor response to ovarian stimulation, but that should be confirmed by an AFC.

Levels of AMH are undetectable at menopause.[11] Antimüllerian hormone levels demonstrate minimal intercycle and intracyle variability, thus it can be measured anytime during the menstrual cycle because the growth of small preantral follicles is continuous and not cyclical. Karyotyping is normally reserved for women with premature menopause (before age 40) and when there have been recurrent pregnancy losses.

In addition to oocyte quantity and quality, the primary determinant of reproductive potential, age-related uterine changes such as fibroids, tubal disease, or endometriosis may contribute to decreased fertility without creating any major change in the hormonal dynamics of the menstrual cycle. Diagnostic laparoscopy is indicated for women with suspected endometriosis or pelvic adhesions. Hysterosalpingogram (HSG) or chromotubation at laparoscopy allow assessment of tubal patency. Hysteroscopy can be used to evaluate the uterine cavity.

Please see Chapter 1 for more on ovarian aging and hormone production.

Fertility-enhancing options

Research related to assisted reproductive technologies has provided significant information regarding aging and fertility. It is thought that *functional ovarian reserve* is the most important indicator of age-related infertility.[12] Ovarian reserve describes a woman's reproductive potential as it relates to follicular depletion and oocyte quality. Although some intercycle variability exists, women with elevations of FSH in one cycle usually have elevations in subsequent cycles. Many other, more direct markers of ovarian function, such as AMH and inhibin B, are currently being evaluated to optimize testing of ovarian reserve.[9]

For women of advanced reproductive age who desire to have children, fertility-enhancing technologies are an option, including controlled ovarian hyperstimulation with intrauterine insemination and IVF. For women with significantly decreased ovarian reserve, IVF with oocyte donation is generally advised. Gestational carriers are recommended for women without a uterus or with significant uterine or endometrial pathology, including severe scarring. Gestational carriers also are recommended for women at high risk for adverse outcomes during pregnancy because of an underlying health problem such as significant cardiac disease.

The success of fertility-enhancing technology depends on a woman's age, general health, reasons for treatment, and the modality used.[13] Many of these treatment options are expensive, involve some risks, and are not always successful; the success rate decreases with increasing age. Women of advanced reproductive age often have a number of underlying health problems as well. In general, fertility treatment with a woman's own oocytes is not advised after age 43 years, and any fertility treatment, including donor oocyte IVF, is not recommended after age 50 years.

The reported success of oocyte donation in women in their 50s and early 60s suggests that pregnancy may be possible in women with a normal uterus, regardless of age or the absence of oocytes. Opponents of donor oocyte IVF in women aged older than 50 years argue that pregnancy in this age group is not in the best interests of older women nor of the children they bear. Others argue that it is unfair to deny women the use of donated oocytes or embryos solely because of their age.[14] If a woman is considering these alternatives, she should be fully apprised of the expected success rates, along with the risks and benefits of each technique. In addition, pregnancy in women aged older than 50 years is associated with an increased risk of pregnancy loss, hypertension, preeclampsia, gestational diabetes, intrauterine fetal demise, and the need for a caesarean delivery.

The American Society for Reproductive Medicine recommends that women aged between 50 and 54 years who are interested in egg donation or embryo donation should be counseled about increased medical risks of conception and pregnancy at an advanced age.[14] Single embryo transfers should be strongly considered because of the additional risks associated with multiple pregnancies. Prospective parents should be counseled to consider the age and health of their partners as well as parenting issues specific to their age.

Birth control options during perimenopause

Despite a decline in fertility during perimenopause, unplanned pregnancy is still possible until menopause (no menstrual periods for 12 consecutive months) or until levels of FSH are consistently elevated (>30 mIU/mL); however, there are no reliable laboratory tests to confirm definitive loss of fertility.[15] Thus, sexually active women aged older than 40 years continue to need an effective method of contraception.[16]

CLINICAL ISSUES

Perimenopausal women have a range of nonhormonal contraception options:

- Sterilization (tubal ligation and vasectomy) is safe and effective and has a very low failure rate (approximately 4-8 per 1,000).[17] The primary disadvantages are the risks associated with anesthesia and the surgical procedure as well as difficulty reversing the process. Sterilization offers no protection from sexually transmitted infections (STIs). Sterilization is a good option for midlife women (or their male partners) if they are in a mutually monogamous, long-term relationship and desire permanent contraception. Permanent female sterilization is available through disruption of the fallopian tubes with laparoscopic fulguration, ligation, or clipping of the tubes.

  In addition, a minimally invasive form of irreversible sterilization is available through a permanent contraceptive tubal occlusion device and delivery system.[18] Using hysteroscopy in the outpatient setting without anesthesia, microinserts are placed into the proximal section of each fallopian tube by a catheter passed from the vagina through the cervix and uterus. Once in place, the device is designed to elicit tissue growth (scarring) in and around the microinsert to form, over a period of 3 months, an occlusion or blockage in the fallopian tubes. This tissue barrier prevents sperm from reaching an egg. During this 3-month period, the patient must use an alternate form of contraception. An HSG is performed after 3 months to confirm the proper location of the device and to document tubal occlusion. Performed correctly, the procedure is considered safe, with minimal postprocedure discomfort and adverse events (AEs). Most clinical data are based on 12 to 24 months of use; the risks of long-term use are not known.[19]

- Another tubal occlusion microinsert permanent contraceptive is a 2-step procedure.[20,21] Through a hysteroscope, radiofrequency energy is delivered to the fallopian tube to remove a thin layer of cells and stimulate tissue response. A soft silicone insert smaller than a grain of rice is implanted at the site. Tissue growth around the implant creates permanent blockage, confirmed by HSG 3 months after the procedure. Successful placement is achieved in 92% to 95% of women, with a 1-year pregnancy rate of 1.1%.

- Other nonhormonal methods of contraception include spermicides and barrier methods, including the male condom, female condom, diaphragm, cervical cap, and cervical sponge. These methods are effective if used correctly and consistently during every act of vaginal sex. Intrauterine devices (IUDs) are highly effective. The long-acting copper IUD provides contraception for up to 10 years. The condom is the only proven effective protection against pregnancy and STIs (during vaginal, oral, and anal sex). Barrier methods can be used in combination with other birth control methods. Disadvantages include potential allergic reaction to latex or spermicides, the need to be used during every act of sex, and (with condoms) the potential to break, leak, or spill when removed. Nonlatex diaphragms and male condoms, as well as polyurethane female condoms, are available. The diaphragm and cervical cap are available only from a healthcare professional.

- Natural family planning (the rhythm method or periodic abstinence) and the withdrawal method are further options. These methods have the advantages of no cost, no need for surgery, and no need to take a drug or use a device. Disadvantages include a high failure rate compared with other methods and no protection against STIs. Natural family planning is not a reliable option during perimenopause because ovulation occurs sporadically and is difficult to predict with irregular menstrual periods. The withdrawal method is never a reliable method of birth control because enough sperm to result in pregnancy may be released from the penis before ejaculation.

Hormonal contraceptive options include:

- The levonorgestrel (synthetic progestin) IUD, releasing 20 µg per day, not only provides contraception for up to 5 years, it significantly decreases menometrorrhagia and dysmenorrhea, which are common in midlife women. The failure rate for IUDs is less than 1% in the first year of typical use.[16]

- A lower-dose levonorgestrel IUD that releases 14 µg per day is smaller than the earlier version and provides contraception for up to 3 years.

- Other hormonal contraceptive products include combination estrogen-progestin oral tablets, transdermal patches, and a vaginal ring. Progestin-only tablets and continuous injectable progestin contraceptives also are available and may be an option for women who have a contraindication to estrogen-containing contraceptives.

Please see Chapter 8 for more information on contraceptives.

It is important for women to know that fertility becomes significantly compromised long before overt clinical signs of perimenopause occur. Exact relationships among the rise in FSH levels, changes in inhibin, accelerated follicular atresia, shortened follicular phase, and oocyte quality remain to be determined. Research in assisted reproductive technologies continues to examine these issues and offers improved options for women with decreased fertility.

Uterine bleeding

Changes in menstrual flow and frequency are the hallmarks of perimenopause. Abnormal uterine bleeding (AUB) encompasses any menstrual flow outside of normal volume, duration, regularity, or frequency.[22] Approximately 90% of women experience 4 to 8 years of menstrual cycle changes before natural menopause. Early perimenopause is characterized by disturbances in timing and regulation of ovulation. Late perimenopause is characterized by a decrease in ovulation because of ovarian follicle depletion.[6] Most women report irregular menses that are attributed to decreased frequency of ovulation and erratic levels of ovarian hormones. Initial menstrual cycle changes as women approach menopause can be subtle, and a variety of menstrual patterns are possible (Table 1).

A large study of midlife women concluded that most subjective menstrual changes before menopause were flow related. These changes included lighter bleeding (32%), heavier bleeding (29%), shorter duration of flow (24%), and longer duration of flow (20%).[23] In the late menopause transition, heavy bleeding is thought to result from ovulatory cycles that follow a prolonged interval of anovulation or from excessive endometrial proliferation after prolonged anovulation.

Abnormal uterine bleeding has an array of consequences, such as heavy or prolonged flow with potential social embarrassment, avoidance of sexual activity, and diminished quality of life (QOL).[24] In some cases, anemia may result, with associated fatigue, pica (unusual food cravings), or headaches. Abnormal uterine bleeding also may be secondary to a number of benign and malignant diseases of the reproductive tract and to systemic diseases (Table 2).

In 2001, the Stages of Reproductive Aging Workshop (STRAW) proposed a summary of a woman's reproductive life in 7 stages that has been adopted as the gold standard.[25] Five main stages occur before the final menstrual period, and 2 occur afterward. Investigators from 4 cohort studies (the ReSTAGE collaboration) analyzed menstrual cycle changes in the transition occurring around menopause to validate the STRAW guidelines and concluded that 60 days of amenorrhea defines the onset of the late menopause transition.[26] Follicular phase hormone levels of estradiol, FSH, inhibin B, and luteinizing hormone are associated with menstrual bleeding patterns and differentiate the earliest stages of the menopause transition. Menstrual history is usually sufficient for determining stage, but hormone level assessment can be used when the clinical picture is not clear. A revised summary was crafted in 2011 that simplifies the bleeding criteria for early and late menopause transitions.[27] Please see Chapter 1 for more on STRAW and ovarian aging and hormone production.

Abnormal uterine bleeding associated with perimenopause

There is inconsistency in the terminology used to describe AUB, and there are a number of potential causes. A classification system based on the causes of AUB, the PALM-COEIN (polyp; adenomyosis; leiomyoma; malignancy and hyperplasia; coagulopathy; ovulatory dysfunction; endometrial; iatrogenic; and not yet classified) system, has been developed and approved by the International Federation of Gynecology and Obstetrics (FIGO) to aid clinicians and patients with communication and with clinical care (Table 3).[28]

If a woman is sexually active, pregnancy should be ruled out. Although rare, pregnancy can still occur until 1 full year without menses.

Anovulatory uterine bleeding. The COEIN portion of the PALM-COEIN system covers nonstructural, hormonal, and systemic causes of AUB. Top among these causes is AUB associated with ovulatory dysfunction or *anovulatory* uterine bleeding, which is defined as menstrual bleeding arising without ovulation or oligoovulation (infrequent ovulation). Anovulatory uterine bleeding presents as noncyclic menstrual blood flow ranging from spotting to heavy. The timing of the bleeding episodes and the amount of blood loss are erratic.

During an anovulatory cycle, the corpus luteum does not form. If the normal cyclical secretion of progesterone does not occur, estrogen stimulates the endometrium unopposed, and it becomes proliferative and eventually outgrows its blood supply. It may slough and bleed irregularly, heavily, or longer than normal.[29] With prolonged anovulation and unopposed estrogen exposure, the endometrium can become hyperplastic and develop atypical or cancerous cells.

Endometrial hyperplasia and carcinoma become more prevalent with age. The incidence of endometrial hyperplasia increases from 13.7 cases per 100,000 women at

Table 1. Terminology for Menstrual Changes During Perimenopause

Term	Definition
Amenorrhea	Absence of menses
Dysmenorrhea	Painful menses
Hypermenorrhea (menorrhagia)	Increased bleeding occurring at regular intervals (a loss of 80 mL or more of blood at each menstrual cycle) or bleeding that lasts >7 days
Hypomenorrhea	Decreased bleeding occurring at regular intervals
Oligomenorrhea	Decreased frequency of menstrual periods (occurring at intervals >35 days, with only 4-9 periods a year)
Polymenorrhea	Bleeding that occurs every ≤21 days
Metrorrhagia	Bleeding that occurs between periods
Menometrorrhagia	Bleeding that is excessive and irregular in amount and duration

age 40 to 44 years to 88.4 cases per 100,000 in women aged 70 to 74 years, decreasing after 75 years.[30]

Thyroid abnormalities, hyperprolactinemia, and polycystic ovary syndrome may cause anovulation and bleeding irregularities, including amenorrhea. Hypothyroidism may result in menorrhagia.

Exogenous hormones. Hormonal contraceptive use may result in a variety of bleeding patterns. Missed oral contraceptive (OC) tablets may cause breakthrough bleeding. Long-cycle or continuous OCs are associated with breakthrough bleeding or spotting, which decreases over time. Progestin-only contraceptives often result in irregular bleeding or spotting, which also diminishes over time. Progestin-releasing IUDs reduce menstrual bleeding overall but may result in a change in pattern, with irregular menses or intermenstrual bleeding. Nonhormonal copper devices may increase menstrual blood loss during regular menses. Certain medications (most notably common anticonvulsants and the antibiotic rifampin) may interfere with absorption of hormonal contraceptives, resulting in spotting or bleeding as well as a potential decrease in efficacy.

Menopausal hormone therapy. Women who use systemic menopausal estrogen-progestogen therapy (EPT) often have progestogen-induced uterine bleeding. If bleeding starts only after initiation of EPT, the bleeding may simply reflect the effect of hormones.

Structural causes. The PALM portion of the PALM-COEIN classification of causes of AUB refers to structural causes such as polyps, adenomyosis, leiomyomas, and malignancies that can often be detected by physical examination, imaging, or biopsy.[28]

Benign uterine fibroid tumors are commonly associated with AUB. Although most fibroids are asymptomatic, others produce dramatic changes in menstrual periods (eg, heavier and prolonged periods) as well as a range of other symptoms such as excessive menstrual cramps, back pain, dyspareunia, and difficulties with bowel movements or urination. Although the cause of fibroids is unknown, hormones can stimulate their growth. Because fibroids are estrogen and progesterone sensitive, they often shrink after menopause when ovarian production of hormones diminishes. Rarely, systemic estrogen therapy (ET) may cause fibroids to resume growth. Fibroids do not usually cause acute pain, but in some cases they can undergo torsion, degenerate, or become necrotic with accompanying pain.

Endometrial abnormalities. Endometrial or endocervical polyps, and possibly endometriosis, can result in AUB.[31]

Cancer. A small percentage of cases of AUB are caused by cancer of the uterus, cervix, or vagina. Please see Chapter 4 for more information on these cancers.

Other causes. Coagulopathies may result in heavy regular uterine bleeding. Women with renal or liver disease may

Table 2. Possible Causes of Abnormal Uterine Bleeding

Benign reproductive tract conditions
- Adenomyosis
- Anovulation
- Endometrial or endocervical polyps
- Endometriosis
- Endometritis
- Fibroids
- Pelvic inflammatory disease
- Pregnancy
- Vaginal/Cervical infection

Endometrial neoplasia
- Endometrial adenocarcinoma
- Endometrial hyperplasia with atypia
- Endometrial hyperplasia without atypia

Systemic causes
- Anorexia
- Extreme stress
- Polycystic ovary syndrome
- Chronic illness
- Coagulation disorders (thrombocytopenia, von Willebrand disease, leukemia)
- Hyperprolactinemia
- Liver disease
- Obesity
- Rapid weight fluctuations
- Thyroid dysfunction

Other causes
- Anticoagulants
- Corticosteroids
- Exogenous progestogen withdrawal
- Hormonal contraceptives (oral, transdermal, vaginal, intrauterine)
- Hormone therapy
- Select herbs
- Tamoxifen

Chapter 3

Table 3. International Federation of Gynecology and Obstetrics PALM-COEIN Classification System for Causes of Abnormal Uterine Bleeding

Structural causes (PALM)	
Polyps	Includes endometrial and endocervical polyps comprised of variable vascular, glandular, and fibromuscular and connective tissue components. Often asymptomatic but at least some contribute to the genesis of AUB. Lesions are usually benign but a small minority may have atypical or malignant features. Polyps are categorized as being either present or absent, as defined by 1 or a combination of ultrasound and hysteroscopic imaging with or without histopathology.
Adenomyosis	Relationship between adenomyosis and AUB is unclear, thus extensive additional research is required. Because there exist sonographic- and MRI-based diagnostic criteria, adenomyosis has been included in the PALM part of the classification system.
Leiomyoma	Benign fibromuscular tumors of the myometrium known by several names, including *leiomyoma, myoma,* and the frequently used *fibroid.* Leiomyoma is generally accepted as the more accurate term. Like polyps and adenomyosis, many leiomyomas are asymptomatic, and frequently their presence is not the cause of AUB.
Malignancy and hyperplasia	Proposed that malignant or premalignant lesions (eg, atypical endometrial hyperplasia, endometrial carcinoma, and leiomyosarcoma) be categorized within this major category but further dealt with using existent WHO and FIGO classification and staging systems.
Nonstructural causes (COEIN)	
Coagulopathy	Encompasses the spectrum of systemic disorders of hemostasis that may be associated with AUB. It is important to consider such disorders because they probably do contribute to some cases of AUB and because evidence indicates that relatively few clinicians consider systemic disorders of hemostasis in the differential diagnosis of women with HMB.
Ovulatory dysfunction	Disorders of ovulation may present as amenorrhea, through extremely light and infrequent bleeding, to episodes of unpredictable and extreme HMB requiring medical or surgical intervention. Ovulatory disorders can be traced to endocrinopathies (PCOS, hypothyroidism, hyperprolactinemia, mental stress, obesity, anorexia, weight loss, or extreme exercise such as that associated with elite athletic training).
Endometrial	When AUB occurs in the context of predictable and cyclic menstrual bleeding, typical of ovulatory cycles, and particularly when no other definable causes are identified, the mechanism is probably a primary disorder of the endometrium.
Iatrogenic	Associated with the use of exogenous gonadal steroids, intrauterine systems or devices, or other systemic or local agents.
Not yet classified	Entities that are rarely encountered or are ill defined.

Abbreviations: AUB, abnormal uterine bleeding; FIGO, International Federation of Gynecology and Obstetrics; HMB, heavy menstrual bleeding; PCOS, polycystic ovary syndrome; WHO, World Health Organization.
Munro MG, et al.[28]

experience AUB. Systemic diseases other than endocrinopathies, such as leukemia, infrequently present with uterine bleeding as the only sign or symptom. Although bleeding usually originates in the uterus, it is possible for the vagina or the cervix to be the source. Vaginal or cervical infections or the genitourinary syndrome of menopause (GSM) may result in postcoital bleeding. In women with cervical stenosis, bleeding may be caused by hematometra or pyometra.

Evaluation of abnormal uterine bleeding

Evaluation of AUB will vary depending on a woman's age, stage of menopause, duration of abnormal bleeding, and presence of risk factors for endometrial cancer, such as obesity and exposure to unopposed estrogen. Although the most common causes of uterine bleeding in a postmenopausal woman not using EPT are benign, any uterine bleeding should be considered abnormal and warrants further investigation.

The history should emphasize the clinical features of menstrual flow, intermenstrual uterine bleeding, contraceptive and other medication use, and systemic diseases. The effect of the bleeding on daily activities also is important.

Charting of uterine bleeding is helpful in assessing reported menstrual abnormalities. Information should include the days of the bleeding, the amount and color of the flow, the presence of clots, and any pain associated with the bleeding. These reports are limited by the subjective nature of each woman's assessment.

A pelvic examination is mandatory in all perimenopausal or postmenopausal women with AUB. Tests should be ordered selectively (Table 4).

For women who start bleeding only after initiation of a continuous-combined EPT regime, and the bleeding is not heavy and stops within several months of EPT initiation, no evaluation is needed. If these parameters are not met or if there is concern regarding the cause of the bleeding, endometrial evaluation is warranted. No evaluation is needed in a woman initiating a cyclic EPT regimen with expected, regular withdrawal bleeding. Likewise, no evaluation is needed in women who experience self-limited bleeding soon after discontinuing EPT. A high index of suspicion of endometrial cancer is appropriate in the case of women who are overweight who experience bleeding during the use of EPT. Pathology should also be suspected in perimenopausal or postmenopausal women using continuous-combined EPT if uterine bleeding persists longer than 6 months or longer than 1 week each month in the first 6 months of therapy.

These strategies represent a prudent approach to endometrial evaluation of the perimenopausal or postmenopausal woman presenting with AUB:

- Begin with transvaginal ultrasonography to measure endometrial thickness and to detect structural abnormalities, including masses, polyps, fibroids, and focal thickening of the endometrium.
- If the endometrial echo is 5 mm or greater or is not adequately visualized, proceed with endometrial biopsy, possibly combined with office hysteroscopy or saline infusion sonohysterography.[32,33] The ability of the endometrial biopsy to determine the cause of AUB is influenced by the underlying etiology. A meta-analysis looking at the sensitivity of office endometrial biopsy showed that it only had a 68% to 78% sensitivity and a 0% to 54% rate of sampling error for cancer.[34] Thus, a nondiagnostic biopsy or continued bleeding warrant further evaluation.

Table 4. Tests to Consider for Abnormal Uterine Bleeding

- Cervical cytology (eg, Pap test)
- Coagulation (if there is a family history or bruising or hemorrhaging seen)
- CBC
- Endometrial sampling
- Hormone measurements (TSH, prolactin, FSH, estradiol)
- Liver function (if a liver disorder suspected)
- Gonorrhea and chlamydia (if STI is suspected)
- Pregnancy
- Progesterone levels during the luteal phase (to confirm ovulation)
- Testosterone and dehydroepiandrosterone sulfate levels (if PCOS is suspected)
- Transvaginal ultrasonography, saline infusion sonohysterography, or office hysteroscopy (if endometrial abnormality is suspected)

Abbreviations: CBC, complete blood count, FSH, follicle-stimulating hormone; PCOS, polycystic ovary syndrome; STI, sexually transmitted infection; TSH, thyroid-stimulating hormone.

- If a focal uterine abnormality is identified on office hysteroscopy or saline infusion sonohysterography, consider surgical management. If the endometrial histology demonstrates benign endometrium, medical or expectant management is appropriate. Further evaluation of persistent abnormal bleeding is indicated because a benign finding cannot completely rule out precancerous or cancerous pathology.[35]

Given the absence of large randomized, controlled trials (RCTs) comparing different AUB evaluation strategies for perimenopausal and postmenopausal women, clinicians—guided by patient preference—should use the techniques with which they are most technically comfortable and that are most accessible and cost-effective in their practices.

Management of abnormal uterine bleeding

For the management of AUB in perimenopausal and postmenopausal women, a number of effective medical and surgical options are available. Before recommending these options, anatomic abnormalities, such as fibroids and polyps, should first be identified and treated.[36]

Approximately 80% of women treated for heavy menstrual bleeding have no underlying pathology; one-third of hysterectomies performed for bleeding show no abnormalities. This makes pharmacologic therapy and the avoidance of possibly unnecessary surgery an attractive alternative.[37,38] Pharmacologic therapy is the least invasive and least expensive option for managing heavy menstrual bleeding and should be the initial treatment of choice. However, lack of evidence-based practice, poor compliance, and AEs can limit the success rates associated with drug therapy.

For perimenopausal women with AUB, management options include hormonal contraceptive products such as combination estrogen-progestin oral tablets, transdermal patches, and the vaginal ring. Continuous injectable or intrauterine progestin contraceptives and cyclic oral progestogen are other available options. Rarely, gonadotropin-releasing hormone (GnRH) agonists have a role, especially if the woman is very anemic. Danazol also may be effective, but both agents are limited by AEs. In patients with an underlying bleeding disorder (eg, von Willebrand disease), intranasal desmopressin may be indicated.

Hormonal treatments. If a woman has no risk factors for endometrial cancer and no laboratory or structural uterine abnormalities, hormone therapy (HT) may be empirically tried to see whether the bleeding responds. Selection of an appropriate agent depends on whether contraception is needed or whether preservation of fertility is a concern. Adverse events frequently limit options or duration of use.

Hormone regimens cause functional and histologic changes to the endometrium, resulting in inhibition of endometrial growth and development. If bleeding is very heavy and associated with significant anemia, patients may require stabilization with intravenous (IV) fluid, blood products, and other measures as needed. For persistent heavy bleeding, a Foley catheter may be inserted into the uterus and inflated with 30 mL of water as a tamponade for the bleeding, or if appropriate, acute management with IV estrogen may be required. Once patients are stable, HT is used to control bleeding. (Please see Chapter 8 for more information on contraceptives and on hormonal therapies.)

- *Estrogen-containing contraceptives.* Use of a low-dose combination (estrogen-progestin) OC is considered the first-line treatment of AUB in otherwise healthy, nonsmoking, perimenopausal women with no history of migraine headaches, regardless of their contraceptive needs. Oral contraceptives are the only combination hormone products assessed in clinical trials for this use, but no OC is government approved in the United States or Canada for treating AUB. Other estrogen-containing contraceptives likely have similar effects. In clinical trials, OCs have normalized irregular bleeding and decreased menstrual flow. Their effectiveness in treating AUB in women with fibroids, however, is variable. Oral contraceptives also offer other benefits, including contraception (if needed) and relief of vasomotor symptoms (VMS).

    Estrogen-containing contraception is not recommended for women with hypertension, a history of deep vein thrombosis, migraine headaches, those with other cardiovascular risk factors, or smokers aged older than 35 years. Some clinicians are reluctant to use these agents in perimenopausal women.

Cycle control is an important issue for perimenopausal women experiencing AUB. The hormone contraceptive formulation selected should result in minimal breakthrough bleeding or irregular bleeding. Different formulations have different effects, depending on the estrogen dose and type of progestin. In a 91-day extended-regimen trial of a low-dose combination OC, less unscheduled bleeding was observed in women taking OCs with lower-dose (≤20 µg) ethinyl estradiol than with higher doses (30-35 µg).[39]

Perimenopausal women with menorrhagia may benefit from less frequent bleeding episodes or even amenorrhea, which often can be achieved with an extended estrogen-progestin OC regimen.[40] The same outcome can often be achieved by using standard OC formulations off label in an extended regimen by skipping the placebo week.

Transdermal and vaginal ring contraceptive systems provide other options to treat AUB.

- *Continuous progestin-only contraceptives.* Depot medroxyprogesterone acetate (DMPA) injections gradually produce amenorrhea and provide contraception if needed. Use of the levonorgestrel-releasing intrauterine system (IUS) also reduces bleeding over time and is effective in the treatment of menorrhagia; contraception (if needed) is provided.[41-43] One RCT found that use of the IUS for 1 year was a cost-effective alternative to hysterectomy in treating AUB, although after 5 years of follow-up, 42% of women assigned to the IUS group eventually underwent hysterectomy.[44-47]

    Progestogen-releasing IUDs are more effective than cyclic oral progestins, with a decrease of dysmenorrhea in 40% of women, although short-term AEs are more common.[48-50] Levonorgestrel can be detected in the circulation within 15 minutes of insertion, reaching maximal plasma levels within a few hours, with a plateau within 1 month and with far lower levels than with progestogen implants or progestogen-only OCs.[51]

    For perimenopausal women with AUB and VMS, menopausal doses of ET can be added to DMPA injections or to an IUS. This combined approach also prevents vaginal atrophy and has a positive effect on bone density while minimizing uterine bleeding, endometrial hyperplasia, and uterine cancer.

- *Progestogen plus low-dose estrogen.* Many perimenopausal women with AUB are not candidates for combination OCs. Cyclic progestogen therapy may be an option, although women with VMS, low bone density, or hypoestrogenism associated with cigarette smoking may benefit from the addition of estrogen in postmenopausal doses.

    It is important to use contraceptive doses of progestogens in perimenopausal women with AUB because the doses in some EPT regimens do not suppress ovulation and could consequently aggravate the bleeding problem.

Continuous-combined regimens using high-dose progestin and low-dose estrogen may initially cause irregular uterine bleeding or spotting, with eventual amenorrhea. Although oral combination EPT formulations that include 1.0 mg or 0.5 mg of norethindrone acetate suppress ovulation, combination formulations with lower doses of norethindrone acetate as well as those formulated with medroxyprogesterone acetate may not. Transdermal EPT formulations likely do not suppress ovulation.

- *Cyclic oral progestogen.* Traditionally, cyclic oral progestogen therapy (progestin or progesterone) has been the standard medical therapy for anovulatory uterine bleeding in perimenopausal women (Table 5). Prescribing it for days 15 to 28 of a woman's cycle, counting the first day of bleeding as day 1, reinforces the luteal phase, which has been found to be low in progesterone in perimenopausal women.[52] For the woman with infrequent, heavy cycles, prescribing the progestogen for the first 14 days of the calendar month may be more convenient and will induce withdrawal bleeding every month. Women should keep a menstrual calendar to assess how well the method is working. This approach is an inexpensive, noninvasive method for the woman with anovulatory bleeding thought to be close to menopause. However, cyclic progestogen does not prevent pregnancy and will not be as effective in the long run for very heavy bleeders as the levonorgestrel IUS. It may be appropriate to add estrogen in postmenopausal doses if VMS occur. Withdrawal bleeding may continue indefinitely in some perimenopausal women treated with cyclic progestogen therapy, particularly those who are overweight and have higher levels of endogenous estrogen. If this occurs, it is appropriate to continue progestogen therapy because of the increased risk of endometrial hyperplasia and neoplasia.[31]

If endometrial proliferation or hyperplasia without atypia is found on endometrial biopsy, cyclic or continuous progestogen is indicated, with follow-up evaluation after 3 or 4 months. If progestogen therapy does not result in histologic regression, dilation and curettage with hysteroscopy should be performed because of the possibility of underlying endometrial malignancy. There is about a 29% chance that complex endometrial hyperplasia with atypia will progress to cancer if untreated; therefore, for women beyond childbearing, hysterectomy represents appropriate surgical management in this setting.

Progestogen therapy for 21 days of the cycle resulted in a significant reduction in menstrual blood loss, although women found the treatment less acceptable than intrauterine levonorgestrel.[53] Limited, uncontrolled data suggest that OCs reduce menstrual blood loss by 40% to 50%.

- *Parenteral estrogen.* In perimenopausal women with acute AUB, treatment with parenteral estrogen can be considered. In 1 controlled study, IV administration of conjugated estrogens (CE) stopped AUB in 71% of women compared with 38% who received placebo.[54] Because high-dose IV estrogen can acutely increase thrombosis risk, therapy is contraindicated in women at high risk of cardiovascular disease (CVD) or venous thromboembolism (VTE), and measures to prevent thrombosis should be considered in this setting.

For severe, acute AUB, IV CE 25 mg every 4 to 6 hours (maximum of 4 doses) may be used. After this, women are given a combination OC until bleeding abates. For less heavy bleeding, combination OCs are used 2 to 3 times a day for 5 to 6 days, then once a day. After acute bleeding is controlled, a combination OC is given continually for about 3 months to prevent recurrence before the first withdrawal bleeding.

- *Gonadotropin-releasing hormone agonists.* Gonadotropin-releasing hormone agonists induce a reversible hypoestrogenic state that causes endometrial atrophy. They are effective in reducing menstrual blood loss in perimenopausal women but limited by their expense and AEs, which include hot flashes and reduction of bone density. Examples include injectable leuprolide acetate and nafarelin acetate nasal spray. Gonadotropin-releasing hormone agonists such as goserelin have been shown to be effective in reducing heavy menstrual bleeding, but hypoestrogenic AEs limit long-term use.[55]

Table 5. Examples of Progestogen-Only Regimens for the Treatment of Anovulatory Uterine Bleeding in Perimenopausal Women

	Available strengths	Recommended doses
Tablet		
Medroxyprogesterone acetate	2.5, 5.0, 10.0 mg	5-10 mg/d, 12-14 d/mo
Norethindrone acetate[a]	5.0 mg	2.5-5.0 mg (.5-1 tablet)/d
Norethindrone	0.35 mg	0.7-1.05 mg (2-3 tablets)/d
Progesterone (micronized)	100, 200 mg	100-400 mg/d, 12-14 d/mo
Intrauterine system		
Levonorgestrel	52 mg	20 μg/d/5y

a. Available in the United States but not Canada.

Chapter 3

- *Desmopressin.* In case reports, surveys, and nonrandomized studies, desmopressin (a synthetic replacement for vasopressin, the hormone that reduces urine production) taken nasally, orally, or intravenously has been used effectively in women with underlying hemostatic disorder (eg, von Willebrand disease).

Nonhormonal treatments. There are nonhormonal options for treatment of AUB:

- *Nonsteroidal anti-inflammatory drugs* (NSAIDs) inhibit cyclooxygenase and reduce endometrial prostaglandin levels. In a review of RCTs, NSAIDs taken at menses decreased menstrual blood loss by 20% to 50% and improved dysmenorrhea in up to 70% of women.[56] Therapy is usually started 24 to 48 hours before menses and then continued for 5 days or until cessation of menstruation. Nonsteroidal anti-inflammatory drugs seem to reduce prostaglandin E_2 through the cylooxygenase enzyme system.[57]

- *Antibiotics.* Chronic endometritis responds well to antibiotic therapy. If pyometra is encountered, antibiotic therapy followed by repeat endometrial sampling to ensure resolution and exclude underlying neoplasia is appropriate. For some women who experience recurrent bleeding because of pyometra or hematometra, repeated cervical dilation to assure drainage may be necessary.

- *Iron.* All women experiencing AUB should be evaluated for iron deficiency (anemia). In addition to medical and surgical treatments, iron supplementation is appropriate for women with AUB who are found to have iron deficiency anemia.

- *Danazol.* This agent is a synthetic steroid with antiestrogenic and antiprogestogenic activity and weak androgenic properties that lead to endometrial atrophy and reduced menstrual loss.[58] However, treatment with danazol caused more AEs than NSAIDs (odds ratio [OR], 7.0; 95% confidence interval [CI], 1.7-28.2) or progestogens (OR, 4.05; 95% CI, 1.6-10.2).

- *Tranexamic acid* is an antifibrinolytic agent that inhibits plasminogen activator and has been associated with a 40% to 60% reduction in menstrual bleeding. The recommended oral dosage is 3.9 g to 4 g per day for 4 to 5 days starting from the first day of the menstrual cycle. No increase in thrombogenic events has been observed, although this remains a theoretical concern.

Promising pharmacologic treatments. There are 3 categories of promising interventions for AUB: steroid hormonal modulators (eg, selective progesterone-receptor (PR) modulators, estrogen-receptor (ER) agonists/antagonists, and aromatase inhibitors), antiangiogenic therapies, and tranexamic acid derivatives/precursors.[59-61]

Surgical treatment. There are several surgical approaches for evaluating and treating perimenopausal women with anovulatory AUB and women with postmenopausal bleeding:

- *Hysteroscopy with dilation and curettage.* Together, these 2 approaches may be therapeutic as well as diagnostic. It may be the treatment of choice when anovulatory bleeding is severe or when HT is ineffective. Structural causes such as polyps or fibroids may be identified and removed with hysteroscopy. This procedure also may decrease bleeding.

- *Dilation and curettage.* Dilation and curettage by itself is considered obsolete for the treatment of AUB because it is a blind procedure, and localized disease, such as polyps, can be missed. Another limiting factor is that dilation and curettage usually requires general anesthesia.

- *Endometrial ablation.* Surgical techniques such as freezing or burning for endometrial resection and ablation have emerged as effective, safe, and cost-effective alternatives to hysterectomy for the treatment of AUB.[62] This procedure is to be used to control cyclical bleeding and is not as effective for AUB. Postprocedure amenorrhea occurs in 20% to 50% of patients. If menses persist, bleeding is improved in 60% to 80% of cases. Adenomyosis is the most common reason for failure to significantly improve bleeding. Newer technologies for endometrial ablation include cryoablation, heated intrauterine fluid, and radio-frequency electrical energy.

Endometrial ablation should be performed only in women after endometrial evaluation has excluded pathology, and preservation of fertility is not desired.[63] Some approaches to ablation (eg, thermal balloon ablation) do not involve visualization of the endometrial cavity and may not effectively treat AUB caused by endometrial polyps or submucous fibroids.[64] Evaluation of the endometrial cavity with diagnostic hysteroscopy or sonohysterography is recommended before endometrial destructive therapy. Clinicians planning hysteroscopic endometrial ablation should be prepared to resect any polypoid lesions encountered intraoperatively.[65-67]

Endometrial ablation may not successfully treat AUB caused by anatomic lesions located in the uterine wall, either intramural fibroids or adenomyosis. The ablation and the scarring the procedure produces may limit the ability to evaluate subsequent AUB with traditional methods. Patients need to be counseled that endometrial changes that occur after endometrial ablation can impede the diagnosis of endometrial cancer later in life because of the inability to sample the endometrium and the masking of abnormal bleeding that can be an initial sign of cancer.

Endometrial ablation offers effective therapy for heavy uterine bleeding without the need for inpatient stay or the time off work usually associated with hysterectomy. Nonetheless, serious complications and even death have resulted, underscoring the need for appropriate surgical training and meticulous patient selection.

The Surgical Treatments Outcomes Project for Dysfunctional Uterine Bleeding multicenter RCT of hysterectomy and endometrial ablation for the treatment of AUB evaluated 237 women and found longer institutional stays and perioperative AEs more common and severe for those randomized to hysterectomy.[68] At 24 months, 94.4% of women randomized to hysterectomy and 84.9% randomized to endometrial ablation considered their major problem to be solved; at 48 months, the numbers were similar at 98.0% and 85%, respectively. Postprocedure QOL improved similarly in both groups, but reoperation was more common for women undergoing ablation (30.9% at 60 months), with most selecting hysterectomy (32 of 34).

The reoperation rates were somewhat consistent with those reported by the Aberdeen Group, another RCT with 4 or more years of follow-up comparing endometrial ablation and hysterectomy.[69] About 40% of patients underwent reoperation, but about half of these women selected ablation. These findings were consistent with Cochrane review findings that patient satisfaction with endometrial ablation is high,[62] although slightly lower than that for hysterectomy.[70]

- *Hysterectomy.* Before the development of newer techniques, hysterectomy was the only definitive cure for benign AUB that failed to respond to medical treatment. Although surgical mortality is low, postoperative complications are not uncommon. In many women with AUB, medical management can prevent the need for hysterectomy. Newer techniques include laparoscopic-assisted vaginal hysterectomy and robotic-assisted hysterectomy. Pros and cons of removal of ovaries at time of surgery should be discussed with patients aged 40 years and older before surgery.

Vasomotor symptoms

The terms *vasomotor symptoms, hot flashes, hot flushes,* and *night sweats* all describe the same phenomenon. Medical literature generally uses the term *vasomotor symptoms* (VMS) to describe recurrent, transient episodes of flushing accompanied by a sensation of warmth to intense heat on the upper body and face. Vasomotor symptoms while sleeping can produce intense perspiration (night sweats). Chills sometimes follow this release of heat. Hot flashes have been shown to adversely affect QOL.[71-73]

The hot flash is the second most frequently reported perimenopausal symptom (after irregular menses). As many as 75% of perimenopausal US women experience hot flashes. It is considered one of the hallmarks of the menopause transition.[74] Most women experience a sudden sensation of heat that spreads over the body, particularly the upper body and face. Sweating begins primarily on the upper body, and it corresponds closely in time with the increase in skin conductance.

An individual hot flash generally lasts 1 to 5 minutes; about 7% are longer and about 17% are shorter. During a hot flash, skin temperature rises as a result of peripheral vasodilation. This change is particularly marked in the fingers and toes, where skin temperature can increase 1°C to 7°C. Modest heart rate increases of about 7 to 15 beats per minute occur at approximately the same time as the peripheral vasodilation and sweating. Heart rate and skin blood flow usually peak within 3 minutes of the onset of a hot flash. Significant elevations in metabolic rate occur simultaneous with sweating and peripheral vasodilation. Skin temperatures return to normal gradually, sometimes taking 30 minutes or longer. Decreases in core body temperature of 0.1°C to 0.9°C approximately 5 to 9 minutes after hot flash onset have been observed, probably because of heat loss through the increased perspiration and peripheral vasodilation. If the heat loss is significant, chills may be experienced.

Hot flashes usually begin in late perimenopause and increase during the menopause transition, reaching greatest frequency and severity within the first 2 years of the final menstrual period and then declining over time. Most women experience hot flashes for 6 months to 2 years, although some reports suggest that the mean duration of symptoms may be considerably longer than what is generally accepted in clinical practice—as long as 10.2 years, depending on menopausal stage at onset.[75] Some women have them for 10 years or longer, and for a small proportion of the population, they never go away.[76] It is not uncommon for women to experience a recurrence of hot flashes more than 10 years after menopause.

Hot flashes can occur infrequently (monthly, weekly) or frequently (hourly), although there is usually a consistent individual pattern. A circadian rhythm has been observed, with hot flash frequency peaking in the early evening hours (about 3 hours after the peak in core body temperature).

Prevalence

Hot flash prevalence varies widely. Reasons for these differences are not known, but they may be influenced by a number of factors, including climate, diet, lifestyle, women's roles, attitudes regarding the end of reproductive life and aging, and genetics. One genetic analysis from the Penn Ovarian Aging Study found that carriers of certain genetic variants who smoked were 6 to 20 times more likely to report severe hot flashes than nonsmoking carriers.[77]

A systematic review of 66 papers addressing the prevalence of VMS around the world concluded that fewer premenopausal women reported having hot flashes than perimenopausal women (21.5% and 41%, respectively).[74] Prevalence of hot flash reporting by postmenopausal women was 41.5%. In addition to demographic reasons for variation in self-reported hot flashes, methodologic differences across studies no doubt come into play. Inconsistent definitions of menopause status, however, plagued some of these studies, making it difficult to pinpoint the longitudinal pattern of hot flashes among individual women.

Hot flash prevalence differs among US racial and ethnic groups. According to the Study of Women's Health Across the Nation (SWAN)—a multiracial, multiethnic sample of 16,065 women aged 40 to 55 years—black women reported VMS most frequently (45.6%), followed by Hispanic (35.4%), white (31.2%), Chinese (20.5%), and Japanese (17.6%) women.[78] However, differences in body mass index (BMI) among these groups of women are an important covariate that may be more predictive than ethnicity for hot flashes. During the menopause transition, a greater proportion of women who are overweight and obese report hot flashes compared with women of normal weight.[79]

Most hot flashes are mild to moderate in intensity. However, approximately 10% to 15% of women have severe or very frequent hot flashes. Hot flashes tend to be more frequent and severe after surgically induced menopause. In US women who undergo bilateral oophorectomy, up to 90% of women will report hot flashes; chemotherapy may also be associated with increased hot flash reporting (rates up to 46%), with more than half of these women reporting moderate or severe symptoms.[80] Over time, symptoms decline to a level similar to those of women who have reached menopause naturally.

Causes and associations

The prevailing theory of the etiology of hot flashes is that core body temperature in humans is regulated between an upper threshold for sweating and a lower threshold for shivering.[81] Between these thresholds, there is a "thermoneutral zone" within which major thermoregulatory responses (sweating, shivering) do not occur. It was observed that this core body temperature thermoneutral zone was vastly reduced or eliminated in symptomatic versus asymptomatic postmenopausal women—measured to be 0.0°C versus 0.4°C, respectively. Further observation demonstrated that most hot flashes are preceded by small but significant elevations in core body temperature. Thus, hot flashes appear to be triggered by small increases in core body temperature acting within a reduced thermoneutral zone in symptomatic postmenopausal women, resulting in a sensation of heat and a heat dissipation response (vasodilation and sweating). These observations are consistent with this theory: 1) hot flashes can be triggered by peripheral heating (eg, a warm room), exercise (raising core body temperature), and core body heating (eg, a hot drink), or conversely, 2) they can be ameliorated by ambient (cold room) and internal (cold drink) cooling. Both clonidine and estrogen have been shown to ameliorate hot flashes and increase the sweating threshold by enlarging the thermoneutral zone.[82,83] Beyond this theory of hot flash etiology, specific mechanisms or brain areas involved in thermogenesis and heat perception remain largely unknown and unexplored.

Other demographic and psychological factors are associated with hot flash reporting. A history of premenstrual complaints is significantly associated with hot flashes in perimenopausal women. Approximately 47% of perimenopausal women with a history of moderate to severe premenstrual complaints experienced hot flashes compared with 32% of women without such a history. Low socioeconomic status has also been associated with more frequent reporting of hot flashes.

Vasomotor symptoms can occur when menopausal HT is discontinued. A large cross-sectional survey showed that even in women aged 70 years and older, 11% experienced VMS after stopping HT.[84] Among women aged 55 to 59 years discontinuing HT, 36% of them experienced VMS. Considering only those women who had VMS at baseline, 57% of those aged 55 to 59 years had a recurrence when discontinuing HT.

Other conditions that can cause hot flashes or symptoms that might masquerade as hot flashes include thyroid disease, epilepsy, infection, insulinoma, pheochromocytoma, carcinoid syndromes, leukemia, pancreatic tumors, autoimmune disorders, new-onset hypertension, diabetic autonomic dysfunction, and mast-cell disorders. Drugs that block estrogen action (eg, tamoxifen and raloxifene) or inhibit estrogen biosynthesis (eg, aromatase inhibitors) frequently cause hot flashes. Other drugs such as the selective serotonin-reuptake inhibitors (SSRIs) and the serotonin norepinephrine-reuptake inhibitors can also cause severe sweating that can be mistaken for menopausal hot flashes. Night sweats also can be associated with more serious diseases such as tuberculosis and lymphoma. In the latter cases, the night sweats are associated with an increase in core body temperature.

Management of vasomotor symptoms

Nearly 25% of US women experience sufficient discomfort from VMS to seek help from healthcare professionals. Although the available treatments do not "cure" hot flashes, they offer symptomatic relief. Hot flashes typically stop eventually without treatment, but there is no reliable method for determining when that will occur. No treatment is necessary unless hot flashes are bothersome. Therapy should be tailored to the individual patient's medical history, goals of treatment, and personal attitudes toward menopause and medication.

Many proposed treatments for VMS have not been evaluated by RCTs. The evaluation of efficacy is also plagued by a relatively high placebo effect of 20% to 40% that has been consistently demonstrated in RCTs.[85]

There are a number of low-risk, nonpharmacologic coping strategies and lifestyle changes that can help manage hot flashes (Table 6). If hot flashes remain significantly disruptive despite these interventions, nonhormone therapy or HT may be considered.

Women with a history of breast cancer or other hormone-sensitive neoplasia require special consideration in the management of VMS. Cancer survivors are more likely to be severely troubled by VMS and report more frequent and more severe hot flashes than other postmenopausal women.[86] Chemotherapy and radiation may induce premature menopause, or menopause symptoms may be an AE of antihormone therapies used in cancer treatment. Systemic HT in women with a hormone-sensitive neoplasia is contraindicated. Lifestyle modifications may be used, or nonhormone prescription therapies may provide relief. Nonprescription remedies that may have or are known to have estrogenic effects (phytoestrogens, black cohosh) should be avoided in women with hormone-sensitive neoplasia.

Data are inadequate to determine whether the physiologic mechanisms for hot flashes in breast cancer survivors (or those electing to use chemoprevention) using tamoxifen differ from hot flashes in women experiencing natural menopause. However, given that the triggers and remedies are similar for women with cancer and those without cancer, it is reasonable to assume that this is the case.[87] Genetic variations associated with tamoxifen metabolism may contribute to differences in severity and frequency of hot flashes in tamoxifen users.[88,89]

Lifestyle changes. For women requesting relief from mild, menopause-related hot flashes, lifestyle changes may provide some relief:

- *Keep core body temperature as cool as possible.* Warm ambient air temperatures increase a woman's core body temperature and make her more likely to reach the sweating threshold for triggering a hot flash. Conversely, cooler air temperatures are associated with a lower incidence of hot flashes.

- *Maintain a healthy body weight.* It was believed that hot flash risk was inversely related to BMI, inasmuch as estradiol is elevated as a result of aromatization in adipose tissue. However, several studies have found that a higher BMI (≥ 27 kg/m^2) to be a predictor of hot flash frequency, particularly in the menopause transition.[79,90] Perimenopausal and postmenopausal increases in body fat are associated with increased frequency of hot flashes.[91] It has been postulated that, at least in premenopausal and perimenopausal women, any increase in estradiol is offset by increased insulation from body fat, resulting in a higher core body temperature and more hot flashes. In women who are obese, weight loss has been associated with a reduction in hot flash frequency.[92,93]

- *Refrain from smoking.* Cigarette smoking (both past and current) increases the relative risk of hot flashes, perhaps because of its effect on estrogen metabolism.[90] One study found that among current smokers, hot flash risk increased with greater amounts smoked. A case-control study showed higher odds of number and severity of hot flashes in current and ever smokers.[94] However, smoking was not associated with lower estradiol or estrone levels.

Table 6. Suggested Nonpharmacologic Strategies to Manage Vasomotor Symptoms

- Enhance relaxation with meditation, yoga, massage, or a leisurely lukewarm bath.
- Exercise regularly to increase fitness, maintain a healthy weight, and promote better, more restorative sleep.
- Keep cool by dressing in layers, using chilling towels, and using a chilling pillow, wicking pajamas and sheets, a bed fan, and sleeping in a cool room at night.
- Maintain a healthy body weight.
- Don't smoke.
- Try paced respiration (deep, slow, abdominal breathing) when a hot flash starts.
- Avoid perceived personal hot flash triggers (hot drinks, caffeine, spicy foods, alcohol, emotional reactions).
- Try nonprescription therapies (soy foods/isoflavones, black cohosh, or vitamin E). Many are available for mild hot flashes; efficacy is generally similar to placebo.

Passive smoke exposure has also been associated with VMS in a non–dose-responsive manner.[95]

- *Exercise regularly.* Although a recent Cochrane review of 6 RCTs of exercise for treatment of menopausal VMS failed to show a significant improvement in VMS with exercise compared with no treatment, HT, or yoga, less physical activity has been shown to increase the relative risk of hot flashes, and daily exercise is associated with an overall decreased incidence.[96,97] Exercise may be associated with a shorter overall duration of hot flashes[76]; however, strenuous exercise has been shown to trigger hot flashes in symptomatic, unconditioned women. Physical activity may trigger hot flashes by raising core body temperature. One study found a significant association between increasing physical activity and decreasing VMS in women with a lifetime history of major depression, but no association was seen in women without this history.[98]

- *Practice relaxation techniques.* Anxiety has been associated with an increased severity and frequency of hot flashes. Anecdotal reports from individual women have suggested a relationship between the frequency and severity of hot flashes and emotional stress or perceived personal hot flash triggers, including consumption of particular types of foods (thermally hot or spicy food) or drinks (caffeine, alcohol). Trial evidence among large groups of women, however, does not support such a relationship. The Melbourne Women's Midlife Health Project found no significant association between alcohol intake and hot flashes.[76]

Chapter 3

Nonprescription remedies. When lifestyle changes are not adequate to achieve the desired level of relief from mild hot flashes, adding a nonprescription remedy may be considered. Trying soy foods or isoflavone supplements, black cohosh, vitamin E, or omega-3 fatty acids may be an option, primarily because these remedies are not associated with serious AEs.[99] A recent review and meta-analysis of 17 RCTs looking at extracted or synthesized soybean isoflavones showed a significant reduction in hot flash frequency and severity compared with placebo.[100] However, RCTs have failed to show efficacy of black cohosh or phytoestrogens for VMS.[101,102] Similarly, scientific data are lacking regarding efficacy and safety of topical progesterone creams for relief of hot flashes.[103] Overall, there is relatively low efficacy but low potential for harm with such remedies. The patient must balance cost and possible harm against the potential for benefit and make an informed choice. (Please see Chapter 6 for more on complementary and alternative medicine and Chapter 7 for more on nonprescription options.)

Prescription therapies: hormonal options. When lifestyle changes and nonprescription approaches do not provide the desired relief, prescription options are available.

Estrogen therapy or estrogen-progestogen therapy. Prescription systemic ET or, for women with a uterus, EPT remains the therapeutic standard for treating moderate to severe menopause-related hot flashes in women who have no contraindications. Until recently, these therapies were the only government-approved treatments in the United States and Canada for this indication.

Moderate to severe menopause-related hot flashes are the primary indication for systemic ET or EPT. Use of these therapies should be limited to the shortest duration consistent with treatment goals, benefits, and risks for the individual woman. Initiating ET or EPT during perimenopause is associated with lower risk than starting therapy several years after menopause.[104] (Please see Chapter 8 for more on estrogen and estrogen-progestogen therapies.)

Progesterone and progestins. Prescription progestogen therapy alone has been used off label to treat hot flashes of varying severity. In clinical trials, oral medroxyprogesterone acetate (MPA), DMPA, megestrol acetate, and micronized progesterone have demonstrated efficacy.[105,106] Short-term use of these drugs seems reasonable in women without contraindications who do not wish to try estrogen but who are not opposed to trying another hormone, although progestogens have been linked to increased breast cancer risk in some studies of HT.[104] (Please see Chapter 8 for more on progestogens.)

Bazedoxifene and conjugated estrogens. Bazedoxifene (BZA) 20 mg paired with CE 0.45 mg and 0.625 mg is the first selective ER modulator (SERM) combination therapy FDA approved to treat moderate to severe hot flashes. This combination of a SERM with an estrogen has been defined as a tissue-selective estrogen complex. SERMs were evaluated for use in combination therapies because of their ability to work selectively in different tissues to activate estrogen receptors in some while inhibiting estrogen activity in others.

Clinical trials in postmenopausal women with a uterus at risk for osteoporosis found that BZA and CE, as an alternative to estrogen combined with a progestogen, reduced menopausal symptoms, including hot flashes, prevented bone loss in postmenopausal women, and had a favorable safety profile on the breast, endometrium, and ovary.[107-110] (Please see Chapter 8 for more on BZA/CE combination therapy.)

Combined oral contraceptives. Perimenopausal women who require hot flash relief and contraception may achieve both goals with a low-dose combined estrogen-progestin OC. This use is suggested for healthy women who do not smoke or have other contraindications. (Please see Chapter 8 for more on contraceptives.)

Bioidentical hormones. The term *bioidentical hormone* typically refers to custom-made HT formulations that are prescribed by a healthcare professional and compounded by a pharmacy for an individual patient. The growing popularity of bioidentical hormones may be related to the public belief that they are more "natural" than FDA-approved HT preparations. However, the lack of regulatory oversight, rigorous safety and efficacy testing, and quality control measures for batch standardization and purity raise concerns regarding the use of these products. Consequently, the use of custom-compounded bioidentical HT is not recommended.[104,111] FDA-approved bioidentical hormones (estradiol and progesterone) are available for women who prefer them. (Please see Chapter 8 for more on bioidentical hormone therapy.)

Prescription therapies: nonhormonal options. The only FDA-approved, nonhormonal medication for menopause hot flashes is the SSRI paroxetine.[112] Paroxetine has been used off label for the treatment of hot flashes in the past; however, a newly approved formulation consists of a lower dose than the standard paroxetine tablets used for psychiatric indications. This approved formulation contains 7.5 mg of paroxetine and is taken once daily at bedtime. It has been shown in 2 RCTs to improve hot flashes at 4 weeks of use compared with placebo. Other medications have been used off label for the treatment of VMS with some benefit. Although several have demonstrated effectiveness in relieving hot flashes, none are as effective as systemic ET. However, there are no comparative trials in similar patient populations to guide clinicians in selecting a particular option. (Please see Chapter 8 for more on SSRIs.)

These drugs are *not* FDA approved for the treatment of vasomotor symptoms:

Selective serotonin-reuptake inhibitors and serotonin norepinephrine-reuptake inhibitors. If there are no contraindications, SSRIs are an option for women who have hot flashes but are not candidates for HT or prefer an alternative. Other SSRIs that have been shown to be more effective than placebo for the treatment of hot flashes include paroxetine 12.5 mg to 25 mg per day, and escitalopram 10 mg to 20 mg per day.

The serotonin norepinephrine-reuptake inhibitors (SNRIs) venlafaxine 37.5 mg to 75 mg per day and desvenlafaxine 100 mg to 150 mg per day have also been evaluated for the treatment of hot flashes and may be considered in women who are not candidates for HT or prefer an alternative. Randomized, controlled trials have demonstrated positive results for treatment of hot flashes using each of these therapies.[113-119] There is limited research about the long-term consequences of SSRIs or SNRIs for hot flashes in the nondepressed population or about the return of hot flashes once the drugs are withdrawn.

Cytochrome P-450 2D6 is involved in the metabolism of tamoxifen to an active metabolite endoxifen. Different SSRIs and SNRIs cause variable inhibition of cytochrome P-450 2D6, with paroxetine and fluoxetine demonstrating the most profound effect and fluvoxamine and citalopram being weak inhibitors.[120] Serum levels of tamoxifen metabolites have been observed to be reduced by 24% to 64% after 4 weeks of paroxetine treatment.[121] This finding has raised concern regarding the efficacy of tamoxifen in women with breast cancer undergoing concomitant treatment with SSRIs. Paroxetine use during tamoxifen treatment for breast cancer has recently been associated with an increased risk of death from breast cancer.[122] In contrast, a Danish population-based study did not observe an increase in breast cancer recurrence among women prescribed an SSRI while on tamoxifen therapy, even among those prescribed paroxetine.[123] Genotyping studies for the cytochrome P-450 2D6 allele have yielded contradictory results regarding the efficacy of tamoxifen, adding to the complexity of the available data.[124] It is probably most prudent to avoid the use of potent cytochrome P-450 2D6 inhibitors, such as paroxetine, in women taking tamoxifen.

The additional antidepressant effects of the SSRI and SNRI class of drugs may benefit some women who suffer from mood disorders in addition to hot flashes.

Hot flash relief, if any, is rapid with these therapies, whereas relief of depression may not be observed for 6 to 8 weeks. This rapid onset of action can be a powerful reinforcement for women who do not find hot flash relief with other, simpler methods. A brief trial of 2 to 4 weeks may determine whether these agents are going to be effective.

Adverse effects for SSRIs and SNRIs, especially nausea and sexual problems, should be monitored. Nausea is dose related and usually subsides within 2 weeks of starting treatment. Women who experience drowsiness should take the drug at night. Caution is advised for women using tamoxifen who decide to take SSRIs or SNRIs.[125]

The SSRI paroxetine can cause weight gain and blurred vision, although this is rare. Fluoxetine is less likely to cause acute withdrawal AEs because of its longer half-life. Clinical studies have implicated SSRIs in reduced bone mass and in clinical fragility fractures.[126] The SNRI venlafaxine is the most likely in its class to promote weight loss by causing anorexia and may be preferred by women who are overweight.

To minimize AEs, very low doses of these antidepressants should be used when starting therapy. If not effective, the dose can be increased after several days to weeks. Higher doses than those used in trials do not seem appropriate, given the lack of additional efficacy and the potential for increased toxicity. Taking the drugs with food may lessen nausea.

These antidepressant medications should not be stopped abruptly, because sudden withdrawal has been associated with headaches and anxiety. Women who have been using an antidepressant for at least 1 week should taper off the drug. Tapering may require up to 2 weeks, and sometimes longer, depending on the initial dosage. Patients should be cautioned to maintain their supply of medication and not to run out, thereby forcing an abrupt withdrawal.

Eszopiclone. This hypnotic is shown to be effective in the treatment of nighttime but not daytime hot flashes and has the additional benefit of reducing depression and anxiety as well as improving overall well-being.[127]

Gabapentin. The anticonvulsant drug gabapentin is another nonhormone option for treating hot flashes. An RCT that compared hot flash composite scores (severity and frequency) in women taking ET, gabapentin, or placebo found a statistically significant decrease in hot flash composite scores for estrogen (P=.016) and gabapentin (P=.004) over placebo.[128] An RCT of gabapentin alone compared with placebo demonstrated similar results.[129] Therapy can be initiated at a daily dose of 300 mg (although starting at 100 mg/d may be advisable in women aged >65 years). Bedtime administration is advised, given the initial AEs of dizziness and drowsiness; these symptoms will often subside by the second week, with complete resolution occurring by the fourth treatment week.[130] In women who continue to have hot flashes, the dose can be increased to 300 mg twice daily and then to 3 times daily at 3- to 4-day intervals. Increased efficacy may be seen at even higher doses, although this has not been well studied. For example, 1 RCT demonstrated efficacy at 900 mg daily but not at 300 mg daily in breast cancer survivors.[131] Antacids may reduce the bioavailability of gabapentin; the drug should be taken at least 2 hours after antacid use. Gabapentin can cause weight gain. Tapering is advised when discontinuing gabapentin therapy.[132]

Combination gabapentin and antidepressants. A 2007 RCT evaluated women with inadequate hot flash control who were taking an antidepressant alone.[132] The investigators compared the addition of gabapentin to the antidepressant versus weaning the antidepressant and starting gabapentin alone. Results showed comparable efficacy in both groups. Both treatments decreased hot flash frequencies and scores by approximately 50%.

Pregabalin. Pregabalin is currently approved for use in patients with fibromyalgia, diabetic neuropathy, postherpetic neuralgias, and partial-onset seizures. A phase 3 RCT showed significant decreases in hot flashes during a 6-week course compared with placebo.[133] Adverse events were similar to those of gabapentin; they included dizziness and cognitive difficulties with coordination and concentration. Although early results seem promising, additional research will be required before recommendations regarding this medication can be made.

Clonidine. The antihypertensive agent clonidine is sometimes used to treat mild hot flashes, although it is less effective than the newer antidepressants or gabapentin. In addition, clonidine has an AE profile that limits its use in many women. Clonidine lowers BP, heart rate, and pulse rate; arrhythmias have been observed at high doses. The initial oral dose for hot flash treatment is 0.05 mg twice daily, but some women may require at least 0.1 mg twice daily. The clonidine patch, delivering 0.1 mg per day, can also be considered. When discontinuing higher-dose therapy, the dose should be gradually tapered to avoid AEs including nervousness, headache, agitation, confusion, and a rapid rise in BP.

Other treatments. Given the limited efficacy data and potential for AEs, methyldopa or the product combining phenobarbital, ergotamine tartrate, and belladonna alkaloids are not recommended as hot flash treatments for most women. The evidence regarding the use of acupuncture to treat hot flashes generally suggests efficacy comparable to sham acupuncture.[134,135]

Ongoing treatment. Any hot flash treatment may need to be adjusted periodically because of gradually lowering levels of ovarian hormones during the menopause transition and the possible appearance of medical conditions unrelated to postmenopause or menopause treatments. New research and changing ideas about treatments may have an effect on health decisions. Before switching from one therapy to another, a washout period may be required.

Regardless of the management option used, treatment should be periodically reevaluated to determine whether it is still necessary, because in almost all women, menopause-related VMS will abate over time. Please see Chapters 6, 7, and 8 for more about available treatments for VMS.

Genitourinary syndrome of menopause

Genitourinary syndrome of menopause is defined as a collection of symptoms and signs associated with decreased estrogen and other sex steroid levels that can involve changes to labia majora/minora, vestibule/introitus, clitoris, vagina, urethra, and bladder. Symptoms include, but are not limited to, dryness, pain with sex that may lead to subsequent sexual dysfunction, bladder and urethral symptoms, frequent urinary tract infections (UTIs), burning, itching, and irritation that are bothersome or distressing. The genitourinary syndrome of menopause is a comprehensive term that includes symptoms associated with menopause affecting the vulvovaginal area as well as the lower urinary tract. Lower urinary tract symptoms associated with menopause include dysuria, urgency, and frequent UTIs. *Symptomatic vulvovaginal atrophy* (VVA) is a component of this syndrome. Women may present with some or all of the symptoms.

Approximately 20% to 50% of US women experience vulvovaginal symptoms sometime during postmenopause. Vulvovaginal dryness and dyspareunia (painful intercourse) are common complaints. These symptoms also can be caused by infectious and noninfectious etiologies (Table 7).[136] In postreproductive-aged women, superimposed vaginal atrophy may need to be addressed for sufficient treatment of any vulvovaginal condition.

Women of any age who have low estrogen levels, perhaps from primary ovarian insufficiency, hypothalamic amenorrhea, hyperprolactinemia, prolonged lactation, or treatment with GnRH agonists or antagonists, may all present with uncomfortable vaginal symptoms that require management.[137] Cancer therapies, either medical (chemotherapy-induced menopause), surgical (removal of ovarian tissue), endocrine, or radiation, may also result in vaginal changes. Some of the estrogen agonists/antagonists that are used as adjuvant therapy in breast cancer may cause increased vaginal discharge from the agonist effects in the vagina, whereas aromatase inhibitors will often increase vaginal dryness and dyspareunia.[87] Vaginal symptoms related to an abrupt menopause induced by surgery or chemotherapy are associated with significantly greater sexual dysfunction and distress as well as poorer QOL outcomes.

Treatment of genitourinary syndrome of menopause

The genitourinary syndrome of menopause should be treated in symptomatic women who are bothered by these symptoms and are interested in intervention. Sexual difficulties and chronic irritating symptoms may result in ongoing discomfort and/or personal or interpersonal distress. Some women may complain of interruption of activities of daily living as a result of severe vaginal dryness, whereas others only complain of painful intercourse. Symptoms should be assessed and treatment goals ascertained for each individual patient.

Nonhormonal over-the-counter (OTC) products such as vaginal moisturizers and lubricants may be used as initial treatment for women with bothersome vaginal dryness. If nonhormonal interventions are not successful in ameliorating symptoms, minimally absorbed vaginal low-dose ET can be considered in women who have no medical contraindications to its use.

CLINICAL ISSUES

In women who are using systemic HT for another indication, the addition of low-dose vaginal estrogen for complete relief of GSM symptoms may be necessary. Systemic HT also may be provided by a vaginal ring, treating vasomotor and vaginal symptoms. In addition to local products, ospemifene, a novel oral estrogen agonist/antagonist, can be considered as treatment for women who suffer from moderate to severe VVA.[138]

Nonmedical treatment. Regular sexual activity promotes blood flow to the genital area and can help maintain vaginal health. Nonpenetrative sexual activity, such as massage or oral stimulation, may increase a couple's intimacy in place of intercourse or while a treatment plan is initiated. Self- or mutual masturbation or use of a vibrator maximizes stimulation and should be encouraged as appropriate. Pelvic floor physical therapy can be very beneficial. Books, movies, or fantasy may increase arousal and also may be incorporated into sexual activity.

Nonhormonal therapy. Mild vaginal dryness or irritation often can be managed with vaginal lubricants and moisturizers available without a prescription (Table 8).[139] Lubricants and moisturizers can decrease the friction on atrophic vulvovaginal structures during sexual activity. The effects of vaginal lubricants are immediate and intended to provide temporary relief from vulvovaginal symptoms during sex. Lubricants are water, silicone, or oil based. In counseling patients about lubricants, concomitant birth control methods and desired fertility should be discussed, if applicable, because certain lubricants may interfere with condom permeability or sperm viability.[140] The clinician should advise menopausal patients to be wary of additives such as colors, flavors, warming agents, bactericides, and spermicides in their moisturizers or lubricants because these products can be irritating to the sensitive atrophic postmenopausal vaginal and vulvar tissues.

In contrast to vaginal lubricants, vaginal moisturizers are applied several times weekly, not just at the time of sexual activity. Moisturizers provide longer-term relief of vaginal dryness and can also reduce uncomfortable symptoms of mild vaginal atrophy by maintaining vaginal moisture and lower vaginal pH.[141]

Although few efficacy studies of these products have been conducted, 1 RCT demonstrated effectiveness of a vaginal gel over placebo in patients with breast cancer.[142] Other studies have shown significant improvement of vulvovaginal symptoms.[143,144]

Hormonal therapies. The North American Menopause Society recommends low-dose vaginal ET when nonhormonal interventions fail to relieve symptoms or in women with severe GSM symptoms.[139] Estrogen restores vaginal blood flow, decreases vaginal pH, and improves the thickness and elasticity of vulvovaginal tissues. Benefits of minimally absorbed low-dose vaginal ET include avoidance of first-pass metabolism in the liver, lower systemic serum hormone levels, and potentially fewer AEs and risks.

Improvements in vulvovaginal health usually occur within a few weeks of starting ET. All administrative vehicles (rings, tablets, creams) have been shown to be effective for the treatment of VVA. The delivery system should be based on patient preference (Table 9).[138,139,145-151]

Table 7. Typical Causes of Vulvar Disorders

Infection
- Candida
- Condylomata acuminatum
- Herpes genitalis
- Herpes zoster
- Lice
- Scabies

Inflammation
- Classic lichen planus
- Contact dermatitis
- Erosive lichen planus
- Postherpetic neuralgia
- Pudendal neuralgia
- Seborrheic keratosis
- Vestibulodynia
- Vulvodynia

Neoplasm
- Acrochordon (skin tags)
- Bartholin gland cyst
- Carcinoma
- Epidermal inclusion cyst
- Fibromas and lipomas
- Follicular cyst
- Hidradenoma
- Nevi
- Paget disease
- Squamous cell hyperplasia
- Intraepithelial neoplasia

Other
- Psoriasis
- Sjögren syndrome
- Vulvar atrophy

Table 8. Nonhormonal Therapeutic Options for Vaginal Atrophy

Lubricants	Moisturizers
Water based	
Astroglide Liquid	Replens, RepHresh
Astroglide Gel Liquid	Vagisil, Feminease
Astroglide	K-Y SILK-E
Just Like Me	Luvena
K-Y Jelly	Silken Secret
Pre-Seed	
Slippery Stuff	
Liquid Silk	
Good Clean Love	
YES Personal Lubricant	
Silicone based	
Astroglide X	
ID Millennium	
K-Y Intrigue	
Pink	
Pjur Eros	
Oil based	
Elégance Women's Lubricants	
Olive oil	

Management of symptomatic vulvovaginal atrophy: 2013 position statement of The North American Menopause Society.[139]

The 17β-estradiol vaginal ring delivers 7.5 μg estradiol per day.[148] The ring is placed into the vagina and should be changed every 3 months. The ring can be removed on a temporary basis, such as during intercourse, depending on the couple's preferences. The estradiol ring also has been FDA approved for treatment of urinary urgency. Estradiol hemihydrate tablets (10 μg) are placed in the vagina twice a week after an initial nightly use of 2 weeks' duration.[150]

Conjugated estrogen cream is approved for VVA and is the only estrogen approved for dyspareunia. The product information sheet states that the dose to treat VVA is 0.5 g to 2 g per day for 21 days then off for 7 days, and to treat dyspareunia, the dosage is either a cyclical dose of 0.5 g per day for 21 days followed by 7 days of no treatment or an ongoing dose of 0.5 g twice a week. The approved dosage of 17β-estradiol to treat VVA is 2 g to 4 g daily for 1 to 2 weeks, then 1 g 1 to 3 times a week. NAMS recommends the lowest dosing of both products (twice-a-week dosing) for either symptomatic VVA or dyspareunia. The higher the dose, the greater the risk of endometrial stimulation.

Systemic absorption of vaginal ET depends on dose and delivery method. A Cochrane review of trials reported no significant differences among the delivery methods of low-dose vaginal estrogen products in terms of hyperplasia, endometrial thickness, or proportion of women with AEs.[152]

The same review concluded that available data cannot answer the question of whether women need progestogen to counter possible AEs on the endometrium. Safety data are available for 1 year only. In women with an intact uterus, addition of a progestogen is generally not indicated. It is the position of NAMS that if a woman is at a high risk for endometrial cancer (ie, obese) or is using a higher dose of ET than is typically recommended, surveillance using transvaginal ultrasound or progestogen withdrawal may be considered. Postmenopausal bleeding should be evaluated by pelvic examination and by either transvaginal ultrasound or endometrial sampling. (Please see Chapter 8 for more on hormonal therapies.)

Ospemifene is an FDA-approved selective ER modulator for the treatment of moderate to severe dyspareunia associated with VVA. It is given as a daily oral dose of 60 mg and has been shown to improve vaginal maturation index (VMI), vaginal pH, and the symptoms of VVA.[153,154] Ospemifene can increase VMS and theoretically may increase the risk of VTE. Studies up to 52 weeks showed no endometrial hyperplasia or cancer.[155] There are insufficient data concerning an effect on breast cancer, although antiestrogenic effects on breast tissue were shown in preclinical models. Preliminary data comparing ospemifene to raloxifene show similar favorable effects on bone.[139,156]

Women who prefer not to use estrogen or ospemifene or have contraindications to their use have few alternatives other than vaginal lubricants or moisturizers or increased vaginal stimulation. Preliminary data show promising results from intravaginal dehydroepiandrosterone with little to no change in serum sex hormone steroid levels (in up to 12 weeks of administration).[157,158] Additionally, no change in lipids, insulin resistance, or endometrial thickness was noted in 52 weeks of oral therapy, during which time serum dehydroepiandrosterone and testosterone levels remained in the postmenopausal range.[159] Without further confirmatory RCT data and evaluation or government approval, dehydroepiandrosterone cannot be recommended at this time.

Inadequate data exist to evaluate the effect on vaginal dryness, if any, of herbal supplements and isoflavone-containing foods and supplements.

Urinary tract infection

A small percentage of postmenopausal women experience recurrent UTIs. After menopause, the vaginal pH increases, leading to greater colonization of bacteria that can act as bladder pathogens. However, in a study comparing postmenopausal women with and without recurrent urinary tract infections, the strongest associated factors were the presence of incontinence, cystocele, elevated postvoid residual, history of premenopausal UTI, type 2 diabetes mellitus (DM), and increasing age.[160]

For women whose urgency and frequency symptoms are attributable to recurrent UTI, the goal after initial antibiotic treatment is prevention. Clinicians should first emphasize

CLINICAL ISSUES

Table 9. Prescription Therapies for Symptomatic Vaginal Atrophy

Composition	Product name	FDA-approved dosage
Vaginal creams		
17β-estradiol	Estrace Vaginal Cream[a]	Initial: 2-4 g/d for 1-2 wk Maintenance: 1 g/1-3 times/wk[c] (0.1 mg active ingredient/g)
Conjugated estrogens	Premarin Vaginal Cream	*For VVA*: 0.5-2 g/d for 21 d then off 7 d[c] *For dyspareunia*: 0.5 g/d for 21 d then off 7 d, or twice/wk[c] (0.625 mg active ingredient/g)
Estrone	Estragyn Vaginal Cream[b]	2-4 g/d (1 mg active ingredient/g) (intended for short-term use; progestogen recommended)
Vaginal rings		
17β-estradiol	Estring	Device containing 2 mg releases approximately 7.5 μg/d for 90 d (for VVA)
Estradiol acetate	Femring[a]	Device containing 12.4 mg or 24.8 mg estradiol acetate releases 0.05 mg/d or 0.10 mg/d estradiol for 90 days (both doses release systemic levels for treatment of VVA and vasomotor symptoms)
Vaginal tablet		
Estradiol hemihydrate	Vagifem	Initial: 1 tablet/d for 2 wk Maintenance: 1 tablet twice/wk (tablet containing 10.3 μg of estradiol hemihydrates, equivalent to 10 μg of estradiol)
Ospemifene	Osphena	60 mg daily oral

Abbreviation: FDA, US Food and Drug Administration; VVA, vulvovaginal atrophy.
Products not noted are available in the United States and in Canada.
a. Available in the United States but not Canada
b. Available in Canada but not the United States
c. Some FDA-approved dosages of conjugated estrogen and estradiol creams are greater than those currently used in clinical practice proven to be effective. Doses of 0.5-1 g of estrogen vaginal cream, used 1-2 times weekly, may be adequate for many women.
Osphena [package insert],[138] Management of symptomatic vulvovaginal atrophy: 2013 position statement of The North American Menopause Society,[139] Estrace [package insert],[145] Premarin vaginal cream [package insert],[146] Estragyn vaginal cream [product monograph],[147] Estring [package insert],[148] Femring [package insert],[149] Vagifem [package insert],[150] Bachmann G, et al.[151]

the importance of nonpharmacologic approaches (Table 10). Although voiding, hygiene, and dietary measures have not been conclusively proven to prevent UTIs, they involve little risk or cost and may be beneficial to many women. Consuming cranberry extract or pure unsweetened cranberry juice may decrease the rate of UTI recurrences.[161,162]

In postmenopausal women with recurrent, symptomatic, lower UTIs caused by common pathogens such as *Escherichia coli*, therapeutic options include vaginal ET or prophylactic antibiotics. The use of low-dose vaginal ET may help reduce the risk of recurrent UTI in a number of ways. Estrogen therapy restores a lactobacillus-predominant flora and more acid environment of the vagina, thus discouraging colonization of the vagina by UTI-associated pathogens. Additionally, estrogen may improve the local immune response by increasing antimicrobial peptides and strengthening intracellular barriers.[163] Clinically, only estrogen administered by the vaginal route has been shown in studies to be effective in reducing the risk of recurrent UTI.[160] Oral HT does not appear to reduce the risk of recurrent UTI.[164] (Please see Chapter 8 for a list of low-dose vaginal estrogens.)

Women who present with unusual bacterial pathogens or whose infection cannot be cleared may require further urologic evaluation. Asymptomatic bacteriuria, on the other hand, most often requires no treatment.

Other vulvar and vaginal clinical issues

Vestibulodynia

Vestibulodynia has variably been called *vulvar vestibulitis* and *vulvodynia*. It is a frequently missed diagnosis in the postmenopausal woman who presents with the common complaint of dyspareunia. Vestibulodynia is often misdiagnosed as VVA because clinicians fail to detect it. The term *vulvodynia* is defined as chronic vulvar pain and discomfort

Chapter 3

> **Table 10.** Nonpharmacologic Strategies for Preventing Urinary Tract Infections
>
> - Void after intercourse
> - Wipe from front to back after a bowel movement to prevent spreading bacteria
> - Do not use soaps or perfumed feminine hygiene products that can irritate the urethra or change the normal vaginal bacterial environment of the vagina
> - Consuming cranberry extract or pure unsweetened cranberry juice may decrease the rate of UTI recurrences

in the absence of gross anatomic or neurologic findings (other than erythema and occasionally small fissures or erosions in the skin). Vulvodynia can be further classified as generalized or localized.[165] Generalized vulvodynia involves chronic, nonlocalized vulvar pain. Localized vulvodynia involves a specific area, most often the vestibule (the area just exterior to the hymeneal ring), hence the term vestibulodynia.

Several potential causes have been proposed (genetic or immune factors), although none have been confirmed. Vulvodynia does not appear to be caused by yeast, human papillomavirus, high urinary oxalates, or sexual abuse. Vulvodynia was previously thought to be infrequent, but studies in a variety of populations suggest that the prevalence ranges from 3% to 15% of women from diverse backgrounds and ethnicities.[166] Vestibulodynia appears to be far more common than generalized vulvodynia. It can occur in reproductive-aged and postmenopausal patients. Research has shown increasing evidence for comorbidity of vulvodynia and other chronic pain conditions such as fibromyalgia, painful bladder syndrome (interstitial cystitis), and irritable bowel syndrome.[167]

The cotton swab test (application of gentle pressure with a moist cotton swab over the various areas of the vulva, clitoris, introitus, and perineum to map the discomfort) is helpful in diagnosing vulvodynia and specifying vestibulodynia. Vulvodynia may have no clinical findings other than patient history, but the well-defined areas of pain mapped by the cotton swab test distinguish this condition. Vulvodynia is a diagnosis of exclusion, and the physical exam should rule out other potential causes of vulvar pain. If the diagnosis is uncertain, a wet mount, vaginal pH, fungal culture, biopsy, or Gram stain can be performed if indicated.

Before initiation of medical treatment, alternate causes should be considered, especially contact or allergic dermatitis. It is very important to ask a woman what products she is using. Irritants such as soap; panty liners; synthetic underwear; moistened wipes; deodorants; douches; lubricants; spermicides; excessive vaginal discharge, urine, and feces; sanitary napkins; colored toilet paper; vaginal sprays; laundry detergents; bubble baths; fragrances; and OTC medications, specifically those that contain benzocaine, should be sought and eliminated.

No treatment for vulvodynia is government approved in the United States or in Canada, and few randomized trials are available to guide treatment algorithms. Current recommendations are based mainly on clinical experience or small clinical trials. They include vulvar care measures (avoiding vulvar irritants), topical estrogen and/or testosterone in combination applied directly to the vestibule or other affected area, topical medications (lidocaine ointment 5%, plain petrolatum), oral medications for chronic pain such as antidepressants and anticonvulsants,[168] biofeedback and physical therapy, intralesional injections, and surgery. Topical lidocaine, used intermittently with sexual activity or applied via soaked cotton ball nightly, is often sufficient for mild symptoms. Topical corticosteroids do not seem to have any benefit.

Off-label use of oral tricyclic antidepressants (amitriptyline, nortriptyline, desipramine) and anticonvulsants (gabapentin, carbamazepine) can decrease neural hypersensitivity and has yielded good clinical results.[168,169] Treatment should begin at the lowest dose, typically much less than the dose required for the approved indications, and titrated upward slowly (see package inserts for contraindications, AEs, and guidance on safely discontinuing treatment). Only 1 drug should be prescribed at a time. Tolerance to AEs (sedation, dry mouth, dizziness) may be achieved over time.

Biofeedback, vaginal dilators, and pelvic floor physical therapy may also be used in the treatment of both localized and generalized vulvar pain, either independently or in conjunction with medical therapies. These techniques are particularly helpful if there is concomitant hypertonic pelvic floor musculature (spasm of the levator muscles of the vagina).

Any therapeutic option requires time to achieve adequate pain control, perhaps 3 to 6 weeks. There is evidence that many cases of vulvodynia improve with time, with or without treatment. For generalized vulvar burning unresponsive to previous behavioral and medical treatments, referral to a pain specialist may be needed. Individual sexual or couples counseling will be helpful to those experiencing other secondary sexual dysfunctions or interpersonal distress. Surgery such as vestibulectomy should be reserved for women with localized symptoms who do not respond to other treatments and who have been comprehensively counseled about the pros and cons of this treatment. Care should be exercised when choosing a surgeon because operator experience with the procedure is critical. Although recurrence is possible after surgery, the literature describes a wide range of postoperative success.

Vulvovaginitis

Vulvovaginitis is most commonly caused by candidal or bacterial vaginosis or a sexually transmitted infection such as trichomoniasis, gonorrhea, or chlamydia. Discharge characteristics including color, odor, pH, and findings on wet prep guide diagnosis (Table 11). Wet preps are helpful in

CLINICAL ISSUES

identifying most yeast, trichomonas, and bacterial vaginosis. Cultures should be reserved for unclear or recurrent cases. A medical history should always include sexual contacts and current medical problems.[170] The use of condoms for protection against STIs should always be discussed with menopausal women, who may feel that barriers are not necessary because pregnancy is no longer a medical concern. Gonorrhea and chlamydia cultures should be considered.

Yeast vaginitis. Yeast vaginitis is most commonly caused by *Candida albicans*. In postmenopause, an increase in candida infection has been associated with HT and systemic diseases such as DM and immunodeficiency states. Yeast vaginitis most often presents with itching and discharge that is thick, clumpy, and white in color. On physical exam, the vulva may be erythematous and inflamed, and excoriations from itching may be present. The discharge will be adherent to the vaginal sidewalls and has a normal pH and no odor. Wet prep shows yeast buds, spores, or hyphae. White blood cells may be present.

Yeast vaginitis is classified as complicated if the infection is present in an immune-compromised host, is caused by a non-albicans species, or presents with severe symptoms or clinical findings. Recurrent yeast is also considered complicated and defined as 4 or more episodes per year.

Treatment includes topical or systemic antifungals. For non-albicans species resistant to azoles, boric acid suppositories (600 mg in gelatin capsules) may be prescribed for 14 nights. Careful patient instruction is necessary, because boric acid can be fatal if swallowed. Complicated yeast vaginitis may need prolonged or suppressive treatment. A common protocol is fluconazole 150 mg every 3 days for 2 or 3 doses, followed by weekly dosing for 6 months.[171] Recurrence after cessation of therapy is common. Decreasing sugar intake may be helpful, but behavioral factors such as vulvar hygiene and tight clothing have not been proven to be causative.

Bacterial vaginosis. Bacterial vaginosis, a microbial imbalance condition, usually presents with gray-yellow discharge with an unpleasant odor, usually worse after sexual intercourse involving ejaculation. Symptoms include irritation or burning; pruritus is generally absent or mild. Bacterial vaginosis is diagnosed using Amsel's criteria and requires that 2 to 3 of these are met: thin, homogeneous vaginal discharge; vaginal pH greater than 4.5; fishy amine odor with the addition of 10% hydrogen peroxide ("whiff" test); and on Gram stain, 20% or more vaginal squamous "clue cells"—cells with borders obscured by adherent coccobacilli.[170,172] In most office settings, the last criterion is met using wet prep and not Gram stain. White blood cells are generally absent. Bacterial vaginosis is treated with oral or vaginal metronidazole or clindamycin.

Recurrent bacterial vaginosis may need prolonged or suppressive treatment. Treatment with intravaginal metronidazole gel 0.75% for a 7- to 10-day course (induction), followed by twice weekly intravaginal application for 4 to 6 months (suppression) has been shown to be superior to placebo.[173] Clindamycin is not recommended as suppressive therapy because of potential toxicity and has not been shown to increase cure rates.

Trichomoniasis. Trichomoniasis is an STI caused by *Trichomonas vaginitis*. Patients will present with copious bubbly, yellow or green discharge. Bladder symptoms such as dysuria or frequency may also be present. Wet prep of the vaginal secretions will reveal the causative organism, seen as a motile round or oval protozoa with an obvious flagellum, often most visible clinging around the edges of clumped squamous cells. Vaginal pH will be 5.5 to 6.0. White blood cells are also usually seen on wet prep. Treatment with oral or vaginal metronidazole or oral tindazole is recommended for the woman and for her sexual contacts. Nonresponders are often recurrent rather than resistant cases, but if

Table 11. Typical Presentation of Vaginitis

Diagnosis	Discharge	pH	Odor	Wet prep	Treatment
Candida infection	Homogeneous White, particulate	4-5	No	Hyphae/Spores Moderate WBCs	Topical/Oral antifungals
Bacterial vaginosis	Homogeneous, gray Low viscosity	>5	Yes (+) Whiff	Clue cells Few to no WBCs	Oral/Topical metronidazole
Trichomonas infection	Yellow, gray Frothy or bubbly Viscous	6-7	Yes	Motile Trichomonads Many WBCs	Metronidazole Tindazole
Allergy	Clear mucus	<4.5	No	Epithelial cells	Removal of irritant Topical steroids Oral antihistamines

Abbreviation: WBCs, white blood cells.

resistance is suspected, tindazole or oral metronidazole at a prolonged high dosage should be considered. If no response is obtained, cultures for sensitivity can be sent to the Centers for Disease Control and Prevention by special arrangement.

Vulvar disorders

Vulvar discomfort in postmenopausal women is not always caused by low estrogen or vaginal atrophy. Similar symptoms can be experienced by postmenopausal women suffering from vaginal infection, trauma, or a vulvar lesion. Also included among the benign disorders of the vulva are contact or allergic dermatitis, eczema, vulvar dystrophy, and vulvodynia, all of which need to be diagnosed and treated. Additionally, vulvar conditions may represent a local manifestation of systemic disease (such as diabetes mellitus or lupus), vulvar intraepithelial neoplasia, or invasive cancer. Infections of the sebaceous, Bartholin, or Skene glands are also possible. If any of these disorders is present, women should also be evaluated for concomitant vaginal atrophy.

Vulvar disorders are often characterized by clinical presentation, most often by the predominant symptom (burning, itching, or pain). Other considerations to differentiate these disorders include chronicity (acute vs chronic), involvement or lack of involvement of mucocutaneous membranes, and the presence or absence of vaginal discharge (Table 7).[136]

Vulvar conditions may present a clinical challenge, even to experienced healthcare professionals. Vulvar biopsy is almost always indicated in the evaluation of vulvar lesions. A biopsy should be considered for long-standing complaints, symptoms not responding to therapeutic interventions, or before initiation of high-dose steroids or prolonged medical therapy.

Vulvar dermatoses

Vulvar dermatoses are pruritic disorders that have various etiologies. Psoriasis, seborrheic keratitis, and contact and allergic dermatitis are examples.

Lichen sclerosus. Lichen sclerosus is a thinning of vulvar squamous epithelium of unknown etiology, with skin and mucous membranes also affected in some patients. Older terms for lichen sclerosus include *kraurosis vulvae, atrophic leukoplakia,* and *lichen sclerosus et atrophicus*. Intense pruritus is the usual presenting symptom. Burning, soreness, dysuria, and dyspareunia also may occur. Clinically, the lesions are white and wrinkled papules and plaques. These parchment-like lesions are seen over the labia, vestibule, and introitus, without involvement of the vaginal mucosa. Plaques may be thickened or hypertrophic (thought secondary to chronic itching), and in 11% of patients, extragenital lesions (thigh, breasts, shoulders) are present. As lichen sclerosus progresses, a figure-8 appearance around the introitus and anus may be seen. Architectural distortion, such as the labia minora adhering to the majora and ultimately becoming indistinguishable, "burying" of the clitoris, fissures, or shrinkage of the introital opening, may occur.

Because lichen sclerosis is associated with squamous cell cancer of the vulva, biopsy is recommended for diagnosis. Treatment is with potent topical corticosteroids such as clobetasol. Initial daily application is followed by a gradual taper, aiming for the lowest dose to relieve symptoms and ultimately as-needed dosing of less potent steroids.[174] Many clinicians advocate annual vulvoscopy because of the higher association with vulvar cancer. The estimated 4.5% incidence of vulvar cancer has prompted guidelines that outline when to refer to a gynecologic oncologist. These guidelines include women who have difficulty with symptom control (requiring potent topical corticosteroids 3 or more times per week or >30 g in 6 months); women previously treated for vulvar intraepithelial neoplasia; women with hyperkeratosis in which biopsy reveals precancerous changes or the lesion does not respond to topical steroids; and biopsies in which the pathologist cannot make a definite diagnosis of vulvar intraepithelial neoplasia but expresses concern.[175] Screening intervals of 3 to 6 months are suggested for women with this diagnosis regardless of the setting in which they are followed.

Squamous cell hyperplasia. Squamous cell hyperplasia, characterized by thickened lesions, is usually the result of chronic irritation or infection. Older terms for squamous cell hyperplasia include *hyperplastic dystrophy, lichen simplex chronicus, hypertrophic vulvitis, chronic reaction vulvitis,* and *neurodermatitis*. Squamous cell hyperplasia is thought to be the result of chronic irritation or infection. The skin develops a white, thickened surface with some cracking. Areas of hyperpigmentation or hypopigmentation may be present. Bleeding and pruritus may occur. Unlike with lichen sclerosus, the labia minora do not atrophy and at times disappear, and the lesion is usually localized. Management is aimed at treating the underlying disorder or finding and eliminating the irritant. Topical steroids and oral antihistamines may aid in symptom control. As in other vulvar disorders, when in doubt of the diagnosis, biopsy should be undertaken.

Lichen planus. Lichen planus affects the skin and the mucosal surfaces of the vulva, especially the vestibule. This condition is an inflammatory dermatosis, characterized by thickening of all layers of the epithelium. The etiology is unknown, although an autoimmune process is suspected, perhaps initiated by certain medications including beta-blockers or angiotensin-converting enzyme inhibitors.

Three types of lichen planus have been described: erosive, classic, and hypertrophic.[174]

- *Erosive lichen planus*, the most common, is associated with vaginal discharge, severe itching, severe pain, and dyspareunia. On examination, the vaginal mucosa is friable and bleeds easily. The vestibule and labia minora may have evidence of erosions or a lacy white mucosal plaque.

Painful erosive areas may be present, and adhesions of opposite mucosal surfaces can cause marked stenosis of the introitus and vagina. Vulvar involvement is minimal.

- *Classical lichen planus*, also called *papulosquamous lichen planus*, appears as a white raised lesion with a reticular, lacy pattern, without mucosal involvement. Clinically, pruritus is the predominant symptom. Extragenital lesions may occur. The 5 Ps (pruritic, planar, purple, polygonal papules) describe the extragenital lesions.

- *Hypertrophic lichen planus* is a variant of papulosquamous, resulting in rough, scaly, hypertrophic brown plaques that affect keratinized skin of the vulva as well as distant sites.

Lichen planus tends to have spontaneous remissions, often after years of relapsing symptoms. Local lesions may be treated by topical corticosteroids such as clobetasol, and intralesional corticosteroids can be used for hypertrophic lesions. Oral corticosteroid treatment may be necessary for symptom relief, whereas oral antihistamines may relieve milder symptoms.

Vulvar psoriasis. Vulvar psoriasis usually coexists with systemic disease, although vulvar plaques tend to be pink, smooth, and glossy and located in intertriginous areas as opposed to dry with a silvery-gray scale as in extragenital manifestations. The vestibule and vagina are not involved. Symptoms of itching and pain are relapsing and remitting. Diagnosis is helped by the presence of extragenital disease, and treatment is with topical corticosteroids, with attention to secondary coinfection.

Seborrheic dermatitis. Seborrheic dermatitis is a chronic skin condition that manifests in areas where sebaceous glands are concentrated. Lesions are pale to yellow-red and covered with an oily scale. Plaques may be seasonal or stress related and respond to topical corticosteroids or ketoconazole.

Contact dermatitis. Contact dermatitis is a vulvar skin reaction to an irritant, which may be nonimmunologic or of truly immunologic (allergic dermatitis) origin. Contact dermatitis occurs when an irritative substance is in fleeting or chronic contact with the vulva, resulting in an immediate reaction such as stinging or pruritus. Resolution usually occurs within a short time of removal of the irritant.

Allergic dermatitis. Allergic dermatitis, by contrast, occurs 36 to 48 hours after exposure to the allergen and may persist for several days. In situ, identification and removal of the offending irritant resolves the problem. Topical lubricating agents and protective barriers such as petroleum may be recommended to lessen symptoms, and topical corticosteroids can be offered to relieve more distressing local symptoms.

Paget disease. Paget disease of the vulva may be diagnosed by biopsy of an itchy, well-demarcated erythematous lesion, most commonly seen on the labia majora, although any vulvar or perineal area may be affected. The lesion will not be relieved with corticosteroid treatment. A coexisting adenocarcinoma of the vulva, breast, gastrointestinal tract, or genitourinary tract will be present 10% to 20% of the time, and appropriate evaluation should be undertaken. Treatment is by excision, but recurrence is common. Referral to appropriate specialists who handle this condition is recommended.

Vulvar masses

Vulvar masses in the postmenopausal woman share the same differential as in a younger population.

- *Epidermal inclusion cysts* are subcutaneous, smooth, mobile, and nontender. Size varies, but growth is generally slow. No treatment is necessary, but if the patient is experiencing discomfort or requests treatment, excision or incision and drainage is recommended. Needle aspiration is not recommended because it may introduce bacteria, causing local abscess or cellulitis, and lesions tend to recur.

- *Bartholin gland cysts and abscesses*. Bartholin glands (greater vestibular glands) are located at both sides of the introitus and provide vaginal lubrication. Bartholin cysts present as swelling in the posterior labia minor, deep to the perineal body. Noninfected cysts are nontender, whereas infected cysts (Bartholin gland abscesses) are extremely tender. Although nontender cysts in young women require no treatment, biopsy is recommended if they develop in postmenopause or if a preexisting cyst exhibits postmenopausal growth. Bartholin abscesses need to be incised and drained at any age, and as in Bartholin cysts, in a postmenopausal population biopsies of any solid region or the cyst wall should be undertaken. Recurrent Bartholin cysts should be excised, and concern for malignancy should be raised when these occur in a postmenopausal woman.

- *Condylomata acuminatum* (genital wart) is caused by human papillomavirus. Genital warts can be asymptomatic or cause itching and irritation. Treatment includes physician-applied topical agents such as trichloracetic acid or podophyllum or patient-applied therapies such as imiquimod or podofilox. Diffuse or recurrent warts may require laser or surgical removal. Sexual contacts should receive treatment if they have visible lesions.

Other vulvar masses include hidradenomas, fibromas, and lipomas. Rare tumors such as syringomas or schwannomas also may be seen. Larger masses need surgical excision for therapeutic or diagnostic purposes. Referral to gynecologic oncologists for wide local excision may be necessary for masses of undetermined etiology.

Vulvovaginal examination

As with all medical encounters, a complete medical history should precede the vulvovaginal examination. In women with vulvovaginal complaints, the history should include

CHAPTER 3

onset, duration, predominant symptom, and prior treatment, including OTC remedies. Discharge should be described, and timing in relation to menopause and sexual activity can help guide diagnosis. Existing medical conditions, medications, and surgical treatment, including prior cancer or cancer treatment, should be reviewed. Sexual history, complaints, activity, and partner status provide important information for diagnosis and may help guide treatment. Prior or current sexual abuse may alert the physician to the need for psychological referral or evaluation. Extragenital lesions or symptoms should be sought. Special attention should be paid to any possible vulvar irritants, such as new hygiene products, including a review of anything that comes into contact with the vulva (Table 12).

A complete physical examination includes evaluation for concomitant disease and a close evaluation for extragenital skin lesions, including those on the oral mucosa. Vulvovaginal inspection begins with evaluation of the external genitalia, introitus, and perineum. Any plaques, skin thickening, discoloration, or lesions are noted. Architectural changes or scars, fissures or erythema, and masses or inflamed or infected glands should be sought. A cotton swab is used to check for vulvodynia. Bleeding or discomfort with speculum insertion should be recorded. Vaginal atrophy is assessed by the presence of vaginal pallor, friability, petechiae, and loss of rugae. Vaginal pH, wet preps, and cultures are obtained as appropriate. Bimanual examination is performed as usual, and tenderness, nodularity, or mass noted.

Biopsy of any white, pigmented, thickened, or nonresponding vulvar lesion is necessary not only for accurate diagnosis but also to rule out a premalignant or malignant condition.

Results from the physical examination and laboratory evaluations guide treatment. Referral to specialists with special expertise in vulvar complaints may be necessary in difficult, resilient, or recurrent cases.

Other urinary tract clinical issues

Urinary complaints become more common during perimenopause and postmenopause. However, these urinary complaints are not an inevitable result of aging and should not be considered normal.

Urinary incontinence

Urinary incontinence is a common, socially restricting, and costly problem, particularly in middle-aged and older women. Prevalence estimates in midlife women range from about 5% for severe incontinence to 60% for mild incontinence. Cross-sectional epidemiologic studies have reported an increase in the prevalence of incontinence among women aged 45 to 55 years, an age range that coincides with the menopause transition.[176,177] However, longitudinal studies have shown that the development or worsening of incontinence is not associated with advancing menopause stages. Although women are more likely to report mild incontinence symptoms in early perimenopause, incontinence symptoms decline in the first 5 years after menopause.[178,179]

Traditionally, incontinence has been considered a symptom of urogenital atrophy related to the reduction in endogenous estrogens during menopause. However, studies do not support this.[180] Estradiol levels and short-term (year-to-year) reductions in estradiol levels have not been shown to be associated with developing incontinence during the menopause transition.[181] Over the entire menopause transition, women who have steeper declines in their endogenous estrogen levels appear less likely to complain of incontinence symptoms.[182] Systemic estrogen treatment in postmenopause has been shown to worsen incontinence.[183,184]

Table 12. Possible Causes of Vulvovaginal Complaints

- Vaginal infection, including candida (yeast) and trichomonas
- Bacterial vaginosis (overgrowth of certain vaginal bacteria)
- Sexually transmitted infections
- Allergic reactions to chemicals in soaps, bubble baths, spermicides, condoms, feminine hygiene sprays, deodorant tampons and pads
- Douching
- Irritation from tampons or birth control devices (eg, diaphragm or cervical cap) left inside the vagina too long
- Trauma
- Foreign body
- Skin conditions such as eczema or lichen sclerosus
- Certain diseases (eg, inflammatory bowel disease, diabetes mellitus, lupus erythematosus)
- Benign and malignant tumors
- Psychological causes
- Injury to pelvic nerve fibers, leading to persistent vulvar pain
- Vulvodynia
- Certain endocrine therapies (eg, aromatase inhibitors)
- Certain medications (eg, antibiotics) that contribute to candida
- Hypoestrogenic states (eg, perimenopause and postmenopause, primary ovarian insufficiency)
- Medically induced menopause (eg, cancer treatment)

Some factors that have been associated with incontinence include age, DM, obesity, weight gain, parity, depression, hysterectomy, and family history.[185-187] Urinary incontinence can be classified into different types:

- **Stress incontinence.** Stress incontinence is defined as involuntary loss of urine that occurs with an activity that increases intra-abdominal pressure such as coughing or sneezing. Leakage is usually in drops, unless it is severe. Stress incontinence is thought to be related to poor urethral support (urethral hypermobility), urethral sphincter weakness (intrinsic sphincter deficiency), and/or dysfunction of the pelvic floor (levator ani) muscles.
- **Urgency incontinence.** Urgency incontinence is defined as involuntary loss of urine preceded by a sensation of urgency to urinate. It is generally associated with losses of larger volumes of urine that soak through pads and clothing. Urgency incontinence results from detrusor (bladder) overactivity—uninhibited contractions of the detrusor muscle (smooth muscle of the bladder wall).
- **Mixed incontinence.** Mixed incontinence includes stress and urgency incontinence symptoms.
- **Extraurethral incontinence.** Extraurethral incontinence is the result of an abnormal opening from the bladder such as a vesicovaginal fistula that might occur as a complication of bladder injury during a hysterectomy. It is the least common type of incontinence.

Although up to half of midlife and older women report having urinary incontinence, less than 50% seek evaluation and treatment. Embarrassment, the misconception that incontinence is a normal part of aging, and lack of awareness about effective treatment options are the main reasons women cite for not seeking care.[188] Even if a cure is not possible, clinicians can offer treatments or advice that can significantly improve incontinence symptoms.

Diagnosing the causes, types, and effects of a woman's urinary incontinence requires a careful assessment of her symptoms, medical history (including medications), surgical history, sexual history, a physical examination (including a pelvic examination), and a urinalysis and urine culture. In some cases, additional specialized studies such as urodynamic testing may be indicated. Every woman with incontinence should be asked specific questions about her symptoms (Table 13).

Additionally, because urinary incontinence is often associated with other pelvic floor disorders that are common in midlife and older women (pelvic organ prolapse and defecatory dysfunction [constipation, fecal urgency, and anal incontinence]), incontinent women should be questioned about whether they have these symptoms or conditions.

One of the best tools to evaluate a woman's complaint of urinary incontinence is a 3-day urinary diary. The diary can help the clinician determine the frequency and type of incontinence symptoms, associated urinary complaints such as urinary frequency, and exacerbating factors such as excessive consumption of fluids or caffeine (Table 14).

Other important information, particularly for frail elderly women who may be at risk of falling, includes proximity to toilet facilities during the day and at night.

The physical examination should include

- Assessment of mental status
- Assessment of mobility (immobility may contribute to a woman's inability to reach the toilet)
- Neurologic screening examination focusing on the sacral nerves, including perineal sensation and assessment of anal sphincter tone (to rule out rare neurologic causes of incontinence)
- Inspection and palpation of the anterior vaginal wall and urethra (screen for urethral abnormalities such as a diverticulum)

Table 13. Standard Questions for Evaluating Urinary Symptoms

- How long have you had urinary incontinence or leaking urine?
- How many times do you urinate during the day? (frequency)
- How often do you wake up at night to urinate? (nocturia)
- Do you worry that you cannot get to the bathroom in time? (urgency)
- Do you ever have the urge to urinate and lose your urine before you are able to reach the toilet? (urgency incontinence)
- Do you leak urine when coughing, sneezing, walking, or lifting? (stress incontinence)

Table 14. Information to Include in a Urinary Diary

- Type and amount of fluid intake and time of day
- Circumstances of each leakage episode (urgency on the way to the toilet or leakage with coughing, sneezing, or exercise) and time of day
- Amount of urine leaked (a few drops, wet underwear, soaked clothing) with each episode
- Use of external protection (pads), including quantity and how wet the pad is when changed
- Amount of urine voided and time of day can be helpful in some situations (normal total 24-h urine volume is 1.0 L to 1.5 L)

- Inspection of the vulva and vagina for infection, discharge, and pelvic organ prolapse
- Assessment of strength and ability to isolate the levator ani muscles (ability to do a Kegel exercise)
- Assessment for urine leakage with provocation, such as coughing or sneezing

Measuring a postvoid residual urine volume within 15 minutes of voiding is recommended, especially with concomitant pelvic organ prolapse, complaints of voiding dysfunction, or abnormal neurologic signs and symptom, to evaluate for incomplete bladder emptying. A urinalysis can help identify potential medical causes for incontinence.[189] For example, the presence of hematuria may suggest bladder pathology (bladder stone or bladder cancer) and should be investigated. A urine culture can identify the presence of infection, which can cause or worsen incontinence symptoms.

Chronic dampness of underwear is sometimes mistaken for incontinence when the cause is an increase or change in vaginal secretions or perineal perspiration. A trial of phenazopyridine HCl, which will color the urine orange, may help differentiate urine from watery vaginal secretions.

Management of urinary incontinence. Most incontinence can be successfully treated or managed on the basis of the clinician's impression of incontinence type from an initial history and physical examination and without the need for urodynamic testing.

After neurologic and intrinsic bladder etiologies for urinary incontinence have been ruled out by a screening neurologic examination and urinalysis, and after any bladder infection has been treated, treatment (Table 15) can be targeted to type of incontinence.

For women with mixed incontinence, the most troublesome type of symptoms should be addressed first. Treatment of incontinence depends on the significance of incontinence to the woman's quality of life, not necessarily on how often she leaks or if she needs to wear pads for protection. Modifiable factors that cause or worsen incontinence (excessive fluid intake, obesity, uncontrolled cough) should be considered and addressed first or at least early in treatment.[190,191]

Strategies for stress and urgency incontinence:

- *Incontinence pads.* Women with severe incontinence should be encouraged to use incontinence pads, not menstrual pads. They provide better absorbency and better skin protection.
- *Fluid restriction.* For women who consume large volumes of fluid, limiting total fluid intake to about 64 oz per day can significantly reduce the number of leakage episodes. However, there is a theoretical risk that concentrated urine is irritating to the bladder, so overrestriction should be discouraged.

Table 15. Medications Approved in North America for the Treatment of Urge Urinary Incontinence

Medication	Dosage
Darifenacin	7.5-15 mg/d
Fesoterodine fumarate[a]	4-8 mg/d
Oxybutynin chloride[a]	2.5-5 mg 1-3 times/d
Extended release	5-15 mg/d
Patch	Change twice weekly
Solifenacin	5-10 mg/d
Tolterodine tartrate	1-2 mg 1-2 times/d
Extended release	2-4 mg/d
Trospium chloride[a]	20 mg 1-2 times/d

a. Available in the United States but not Canada.

- *Weight loss.* For overweight or obese women, weight loss has been shown to reduce the frequency of incontinence episodes by up to 70%.[192]
- *Timed voiding.* A woman is instructed to void at regular intervals by the clock rather than waiting for the physical sensation of the urge to urinate. This can avoid the urgency incontinence episodes and reduce the amount of urine in the bladder, which may decrease the frequency of stress incontinence episodes. This technique is especially useful for women who void infrequently or who have dementia.

Strategies and treatments for stress incontinence:

- *Cough suppression.* Smokers should be encouraged to quit smoking, and women with poorly controlled asthma or allergies should have these conditions optimally treated.
- *Incontinence pessaries.* Some women have excellent results from being fitted with incontinence pessaries. These can be worn at all times or just during the activities that induce incontinence (running or aerobics).
- *Pelvic floor exercises.* Pelvic floor muscle (levator ani) strengthening exercises, commonly called Kegels, can improve stress incontinence by increasing the strength, bulk, and coordination of the levator ani. Women have reported up to 70% improvement in incontinence episodes when doing these exercises. For Kegel instruction, women should not be asked to stop their urine flow but rather to contract the muscles they would use to delay a bowel movement. To help women who have difficulty isolating the pelvic floor muscles, Kegels can also be taught by trained clinicians (physical therapists, nurse continence advisors, or nurse practitioners) with the use of biofeedback, electrical stimulation, or vaginal cones. Women should also be taught to coordinate a pelvic floor

muscle contraction at the time of a cough or sneeze. This maneuver can also prevent stress incontinence episodes.

- *Medications.* There are no FDA-approved medications for the treatment of stress incontinence. Duloxetine, a serotonin and noradrenaline reuptake inhibitor, is approved in Canada and European countries for this use but has been used off label in the United States; the effectiveness of this medication is limited.[193] Systemic menopausal HT or local ET does not help stress incontinence and may exacerbate it by uncertain mechanisms, including uterine weight or remodeling of suburethral collagen.[194]
- *Surgery.* For women who have the diagnosed sign of stress incontinence and have failed more conservative treatments, surgery is an option.[195] Several surgical procedures are currently available. The most effective surgical treatment has an approximate 85% success rate (either cured or significantly improved). The long-term outcomes (>5 years) of stress incontinence surgeries have not been well studied.

Strategies and treatments for urgency incontinence:

- *Avoid caffeine.* Beverages high in caffeine (coffee, cola soft drinks) can contribute to urgency incontinence by their diuretic effect and possibly by irritating the bladder mucosa.
- *Improving mobility or toilet access.* In frail elderly persons, urgency incontinence has been associated with falls and fractures. Working to either improve mobility or providing a bedside commode may help reduce leaking accidents and prevent other morbidity.
- *Bladder retraining.* First, women must be able to isolate and contract their pelvic floor muscles, so training in Kegel exercises is required. Women are then taught to contract these muscles at the first sensation of urge. Because a levator ani contraction sends negative feedback to the detrusor muscle, this technique can suppress the detrusor contraction and prevent leakage. Women who have urinary frequency can also suppress the urge to urinate, thus extending the intervals between voids. Bladder retraining has been found to be the most effective method for treating urgency incontinence.[196]
- *Medications.* The most effective medications to treat urgency incontinence are anticholinergic agents, all government approved for this indication (Table 15). These agents work to decrease the frequency and intensity of detrusor contractions. The main AEs of these medications are dry mouth and constipation. If urgency incontinence is not adequately controlled, the drug dosage can be increased every 3 to 5 days until clinical improvement is seen or until the woman experiences AEs. Caution should be used when prescribing anticholinergic drugs to older women because these drugs have been shown to increase cognitive impairment. Imipramine HCl (10-25 mg 1-3 times/d) is a medication used off label to control nocturnal urgency incontinence but should be used with caution in older women because of possible drowsiness and dizziness (which could be concerning if patient gets up in the middle of the night), as well as mental cloudiness and confusion. Local vaginal ET is used by many clinicians in women with urgency incontinence and vaginal atrophy, although the evidence of benefit is not clear.
- *Sacral neuromodulation stimulation.* For women whose urgency incontinence does not respond to other treatments, sacral neuromodulation stimulation (InterStim) is another option. This system stimulates the sacral nerve root to modulate neural reflexes influencing bladder storage and emptying. An impulse generator is surgically implanted under the skin in the upper buttock area and attached to 4 leads placed into the sacral nerve space at S3. The effectiveness of InterStim for urgency incontinence ranges from about 39% to 65%, depending on the definition of improvement.[197]
- *Botulinum A injections.* Another option for women whose urge incontinence does not respond to basic treatments is injection of botulinum A via cystoscopy, a newer option. Improvement is noted in about 60% of women.[198]

Referral to a urologist or urogynecologist is appropriate for women with

- Complex problems, such as neurologic conditions, pelvic organ prolapse, or a history of previous incontinence surgery
- Combined incontinence and recurrent bladder infections
- Extreme personal distress secondary to incontinence
- Failure of nonsurgical treatments

Overactive bladder syndrome

Overactive bladder (OAB) syndrome consists of idiopathic urinary urgency (with or without incontinence), usually with urinary frequency (>8 voids/24 h) and nocturia (awakening to urinate >2 times/night), without a clear cause. Because OAB is a diagnosis based on patient-reported symptoms and exclusion of other etiologies, the evaluation includes ruling out specific causes of urgency, frequency, and nocturia symptoms.

The estimated prevalence of these symptoms in population-based studies of men and women is about 12%. The incidence increases with age and is associated with urinary incontinence; up to 50% of women aged older than 50 years with urinary incontinence report OAB symptoms.[199] These symptoms have a negative effect on a woman's quality of life and lead to coping behaviors such as always knowing the location of a toilet (toilet mapping) and decreased fluid intake. Women with nocturia can have poor sleep.

Because OAB is a diagnosis based on symptoms, it can have a number of etiologies. The differential diagnosis for symptoms includes behavioral causes, neuromuscular

Chapter 3

disorders, UTIs, interstitial cystitis (also called painful bladder syndrome), urethral causes, polyuria, and other bladder causes (Table 16).[200,201]

Interstitial cystitis most commonly presents in women aged 30 to 40 years and is characterized by bladder pain in conjunction with urgency and frequency symptoms. The cause of this condition is unclear, although many treatments are targeted at what seems to be a deficient/damaged bladder epithelium. With interstitial cystitis, bladder capacity is often small (maximal <350 mL), and the bladder walls can become noncompliant. Evidence of inflammation or bleeding into the bladder walls can be seen on cystoscopy.[202]

Urethral diverticulum is a rare cause of urinary symptoms. Isolated urethritis is uncommon in women; causes of urethritis include infections (particularly sexually transmitted infections) and trauma (such as after catheterization). Also, the urethra shortens with age, decreasing its defense against bacteria. Urethral syndrome is a diagnosis given for chronic urethral irritation without a clear etiology and can include symptoms of urinary urgency and frequency.

Evaluation for OAB is similar to the evaluation for urinary incontinence (Table 13).

A urinary diary that details the type and amount of fluid intake and the number of voids during the day and night and that measures the amount of urine produced in a day can help diagnose urgency and frequency symptoms related to behavior, such as excessive fluid and/or caffeine intake (Table 14). Asking women about bladder pain can help to distinguish OAB from interstitial cystitis. Women with interstitial cystitis generally have chronic midline pelvic pain or pain with a full bladder (Table 17).

As with incontinence, measuring a postvoid residual within 15 minutes of voiding is recommended, especially with concomitant pelvic organ prolapse or abnormal neurologic signs and symptoms, to evaluate for incomplete bladder emptying. A urinalysis can help identify potential medical causes for the symptom of urinary urgency. For example, the presence of hematuria may suggest bladder pathology (a stone or bladder cancer) and should be investigated. A urine culture can identify the presence of infection, which can be a cause of urgency and frequency symptoms or worsen OAB. Other investigations, such as cystoscopy, may be used in some women who do not respond to treatment or who have unusual symptoms or signs.

Management of overactive bladder. Once a woman has been screened for common and serious causes of urinary urgency, frequency, and nocturia symptoms, treatment of OAB can be initiated. Because urge incontinence is considered a symptom of OAB (sometimes called "OAB wet"), refer to specific treatments for urge incontinence to treat OAB. Treatment for OAB without incontinence (sometimes called "OAB dry") has similar treatment recommendations. All the anticholinergic medications available for urge incontinence can be used for overactive bladder without incontinence in the same dosages and schedule.[203] In one study, an estradiol ring compared favorably with oxybutynin.[204] Treatment options for OAB with urinary urgency incontinence refractory to oral antimuscarinics include botulinum toxin type A, sacral neuromodulation, and augmentation cystoplasty.[205]

Table 16. Differential Diagnosis for Urinary Urgency, Frequency, and Nocturia Symptoms

Behavioral	Excessive fluid (often associated with dieting) or caffeine intake. Caffeine is a diuretic and may increase detrusor muscle excitability. Drinking fluids just before bedtime can lead to nocturia.
Neuromuscular disorders	Because women with OAB symptoms respond to pelvic floor physical therapy suggests a musculoskeletal etiology. Rarely, neurologic diseases such as multiple sclerosis can present with urgency and frequency symptoms.
Urinary tract infection	Recurrent UTIs, bladder infection, and infectious cystitis are the most common diagnoses.
Interstitial cystitis (painful bladder syndrome)	Characterized by bladder pain in conjunction with urgency and frequency symptoms.
Urethral causes	Urethral diverticulum, isolated urethritis, urethral syndrome.
Polyuria	Causes of excessive urine production include diuretic use, uncontrolled type 2 DM, psychogenic polydipsia, and hypercalcemia.
Other bladder causes	Bladder stones, intrinsic bladder tumors, or extrinsic pelvic masses (uterine fibroids, ovarian tumors) that may be causing compression of the bladder.

Abbreviations: DM, diabetes mellitus; OAB, overactive bladder; UTIs, urinary tract infections.

Nonpharmacologic strategies include fluid restriction, avoiding bladder irritants, pelvic floor physical therapy,[206] and bladder retraining. At least 1 study suggests that acupuncture may improve OAB symptoms.[207]

Whether estrogen by any route is effective in treating OAB is not clear.[208]

Anal incontinence

Approximately 11% of all women report anal incontinence—defined as the loss of anal sphincter control leading to involuntary leakage of gas or solid or liquid stool sufficient to impair the individual's quality of life.[164] Up to 17% of midlife women with other pelvic floor disorders, such as urinary incontinence, also report anal incontinence.

Anatomic defects (incompletely healed anal sphincter tears usually from third- or fourth-degree obstetric lacerations) and neurologic damage (denervation of the anal sphincter related to childbirth and aging) can lead to anal incontinence. Loss of solid or liquid stool may also arise from intrinsic bowel problems such as inflammatory bowel disease, malabsorption syndromes, colonic polyps, and hemorrhoids.

In midlife women, evaluation of anal incontinence starts with a diet review and may include colonoscopy, endoanal ultrasonography, and evaluation for anal sphincter denervation.

Treatment for anal incontinence should be approached initially with dietary changes (bulking stool with fiber), antidiarrheal agents (loperamide, diphenoxylate/atropine), and pelvic floor physical therapy. Most women respond to these measures.[209] Refractory anal incontinence may require sacral nerve stimulation or anal sphincter repair.[210]

Sexual function

Sexual desire decreases with age in both sexes, and low desire is particularly common in women aged in their late 40s and 50s. Sexual concerns are often an issue for women at midlife and beyond, although they frequently are not reported to healthcare professionals. Data from the PRESIDE (Prevalence of Female Sexual Problems Associated with Distress and Determinants of Treatment Seeking) study confirm that sexual problems are highly prevalent. They are reported in approximately 40% of US women, with 12% reporting a sexual problem associated with personal distress.[211] Although sexual problems generally increase with age, distressing sexual problems peak in midlife women and are lowest in women aged 65 years and older.[212]

Epidemiologic data indicate that between one-third and one-half of perimenopausal and postmenopausal women experience a problem with 1 or more aspects of sexual functioning. These include problems with sexual desire, arousal, orgasmic response, and sexual pain. When these difficulties are associated with clinically significant personal distress, they are classified in the *Diagnostic and Statistical Manual of Mental Disorders*, 5th edition (DSM-5), as female interest/arousal disorder (formerly categorized as *hypoactive sexual desire disorder* and *female sexual arousal disorder* in the fourth edition; Table 18).[213]

Menopause contributes to sexual function changes through decreases in ovarian hormone production. The effect of lower hormone levels varies from woman to woman, presumably because changes in sexual function are multifactorial in nature. A range of psychological, sociocultural, interpersonal, and biologic factors also contribute to sexual disorders at midlife (Table 19).

Some perimenopausal and postmenopausal women experience symptoms such as vaginal dryness, dyspareunia, and urinary urgency (GSM), with urogenital atrophy.[139]

Changes in the epithelial lining of the vagina occur relatively rapidly as estrogen levels decline with menopause. Subsequent changes in glandular, vascular, nervous, muscular, and connective tissues of the internal and external genitalia and pelvic floor occur over time, which can adversely affect sexual function. Decreased secretions from vaginal glands and transudate from the subepithelial vasculature reduce engorgement and lubrication. The vagina loses its elasticity, which can result in discomfort during sexual activity.[139] Decreased clitoral blood flow and neuronal changes with impaired perception of touch and vibration may cause delayed or absent orgasms and a reduction in overall sexual satisfaction.

Decreased estrogen is responsible for most of these changes, but testosterone also is an important factor in midlife sexual changes for women. Testosterone contributes to sex drive in women, playing a role in motivation, desire, and sexual sensation. Testosterone levels decline gradually with age, so that by the time women reach age 70, their

Table 17. Screening for Causes of Urgency and Frequency Symptoms

- Neurologic screening examination focusing on the sacral nerves, including perineal sensation and assessment of anal sphincter tone (to rule out rare neurologic causes of incontinence).
- Inspection and palpation of the anterior vaginal wall and urethra (screen for urethral abnormalities such as a diverticulum and urethritis). Pain on palpation of the anterior vaginal wall (bladder) is suggestive of interstitial cystitis.
- Inspection of the urethra, vulva, and vagina for infection, discharge, and pelvic organ prolapse.
- Bimanual examination to rule out a pelvic mass.
- Assessment of pelvic floor muscles: tenderness, strength, and ability to isolate the levator ani muscles (ability to do a Kegel exercise).

testosterone levels are approximately half of what they were in their early 20s.[214] There is no abrupt decline in testosterone at menopause.

As estrogen levels decrease at menopause, so do levels of sex hormone-binding globulin (SHBG), which binds estrogen and testosterone in the circulation. As a result, some women may experience increased sexual desire and activity, perhaps because the declining levels of SHBG increase concentrations of free testosterone.

Desire and other components of sexual health

One of the most significant and universal changes that occurs with age is a decrease in the drive component of sexual desire. Desire refers to a person's interest in being sexual and is determined by the interaction of 3 related but separate components: drive; beliefs, values, and expectations; and motivation.

- **Drive.** The biologic component of desire is drive, resulting from neuroendocrine mechanisms. Drive is typically manifested by sexual thoughts, feelings, fantasies, or dreams; increased erotic attraction to others in proximity; seeking out sexual activity (alone or with a partner); and genital tingling or increased genital sensitivity. Drive declines in men and women as a function of aging, although the exact neuroendocrine mechanisms responsible for drive are not fully understood.

  For some women, lower levels of free testosterone, related to reduced ovarian and adrenal function with aging or surgical menopause, may result in a noticeable decrease in sexual drive, although this effect is not clearly supported by research. Other hormones and neurotransmitters that may be implicated in the sexual response cycle include dopamine, serotonin, norepinephrine, melanocortins, oxytocin, and opioids. Further data are needed to elucidate the exact role of these components.

- **Beliefs, values, and expectations.** The second component of desire reflects a person's beliefs, values, and expectations about sexual activity. The more positive a person's beliefs and values are about sexuality, the greater his or her desire to behave sexually.

- **Motivation.** The third component, psychological and interpersonal motivation, is driven by emotional and relationship factors and is characterized by the willingness of a person to behave sexually with a given partner. This component tends to have the greatest effect overall on desire and is the most complex and elusive.

For many women, particularly postmenopausal women, drive diminishes and may no longer be the initial step in the sexual response cycle. The classic Masters and Johnson model first developed in 1966 describes a linear model of sexual response—desire leading to arousal and plateau, then to orgasm and resolution.[215] An alternative model to understanding the sexual response cycle suggests that for many women desire comes after arousal and that many women begin sexual encounters from a point of sexual neutrality.[216] Arousal may come from a conscious decision or as a result of an environmental cue, including seduction or suggestion from a partner. A woman's sexual response patterns may vary between models, depending on the duration of the relationship and stage of life.

The Massachusetts Women's Health Study II, a large, population-based study, showed that a woman's menopause status has a smaller effect on sexual functioning than such

Table 18. *DSM-5* Diagnostic Criteria for Female Sexual Interest/Arousal Disorder

Criterion	Symptom
A	• Absent or reduced interest in sexual activity • Absent or reduced sexual thoughts or fantasies • No or reduced initiation of sexual activity; unreceptive to partner's attempts • Absent or reduced sexual excitement or pleasure during sexual activity in almost all (75%-100%) sexual encounters • Absent or reduced sexual interest to any internal or external sexual cues (written, verbal, visual) • Absent or reduced genital or nongenital sensations during sexual activity in almost all (75%-100%) sexual encounters
B	Symptoms in criterion A have persisted for approximately 6 months
C	Symptoms in criterion A cause clinically significant distress
D	The sexual dysfunction is not better explained by a nonsexual mental disorder or as a consequence of severe relationship distress (eg, partner violence) and is not attributable to a medical condition

Abbreviation: *DSM-5, Diagnostic and Statistical Manual of Mental Disorders*, 5th edition.
American Psychiatric Association.[213]

Clinical Issues

Table 19. Potential Factors Influencing a Woman's Sexual Function

- *Previous attitudes toward sex.* In general, women who enjoyed sex in their younger years will continue to do so during perimenopause and postmenopause. Those who have not enjoyed sex previously may view any midlife reduction in sexual activity as a relief rather than a loss. Some women, however, have an increased interest in sex as they reach menopause.
- *No available partner.* Women may lose a partner through illness, death, or divorce.
- *Partner's loss of interest in sex.* A partner may have decreased interest in or capacity for sexual activity because of illness, aging, or erectile dysfunction.
- *Partner's renewed interest in sex.* A male partner's ability to once again achieve erections with erectile dysfunction therapy (sildenafil, tadalafil, vardenafil) may result in improved sexual satisfaction for some women but also may cause extreme vaginal discomfort because of lack of vaginal lubrication and elasticity resulting from having had no intercourse for months or years.
- *Age-related changes.* With aging, sexual drive generally decreases gradually in men and women. However, a lower sex drive does not mean sexual activity ceases, and the rate and extent of any decline and its effect on sexual activity are individual.
- *Body image.* Menopause usually occurs at a time when women are experiencing changes in their physical appearance. Women who accept these changes and maintain a positive outlook about their bodies may not experience related sexual changes. In contrast, those who perceive aging as unattractive often feel undesirable, with decreased interest in sex.
- *Health concerns.* Women with cancer, heart disease, arthritis, diabetes mellitus, or any major medical illness often experience fatigue, discomfort, and anxiety related to their health problems, adversely affecting sex. After surgical procedures such as removal of a breast or the uterus, radiation, or chemotherapy, a woman may feel less feminine or unattractive and may avoid initiating sexual encounters. Also, her partner may be affected by changes in her body and/or fearful that sexual activity will cause her pain.
- *Psychological problems.* Depression, and anxiety are common causes of decreased sexual interest and response. Past physical or sexual abuse and substance abuse also adversely affect sexual function.
- *Weight gain.* Many midlife women gain weight unless they are careful about their diet and exercise regularly. This change in appearance may decrease sexual interest.
- *Incontinence.* Involuntary loss of urine or stool, especially during sexual activity, can lead to sexual avoidance.
- *Sleep disturbances.* Sleep problems, sometimes secondary to vasomotor symptoms and night sweats, often result in fatigue and irritability, reducing sexual desire.
- *Stressors.* Midlife women often experience significant stress from work, relationships, and family (adolescent children, midlife partners, and aging parents).
- *Medications.* Some drugs, such as antidepressants (especially SSRIs) and possibly antihypertensives, can decrease sexual desire and orgasmic capacity.
- *Diminished estrogen and androgen levels.* Low estrogen levels with menopause may reduce sexual interest and pleasure by causing vaginal dryness and/or bothersome vasomotor symptoms. Reduced androgen levels with aging also may adversely affect sexual function.

Abbreviation: SSRIs, selective serotonin-reuptake inhibitors.

factors as health, sociodemographic variables, psychological issues, a partner's health and sexual disorders, and lifestyle.[217] Although menopause was significantly associated with several aspects of sexual function, including reduced sexual desire and arousal, the effect was not as great as that of other factors.

The Melbourne Women's Midlife Health Project found that the major factors affecting women's sexuality were feelings for their partners and sexual difficulties experienced by their partners.[218] Other variables such as work or interpersonal stress and educational level also affect sexual function.

Low estrogen levels at menopause have been associated with a decline in sexual function. Estrogen loss often leads to GSM, which consists of urogenital atrophy, vaginal dryness, and dyspareunia.[139] These changes typically appear during perimenopause but are more common during the first few years after menopause and progress with time if untreated. During the menopause transition, hot flashes can

Chapter 3

result in chronic sleep disturbance, with resulting fatigue and psychological disturbances. Negative changes in mood and well-being likely contribute to the sexual disorders associated with menopause. During perimenopause and postmenopause, untreated anxiety or depression, whether new or preexisting, may have a negative effect on sexual function. During midlife, many social issues also may affect sexual function (ie, personal or partner retirement or career change, "empty nest syndrome" [after children leave the home], or divorce or separation).

Some experts believe that diminished estrogen effects on the cardiovascular system (impairing arterial blood flow) or central and peripheral nervous systems (impairing touch and vibration perception) contribute to reduced sexual desire and responsiveness in menopausal women.

Although declining androgens are often thought to be a cause of sexual problems for women, a clear association between decreased androgen levels and impaired female sexual function is not supported by evidence. Not all women with low testosterone levels experience symptoms, and many women with sexual problems have normal androgen levels. Several large studies using quality hormone assays and validated sexual function measures have not identified an association between testosterone levels and sexual problems.[219] This lack of an association should not be unexpected, because female sexuality and female sexual interest/arousal disorder are complex and cannot be summed up by a single biologic marker. Even when low androgen levels may contribute to a sexual problem, lifestyle, relationship, medical, and psychological factors remain critically important.[220]

Low progesterone levels at menopause seem to have no AEs on sexual function, although some types of progestogen therapy can indirectly affect sexual function and sexual activity by negatively influencing mood or by causing irregular uterine bleeding.

Evaluation of sexual function

It is important that healthcare professionals encourage their patients to discuss any sexual concerns. A sexual history should focus on the conditions or circumstances that affect sexual function and should be confidential and nonjudgmental (Table 20). Clinicians should phrase questions carefully and not assume that a woman is necessarily heterosexual or monogamous. For example, the NAMS Menopause Health Questionnaire contains several questions addressing sexuality and may assist healthcare professionals in gathering critical information (Table 21).[221]

In addition to a thorough history, clinicians may obtain more detailed sexual function information by using 1 of a wide variety of validated instruments.[222] The Watts Sexual Function Questionnaire focuses on 4 subscales: desire, arousal, orgasm, and satisfaction.[223] The Female Sexual Function Index is a brief, self-report measure of 6 domains including desire, subjective arousal, lubrication, orgasm, satisfaction, and pain associated with intercourse.[224] Several other instruments of varying quality and validity to measure sexual function, interest, or desire are available.[225]

Improving all potential physical, psychological, relationship, and lifestyle factors amenable to intervention should be the primary therapeutic goal for women with sexual concerns. Clinicians should evaluate and address potential causes of decreased libido and response, including depression, anxiety, fatigue, stress, relationship conflict, vaginal

---

Table 20. Areas of Focus for a Sexual History

- Gynecologic history
  - Menstrual history
  - Bleeding patterns
  - Incontinence
  - Pelvic pain
  - Vulvodynia
  - Vaginal dryness, dyspareunia, sexual pain
- Obstetric history
- Major medical problems
- Psychological problems
- Surgical procedures (especially involving breasts, genitalia, and pelvic organs
- Sexually transmitted infections
- Safer sex practices
- Medications (including adverse events)
- Relationships (current and past; quality and conflict)
- Sexual orientation (sexual activity with men, women, or both)
- Partner sexual function
- Substance abuse (tobacco, alcohol, illicit drugs)
- Social issues (life stress; work and family issues)
- History of physical , emotional or sexual abuse
- Concerns about aging (body image, weight gain)
- Sexual satisfaction (prior and current level of interest, arousal, orgasmic response, pleasure)
  - Factors associated with improved sexual satisfaction (vacations, date night)
  - Factors associated with reduced sexual satisfaction (fatigue, illness, lack of privacy)
  - Interventions tried to address sexual concerns and result (improved sexual satisfaction after counseling or after initiation of lubricants with intercourse)

atrophy, underlying medical problems, medications, and a partner's sexual disorders.

A physical examination, with a focus on the pelvic exam, is required as part of a thorough evaluation of any sexual concern. As vaginal changes are highly prevalent at the menopause transition and contribute to many sexual problems, all women of perimenopausal age and beyond should have an assessment of vulvovaginal health, regardless of symptoms or sexual activity. Of note, some women using low-dose systemic ET may have sexual problems related to inadequate estrogenization of the vulvovaginal tissues and may benefit from use of low-dose vaginal ET in addition to systemic ET.[104]

Management of female sexual interest/arousal disorder

Many sexual problems can be successfully treated (Table 22). Nonprescription vaginal lubricants and moisturizers are available to treat mild vaginal dryness and resulting dyspareunia; however, stimulating agents and flavors added to lubricants may be irritating to a sensitive atrophic mucosa.[139] Prescription low-dose vaginal ET is a highly effective option for moderate to severe vaginal atrophy. Vaginal ET is available by prescription as a cream, tablet, or ring. Treatment of GSM will not only address a sexual problem related to atrophy but also may prevent other problems such as secondary pelvic floor hypertonus, shortening of the vagina, and distressing problems of sexual interest, arousal, and orgasmic response from developing. Nonhormonal ospemifene (an estrogen agonist/antagonist) has been approved to treat symptoms of moderate to severe dyspareunia associated with GSM.[154]

Counseling and sex therapy. Continued sexual activity is a natural part of aging for many women. Healthcare professionals must be sensitive and informed about changes in sexual function with aging and menopause to better counsel women about recognizing and adjusting to these changes (Table 23). Confidentiality is a special concern when discussing sexual function.

A 1993 study found that only 3% of US women with sexual problems initiated discussion with their physicians.[226] However, when asked specifically about sexual function, 19% reported a problem.[212,226] A 1999 survey reinforced the importance of clinicians initiating a discussion about sexual health.[227] This survey showed that 71% of patients believed that their physicians would dismiss any mention of sexual concerns, 68% believed that their physicians would be embarrassed by any discussion of sexual problems, and 76% did not think there were any treatments available to help with sexual problems.

Counseling, cognitive behavioral therapy, and sex therapy are effective interventions for many women and couples with sexual concerns.[228] Women without sexual partners also engage in sexual activities and will benefit similarly from counseling about changes in sexual function with aging. The

Table 21. Sex-History Questions from the North American Menopause Society Health Questionnaire

Are you currently sexually active?

If yes, are you currently having sex with a man (or men)? A woman (or women)? Both men and women?

How long have you been with your current sex partner?

Are you in a committed, mutually monogamous relationship?

If not, do you use condoms (practice safe sex)?

In the past, have you had sex with a man (or men)? A woman (or women)?

Have you had any sexually transmitted infections?

Do you have concerns about your sex life?

Do you have a loss of interest in sexual activities (libido, desire)?

Do you have a loss of arousal (tingling in the genitals or breasts; vaginal moisture, warmth)?

Do you have a loss of response (weaker or absent orgasm)?

Do you have any pain with intercourse (vaginal penetration)?

If yes, how long ago did the pain start?

Please describe the pain: pain with penetration; pain inside; feels dry.

Menopause Health Questionnaire.[221]

addition of therapy often provides further benefit even when medication is being prescribed.

When counseling about hysterectomy, women and their partners need to be assured that losing the uterus does not impair sexual desire or response. After hysterectomy, some women may notice changes in sensation or orgasm during sexual activity, but most women report improved sex lives after hysterectomy because of pain relief, absence of uterine bleeding, and the lack of need for birth control. Women facing chemotherapy or pelvic radiation therapy should be counseled about the potential AEs that a cancer diagnosis and its treatments often have on sexual function.

Nonpharmacologic interventions. Modifying sexual technique, increasing sexual novelty, enhancing the partner relationship and communication, and improving health and body image are effective nonpharmacologic interventions to address sexual problems (Table 23). One study showed that a 12-week yoga program significantly improved sexual desire, arousal, orgasm, pain, and satisfaction.[229]

Pharmacologic interventions. Although ET (local and systemic) improves vaginal health and may improve sexual

Chapter 3

Table 22. Strategies for Treatment of Sexual Disorders

Nonpharmacologic interventions

- Modify sexual technique
  - Allow more time for foreplay, including manual or oral stimulation
  - Use vaginal lubricants or moisturizers
  - Explore noncoital sexual activity such as oral sex or mutual masturbation
- Increase sexual novelty
  - Experiment with erotic materials (books, videos), sexual fantasies
  - Try a sensual massage or a warm bath
  - Change the sexual routine, such as the location, position, or the time of day
  - Experiment with sexual devices (vibrators, dildos, Eros CTD)
  - Try a topical stimulating lubricant (may be irritating if urogenital atrophy)
- Enhance relationship with partner
  - Increase communication about sexual and other concerns
  - Seek counseling and/or sex therapy
  - Date nights, overnight outings, vacations
- Improve health and body image
  - Exercise
  - Healthy diet
  - Optimize weight
  - Stress reduction
  - Treat medical problems (physical therapy for incontinence, arthritis)
  - Treat psychological problems (counseling for anxiety, depression)

Pharmacologic interventions

- Treat medical problems
- Treat psychological problems
- Modify type and/or dosage of drugs that adversely affect sexual function (eg, SSRIs)
- Systemic estrogen therapy (for bothersome vasomotor symptoms)[a]
- Local vaginal estrogen therapy (for vaginal dryness and dyspareunia)
- Ospemifene (for dyspareunia secondary to vaginal atrophy)
- Androgen therapy[a]

Abbreviations: CTD, clitoral therapy device; SSRIs, selective serotonin-reuptake inhibitors.
a. Used off label for female sexual interest/arousal disorder.

function by restoring vaginal lubrication and reducing dyspareunia, its effect on libido is uncertain. No studies have confirmed a beneficial effect of ET on sexual desire. Oral estrogens, unlike transdermal estrogens, increase SHBG levels, resulting in decreased levels of free testosterone.[230] Women who experience decreased libido after initiating oral ET may benefit from switching to transdermal ET. Androgen therapy is receiving increased attention for treating postmenopausal women with sexual disorders, although its role remains unclear.

Underlying depression and anxiety should be treated, and antidepressant medication may need adjustment. Selective serotonin-reuptake inhibitors have been associated with an increase in female sexual interest/arousal disorder. Bupropion may be an effective alternative in women with sexual disorders associated with SSRIs. Although not FDA approved for this indication, bupropion also may be an effective pharmacologic agent for nondepressed women with sexual disorders. Two small, double-blind studies reported increased sexual pleasure, arousal, and orgasm in nondepressed women with distressing low desire treated with bupropion.[231,232]

Sildenafil at daily doses of 10 mg, 50 mg, and 100 mg did not improve sexual response in perimenopausal or postmenopausal women with sexual disorders, although sildenafil may benefit women who develop problems with arousal and orgasmic response on SSRIs.[233] Headaches and hot flashes are AEs of sildenafil use.[234] Women electing sildenafil to treat sexual disorders must be informed of potential risks, AEs, and off-label nature of use. Sildenafil should not be used concurrently with nitrate therapy.

Treatment of a male partner's sexual disorders may be critically important in improving a woman's sexual satisfaction. In addition, a male partner's sexual function may be directly affected by his partner's vaginal dryness and dyspareunia.

Alternatively, a couple's sexual problems may be exacerbated when the male partner is successfully treated for erectile dysfunction. If the couple has not had intercourse for months or years, the woman may have extreme vaginal discomfort because of lack of lubrication and elasticity. In some cases, a combination of vaginal ET, vaginal dilator exercises, and pelvic floor physical therapy may be required before pleasurable sexual activity can resume.

In addition to drug therapies, devices have been developed that may be helpful for some women with sexual disorders. The suction vacuum device Eros CTD is cleared by FDA for treatment of female sexual disorder.[235] Its design is similar to that of vacuum devices used for male erectile dysfunction. Theoretically, it may improve arousal and response by improving clitoral blood flow. The device is expensive and likely no more effective than less-costly devices such as vibrators, available to women without a prescription.

> **Table 23.** Suggestions for Sexual Counseling
>
> - Educate women and their partners
>   - Normal, age-related, sexual response changes in women, including diminished lubrication, need for increased time and stimulation for arousal, decreased orgasmic contractions, decreased breast fullness and nipple erection, reduced clitoral sensitivity
>   - Normal, age-related, sexual response changes in men, including decreased penile rigidity, need for increased time and stimulation for erection and orgasm, longer refractory time, and available medications for erectile dysfunction
>   - Decreased sexual interest with relationship duration and benefit of increasing novelty
> - Advise interventions to reduce effect of age-related changes on sexual pleasure and to increase novelty
>   - Warm baths before genital sexual activity
>   - Extended foreplay time to accommodate longer sexual arousal time
>   - Sexual fantasies, erotic clothing or materials (movies, literature), vibrators
>   - Experimentation with noncoital activities such as massage, oral stimulation
>   - Masturbation as an alternative to intercourse
>   - Changing sexual routines, such as having sex in the morning when energy levels are higher
>   - Positions other than the missionary position

Sleep disturbances

About 46% of US women aged 40 to 54 years and 48% aged 55 to 64 years report sleep problems, according to a 2007 National Sleep Foundation survey.[236] This survey revealed that perimenopausal and postmenopausal women sleep less, have more frequent insomnia symptoms, and are more than twice as likely to use prescription sleeping aids as premenopausal women. Most people do not voluntarily report sleep disturbances to their healthcare professionals, nor do most clinicians ask about sleep disturbances.

In a multiethnic sample of 12,603 US women aged 40 to 55 years in a community-based survey, difficulty sleeping was reported by 38% of respondents.[237] Age-adjusted rates were highest in the late perimenopausal (45.4%) and surgically postmenopausal (47.6%) groups. Among ethnic groups, rates ranged from 28% in Japanese women to 40% in white women. In the multivariate analysis, menopause status, ethnicity, VMS, psychological symptoms, self-perceived health and health behaviors, arthritis, and education were significantly associated with difficulty sleeping. Older age per se was not significantly associated with insomnia. A report based on the National Sleep Foundation survey found that sleepiness along with depressive symptoms, medical comorbidities, obesity, and less education were associated with poor self-rated health, whereas menopause status (premenopause, perimenopause, or postmenopause) was not.[238]

Poor sleep (inadequate quantity or poor quality) is associated with somatic, mood, and cognitive symptoms and performance deficits. Related symptoms include muscle aches, dysphoria, tension, irritability, fatigue, lethargy, inability to concentrate, lack of motivation, and difficulty performing tasks. It also has been linked to risk of chronic illness, especially cardiac problems and mood disorders such as depression. Increased automobile and work-related injuries are associated with excessive daytime (waking) sleepiness from multiple causes.

Insomnia includes lengthy time to fall asleep, inability to stay asleep through the night, or premature awakening without being able to resume sleep. It can be transient (a few days) or short term (no more than 3-4 wk), usually accompanying acute emotional life situations or environmental changes. Chronic or persistent insomnia (defined as occurring ≥3 nights/wk/mo or longer) may benefit from medical intervention.

Reports of insomnia increase as women transition through midlife. Perceived declines in sleep quality may be attributed to general aging effects (eg, nocturnal urination), the onset of sleep-related disorders (eg, apnea) or other illness-related disorders (eg, chronic pain conditions, depression), stress and social strain, negative mood, or ovarian hormone changes. Women in midlife are as likely to report concern about sleep difficulties as they are to report concerns about weight gain.

Menopause, hot flashes, and sleep

Although women in the menopause transition are more likely to report perceived sleep disturbance, some objective reports on sleep patterns do not indicate that perimenopause and postmenopause are associated with sleep disruption.[239-241] Sleep efficiency, a global measure representing the proportion of achieved intended sleep, rarely varies by menopause status. Most studies of menopause status and physiologic sleep reveal that disturbances emerging during the menopause transition occur mainly in women bothered by nighttime hot flashes, even though actual awake time is low. However, laboratory studies have been conflicting.

A study using a model of menopausal hot flashes reported a correlation between subjective and objective indicators of sleep disturbance.[242] Researchers used gonadotropin-releasing hormone agonist model to induce a low-estrogen state with hot flashes. The menopause model showed that nighttime VMS correlate with sleep fragmentation and are consistent with polysomnography-measured sleep interruption in the setting of menopause.

Chapter 3

The Wisconsin Sleep Cohort Study of 589 premenopausal, perimenopausal, and postmenopausal women found that postmenopausal women had the best physiologically recorded sleep and that this was somewhat worse in women who were using HT.[240] Researchers did not find evidence that hot flashes caused sleep disturbances.

Although previous studies found that hot flashes interrupt objectively measured sleep, results of other studies suggest that hot flashes may have a more limited effect on awakenings and the amount of time spent asleep. Women may perceive poor sleep quality in association with hot flashes even if there are relatively few changes in measured sleep. This type of discrepancy is common with sleep disorders and has been observed in patients with chronic insomnia unrelated to hot flashes.

The effect of hot flashes on sleep may vary according to when they occur. Hot flashes can trigger awakenings and arousals in the first, but not the second, half of the night. The lack of arousals during the second half of the night might be attributed to the predominance of rapid eye movement sleep, which occurs at that time and suppresses thermoregulation. Motor movements expend energy, which also elicits a thermoregulatory response. Awakenings increase norepinephrine levels, which also alter the thermoneutral zone in which body temperature changes occur without eliciting a thermoregulatory response. Thus, there may be an interaction among hot flashes, thermoregulation, and related neural activity.

Two studies support the role of the sympathetic system in the etiology of hot flashes and their effects on sleep. In the first investigation, researchers found increased spectral power in the frequency bin of 0 Hz to .15 Hz, indicating increased sympathetic activation during hot flashes compared with nonflash periods.[243] This occurred mainly during waking and stage 1 sleep. A second study also analyzing heart rate variability found reduced high-frequency power, indicating a decrease in vagal activity.[244]

Studies investigating common causes of sleep disturbance in midlife women have shown that primary sleep disorders (sleep apnea, restless leg syndrome—crawly and strong urge-to-move sensations) are common in this population. In a study conducted in 102 perimenopausal and postmenopausal women complaining of poor sleep, laboratory sleep recordings showed that 53% of the women had apnea, restless legs, or both.[245] The best predictors of poor objective sleep quality (sleep efficiency) were apneas, periodic limb movements (jerky, rhythmic movements of legs), and arousals. The best predictors of poor subjective sleep quality (Pittsburgh Sleep Quality Index global score) were anxiety and the number of hot flashes in the first half of the night. Amelioration of hot flashes may reduce some complaints of poor sleep but will not necessarily alleviate underlying primary sleep disorders. Because these can cause significant morbidity and mortality, they require careful evaluation and attention in this patient population.

In addition to hot flashes, there are other important causes of sleep disturbances during midlife. Women and their healthcare professionals frequently attribute sleep disturbances during perimenopause to VMS when in fact they may be the result of a primary sleep disorder or psychiatric conditions, for example. Stress and insomnia are closely linked.

Many midlife women experience significant life challenges (job-related stress, loss of life partners through divorce or death, caregiving for young or old family members, development of chronic illness).[246] Insomnia has been associated with painful chronic illnesses such as arthritis, fibromyalgia, and gastrointestinal disturbances as well as with CVD, respiratory disease, neurologic and psychiatric conditions, thyroid abnormalities, and allergies. Drugs that can disturb sleep include thyroid medication, theophylline, phenytoin, levodopa, bupropion, and SSRIs.

Sleep-disordered breathing

Characterized as the sleep apnea/hypopnea syndrome, sleep-disordered breathing (SDB) can emerge in midlife for women.[247] Symptoms occur on a continuum from increased airway resistance (manifested as snoring or airflow reductions [hypopneas]) to periodic cessation of breathing effort or airflow (apneas). Severe or long-standing manifestations have been linked to CVD. Episodes of SDB are associated with loud snoring, sleep arousals, and varying blood desaturated oxygen levels. These episodes lead to fragmented sleep, reports of waking from sleep unrefreshed, and excessive daytime sleepiness.

More postmenopausal women experience SDB episodes than premenopausal women, but comparisons of premenopausal, perimenopausal, and postmenopausal women have shown no clear differences in apnea/hypopnea, sleep arousal, or arterial oxygen desaturation episodes among the groups. Heavy body weight and facial morphology, with a crowded oropharynx (with or without obesity), have more importance than ovarian hormone factors in the SDB patterns of midlife women, but a functional breathing difference over and above the anatomic factors also has been associated with menopause status.

Women with apnea seem similar to men in reporting snoring and daytime sleepiness, but they report less restless sleep or witnessed apneas. Women with SDB are more likely than men to report morning headaches, fatigue, and mood changes. They are more likely to exhibit upper airway resistance than breathing pauses. Consequently, they may be less likely to be referred to sleep centers for evaluation. Explanations for the sex differences in SDB are being pursued. Research includes upper airway dynamics, fat distribution patterns, effects of sex-related hormones, and obesity-hypoventilation syndrome.[248,249]

Management of sleep disturbances

Healthcare professionals are encouraged to assess sleep quality in all women during perimenopause and beyond.

The decision to use behavior or drug treatments, or both, for insomnia depends on the type of sleep disturbance (acute or chronic, primary or secondary to other conditions), the context of the sleep problem (high VMS or life strain), and the severity of daytime consequences. Apnea, restless leg syndrome, anxiety, and depression need to be addressed.[246] Because SDB is associated with increased risk of hypertension and sudden cardiac death, prompt evaluation in a sleep center is recommended.

Behavior therapies. For people with sustained sleep problems, behavior therapies aim to eliminate patterns that interfere with sleep and reinforce those that promote sleep (eg, sleep hygiene measures). Strategies include ritualizing environmental cues, regularizing the sleep-wake schedule, and relaxation techniques to control tension.[250] Behavior therapies can be used alone or with pharmacologic or botanical therapies.

Caffeine, alcohol, and nicotine should be avoided close to bedtime if sleep induction is difficult. About 15 to 30 minutes are required for caffeine from a cup of coffee (80 mg-115 mg) to affect the brain, and up to 7 hours are required to rid the system of caffeine; its stimulant effects have lasted up to 20 hours as they accumulate during the day.[251] Besides being found in coffee, tea, "energy drinks," cola drinks, and chocolate, caffeine is also present in nonprescription pain relievers, premenstrual syndrome (PMS) remedies, diuretics, alertness and allergy/cold medications, and weight-control aids.

Alcohol initially promotes drowsiness, thus assisting with falling asleep. However, it often results in rebound early awakening and fragmented sleep, leading to feeling unrefreshed on awakening (unrestorative sleep). Alcohol also affects breathing and tends to swell oral and nasal mucous membranes, which may worsen SDB. Nicotine is frequently overlooked as contributing to sleep disturbances, but it has been observed to prolong sleep onset and decrease sleep duration. Illicit drugs, such as marijuana, morphine, and heroin, also disrupt normal sleep patterns.

Although eating a large, heavy meal before bed can interfere with sleep, a snack with protein (to support central nervous system neurochemical production, especially serotonin) and carbohydrates (to promote blood-brain barrier entry) is recommended. Strenuous exercise close to a desired sleep time amplifies arousal, making it difficult to fall asleep; however, regular daily exercise is considered beneficial.

Nightly rituals and establishing a sleep-conducive environment (quiet, cool, dark, and safe) can "condition" better sleep.[250] The bedroom should be reserved only for sleep, sex, and perhaps relaxation activities. If people are not asleep within 10 to 15 minutes, they should leave the bedroom to engage in relaxing activities elsewhere until drowsy, then return to bed again for sleep. This should be repeated as necessary. Resisting the temptation to check the clock will help avoid habitual awakenings.

A regular sleep schedule promotes sleep induction and stability. Choosing a consistent time to get up (regardless of time to bed and even on weekends) promotes synchrony with the light-dark cycle, which is important to a restorative sleep pattern.

Sleep-restriction therapy is another technique that can help reestablish a restorative sleep pattern for those unable to get quality hours of sleep.

Relaxation techniques can help patients with insomnia. Several modalities facilitate learning how to enter and adopt a deeply relaxed state, including instructional or mood-inducing tapes, concentration techniques such as meditation or creative imagery, or combining mind with movement techniques such as yoga or tai chi.

Two recent studies found that yoga and acupuncture improved reported sleep in menopausal women complaining of sleep disturbance.[252,253]

Cognitive-behavior therapy for insomnia has demonstrated comparable efficacy with other treatments. The National Institutes of Health Consensus and the American Academy of Sleep Medicine practice parameters recommend that cognitive-behavior therapy be considered standard treatment.[254]

Prescription remedies. Several prescription options can be used to improve sleep.

Sedatives and hypnotics. Sleeping pills may be used to break a cycle of insomnia and are typically used for brief periods of time.

- Short-acting nonbenzodiazepine hypnotic sleeping aids, such as zolpidem, zaleplon, or eszopiclone may be prescribed to improve sleep patterns. Compared with benzodiazepines, they show fewer withdrawal effects, less tolerance or addictive issues, and less loss of effectiveness over time, but long-term data are sparse and equivocal.

- Benzodiazepines such as lorazepam, clonazepam, diazepam, or alprazolam can be used to initiate or maintain sleep or both. However, AEs (such as next-day sedation, rebound insomnia when drug is discontinued, tolerance, and dependence) underlie recommendations that they be used for only brief periods of time if possible.

- Ramelteon, a melatonin receptor agonist, is a hypnotic sleep aid; it is government approved to assist in falling asleep.

Menopausal hormone therapy. Neither ET nor EPT is government approved as treatment for insomnia. However, oral ET has been shown to improve nighttime restlessness and awakening in women with VMS. Both ET and EPT seem to affect perceived and polysomnographic sleep positively, mainly in conjunction with reducing hot flash and night sweat activity. However, reducing hot flashes may not treat the underlying sleep disturbance.

Estrogen-progestogen therapy was thought to lessen SDB, although small-sample studies have not confirmed these effects. Using natural progesterone instead of a synthetic progestin may improve sleep because progesterone is a mild soporific. Bedtime dosing of progesterone is recommended.

Nonprescription remedies. Botanical sedatives and melatonin are sometimes considered as nonprescription options to improve sleep. Over-the-counter products containing these ingredients are government regulated in the United States as dietary supplements; in Canada, they are regulated as natural health products.

- *Botanicals*. Some sufferers use botanical sedatives to improve sleep quality. Valerian has been observed to promote sleep onset and deeper sleep. German chamomile, lavender, hops, lemon balm, and passion flower are said to be mild sedatives, although scientific data are scant.
- *Melatonin*. Some women self-medicate with melatonin, an endogenous pineal gland hormone, but its effects on sleep and sedation are inconsistent in studies. There are no data addressing the effects of melatonin on women with menopause-related sleep disturbances. Although melatonin is a hormone, it is not government regulated as a drug.

Ask patients about sleep disturbances. Refer to sleep centers women with SDB manifestations or other sleep-related disorders such as restless leg syndrome, periodic limb movements during sleep, or narcolepsy (uncontrollable sleep bouts during waking hours, loss of muscle tone known as cataplexy, hypnologic hallucinations, excessive daytime sleepiness, fragmented sleep, and automatic behaviors). Refer to psychiatrists and other mental health professionals when anxiety or depression is a pronounced component of the sleep problem.

Headache

Approximately one-half of the adult population worldwide is affected by a headache disorder.[255] The World Health Organization ranks headache disorders in the top 5 most disabling conditions for women.[256]

The Headache Classification Committee of the International Headache Society recently updated the classification of the common types of primary headache into these categories: 1) tension-type headache (TTH); 2) trigeminal autonomic cephalgias (*cluster headache* now falls into this category, as does short-lasting unilateral neuralgiform headache attacks with conjunctival injection and tearing and paroxysmal hemicranias; 3) migraine; and 4) "other" primary headache disorders (includes cough-, exercise-, cold-, or sex-induced headaches, thunderclap headaches, and primary stabbing headaches).[257] Ninety percent of headaches seen in outpatient practice are primary headaches, whereas less than 10% are secondary headaches. Secondary headaches have a definite underlying cause (brain tumor, meningitis, subarachnoid hemorrhage).[258]

Globally, within the adult population, 42% of the primary headaches are tension-type, 11% are migraines, and 3% are chronic daily headache.[256] Most patients who present to an outpatient clinic with a chief complaint of headache meet the criteria for migraines. Patients with TTHs, although statistically most common, rarely seek help. Unfortunately, about half of those who request treatment for tension-type or migraine headaches either do not receive appropriate treatment or are dissatisfied with their treatment.[259]

Although most primary headaches are not life threatening, these characteristics may be an indication of a more serious problem, such as a brain tumor:

- Occurrence of a "first or worst" headache
- Progressively worsening headache
- Acute or sudden onset (during sex, exercise, coughing/sneezing)
- Onset at age 50 years or older
- Change in headache pattern (frequency or severity)
- Headache that causes nocturnal awakening
- Stiff neck accompanied by a high fever
- Confusion, dizziness, weakness, or systemic symptoms (fever, chills, weight loss, cough)
- Presence of focal neurologic symptoms or signs

Headache management

Many primary headaches such as migraine are caused by genetic factors. Three genes that modulate various cell types within the brain have been linked to carrying a 10% to 15% greater risk of migraines.[260] Causes of headaches include sinus infections, dental problems, allergies, or colds. These are the 4 primary headache types and their management:

Tension-type headache. is the most prevalent headache in the general population.[256] The term *tension-type headache* (TTH) replaces previous terms such as *stress* or *tension headache*, *muscle-contraction headache*, and *psychogenic headache*.[261]

The typical presentation of a TTH attack is a bilateral, mild to moderate intensity, nonthrobbing (often described as a steady squeezing or pressing pain in the head or neck) headache typically lasting between 30 minutes and 7 days. There is no worsening of the headache with normal physical activity and no aura associated with it. Tension-type headache can be acute (frequent or infrequent) or chronic (>15 d/mo). The current pathophysiologic model of TTH suggests that pericranial myofascial pain receptor sensitivity causes episodic TTH, whereas central sensitization of pain caused by prolonged nociceptive stimuli from pericranial myofascial tissues seems to be responsible for chronic TTH.[262] Genetic factors may play a role in the development of chronic TTH, and women have a slightly higher prevalence of TTH than do men. Stress and mental tension are reported to be the most common precipitants for TTH.[263]

The diagnosis is based on clinical impression, and there are no diagnostic tests specific for TTH.

Most TTHs can be effectively treated with nonprescription analgesics such as aspirin 500 mg to 1,000 mg or acetaminophen 1,000 mg and nonsteroidal anti-inflammatory drugs (NSAIDs) such as naproxen 375 mg to 550 mg or ibuprofen 200 mg to 400 mg. Nonsteroidal anti-inflammatory drugs are probably the most effective. Evidence for efficacy of muscle relaxants (aside from tizanidine) is weak, and these, as well as combination medications (ie, those containing caffeine or codeine), should be avoided because of risk of habituation and development of chronic-daily headaches or medication-overuse headaches.[261]

Nonpharmacologic therapies, including physical therapy, stress management, relaxation therapy, and biofeedback, are also helpful for some people. For those who need prophylactic treatment, evidence suggests that tricyclic antidepressants are probably the most effective. Other medications that may be useful include the antidepressants mirtazapine and venlafaxine, the anticonvulsants topiramate and gabapentin, and the muscle relaxant tizanidine. In contrast, the available evidence suggests that SSRIs are not effective for TTH prophylaxis.[261]

Trigeminal autonomic cephalgias. are characterized by unilateral head pain in the distribution of the trigeminal nerve with ipsilateral autonomic features (ptosis, miosis, lacrimation, rhinorrhea, and nasal congestion). Included in this group are cluster headaches (that last minutes to hours, typically <10 episodes daily for several weeks at a time, often followed by periods of remission), paroxysmal hemicrania (usual duration 2-30 min, with 5-40 episodes/d), and short-lasting unilateral neuralgiform headache attacks with cranial autonomic symptoms. Short-lasting unilateral neuralgiform headache attacks with conjunctival injection and tearing and short-lasting unilateral neuralgiform headache attacks with cranial autonomic symptoms headaches can occur up to 200 times per day and last seconds or minutes.

In addition to their differences in duration and frequency, trigeminal autonomic cephalgias also differ in their response to treatment. Cluster headaches respond to oxygen therapy as well as subcutaneous sumatriptan for abortive therapy, and verapamil is first-line for preventive therapy. Paroxysmal hemicrania is exquisitely responsive to indomethacin, and because of the short duration of symptoms, it is most effectively used prophylactically.[264]

Short-lasting unilateral neuralgiform headache attacks with conjunctival injection and tearing and short-lasting unilateral neuralgiform headache attacks with cranial autonomic symptoms are responsive acutely to treatment with intravenous lidocaine and lamotrigine, whereas topiramate and gabapentin are the most effective medications available for prevention.[265]

Migraine headache. Migraines often begin in the mid-third decade, with peak prevalence in midlife.[257] Typically, migraines cause a moderate to severe throbbing pain that is worse on one side of the head and is usually aggravated by physical activity. The International Headache Society's diagnostic criterion for migraine includes a history of at least 5 headaches of this nature, lasting 4 to 72 hours, with at least 1 of these symptoms: phonophobia, photophobia, and nausea or vomiting.

There are 2 types of migraine headaches: those with aura and those without aura. An aura is a neurologic symptom that occurs just before or at the onset of a migraine. Aura symptoms usually begin less than an hour before the headache and are typically visual, characterized by flashing lights or wavy lines or even temporary loss of vision (scotomata), often in the peripheral visual fields. A person may also have speech problems or experience numbness, tingling, or weakness in an extremity, although this is rare. Such sensory deficits occur gradually over 5 or more minutes, last less than 1 hour, and are completely reversible. Several different symptoms or deficits can occur in succession.[258]

Migraines without aura are much more common than migraines with aura. Both types of migraines may have accompanying premonitory symptoms, such as mood changes, fatigue, nausea, vomiting, hyperactivity, hypoactivity, depression, food cravings, repetitive yawning, and neck stiffness, diarrhea, and facial congestion.[257] These symptoms may occur up to hours or several days before a headache. Patients with facial congestion are often misdiagnosed with sinus headache because many of these headaches meet the criteria for migraines. Research indicates that migraines may also be accompanied by cutaneous allodynia or excessive skin sensitivity (eg, pain when brushing the hair or touching the scalp).[266] Patients with cutaneous allodynia should be treated as early as possible in the course of the migraine because their headaches may be less responsive to medication if treatment is delayed.

Most presumed migraine triggers have not been well studied. Common factors that may be migraine triggers for susceptible patients include[258]

- Consumption of alcoholic beverages, caffeine, tyramine-containing foods (chocolate, yogurt, sour cream, aged cheese, red wine); foods containing nitrite preservatives (hot dogs, sausage, bacon, bologna, smoked fish); and foods containing monosodium glutamate (a flavor-enhancer sometimes added to Chinese and processed or frozen foods)

- Change in eating pattern (fasting or skipping meals, not drinking enough water)

- Change in sleeping pattern (varying sleep onset or cessation by more than 1 h)

- Emotional changes (stress, anxiety, anger, excitement)

- Environmental changes (noise, bright lights, changes in barometric pressure, fumes)
- Decline in endogenous or exogenous estrogen level (menstrual migraines)
- Use of any type of systemic ovarian hormone (for menopause or contraception), especially with a progestogen

Role of hormones. In the United States, migraines affect about 18% of women and 6% of men aged between 25 and 55 years. However, before puberty and after menopause, the incidence of headache is approximately the same in both men and women, suggesting some role for estrogen.[267]

A drop in estrogen level as seen with natural menses and with the placebo week of hormonal contraception appears to be a trigger for migraines in some women.

Studies have clearly established a connection between headaches and menstrual periods (called menstrual migraines) in susceptible women, with 70% of women with migraines reporting some association with their menstrual cycles.[268] In these women, the incidence of migraines often declines during pregnancy, when estrogen levels are more stable. Women with migraine without aura often see a decrease in migraines with natural menopause by approximately one-half; women who experienced only menstrual migraines can expect complete resolution of their migraines. However, the use of cyclic HT with monthly estrogen withdrawal might also trigger migraines. If these women are candidates for HT, they would be better served with a continuous regimen. This migraine abatement at the time of menopause may not be experienced by those with aura, and the history of aura could be a contraindication for HT.[267,269]

It remains unclear whether a validated association between migraine and menopausal VMS exists, but growing evidence suggests serotonin may be the common link because estrogen levels affect serotonin levels and metabolism.[267,269] Although progesterone also influences neuronal activity, less is known about the exact role of progestogens in migraine.

Migraine therapy. is traditionally divided into abortive therapy for acute pain and preventive therapy to decrease recurrences. Using a headache diary to identify (and avoid) triggers can be very helpful in headache management.[257] Data that should be recorded include the time a headache was experienced, the symptoms, and the potential triggers (particular foods, menses, or stress). For mild to moderately painful migraines, nonprescription pharmacologics such as aspirin or acetaminophen combinations with caffeine can be effective as abortive agents. Paradoxically, caffeine can also be a migraine trigger for some patients and also can increase withdrawal headaches, thus usually is not favored.[261] Older medications such as butalbital and isometheptene mucate-dichloralphenazone-acetaminophen are no longer recommended for migraine therapy because of the lack of clear evidence of effect and also their risk of habituation and abuse.

The advent of the triptan prescription medications (almotriptan, frovatriptan, rizatriptan, sumatriptan, eletriptan, naratriptan, and zolmitriptan) has greatly enhanced abortive migraine therapy. Triptans have made it possible for many migraine sufferers to lead relatively normal and productive lives despite severe or debilitating headaches. The triptans are extremely effective and safe, although they are contraindicated in patients with coronary heart disease. Nonsteroidal anti-inflammatory drugs are often recommended in combination with a triptan. For women with menstrual migraines, an NSAID or a triptan may be used preventively, beginning up to 2 days before the expected onset of symptoms.[270]

Daily preventive medication should be considered when a patient has headaches more than 2 days per week or if headache severity affects QOL. Any preventive medication is about 60% likely to be effective for any given patient. Prescription drugs found to be effective in preventing migraines include beta-blockers such as propranolol and timolol, calcium channel blockers such as verapamil, antidepressants such as amitriptyline, and anticonvulsants such as topiramate and divalproex. With a preventive drug, starting doses should be low and increased slowly. Drugs should be taken for at least 2 months to judge effectiveness.

For women who experience menstrual migraines, some studies suggest benefit to boosting doses of these conventional medications during the perimenstrual-menstrual period or actually limiting their use only related to the menstrual cycle instead of daily dosing. Medications studied but not FDA approved for use in this way are magnesium, NSAIDs, triptans, ergots, and hormones. Menstrual cycle irregularity, especially that commonly experienced in perimenopause, can limit this strategy because women may be unable to predict their cycle onset and thus when to start the medications.[271]

Magnesium, riboflavin, butterbur, and coenzyme Q10 are nonprescription preventive medications that, when taken daily, may be effective and safe for many migraine sufferers.[272,273] They can be used as baseline preventive treatment that may diminish the need for other preventive medications.

Hormonal treatment has been found to exacerbate migraines in some women and ease them in others. No hormone product is FDA approved to prevent or treat headaches. Benefit is more likely if hormonal fluctuations with therapy can be avoided (eg, adding a low-dose estrogen supplement during the withdrawal phase of OCs; using continuous menopausal HT; using continuous-release transdermal estrogen).[259] Migraine with aura may be adversely affected by HT. Reducing the dosage or changing the route may resolve the problem. Some evidence suggests that progestogens can prevent or aggravate headaches.[268] If headaches are worsened by a progestogen such as MPA, switching to micronized progesterone may help.

Caution should be used when prescribing estrogen-containing OCs for a woman who has migraine with aura, because studies suggest that these women have a small increased risk of ischemic stroke, especially in those who also smoke.[269,274,275] However, studies have been variable because such risk is confounded by numerous risk factors that are likely synergistic, such as smoking, hypertension, DM, and hyperlipidemia, as well as the dose of estrogen.[275] Additionally, migraine alone has been variably reported to be an independent risk factor for stroke. Evidence is inconsistent linking migraine and stroke in older women and in men.[275,276] Despite this increased risk, the absolute risk to any one person remains fairly low.[276,277] It remains unclear whether treating migraines and preventing attacks can affect potential ischemic stroke risk.[278]

The World Health Organization recommends that women with migraine with aura at any age and those with migraine without aura aged 35 years and older avoid using OC estrogen doses (20-50 µg estradiol).[279] A similar recommendation has been made by ACOG for women with migraine with aura, as well as those with migraine who smoke or have significant comorbidities for stroke.[43] A similar contraindication has not been identified for those with migraine with aura who need postmenopausal HT doses.[269,275,280] However, for some women with menstrual migraines, stabilization of hormone levels is a necessity to control their symptoms and an understanding of the related risks and associated discussion with the patient is critical. Nonpharmacologic migraine interventions, including greater occipital nerve blocks and acupuncture, are gathering evidence.[281,282]

"Other" primary headache disorders are relatively uncommon and include primary stabbing headache (icepick headache); headache precipitated by cough, exertion, or sexual intercourse; thunderclap headache; hypnic headache; daily-persistent headaches; and hemicrania continua. The pathogenesis of these headaches is still poorly understood and treatment is suggested on the basis of anecdotal reports and uncontrolled trials.

Ongoing treatment

Over-the-counter and prescription drugs used for acute treatment of all these primary headaches can result in more frequent headaches, known as chronic daily headaches. Care should be taken to monitor the use of these drugs and, if headaches occur more than twice a week, preventive medications should be considered. For many midlife women, headaches are debilitating and frustrating, greatly interfering with QOL at a time when career and family responsibilities are already stressful.[283] A supportive relationship between the chronic headache sufferer and her healthcare professional can be extremely effective in determining the appropriate individual interventions.

Cognition

The term *cognition* describes the group of mental processes by which knowledge is acquired and used. It encompasses mental skills such as attention and concentration, learning and memory, language, spatial abilities, judgment, problem solving, and reasoning.

Sex hormones—estrogens, progesterone, and testosterone—modulate aspects of brain function, and subsets of nerve cells within the brain have receptors for these hormones. Effects of estradiol on several neurotransmitter systems involving acetylcholine, serotonin, norepinephrine, and dopamine can potentially influence neural networks involved in concentration, memory, and other cognitive functions. Other estrogen actions within the hippocampus (a brain region essential to the formation of conscious memories) might affect learning and memory. Still other actions may have an effect on physiologic and pathologic processes implicated in Alzheimer disease and other brain disorders. However, the clinical importance of these brain effects during the menopause transition and in postmenopause is not always clear.

Cognitive aging, mild cognitive impairment, and dementia

Memory and other cognitive abilities change throughout life. With advancing age, performance tends to decline somewhat on many, but not all, cognitive tests. Difficulty concentrating and remembering are common during the menopause transition and early postmenopause.[284]

The ability to concentrate is reduced by sleep disturbances, hot flashes, fatigue, depressed mood, physical symptoms, medication use, and a variety of midlife stressors.[285] Poor concentration can in turn exert an effect on how efficiently and accurately other cognitive tasks are performed. Small reductions in mental ability, usually below the detection threshold with standard mental status tests, might be expected on the basis of age alone in the presence of other physical and psychological factors that reduce the ability to focus and maintain attention. There may be an association between hot flashes and memory difficulty.[286] It is worthwhile to look for and treat these contributing factors. Any obvious change in cognitive ability, particularly in patients older than 65 years, suggests the need to consider an underlying medical or neurologic disorder.

Some cross-sectional data imply that memory may be worse after the natural menopause transition than before.[287] However, in the longitudinal SWAN, there was a weak trend for memory to be worse during the menopause transition, but memory after the transition was as good as it was before.[288] Moreover, depression, anxiety, sleep disturbance, and VMS did not account for the transient decrement in cognitive performance observed during late perimenopause.[289] Serum estradiol concentrations in midlife are not associated with scores on memory tests,[290] and the extent to which memory is substantially affected by natural menopause remains controversial. Some problems that women experience may be more related to normal cognitive aging, mood, and other factors than to menopause or the menopause transition.[285]

Chapter 3

Early or rapid transition to menopause may affect cognitive performance.[291] Menopause-related symptoms are more frequent and intense after surgical menopause than after natural menopause, and there is some evidence that cognitive skills such as memory for verbal information can be compromised in the immediate period after surgical menopause.[292,293]

Dementia refers to the loss of memory and other intellectual abilities severe enough to interfere substantially with independence or usual daily activities. It is perhaps the most-feared consequence of aging. Alzheimer disease, the most common cause of dementia, accounts for well over half of cases.[294] More women are affected than men, primarily because women tend to live longer. Alzheimer disease and other forms of dementia may be preceded by a period of moderate difficulty with memory or other cognitive abilities. The term *mild cognitive impairment* is sometimes used to refer to excessive difficulty with memory or other aspects of cognition that fall short of dementia but may presage its development.[295]

Management of cognition symptoms

Observational data indicate that some activities and lifestyle choices may benefit memory or help protect against dementia. These include maintaining an extensive social network, remaining physically and mentally active, increasing dietary intake of omega-3 fatty acids and certain vitamins from natural foods, not smoking, consuming alcohol only in moderation, and reducing cardiovascular risk factors such as hypertension, DM, and high cholesterol.

These are reasonable goals worth pursuing, even though few have been rigorously confirmed by RCTs.[296] Evidence is perhaps strongest for a role of regular aerobic exercise in preventing cognitive decline.[297] Trials of dietary supplements with vitamin E, B-vitamins, gingko biloba, dehydroepiandrosterone, soy isoflavones, and omega-3 fatty acids have generally failed to show significant cognitive benefit.[298-305]

Hypertension is a direct risk factor for vascular dementia, and studies have suggested that hypertension also affects the prevalence of Alzheimer disease. A Cochrane systematic review concluded, however, that there was no convincing evidence that lowering BP in later life prevents the development of dementia or cognitive impairment in patients with hypertension who have had no prior cerebrovascular disease.[306] For many factors, the optimal time for effective intervention is likely to be during midlife rather than during old age.

Effects of menopausal HT on Alzheimer disease and cognition are beginning to be better understood.[307] In the Women's Health Initiative (WHI) Memory Study, an RCT conducted in relatively healthy postmenopausal women aged 65 to 79 years, the risk of dementia was doubled for women using EPT.[308] The increase in risk for women without a uterus who used ET was not significant.[309] On the basis of this evidence, initiating menopausal HT after age 65 cannot be recommended for primary prevention of dementia.[104,310,311]

Menopausal HT is not recommended for the prevention of Alzheimer disease even before this age. Observational studies imply potential reductions in Alzheimer disease risk when menopausal HT is used at younger ages.[312-315] However, given the absence of trial data and concerns about dementia risk later in life, the evidence is insufficient to conclude that menopausal HT helps prevent late-life dementia, even when initiated during perimenopause or early postmenopause.

Among older women in late postmenopause, menopausal HT has small or no overall effect on cognition. In the ancillary WHI Study of Cognitive Aging and in other large trials involving older postmenopausal women, menopausal HT had no consistent effect on cognition.[290,316,317] Menopausal HT effects, when reported, are small. In the WHI Study of Cognitive Aging, there was a small negative effect on verbal memory and a small positive effect on figural (nonverbal) memory in women with a uterus using EPT.[316] In women without a uterus who were assigned to ET, there was a small negative effect on a visual task (the ability to identify rotation in space).[317]

Two large RCTs focused on early postmenopausal women: the Kronos Early Estrogen Prevention Study (KEEPS) and the Early Versus Late Intervention Trial With Estradiol (ELITE). Results are pending, but preliminary analyses from KEEPS suggest no cognitive benefit or harm of oral or transdermal estrogens.[318] Follow-up results after trial completion in women from the WHI aged 50 to 55 years at the time of enrollment are consistent. These indicate no sustained oral estrogen benefit or risk to cognitive function.[319] When available, the ELITE results will allow direct comparison of cognitive effects of oral estradiol given to women close to or more remote from the menopause.

Based on trial evidence, menopausal HT should not be recommended to improve cognition after age 65.[290] For women in their late 40s and early 50s undergoing natural menopause, there is insufficient evidence to recommend menopausal HT for cognitive function; clearer recommendations will be possible after peer-review publication of results from KEEPS and ELITE trials. None of these recommendations apply to women with premature menopause, who have not yet been adequately studied and may be uniquely vulnerable.

Cognitive consequences of induced menopause may differ from those of natural menopause. For women undergoing surgical menopause, there is limited clinical trial evidence that HT begun soon after surgery may benefit cognitive skills such as verbal memory, at least in the short term.[293] Early hysterectomy (with or without oophorectomy) is linked to early onset dementia before age 50[320]; fortunately, the absolute risk of dementia before age 65 is rare. Oophorectomy before age 46 is also associated with increased risk of cognitive decline or dementia in late life, although other research has not observed long-term cognitive sequelae of hysterectomy or oophorectomy.[321,322]

Few studies have focused on menopausal HT and vascular dementia, which is most often caused by multiple ischemic strokes. However, consistent evidence from clinical trials (including WHI) and observational research (including the Nurses' Health Study) indicates that standard-dose menopausal HT increases the risk of ischemic stroke for postmenopausal women by about one-third.[323-325] This risk is not modified by age or timing with respect to menopause.[325] For younger postmenopausal women, the absolute risk of stroke from standard-dose menopausal HT is rare, but risk is more substantial for older women. Although evidence is limited, low doses of transdermal estradiol (≤50 µg/d) appear not to alter stroke risk.[326]

For women with dementia caused by Alzheimer disease, there are still no therapies that lead to consistent improvement in symptoms or halt the degenerative course of the illness. Limited clinical trial evidence suggests that menopausal HT does not have a role in the treatment of women with Alzheimer disease.[307] Other agents or medications assessed in RCTs that do not seem to benefit Alzheimer disease include aspirin, B vitamins, vitamin E, steroids, traditional NSAIDs, selective cyclooxygenase-2 inhibitor anti-inflammatory drugs, omega-3 fatty acids, and statins.[327-330]

Several medications for treating patients with symptoms of Alzheimer disease are government approved in the United States and Canada. One class of drugs (cholinesterase inhibitors) increases levels of acetylcholine (a chemical transmitter) in the brain by blocking its breakdown. This class includes donepezil, rivastigmine, and galantamine. These agents can have a modest beneficial effect on the disease.[331] Memantine, a drug thought to reduce nerve damage caused by excitatory neurotransmitters, is approved for patients with moderate or severe Alzheimer disease symptoms. The clinical effect of this medication is also modest.

There is no evidence that use of these medications by healthy people or people with mild cognitive impairment will enhance cognition or help to prevent Alzheimer disease.

Psychological symptoms

Although most women make the transition into menopause without experiencing depression, many women report symptoms of depressed mood, anxiety, stress, and a decreased sense of well-being. Common and distressing symptoms include sadness, irritability, tearfulness, insomnia, fatigue, decreased memory and concentration, and depression. Mood changes have been observed in up to 23% of perimenopausal and postmenopausal women.[332] Epidemiologic studies suggest a greater prevalence of clinical depression in perimenopausal women than in premenopausal women during midlife.[333,334] Women with a history of clinical depression or a history of PMS or postpartum depression seem to be particularly vulnerable to recurrent depression during perimenopause, as are women who report significant stress, sexual dysfunction, physical inactivity, or hot flashes.[335,336]

Depression

The term *depression* can sometimes be misleading because it may refer to a symptom or a clinical disorder, each of which is managed differently. Depression is commonly used to mean

- *Depressed mood.* Sometimes called dysphoria, this is a normal, brief period of feeling blue or sad that is commonly experienced and rarely requires treatment.

- *Depression as an adjustment reaction.* This type of depression may be because of a wide variety of medical or psychological problems or intense reactions to life events (eg, divorce, losing a job, death of a loved one). It is usually short term and most often does not require treatment, although it can progress to clinical depression.

- *Clinical depression.* A clinical depression or *major depressive disorder* (in contrast to dysphoria and adjustment reactions) is a pathologic disorder that results from a chemical imbalance in the brain (Table 24).[213] A clinical depression impairs function and requires treatment.

- *Dysthymia.* Dysthymia or *persistent depressive disorder* is a chronic depression that occurs most of the day, more days than not, for at least 2 years. This chronic mood disorder is in contrast to the more acute and more intensive symptomatology of a clinical depression and can be more difficult to recognize and treat.

Several clinical findings indicate that a woman may require further psychiatric or psychosocial evaluation. Women exhibiting relevant symptoms can be screened for clinical depression using a clinical interview together with self-rated tools such as the Beck Depression Inventory or the Center for Epidemiologic Studies Depression Scale. Structured diagnostic interviews may also be used.

Anxiety

The term *anxiety* refers to such symptoms such as tension, nervousness, panic, and worry. These symptoms are reported more frequently during the perimenopausal period than during premenopause, independent of depressive symptoms. Although it was believed that bilateral oophorectomy increased the risk of anxiety symptoms, particularly when surgery occurs before age 48,[337] findings inconsistent with this from SWAN have made this controversial.[338]

An evaluation of anxiety is needed to differentiate normal day-to-day anxiety from pathologic states. Women with anxiety conditions such as panic disorder, generalized anxiety disorder, social phobia, and obsessive-compulsive and posttraumatic stress disorders may benefit from pharmacologic or psychotherapy interventions or both. Anxiety is often associated with depression but may also indicate a distinct clinical disorder.

Table 24. *DSM-5* Criteria for Clinical Depression

Clinical depression is confirmed when these criteria are met:

Criterion A. Five or more of these symptoms have been present during the same 2-week period and represent a change from previous functioning; at least 1 of the symptoms is either 1) depressed mood or 2) loss of interest or pleasure. Do not include symptoms that are clearly attributable to another medical condition.

1. Depressed mood most of the day, nearly every day, as indicated by either subjective report (feels sad, empty, hopeless) or observation made by others (appears tearful).
2. Markedly diminished interest or pleasure in all, or almost all, activities most of the day, nearly every day (as indicated by either subjective account or observation).
3. Significant weight loss when not dieting, or weight gain (a change of more than 5% of body weight in a month), or decrease or increase in appetite nearly every day
4. Insomnia or hypersomnia nearly every day.
5. Psychomotor agitation or retardation nearly every day (observable by others, not merely subjective feelings of restlessness or being slowed down).
6. Fatigue or loss of energy nearly every day.
7. Feelings of worthlessness or excessive or inappropriate guilt (which may be delusional) nearly every day (not merely self-reproach or guilt about being sick).
8. Diminished ability to think or concentrate or indecisiveness nearly every day (either by subjective account or as observed by others).
9. Recurrent thoughts of death (not just fear of dying), recurrent suicidal ideation without a specific plan, or a suicide attempt, or a specific plan for committing suicide.

Criterion B. The symptoms cause clinically significant distress or impairment in social, occupational, or other important areas of functioning.

Criterion C. The episode is not attributable to the physiological effects of a substance or to another medical condition.

See *DSM-5* for exclusionary criteria.
Abbreviation: *DSM-5, Diagnostic and Statistical Manual of Mental Disorders.* 5th edition.
American Psychiatric Association.[213]

In a NAMS-sponsored Gallup Poll of recently postmenopausal US women, respondents indicated that they felt happier and more fulfilled at this time of their life than at any other.[339] Nevertheless, growing older may be difficult for some women. Often, hormone-related changes coincide with other stressors and losses in their lives (Table 25).[340] Although stressful life transitions may coincide with the menopause transition, the "empty nest" syndrome is not associated with depression in this population.

Women with histories of early stressful life events (eg, maltreatment, poverty, chronic illness) are particularly vulnerable to depression that may be exacerbated during perimenopause.

Many women begin to think about aging, becoming introspective about the meaning and purpose of their lives. Although these changes may provide an opportunity for positive transformation and growth, some women may need support to successfully adapt. Healthcare professionals may be able to diminish or prevent some minor psychological symptoms by counseling women on what to expect physically and psychologically at menopause.

Mood disturbance during perimenopause

Most women become accustomed to their own hormonal rhythm during their reproductive years. During perimenopause, however, this rhythm changes and becomes less stable. Hormonal fluctuations, although a normal consequence of declining ovarian activity, may still provoke stress. The unexpected timing and extent of these changes may create feelings of upset and loss of control. Reports of irritability, fatigue, and "blue" moods (dysphoria) are common. Although adjustment to bodily changes may be a factor for some, the hormonal fluctuations can also result in depressive and anxiety symptoms because erratically changing levels may perturb neural systems that affect mood. Women with a history of bipolar disorder may report an increase in depressive symptoms, increased irritability, hypomania or mania, and more rapid cycling.

CLINICAL ISSUES

Women often do not recognize that numerous physical and psychological symptoms are related to perimenopause. Because perimenopausal symptoms may occur as early as age 35, education and anticipatory guidance about common perimenopausal symptoms are best addressed when women are in their early- to mid-30s. Transient depressed mood during perimenopause is often associated with a history of depression, a longer perimenopause, or more severe menopause-related symptoms.

Compared with perimenopausal women without mood changes, perimenopausal women seeking help for mood changes are usually less healthy, have more hot flashes and psychosomatic complaints, and are more likely to have a history of PMS. Some women of reproductive age report symptoms such as irritability, tension, dysphoria, and lability of mood that may indicate the beginning of perimenopause or the beginning or worsening of PMS. Extreme symptoms that are isolated during the premenstrual phase of the cycle may indicate premenstrual dysphoric disorder (PMDD; Table 26). Women reporting PMS should be thoroughly evaluated for depression because of the overlap between PMS symptoms and an underlying depressive disorder.[336,341,342]

There has been considerable controversy in the scientific literature regarding the direct effect of changing estrogen levels on perimenopausal mood symptoms, and the interaction between estrogen and mood is complex. Some epidemiologic studies have suggested that as estrogen levels vary widely and decline, susceptibility to major depression increases.[334] It is hypothesized that mood symptoms may be related to marked and erratic fluctuations in estrogen levels, but limited data exist on the precise mechanism. Others hypothesize that hot flashes and associated sleep disturbance play an intermediary role in the causal pathway between changing estradiol levels and mood, but there is little direct evidence to support this *domino hypothesis*.[72] Perimenopausal depression appears to be a complex interplay between hormonal vulnerability, psychosocial resources, lifestyle factors, and stressful events.[343]

Evaluation

Most women present to their primary care clinicians with psychological symptoms instead of consulting or before they consult a mental health professional. Therefore, primary care clinicians should conduct an initial assessment of psychological health such as screening for clinical depression and significant anxiety. Even minor depression is associated with social dysfunction and disability, and long-lasting anxiety symptoms may interfere with daily activities. Referral to mental health professionals is advised when significant symptoms of depression or anxiety are suspected. Studies provide evidence of higher cardiovascular risk in women with depressive symptoms, particularly the symptom of hopelessness.[344] Additionally, women with psychiatric symptoms in midlife and beyond are shown to be at higher risk of cognitive decline.[345] Referral to physicians with expertise in CVD or neurologic disorders may also be warranted.

Table 25. Potential Stressors at Midlife

- Undesired childlessness
- Difficulties in relationship with a partner
- Development of personal or family medical problems
- Changes in self-concept, self-esteem, and body image
- Divorce or widowhood
- Care of young children, struggles with adolescents, or return of grown children to the home
- Concerns about aging parents or other family members
- "Sandwich generation" phenomena (responsibility for children and elders)
- Career and education issues
- Socioeconomic status/Financial concerns

Schmidt PJ, et al.[340]

A constellation of symptoms associated with distress or impairment must be present and persistent for a certain period of time for a clinician to make a clinical diagnosis. The *DSM-5* outlines valid and reliable criteria for determining specific psychiatric diagnoses.[213] A psychosocial history is the first step in identifying mental health problems. This assessment includes taking a history of prior mental health problems as well as asking about current symptoms. Assessment of mood episodes includes evaluating for changes in mood, appetite, sleep, energy, sexual function, concentration, memory, and suicidal thoughts.

Symptoms such as depressed mood, prolonged tiredness, low energy, loss of interest in normal activities, increased levels of guilt, anhedonia (inability to experience pleasure in normally pleasurable acts), irritability, psychomotor retardation or agitation, or other symptoms that may persist 2 weeks or longer are likely to indicate a clinical depression. Symptoms such as decreased need for sleep, pressured speech, racing thoughts, distractibility, increased goal-directed activity, and excessive involvement in pleasurable activities may suggest a manic or hypomanic mood episode of bipolar disorder.

Assessment of anxiety includes evaluating for excessive worry, physiologic symptoms (eg, fatigue, muscle tension, restlessness, and other somatic complaints), panic, or obsessive-compulsive symptoms. Anxiety can be a trigger for VMS.

Gathering information on family or personal history of depression, other psychiatric disorders, substance abuse, psychiatric hospitalizations, and suicide attempts, as well

Chapter 3

> **Table 26.** *DSM-5* Criteria for for Premenstrual Dysphoric Disorder
>
> *Premenstrual dysphoric disorder is confirmed when Criteria A-G are met:*
>
> *Criterion A.* In most menstrual cycles, at least 5 symptoms must be present in the final week before the onset of menses, start to improve within a few days after the onset of menses, and become minimal or absent in the week postmenses.
>
> *Criterion B.* One (or more) of these symptoms must be present:
>
> 1. Marked affective lability (mood swings; feeling suddenly sad or tearful, or increased sensitivity to rejection).
> 2. Marked irritability or anger or increased interpersonal conflicts.
> 3. Marked depressed mood, feelings of hopelessness, or self-deprecating thoughts.
> 4. Marked anxiety, tension, and/or feelings of being keyed up or on edge.
>
> *Criterion C.* One (or more) of these symptoms must additionally be present to reach a total of 5 symptoms when combined with symptoms from Criterion B:
>
> 1. Decreased interest in usual activities (work, school, friends, hobbies).
> 2. Subjective difficulty in concentration.
> 3. Lethargy, easy fatigability, or marked lack of energy.
> 4. Marked change in appetite; overeating; or specific food cravings.
> 5. Hypersomnia or insomnia.
> 6. A sense of being overwhelmed or out of control.
> 7. Physical symptoms such as breast tenderness or swelling, joint or muscle pain, a sensation of "bloating" or weight gain.
>
> The symptoms in Criteria A-C must have been met for most menstrual cycles that occurred in the preceding year.
>
> *Criterion D.* Symptoms are associated with clinically significant distress or interference with work, school, usual social activities, or relationships with others (avoidance of social activities; decreased productivity and efficiency at work, school, or home).
>
> *Criterion E.* Disturbance is not merely an exacerbation of the symptoms of another disorder, such as major depressive disorder, panic disorder, persistent depressive disorder (dysthymia), or a personality disorder (although it may co-occur with any of these disorders).
>
> *Criterion F.* Criterion A should be confirmed by prospective daily ratings during at least 2 symptomatic cycles.
>
> *Criterion G.* Symptoms are not attributable to the physiological effects of a substance (a drug of abuse, a medication, other treatment) or another medical condition (eg, hyperthyroidism).
>
> Abbreviations: *DSM-5, Diagnostic and Statistical Manual of Mental Disorders.* 5th edition. American Psychiatric Association.[213]

as previous responses to psychopharmacologic medication and psychotherapy, is also useful. Use of alcohol or other stimulants may mask mood or anxiety problems. A medical history, physical examination, and routine laboratory tests can rule out nutritional deficiencies and medical illnesses that are frequently associated with depression and anxiety (eg, endocrine disorders such as hypothyroidism). Depression may be an AE of medications, including beta-blockers, corticosteroids, and hormonal contraceptives (Table 27).[346] Although hormonal contraceptives can result in mood deterioration, most women do not experience this AE, and others experience mood improvement.[347]

Similarly, anxiety also may be an AE to a medication or medication withdrawal (Table 28).[213] Only when the exact causes of psychiatric symptoms are determined can an appropriate treatment plan be developed.

The most predictive factor for depression during midlife and beyond is a history of clinical depression. Women who have been diagnosed with depression in their younger reproductive years may experience recurrence of symptoms during perimenopause. Identifying a history of depression at other times related to hormonal fluctuations (eg, premenstrual, pregnancy, or postpartum) or related to use of hormonal contraception may help to determine whether a woman is vulnerable to depressive episodes caused by changes in hormone levels.[348,349] If a perimenopausal woman does not have a history of depression and she develops depressive symptoms while experiencing

Clinical Issues

Table 27. Medications Associated With Depression

- Analgesics (ibuprofen, indomethacin, opiates)
- Anticonvulsants (phenytoin, carbamazepine)
- Antihypertensives (reserpine, clonidine, thiazides, beta-blockers, hydralazine)
- Dopamine agonists (levodopa, bromocriptine, amantadine)
- H_2 receptor antagonists (cimetidine, ranitidine)
- Sedatives (alcohol, barbiturates, benzodiazepines, chloral hydrate)
- Steroids (corticosteroids, oral contraceptives)
- Stimulant withdrawal (amphetamines, cocaine)

Landau C, et al.[346]

menopausal symptoms and significant sleep disturbance, her primary problem may be the domino effect in which estrogen fluctuations result in VMS, leading to sleep disturbances, which in turn precipitate psychological and cognitive symptoms of depression.[350] Studies finding a strong association between hot flashes and depression support this hypothesis, but others suggest that sleep disturbance does not play an intermediary role in the association between VMS and depression.[72,333,351,352]

In addition, other evidence indicates that depressive symptoms more commonly precede rather than follow the onset of VMS in women who experience both symptoms, suggesting that VMS are not necessarily causally related to depression during the menopause transition.[353]

Management

Psychotherapy alone is useful for mild depression, especially when there are psychosocial stressors associated with

Table 28. Medications Associated With Anxiety

- Alcohol
- Antidepressants
- Caffeine
- Cannabis
- Hallucinogens
- Phencyclidine
- Sedative and anxiolytic withdrawal
- Stimulants (amphetamines, cocaine)

American Psychiatric Association.[213]

the onset of depression, but when depressive symptoms are moderate to severe, antidepressants are indicated. Serotonin-based antidepressants are also highly effective for anxiety and depressive disorders, as can be anxiolytic medications. Cognitive-behavior and other types of therapies, including supportive psychotherapy, might be added.

Nonpharmacologic methods. Relaxation and stress-reduction techniques, including lifestyle modification, may help women cope with stress-producing factors during this time of hormonal fluctuation (Table 29). Some women attempt to self-treat their depression symptoms by using OTC products such as St. John's wort or omega-3. Always ask what medications and OTC products women are taking and for what reason.

Pharmacologic treatment. Any time a woman meets the criteria for clinical depression, regardless of where she is in the menopause transition, treatment is indicated with antidepressant medication, psychotherapy, or a combination. Women may also experience symptoms of mild depression, such as depressed mood, irritability, poor concentration, and fatigue, in association with marked sleep deprivation resulting from hot flashes and night sweats. These symptoms often improve when hot flashes are treated and sleep patterns return to baseline. Cognitive-behavior therapies may be useful in the treatment of menopausal sleep disturbances.[354,355]

For premenstrual dysphoric disorder. If the diagnosis is PMDD, 4 prescription drugs are government approved to treat the condition: 3 selective SSRIs—fluoxetine, controlled-release paroxetine, and sertraline—and the sole OC with ethinyl estradiol plus drospirenone.[356-359] Refer to the product labeling before prescribing. Over-the-counter pain medications will not relieve the most extreme physical symptoms of PMDD. Augmentation of an antidepressant with an OC might play a role in treating premenstrual worsening of depression.[360]

For menopause-related depression. Antidepressants are the primary pharmacologic treatment for menopause-associated

Table 29. Nonpharmacologic Methods for Coping With Stress at Midlife

- Stress reduction exercises (deep breathing exercises, progressive muscle relaxation, meditation)
- Daily exercise (yoga may be particularly helpful)
- Healthy diet (plant-based, low-fat, low-caffeine, and low-alcohol)
- Sufficient self-care and enjoyable self-nurturing activities (eg, massage)
- Psychological support/therapy (psychotherapy, menopause support group)
- Creative outlets that enhance quality of life

depression. Menopausal HT and hormonal contraceptives can be used as off-label therapies, especially in women with concurrent hot flashes. Hypnotic agents can be coadministered with antidepressants or menopausal HT, especially when prominent sleep disturbance is present and is not treated by primary medication and/or psychotherapy. Studies using the hypnotic agent eszopiclone to treat insomnia in perimenopausal and postmenopausal women with mild subthreshold depressive symptoms have shown benefits in reducing depression and anxiety as well as improving overall well-being.[125]

- *Antidepressants.* Selective serotonin-reuptake inhibitors and other antidepressants are highly effective treatments of depression in perimenopausal and postmenopausal women. Open-label studies and randomized trial data show the benefits of using antidepressants to treat depression in this population and include citalopram, escitalopram, duloxetine, and mirtazapine.[347,360-362] Preliminary evidence from epidemiologic studies suggests that SSRI use is associated with reduced bone mass and with clinical fragility fractures.[124] However, a more recent study using data from SWAN found no significant bone loss in midlife women taking an SSRI.[363]

- *Hormonal therapy.* There is evidence that estrogen has a positive effect on neural functions that regulate mood and behavior, thus producing a mood-enhancing effect. In prospective, controlled clinical trials with perimenopausal women who have depression, HT has been shown to be consistently effective in relieving depression.[364-366] Hormonal therapy or hormonal contraceptives in doses that are conventionally used to treat hot flashes will often reduce or eliminate mood swings, tearfulness, irritability, and feelings of sadness.[367] Hormonal therapies are especially, but not exclusively, effective in treating depression when coexisting hot flashes are present. In contrast, estrogen has not been shown to be more effective than placebo in treating older postmenopausal women with depression.[368] Given these different findings, it has been suggested that the antidepressant response to estrogen may be most effective during the changing hormonal milieu but not when hormonal levels have finally stabilized.[334]

The wide range of psychological symptoms reported during the menopause transition, from irritability and blue moods to the recurrence of major depression, can be identified and often treated by a woman's primary care or menopause practitioner. The practitioner should know, however, when it is appropriate to refer a woman to a mental health professional for further evaluation. Practitioners who are uncomfortable assessing or treating psychological symptoms should make a referral earlier in the process.

Sexually transmitted infections

Although 50% of sexually transmitted infections (STIs) occur in women aged 15 to 24 years, perimenopausal and postmenopausal women are still at risk of contracting them. The risk of STIs—including syphilis, gonorrhea, chlamydia, genital herpes, human papillomavirus (HPV; genital warts), hepatitis B, hepatitis C, and human immunodeficiency virus (HIV)—should be a lifelong concern for women not in long-term, mutually monogamous relationships (defined as only 1 sexual partner for at least 6 months). The incidence of STIs in the United States is greatest for HPV, chlamydia, and trichomoniasis (Table 30).[369]

Older women at high risk for STIs include those with a new sexual partner, multiple sexual partners, or a partner who has multiple sexual partners.[370] Most STIs are more easily transmitted from man to woman than from woman to man. Women are twice as likely as men to contract gonorrhea, hepatitis B, and HIV, if exposed. Moreover, STIs are less likely to produce symptoms in women and are therefore more difficult to diagnose until serious complications develop.

Sexually active postmenopausal women with genital atrophy may be at increased risk for STIs because the delicate genital tissue is prone to small tears and cuts that can act as pathways for infection.[371] Also, once infected, symptoms of STIs may be misinterpreted in this population, and the diagnosis delayed.

Safer sex guidelines

Avoidance of STIs is an important behavior to reinforce, especially among women who are no longer at risk for pregnancy and who therefore may not be thinking about safer sex practices.[372,373]

Women who have sex with women tend to have fewer STIs than heterosexual women, but STIs can still be passed from woman to woman.[370] Lesbians and bisexual women not in long-term, mutually monogamous relationships are at an increased risk. Clinicians can provide counseling to lower this risk (Tables 31[374,375] and 32).

Screening

Clinicians should not assume that older women are not at risk for STIs. In addition, older women may not be as

Table 30. Estimated Number of New Sexually Transmitted Infections in the United States, 2008

HPV	14,100,000
Chlamydia	2,860,000
Trichomoniasis	1,090,000
Gonorrhea	820,000
HSV	776,000
HIV	41,400
Hepatitis B	19,000

Abbreviations: HIV, human immunodeficiency virus; HPV, human papillomavirus; HSV, herpes simplex virus.
Satterwhite CL, et al.[369]

CLINICAL ISSUES

Table 31. Safer Sex Guidelines for All Women

- Choose sex partners carefully.
- Discuss sexual history with a partner; do not let embarrassment compromise health.
- Always insist that male partners use a latex condom for genital, oral, and anal sex, unless in a long-standing, mutually monogamous relationship. Never use petroleum-based oils as lubrication for latex condoms because they can damage the condom, potentially causing a break. Polyurethane condoms are available for persons who are allergic to latex and are equal to latex condoms in protecting against pregnancy and STIs or HIV. Natural membrane condoms are not recommended for prevention of STIs or HIV.
- Have an annual physical examination, including (when indicated) Pap and HPV tests, as well as tests to identify STIs when suspected. Ensure that vaccinations are up-to-date (eg, hepatitis B vaccine).
- After learning of exposure to an STI or after a confirmed diagnosis, urge any partners to be examined and treated.
- Consider having you and your partner checked for STIs before initiating a sexual relationship.

Abbreviations: HPV, human papillomavirus; Pap, Papanicolaou; STI, sexually transmitted infection.

knowledgeable about infection risks or accustomed to taking steps to minimize these risks compared with younger women who have lived with the threat of HIV and acquired immune deficiency syndrome (AIDS) their entire sexual lives. Patients diagnosed with one STI may have other STIs; additional testing is appropriate.

Expedited partner therapy. Expedited partner therapy is the clinical practice of treating the sex partners of women diagnosed with chlamydia or gonorrhea by providing prescriptions or medications to the patient to take to her partner without the healthcare professional first examining the partner.[376] This strategy has been endorsed by the Centers for Disease Control and Prevention (CDC) as another way to ensure treatment of partners when women are diagnosed with an STI. Although examination and treatment of the partner or referral of the partner to a men's healthcare professional is still the preferred method to avoid spreading the STI, the CDC realizes that this is not always possible. The legal status of expedited partner therapy varies by state. The CDC has resources that can assist healthcare professionals in determining whether their state allows this practice (www.cdc.gov/std/ept/legal/default.htm).

Bacterial vaginosis. The most common abnormal vaginal flora condition in women of childbearing age is bacterial vag-inosis (BV). Perimenopausal and postmenopausal women are also susceptible. However, BV is not an STI. Although the cause is not fully understood, BV is associated with an imbalance in the vaginal bacterial flora in which the normal lactobacilli are replaced by *Gardnerella vaginalis* and other anaerobic bacteria. The risk for BV increases by having a new sex partner or multiple sex partners, douching, and smoking.

Symptoms of BV include a thin, white or gray vaginal discharge with a high pH and a strong fishy odor, but some women have no signs or symptoms.[370] Complications for perimenopausal and postmenopausal women include an increased susceptibility to other STIs and pelvic inflammatory disease. Bacterial vaginosis is diagnosed through microscopic examination of the vaginal fluid looking for the characteristic clue cells, more than 20% per high-power field (squamous epithelial cells studded with bacteria appearing as though they were sprinkled with coarse pepper), pH higher than 4.5, and potassium hydroxide (10% KOH) "whiff" test positive for the characteristic fishy odor. Bacterial vaginosis can also be diagnosed with point-of-care tests that use nucleic acid probes to detect high concentrations of *G vaginalis*.

The CDC recommends treatment with vaginal or oral metronidazole or clindamycin. Bacterial vaginosis recurs in up to 30% of cases, and repeated antibiotic courses may be required.

Chlamydia. Most *Chlamydia trachomatis* infections occur in women aged younger than 25 years. In perimenopausal and postmenopausal women, testing is recommended only for those at high risk for STIs. These include women with new or multiple sex partners, a sex partner who has had multiple sexual contacts, or a sex partner who has a chlamydial infection.[370] Most women who have chlamydia are asymptomatic; therefore, screening is required to detect and diagnose the condition. However, women who present with symptoms and signs of chlamydia such as fever, pelvic pain, and purulent cervical discharge should also be screened.

Table 32. Preventing Sexually Transmitted Infections in a Woman-to-Woman Sexual Relationship

- Prevent transfer of any body fluids, including menstrual blood and vaginal fluids, into bodily openings, including cuts and abrasions.
- During oral sex, cover the partner's vaginal area with a barrier impermeable to fluid to avoid contact with vaginal secretions.
- Use a latex barrier between vaginas during vulva-to-vulva sex.
- Avoid sharing sex toys. Either clean them in hot, soapy water or cover them with a new condom before switching users.

Chapter 3

Infections of *C trachomatis* can be diagnosed by testing urine or vaginal/endocervical swabs. Nucleic acid amplification tests are recommended because of their sensitivity, availability, and lower cost than cell cultures. According to the CDC, a self- or clinician-collected vaginal swab is the preferred sample type and an option for screening women when a pelvic exam is not otherwise indicated. However, an endocervical swab is acceptable when a pelvic examination is indicated. Urine testing is acceptable but is estimated to detect up to 10% fewer infections when compared with vaginal and endocervical swab samples.[377]

Guidelines advise treatment with antibiotics; a single dose of azithromycin or a week of doxycycline twice daily are most common.[370] Except in pregnant women, test of cure is not advised after the treatment of chlamydia. However, women with chlamydia should be rescreened in 3 months to detect the possibility of failure to treat their partner or reinfection with a new partner. Untreated chlamydia can cause pelvic inflammatory disease and serious sequelae, including long-lasting pelvic pain and infertility

Genital herpes. Genital herpes is caused by the herpes simplex viruses type 1 (HSV-1) and type 2 (HSV-2). Currently, the overall seroprevalence of HSV-2 infection in the general US population is 16.2% of adults aged 14 to 49 years.[369] Infection with HSV-2 is more common in women (1 in 4) than in men (1 in 5), possibly because of male-to-female transmission being more efficient than female to male. Also, most persons infected with HSV-2 have not been diagnosed with genital herpes. Nevertheless, most, if not all, shed virus from the genital area intermittently.[378]

Most genital herpes is caused by HSV-2, and infection typically occurs during sexual contact. Genital herpes can be caused by HSV-1, but it more commonly causes infections of the mouth and lips ("fever blisters"). Infection with HSV-1 of the genitals can be caused by oral-genital contact. Although HSV-1 is less likely to result in severe recurrent outbreaks, it is possible to genitally transmit HSV-1 as well as HSV-2. Because almost all HSV-2 infections are sexually acquired, type-specific HSV-2 antibody indicates anogenital infection. However, the presence of HSV-1 antibody does not distinguish anogenital from orolabial infection. Anyone with a history of either type should be aware of the transmissibility of the infection through genital, oral, and anal contact.

Most patients have no or only minimal signs or symptoms from HSV-1 or HSV-2 infection. When signs do occur, they typically appear as one or more painful blisters on or around the genitals or rectum. The blisters break, leaving tender ulcers that may require 2 to 4 weeks to heal the first time they occur. Other signs and symptoms during the primary episode may include flulike symptoms, including fever and swollen inguinal lymph nodes. Typically, another outbreak can appear weeks or months after the first, although it is almost always less severe and of shorter duration. In some patients, the first clinical episode is actually a recurrence because the primary infection was not recognized.[379] Complications include an increased susceptibility to other STIs, including HIV.[378]

The clinical diagnosis of genital herpes is insensitive and nonspecific. Up to 30% of first-episode cases of genital herpes are caused by HSV-1, but recurrences are much less frequent for genital HSV-1 infection than for genital HSV-2 infection. Therefore, the distinction between HSV serotypes influences prognosis and counseling. For these reasons, some experts believe that the clinical diagnosis of genital herpes should be confirmed by laboratory testing. Virologic tests and type-specific serologic tests for HSV are often used because the sensitivity of the culture methods decline rapidly as lesions begin to heal. Nevertheless, if an ulcer is present, virologic culture is considered the gold standard for diagnosis. According to the CDC, type-specific serologic assays might be useful

- When there is recurrent or atypical genital symptoms with negative cultures
- When there is a clinical diagnosis of genital herpes without laboratory confirmation
- When a sex partner has genital herpes
- As part of a comprehensive evaluation for STDs among persons with multiple sex partners and HIV infection

There is no treatment that can cure herpes, but antiviral medications can shorten and prevent outbreaks. Oral HSV therapy includes acyclovir, valacyclovir, and famciclovir.[370] Topical antiviral treatment is of minimal clinical benefit, and it is not recommended. The CDC recommends daily suppressive therapy for symptomatic herpes to reduce transmission among discordant, heterosexual partners. Suppressive therapy is also an option for women who have frequent outbreaks (6 or more recurrences per year). Suppressive therapy can reduce the frequency of genital herpes recurrences by 70% to 80%, improving quality of life.

Gonorrhea. Caused by the bacterium *Neisseria gonorrhoeae* that multiplies easily in warm, moist areas, gonorrhea infection can be found in the reproductive tract, anus, urethra, mouth, throat, and eyes. Gonorrhea is easily transmitted, primarily through sexual contact. Screening should be performed in those at high risk for gonorrhea infection (women with previous gonorrhea infection or other STIs or with a new or multiple sexual partners).[370]

In women, symptoms are often mild and so nonspecific as to be mistaken for a bladder or vaginal infection. Initial symptoms may include a painful or burning sensation when urinating, increased vaginal discharge, or vaginal bleeding between periods. Many women who are infected have no symptoms but are still at risk of developing serious complications. Symptoms of rectal infection may include discharge, anal itching, soreness, bleeding, or painful bowel movements. Untreated gonorrhea can cause pelvic inflammatory disease and serious sequelae, including long-lasting pelvic pain and infertility. Gonorrhea can spread to the blood or joints and can become life threatening.

Several laboratory tests are available to confirm the diagnosis of gonorrhea. Testing of urine or vaginal/endocervical samples with nucleic acid amplification tests is the preferred method. As with chlamydia, a self- or clinician-collected vaginal swab is the preferred sample type.[377]

Several antibiotics can cure gonorrhea. First-line treatment is a cephalosporin plus azithromycin or doxycycline.[370] Because persons infected with gonorrhea are commonly coinfected with chlamydia, dual treatment is advised. However, drug-resistant strains of gonorrhea are increasing in many areas of the world; for example, quinolones are no longer recommended to treat gonorrhea.[380]

Hepatitis B virus. Hepatitis B is transmitted via percutaneous or mucous membrane exposure to infectious body fluids. Hepatitis B attacks the liver and may cause acute or chronic hepatitis. Although 90% of those infected at birth develop chronic hepatitis, less than 10% of those infected as adults will do so.[381] Acute hepatitis is self-limiting, whereas chronic hepatitis can result in cirrhosis and liver cancer. Although mother-to-infant transmission is most common worldwide, routine screening and vaccination in the United States make this uncommon, and two-thirds of hepatitis B infections in the United States currently are sexually transmitted.[382]

Hepatitis B is found in blood, semen, and vaginal secretions and is 50 to 100 times more infectious than HIV. Infants and adolescents are now routinely vaccinated against hepatitis B, but many perimenopausal and postmenopausal women have not received vaccination because it was not introduced until 1982. However, the CDC recommends that all high-risk adults receive hepatitis B vaccination—this includes all adults with more than one sex partner—however, any adult concerned about hepatitis B can receive the vaccine.[382] Adults with diabetes and chronic liver disease should also be given the hepatitis B vaccine. If infection is suspected, serologic testing can be used to identify both acute and chronic HBV infection.[383]

Hepatitis C virus. Similar to the hepatitis B virus, hepatitis C is a virus that attacks the liver. Unlike hepatitis B, which may resolve spontaneously, most hepatitis C infections become chronic, incurring a risk of cirrhosis and liver cancer. Hepatitis C is most often spread through contact with blood, although sexual transmission also rarely occurs. Baby boomers are at the highest risk of hepatitis C infection, with infection rates 5 times that of other birth cohorts. The CDC recommends that all women and men born between 1945 and 1965 be screened for hepatitis C with a blood-test screening for the antibody to the virus.[384] The reason for high hepatitis C rates among baby boomers is not clear but may result from sexual transmission during the 1970s and 1980s, when national hepatitis C virus rates were highest, as well as contact with contaminated blood products. Routine screening of the blood supply was instituted in 1992, so women who received blood transfusions, blood products, and/or organ transplants or who were on kidney dialysis before 1992 may have acquired hepatitis C in this way. The most common mode of transmission is through sharing intravenous (IV) drug equipment.

HIV. All adults (up to age 64) should be tested at least once for HIV (the AIDS virus).[370] For perimenopausal and postmenopausal women who have already been tested at least once for HIV, routine screening is recommended only in women seeking treatment for an STI, past or present IV drug users, women with multiple sex partners or whose partners have multiple sexual partners, and women having sexual contact with partners who are HIV-infected bisexual or IV drug users. Little is known about HIV risk and older women; however, the potential for infection should not be underestimated. Approximately 11% of new HIV infections in the United States occur in persons aged 50 years and older.[371]

The initial screening test to detect antibodies to HIV is the enzyme-linked immunosorbent assay (ELISA).[370] This test has high sensitivity and specificity; however, false-negative results can occur in the first 6 to 12 weeks after infection, before antibodies develop. Some immunologic disorders may cause a false-positive test result; thus, a second test is warranted in women with a positive HIV result using ELISA. A confirmatory test with the Western blot method should be performed. The Western blot test is the most accurate test and has a false-positive rate of less than 0.001%.[385] Rapid HIV tests are also available for use on saliva or blood, but their results must be confirmed with regular testing. In developed countries, the median time from diagnosis to clinical AIDS is 10 years. Guidelines recommend antiretroviral therapy for all HIV-infected patients to reduce the risk of disease progression and transmission.[386] Referral to an infectious disease specialist for management is appropriate. It has been demonstrated that perimenopausal women with HIV may be at higher risk for depression; therefore, appropriate depression screening should be initiated in these women.[387] In addition, there is evidence that menopause occurs earlier in women with HIV and is associated with more symptoms.[388]

Human papillomavirus. By age 50, at least 80% of US women will have acquired genital HPV infection, a group of viruses that includes more than 100 different strains or types. More than 30 of these viruses are sexually transmitted, living in the skin or mucous membranes of the reproductive tract, vulva, penis, anus, and oropharynx. Most people with HPV will not have any symptoms, and the virus may remain dormant for decades. However, recent evidence indicates that

Chapter 3

HPV infections can reactivate later in life, and more detectable HPV infections in perimenopausal and postmenopausal women are because of reactivations of old infections than newly acquired infections.[389,390] High-risk HPV types are associated with cervical, vaginal, vulvar, anal, and oral cancers, whereas low-risk types are associated with genital warts.

Nearly all cervical cancers are caused by HPV.[391] There is no treatment for HPV, although women aged younger than 26 years are eligible to receive prophylactic vaccination against the most highly oncogenic strains. However, perimenopausal and postmenopausal women are not eligible for HPV vaccination and are the group at highest risk for cervical cancer. The median age of cervical cancer diagnosis is 49 years.[392] Treatments do exist for the lesions that HPV causes, such as genital condyloma, cervical intraepithelial neoplasia, and cancer. Guidelines published in 2012 by the American Society of Colposcopy and Cervical Pathology and endorsed by other organizations recommend Pap screening every 3 years or Pap and HPV co-testing every 5 years for women aged 30 to 65 years.[393] Women aged older than 65 years may discontinue screening only if they have no history of a high-grade cervical lesion, they are not immunosuppressed (HIV, organ transplant, or autoimmune disease requiring immune suppressing medications), they were not diethylstilbestrol exposed, and they have had at least 2 normal screens (either Pap or Pap-HPV co-tests) and no abnormal screens since age 55. Nearly 20% of cervical cancers are diagnosed in women aged older than 65 years, most of whom did not have adequate screening, so ensuring that patients meet all of the above criteria before discontinuing screening is critical to avoiding late-onset cancers.

Syphilis. This STI, caused by the bacterium *Treponema pallidum*, is often called the "great imitator" because so many of its signs and symptoms are indistinguishable from those of other diseases. Many people infected with syphilis have no symptoms for years, yet remain at risk for complications. The primary stage is usually marked by a single or multiple painless chancres, which heal within 3 to 6 weeks. Skin rash and mucous membrane lesions characterize the second stage, followed by the latent stage when symptoms disappear. Untreated, death can result from progressive syphilitic infection.

Syphilis should be diagnosed by examining the exudate from a chancre with dark-field microscopy; however, no commercially available *T pallidum* detection tests are available. Therefore, syphilis can be presumptively diagnosed using 2 serologic tests: 1) Nontreponemal screening tests (rapid plasma regain, Venereal Disease Research Laboratory); and 2) diagnostic treponemal antibody tests (microhemagglutination, fluorescent treponemal antibody absorbed).[370] Because of the possibility of false positives in the presence of certain medical conditions, women with reactive nontreponemal tests should have the diagnosis confirmed with a treponemal test.

Routine screening of women is not recommended, based on the low incidence of syphilis in the general population. However, screening is justified in women who engage in sex with multiple partners, have another STI, live in areas where syphilis is prevalent, or who have had sexual contact with persons with syphilis. In early stages, syphilis can be cured with a single injection of penicillin G. Additional doses are needed to treat someone who has had syphilis for longer than a year.[370] All patients who have syphilis should be screened for HIV infection.

Trichomoniasis. This is the most common curable STI in sexually active women, and unlike other STIs, occurs equally in older and younger women.[394] Caused by the single-cell protozoan parasite, *Trichomonas vaginalis*, trichomoniasis infects the vagina, Bartholin glands, and urethra. Nearly 50% of women are asymptomatic. When women have symptoms, they usually appear within 5 to 28 days of exposure. Many infected women exhibit a heavy, yellow-green, or gray vaginal discharge, sometimes with a strong unpleasant odor, possibly with discomfort during intercourse and urination, as well as genital irritation and itching. On rare occasions, lower abdominal pain can be present. In about two-thirds of infected women, there is edema and inflammation. Diagnosis is confirmed with wet mount or point-of-care tests that use nucleic acid probes to detect *T vaginalis*. Culture is usually only available in research settings.

Trichomoniasis can usually be cured with prescription drugs, either metronidazole or tinidazole, given by mouth for a single dose.[370] Treatment of sex partners is important; up to 20% of patients will be reinfected within 3 months. Untreated infections can last for months to years.

References

1. Committee on Gynecologic Practice of American College of Obstetricians and Gynecologists; Practice Committee of American Society for Reproductive Medicine. Age-related fertility decline: a committee opinion. *Fertil Steril*. 2008;90(3):486-487.
2. Nugent D. The effects of female age on fecundity and pregnancy outcome. *Hum Fertil* (Camb). 2001;4(1):43-48.
3. Pal L, Santoro N. Age-related decline in fertility. *Endocrinol Metab Clin North Am*. 2003;32(3):669-698.
4. Pellestor F, Andréo B, Arnal F. Humeau C, Demaille J. Maternal aging and chromosomal abnormalities: new data drawn from in vitro fertilized human oocytes. *Hum Genet*. 2003;112(2):195-203.
5. Abdalla H, Thum MY. An elevated basal FSH reflects a quantitative rather than qualitative decline of the ovarian reserve. *Hum Reprod*. 2004;19(4):893-898.
6. Hale GE, Robertson DM, Burger HG. The perimenopausal woman: endocrinology and management. *J Steroid Biochem Mol Biol*. 2014;142C:121-131.
7. Klein NA, Houmard BS, Hansen KR, et al. Age-related analysis of inhibin A, inhibin B, and activin a relative to the intercycle monotropic follicle-stimulating hormone rise in normal ovulatory women. *J Clin Endocrinol Metab*. 2004;89(6):2977-2981.
8. Hsu A, Arny M, Knee AB, et al. Antral follicle count in clinical practice: analyzing clinical relevance. *Fertil Steril*. 2011;95(2):474-479.
9. Roudebush WE, Kivens WJ, Mattke JM. Biomarkers of ovarian reserve. *Biomark Insights*. 2008;3:259-268.

10. Seifer DB, Baker VL, Leader B. Age-specific serum anti-Müllerian hormone values for 17,120 women presenting to fertility centers within the United States. *Fertil Steril*. 2011;95(2):747-750.
11. Broekmans FJ, Kwee J, Hendriks DJ, Mol BW, Lambalk CB. A systematic review of tests predicting ovarian reserve and IVF outcome. *Hum Reprod Update*. 2006;12(6):685-718.
12. Rebar RW. Premature ovarian failure. *Obstet Gynecol*. 2009;113(6):1355-1363.
13. Farr SL, Schieve LA, Jamieson DJ. Pregnancy loss among pregnancies conceived through assisted reproductive technology, United States, 1999-2002. *Am J Epidemiol*. 2007;165(12):1380-1388.
14. Ethics Committee of the American Society for Reproductive Medicine. Oocyte or embryo donation to women of advanced age: a committee opinion. *Fertil Steril*. 2013;100(2):337-340.
15. Division of Reproductive Health, National Center for Chronic Disease Prevention and Health Promotion, Centers for Disease Control and Prevention (CDC). US Selected Practice Recommendations for Contraceptive Use, 2013: adapted from the World Health Organization selected practice recommendations for contraceptive use, 2nd edition. *MMWR Recomm Rep*. 2013;62(RR-05):1-60.
16. ESHRE Capri Workshop Group. Female contraception over 40. *Hum Reprod Update*. 2009;15(6):599-612.
17. Pollack A; ACOG Committee on Practice Bulletins-Gynecology. ACOG Practice Bulletin. Clinical management guidelines for obstetrician-gynecologists. Number 46, September 2003. (Replaces technical bulletin number 222, April 1996). *Obstet Gynecol*. 2003;102(3):647-658.
18. Kerin JF, Cooper JM, Price T, et al. Hysteroscopic sterilization using a micro-insert device: results of a multicentre phase II study. *Hum Reprod*. 2003;18(6):1223-1230.
19. Litta P, Cosmi E, Sacco G, Saccardi C, Ciavattini A, Ambrosini G. Hysteroscopic permanent tubal sterilization using a nitinol-dacron intratubal device without anaesthesia in the outpatient setting: procedure feasibility and effectiveness. *Hum Reprod*. 2005;20(12):3419-3422.
20. Cooper JM, Carignan CS, Cher D, Kerin JF; Selective Tubal Occlusion Procedure 2000 Investigators Group. Microinsert nonincisional hysteroscopic sterilization. *Obstet Gynecol*. 2003;102(1):59-67.
21. Vancaillie TG, Anderson TL, Johns DA. A 12-month prospective evaluation of transcervical sterilization using implantable polymer matrices. *Obstet Gynecol*. 2008;112(6):1270-1277.
22. Committee on Practice Bulletins—Gynecology. Practice bulletin no. 128: diagnosis of abnormal uterine bleeding in reproductive-aged women. *Obstet Gynecol*. 2012;120(1):197-206.
23. Mitchell ES, Woods NF, Mariella A. Three stages of the menopausal transition from the Seattle Midlife Women's Health Study: toward a more precise definition. *Menopause*. 2000;7(5):334-349.
24. Greendale GA, Ishii S, Huang MH, Karlamangla AS. Predicting the timeline to the final menstrual period: the study of women's health across the nation. *J Clin Endocrinol Metab*. 2013;98(4):1483-1491.
25. Soules MR, Sherman S, Parrott E, et al. Executive summary: Stages of Reproductive Aging Workshop (STRAW) Park City, Utah, July, 2001. *Menopause*. 2001;8(6):402-407.
26. Harlow SD, Cain K, Crawford S, et al. Evaluation of four proposed bleeding criteria for the onset of late menopausal transition. *J Clin Endocrinol Metab*. 2006;91(9):3432-3438.
27. Harlow SD, Gass M, Hall JE; STRAW 10 Collaborative Group. Executive summary of the Stages of Reproductive Aging Workshop + 10: addressing the unfinished agenda of staging reproductive aging. *Menopause*. 2012;19(4):387-395.
28. Munro MG, Critchley HO, Broder MS, Fraser IS; FIGO Working Group on Menstrual Disorders. FIGO classification system (PALM-COEIN) for causes of abnormal uterine bleeding in nongravid women of reproductive age. *Int J Gynaecol Obstet*. 2011;113(1):3-13.
29. Chaudhry S, Berkley C, Warren M. Perimenopausal vaginal bleeding: diagnostic evaluation and therapeutic options. *J Womens Health (Larchmt)*. 2012;21(3):302-310.
30. Howlader N, Noone AM, Krapcho M, et al, eds. *SEER Stat Fact Sheets: Cervix Uteri Cancer*. Bethesda, MD: National Cancer Institute; 2014. http://seer.cancer.gov/statfacts/html/cervix.html. Accessed May 13, 2014.
31. Baak JP, Mutter GL, Robboy S, et al. The molecular genetics and morphometry-based endometrial intraepithelial neoplasia classification system predicts disease progression in endometrial hyperplasia more accurately than the 1994 World Health Organization classification system. *Cancer*. 2005;103(11):2304-2312.
32. American College of Obstetricians and Gynecologists. ACOG Technology Assessment in Obstetrics and Gynecology No. 5: sonohysterography. *Obstet Gynecol*. 2008;112(6):1467-1469.
33. Grimbizis GF, Tsolakidis D, Mikos T, et al. A prospective comparison of transvaginal ultrasound, saline infusion sonohysterography, and diagnostic hysteroscopy in the evaluation of endometrial pathology. *Fertil Steril*. 2010;94(7):2720-2725.
34. Dijkhuizen FP, DeVries LD, Mol BW, et.al. Comparison of transvaginal ultrasonography and saline infusion sonography for the detection of intracavitary abnormalities in premenopausal women. *Ultrasound Obstet Gynecol*. 2000;15(5):372-376.
35. Moschos E, Ashfaq R, McIntire DD, Liriano B, Twickler DM. Saline-infusion sonography endometrial sampling compared with endometrial biopsy in diagnosing endometrial pathology. *Obstet Gynecol*. 2009;113(4):881-887.
36. Telner DE, Jakubovicz. Approach to diagnosis and management of abnormal uterine bleeding. *Can Fam Physician*. 2007;53(1):58-64.
37. Marjoribanks J, Lethaby A, Farquhar C. Surgery versus medical therapy for heavy menstrual bleeding. *Cochrane Database Syst Rev*. 2006;19;(2):CD003855.
38. Casablanca Y. Management of dysfunctional uterine bleeding. *Obstet Gynecol Clin North Am*. 2008;35(2):219-234.
39. Kroll R, Reape KZ, Margolis M. The efficacy and safety of a low-dose, 91-day, extended-regimen oral contraceptive with continuous ethinyl estradiol. *Contraception*. 2010;81(1):41-48.
40. Anderson FD, Gibbons W, Portman D. Long-term safety of an extended-cycle oral contraceptive (Seasonale): a 2-year multicenter open-label extension trial. *Am J Obstet Gynecol*. 2006;195(1):92-96.
41. Irvine GA, Campbell-Brown MB, Lumsden MA, Heikkilä A, Walker JJ, Cameron IT. Randomised comparative trial of the levonorgestrel intrauterine system and norethisterone for treatment of idiopathic menorrhagia. *Br J Obstet Gynaecol*. 1998;105(6):592-598.
42. Bahamondes L, Bahamondes MV, Monteiro I. Levonorgestrel-releasing intrauterine system: uses and controversies. *Expert Rev Med Devices*. 2008;5(4):437-445.
43. ACOG Committee on Practice Bulletins-Gynecology. ACOG practice bulletin. No. 73: Use of hormonal contraception in women with coexisting medical conditions. *Obstet Gynecol*. 2006;107(6):1453-1472.
44. Hurskainen R, Teperi J, Rissanen P, et al. Clinical outcomes and costs with the levonorgestrel-releasing intrauterine system or hysterectomy for treatment of menorrhagia: randomized trial 5-year follow-up. *JAMA*. 2004;291(12):1456-1463.
45. Hurskainen R, Teperi J, Rissanen P, et al. Quality of life and cost-effectiveness of levonorgestrel-releasing intrauterine system versus hysterectomy for treatment of menorrhagia: a randomized trial. *Lancet*. 2001;357(9252):273-277.
46. Raudaskoski T, Tapanainen J, Tomás E, et al. Intrauterine 10 microg and 20 microg levonorgestrel systems in postmenopausal women receiving oral oestrogen replacement therapy: clinical, endometrial and metabolic response. *BJOG*. 2002;109(2):136-144.
47. Varila E, Wahlstrom T, Rauramo I. A 5-year follow-up study on the use of a levonorgestrel intrauterine system in women receiving hormone replacement therapy. *Fertil Steril*. 2001;76(5):969-973.
48. Kaunitz AM, Inki P. The levonorgestrel-releasing intrauterine system in heavy menstrual bleeding: a benefit-risk review. *Drugs*. 2012;72(2):193-215.
49. Mansour D. Modern management of abnormal uterine bleeding: the levonorgestrel intra-uterine system. *Best Pract Res Clin Obstet Gynaecol*. 2007;21(6):1007-1021.
50. Hickey M, Higham J, Fraser IS. Progestogens versus oestrogens and progestogens for irregular uterine bleeding associated with anovulation. *Cochrane Database Syst Rev*. 2007;(4):CD001895.
51. Desai RM. Efficacy of levonorgestrel releasing intrauterine system for the treatment of menorrhagia due to benign uterine lesions in perimenopausal women. *J Midlife Health*. 2012;3(1):20-23.
52. Hale GE, Hughes CL, Burger HG, Robertson DM, Fraser IS. Atypical estradiol secretion and ovulation patterns caused by luteal out-of-phase (LOOP) events underlying irregular ovulatory menstrual cycles in the menopausal transition. *Menopause*. 2009;16(1):50-59.
53. Lethaby A, Irvine G, Cameron I. Cyclical progestogens for heavy menstrual bleeding. *Cochrane Database Syst Rev*. 2008;(1):CD001016.
54. DeVore GR, Owens O, Kase N. Use of intravenous Premarin in the treatment of dysfunctional uterine bleeding—a double-blind randomized control study. *Obstet Gynecol*. 1982;59(3):285-291.

55. Kouides PA, Byams VR, Philipp CS, et al. Multisite management study of menorrhagia with abnormal laboratory haemostasis: a prospective crossover study of intranasal desmopressin and oral tranexamic acid. *Br J Haematol.* 2009;145(2):212-220.
56. Lethaby A, Duckitt K, Farquhar C. Non-steroidal anti-inflammatory drugs for heavy menstrual bleeding. *Cochrane Database Syst Rev.* 2013;1:CD000400.
57. Jabbour HN, Sales KJ. Prostaglandin receptor signalling and function in human endometrial pathology. *Trends Endocrinol Metab.* 2004;15(8):398-404.
58. Beaumont H, Augood C, Duckitt K, Lethaby A. Danazol for heavy menstrual bleeding. *Cochrane Database Syst Rev.* 2007;(3):CD001017.
59. Samuel NC, Clark TJ. Future research into abnormal uterine bleeding. *Best Pract Res Clin Obstet Gynaecol.* 2007;21(6):1023-1040.
60. Lockwood CJ, Krikun G, Hickey M, Huang SJ, Schatz F. Decidualized human endometrial stromal cells mediate hemostasis, angiogenesis, and abnormal uterine bleeding. *Reprod Sci.* 2009;16(2):162-170.
61. Senthong AJ, Taneepanichskul S. The effect of tranexamic acid for treatment irregular uterine bleeding secondary to DMPA use. *J Med Assoc Thai.* 2009;92(4):461-465.
62. Lethaby A, Pennix J, Hickey M, Garry R, Marjoribanks J. Endometrial resection and ablation techniques for heavy menstrual bleeding. *Cochrane Database Syst Rev.* 2013;8:CD001501.
63. ACOG Committee on Practice Bulletins. ACOG Practice Bulletin. Clinical management guidelines for obstetrician-gynecologists. Number 81, May 2007. *Obstet Gynecol.* 2007;109(5):1233-1248.
64. Bongers MY, Mol BW. Thermal balloon ablation versus endometrial resection for the treatment of abnormal uterine bleeding. *Hum Reprod.* 2000;15(6):1424-1425.
65. American Institute of Ultrasound in Medicine; American College of Obstetricians and Gynecologists; American College of Radiology. AIUM standard for the performance of saline infusion sonohysterography. *J Ultrasound Med.* 2003;22(1):121-126.
66. Breitkopf D, Goldstein SR, Seeds JW; ACOG Committee on Gynecologic Practice. ACOG technology assessment in obstetrics and gynecology. Number 3, September 2003. Saline infusion sonohysterography. *Obstet Gynecol.* 2003;102(3):659-662.
67. Busfield RA, Farquhar CM, Sowter MC, et al. A randomised trial comparing the levonorgestrel intrauterine system and thermal balloon ablation for heavy menstrual bleeding. *BJOG.* 2006;113(3):257-263.
68. Dickersin K, Munro MG, Clark M, et al; Surgical Treatments Outcomes Project for Dysfunctional Uterine Bleeding (STOP-DUB) Research Group. Hysterectomy compared with endometrial ablation for dysfunctional uterine bleeding: a randomized controlled trial. *Obstet Gynecol.* 2007;110(6):1279-1289.
69. A randomized trial of endometrial ablation versus hysterectomy for the treatment of dysfunctional uterine bleeding: outcome at four years. Aberdeen Endometrial Ablation Trials Group. *Br J Obstet Gynaecol.* 1999;106(4):360-366. Erratum in: *Br J Obstet Gynaecol.* 1999;106(8):876.
70. Longinotti MK, Jacobson GF, Hung YY, Learman LA. Probability of hysterectomy after endometrial ablation. *Obstet Gynecol.* 2008;112(6):1214-1220.
71. Avis NE, Colvin A, Bromberger JT, et al. Change in health-related quality of life over the menopausal transition in a multiethnic cohort of middle-aged women: Study of Women's Health Across the Nation. *Menopause.* 2009;16(5):860-869.
72. Burleson MH, Todd M, Trevathan WR. Daily vasomotor symptoms, sleep problems, and mood: using daily data to evaluate the domino hypothesis in middle-aged women. *Menopause.* 2010;17(1):87-95.
73. Williams RE, Levine KB, Kalilani L, Lewis J, Clark RV. Menopause-specific questionnaire assessment in US population-based study shows negative impact on health-related quality of life. *Maturitas.* 2009;62(2):153-159.
74. Freeman EW, Sherif K. Prevalence of hot flushes and night sweats around the world: a systematic review. *Climacteric.* 2007;10(3):197-214.
75. Freeman EW, Sammel MD, Lin H, Liu Z, Gracia CR. Duration of menopausal hot flushes and associated risk factors. *Obstet Gynecol.* 2011;117(5):1095-1104.
76. Col NF, Guthrie JR, Politi M, Dennerstein L. Duration of vasomotor symptoms in middle-aged women: a longitudinal study. *Menopause.* 2009;16(3):453-457.
77. Butts SF, Freeman EW, Sammel MD, Queen K, Lin H, Rebbeck TR. Joint effects of smoking and gene variants involved in sex steroid metabolism on hot flashes in late reproductive-age women. *J Clin Endocrinol Metab.* 2012;97(6):E1032-E1042.
78. Gold EB, Sternfeld B, Kelsey JL, et al. Relation of demographic and lifestyle factors to symptoms in a multi-racial/ethnic population of women 40-55 years of age. *Am J Epidemiol.* 2000;152(5):463-473.
79. Randolph JF Jr, Sowers M, Gold EB, et al. Reproductive hormones in the early menopausal transition: relationship to ethnicity, body size, and menopausal status. *J Clin Endocrinol Metab.* 2003;88(4):1516-1522.
80. Tierney KD, Facione N, Padilla G, Blume K, Dodd M. Altered sexual health and quality of life in women prior to hematopoietic cell transplantation. *Eur J Oncol Nurs.* 2007;11(4):298-308.
81. Freedman RR, Krell W. Reduced thermoregulatory null zone in postmenopausal women with hot flashes. *Am J Obstet Gynecol.* 1999;181(1):66-70.
82. Freedman RR, Dinsay R. Clonidine raises the sweating threshold in symptomatic but not in asymptomatic post-menopausal women. *Fertil Steril.* 2000;74(1):20-23.
83. Freedman RR, Blacker CM. Estrogen raises the sweating threshold in postmenopausal women with hot flashes. *Fertil Steril.* 2002;77(3):487-490.
84. Ockene JK, Barad DH, Cochrane BB, et al. Symptom experience after discontinuing use of estrogen plus progestin. *JAMA.* 2005;294(2):183-193.
85. Stearns V, Ullmer L, López JF, Smith Y, Isaacs C, Hayes DF. Hot flushes. *Lancet.* 2002;360(9348):1851-1861.
86. Marino JL, Saunders CM, Emery LI, Green H, Doherty DA, Hickey M. Nature and severity of menopausal symptoms and their impact on quality of life and sexual function in cancer survivors compared with women without a cancer history. *Menopause.* 2014;21(3):267-274.
87. Loprinzi CL, Wolf SL, Barton DL, Laack NN. Symptom management in premenopausal patients with breast cancer. *Lancet Oncol.* 2008;9(10):993-1001.
88. Jin Y, Hayes DF, Li L, et al. Estrogen receptor genotypes influence hot flash prevalence and composite score before and after tamoxifen therapy. *J Clin Oncol.* 2008;26(36):5849-5854.
89. Henry NL, Rae JM, Li L, et al; Consortium on Breast Cancer Pharmacogenomics Investigators. Association between CYP2D6 genotype and tamoxifen-induced hot flashes in a prospective cohort. *Breast Cancer Res Treat.* 2009;117(3):571-575.
90. Whiteman MK, Staropoli CA, Lengenberg PW, McCarter RJ, Kjerulff KH, Flaws JH. Smoking, body mass, and hot flashes in midlife women. *Obstet Gynecol.* 2003;101(2):264-272.
91. Thurston RC, Sowers MR, Sternfeld B, et al. Gains in body fat and vasomotor symptom reporting over the menopausal transition: the study of women's health across the nation. *Am J Epidemiol.* 2009;170(6):766-774.
92. Kroenke CH, Caan BJ, Stefanick ML, et al. Effects of a dietary intervention and weight change on vasomotor symptoms in the Women's Health Initiative. *Menopause.* 2012;19(9):980-988.
93. Huang AJ, Subak LL, Wing R, et al; Program to Reduce Incontinence by Diet and Exercise Investigators. An intensive behavioral weight loss intervention and hot flashes in women. *Arch Intern Med.* 2010;170(13):1161-1167.
94. Gallicchio L, Miller SR, Visvanathan K, et al. Cigarette smoking, estrogen levels, and hot flashes in midlife women. *Maturitas.* 2006;53(2):133-143.
95. Gold EB, Block G, Crawford S, et al. Lifestyle and demographic factors in relation to vasomotor symptoms: baseline results from the Study of Women's Health Across the Nation. *Am J Epidemiol.* 2004;159(12):1189-1199.
96. Daley A, Stokes-Lampard H, Macarthur C. Exercise for vasomotor menopausal symptoms. *Cochrane Database Syst Rev.* 2011;(5):CD006108.
97. Woods NF. Exercise and hot flashes: toward a research agenda. *Menopause.* 2006;13(4):541-543.
98. Thurston RC, Joffe H, Soares CN, Harlow BL. Physical activity and risk of vasomotor symptoms in women with and without a history of depression: results from the Harvard Study of Moods and Cycles. *Menopause.* 2006;13(4):553-560.
99. Scambia G, Mango D, Signorile PG, et al. Clinical effects of a standardized soy extract in postmenopausal women: a pilot study. *Menopause.* 2000;7(2):105-111.
100. Taku K, Melby MK, Kronenberg F, Kurzer MS, Messina M. Extracted or synthesized soybean isoflavones reduce menopausal hot flash frequency and severity: systematic review and meta-analysis of randomized controlled trials. *Menopause.* 2012;19(7):776-790.

101. Leach MJ, Moore V. Black cohosh (Cimicifuga spp.) for menopausal symptoms. *Cochrane Database Syst Rev.* 2012;9:CD007244.
102. Lethaby AE, Brown J, Marjoribanks J, Kronenberg F, Roberts H, Eden J. Phytoestrogens for vasomotor menopausal symptoms. *Cochrane Database Syst Rev.* 2007;(4):CD001395.
103. Wren BG, Champion SM, Willetts K, Manga RZ, Eden JA. Transdermal progesterone and its effect on vasomotor symptoms, blood lipid levels, bone metabolic markers, moods, and quality of life for postmenopausal women. *Menopause.* 2003;10(1):13-18.
104. North American Menopause Society. The 2012 hormone therapy position statement of: The North American Menopause Society. *Menopause.* 2012; 19(3):257-271.
105. Barton D, Loprinzi C, Quella S, Sloan J, Pruthi S, Novotny P. Depomedroxyprogesterone acetate for hot flashes. *J Pain Symptom Manage.* 2002;24(6):603-607.
106. Prior JC, Hitchcock CL. Progesterone for hot flush and night sweat treatment—effectiveness for severe vasomotor symptoms and lack of withdrawal rebound. *Gynecol Endocrinol.* 2012;28(suppl 2):7-11.
107. Pinkerton JV, Utian WH, Constantine GD, Olivier S, Pickar JH. Relief of vasomotor symptoms with the tissue-selective estrogen complex containing bazedoxifene/conjugated estrogens: a randomized, controlled trial. *Menopause.* 2009;16(6):1116-1124.
108. Lobo RA, Pinkerton JV, Gass ML, et al. Evaluation of bazedoxifene/conjugated estrogens for the treatment of menopausal symptoms and effects on metabolic parameters and overall safety profile. *Fertil Steril.* 2009;92(3):1025-1038.
109. Pickar JH, Yeh IT, Bachmann G, Speroff L. Endometrial effects of a tissue selective estrogen complex containing bazedoxifene/conjugated estrogens as a menopausal therapy. *Fertil Steril.* 2009;92(3):1018-1024.
110. Lindsay R, Gallagher JC, Kagan R, Pickar JH, Constantine G. Efficacy of tissue-selective estrogen complex of bazedoxifene/conjugated estrogens for osteoporosis prevention in at-risk postmenopausal women. *Fertil Steril.* 2009;92(3):1045-1052.
111. de Villiers TJ, Gass ML, Haines CJ, et al. Global consensus statement on menopausal hormone therapy. *Climacteric.* 2013;16(2):203-204.
112. US Food and Drug Administration. FDA approves the first non-hormonal treatment for hot flashes associated with menopause [press release]. FDA Web site. www.fda.gov/newsevents/newsroom/pressannouncements/ucm359030.htm. Last update July 2, 2013. Accessed May 15, 2014.
113. Kimmick GG, Lovato J, McQuellon R, Robinson E, Muss HB. Randomized, double-blind, placebo-controlled, crossover study of sertraline (Zoloft) for the treatment of hot flashes in women with early stage breast cancer taking tamoxifen. *Breast J.* 2006;12(2):114-122.
114. Loprinzi CL, Sloan JA, Perez EA, et al. Phase III evaluation of fluoxetine for treatment of hot flashes. *J Clin Oncol.* 2002;20(6):1578-1583.
115. Nelson HD, Vesco KK, Haney E, et al. Nonhormonal therapies for menopausal hot flashes; systemic review and meta-analysis. *JAMA.* 2006; 295(17):2057-2071.
116. Stearns V, Beebe KL, Iyengar M, Dube E. Paroxetine controlled release in the treatment of menopausal hot flashes: a randomized controlled trial. *JAMA.* 2003;289(21):2827-2834.
117. Sun Z, Hao Y, Zhang M. Efficacy and safety of desvenlafaxine treatment for hot flashes associated with menopause: a meta-analysis of randomized controlled trials. *Gynecol Obstet Invest.* 2013;75(4):255-262.
118. Carpenter JS, Guthrie KA, Larson JC, et al. Effect of escitalopram on hot flash interference: a randomized, controlled trial. *Fertil Steril.* 2012;97(6):1399-1404.
119. Barton DL, LaVasseur BI, Sloan JA, et al. Phase III, placebo-controlled trial of three doses of citalopram for the treatment of hot flashes: NCCTG trial N05C9. *J Clin Oncol.* 2010;28(20):3278-3283.
120. Cronin-Fenton D, Lash TL, Sorensen HT. Selective serotonin reuptake inhibitors and adjuvant tamoxifen therapy: risk of breast cancer recurrence and mortality. *Future Oncol.* 2010;6(6):877-880.
121. Stearns V, Johnson MD, Rae JM, et al. Active tamoxifen metabolite plasma concentrations after coadministration of tamoxifen and the selective serotonin reuptake inhibitor paroxetine. *J Natl Cancer Inst.* 2003;95(23):1758-1764.
122. Kelly CM, Juurlink DN, Gomes T, et al. Selective serotonin reuptake inhibitors and breast cancer mortality in women receiving tamoxifen: a population based cohort study. *BMJ.* 2010;340:c693.
123. Lash TL, Cronin-Fenton D, Ahern TP, et al. Breast cancer recurrence risk related to concurrent use of SSRI antidepressants and tamoxifen. *Acta Oncol.* 2010;49(3):305-312.
124. Rae JM. CYP2D6 genotype should not be used to determine endocrine therapy in postmenopausal breast cancer patients. *Clin Pharmacol Ther.* 2013;94(2):183-185.
125. Gordon PR, Kerwin JP, Boesen KG, Senf J. Sertraline to treat hot flashes: a randomized controlled, double-blind, crossover trial in a general population. *Menopause.* 2006;13(4):568-575.
126. Diem SJ, Blackwell TL, Stone KL, et al. Use of antidepressants and rates of hip bone loss in older women: the study of osteoporotic fractures. *Arch Intern Med.* 2007;167(12):1240-1245.
127. Joffe H, Petrillo L, Viguera A, et al. Eszopiclone improves insomnia and depressive and anxious symptoms in perimenopausal and postmenopausal women with hot flashes: a randomized, double-blinded, placebo-controlled crossover trial. *Am J Obstet Gynecol.* 2010;202(2):171.e1-171.e11.
128. Reddy SY, Warner H, Guttuso T Jr, et al. Gabapentin, estrogen, and placebo for treating hot flashes: a randomized controlled trial. *Obstet Gynecol.* 2006;108(1):41-48.
129. Guttuso T Jr, Kurlan R, McDermott MP, Kieburtz K. Gabapentin's effects on hot flashes in postmenopausal women: a randomized controlled trial. *Obstet Gynecol.* 2003;101(2):337-345.
130. Butt DA, Lock M, Lewis JE, Ross S, Moineddin R. Gabapentin for the treatment of menopausal hot flashes: a randomized controlled trial. *Menopause.* 2008;15(2):310-318.
131. Pandya KJ, Morrow GR, Roscoe JA, et al. Gabapentin for hot flashes in 420 women with breast cancer: a randomised double-blind placebo-controlled trial. *Lancet.* 2005;366(9488):818-824.
132. Loprinzi CL, Kugler JW, Barton DL, et al. Phase III trial of gabapentin alone or in conjunction with an antidepressant in the management of hot flashes in women who have inadequate control with an antidepressant alone: NCCTG N03C5. *J Clin Oncol.* 2007;25(3):308-312.
133. Loprinzi CL, Qin R, Baclueva EP, et al. Phase III, randomized, double-blind, placebo-controlled evaluation of pregabalin for alleviating hot flashes, N07C1. *J Clin Oncol.* 2010;28(4):641-647. Erratum in: *J Clin Oncol.* 2010;28(10):1808.
134. Huang MI, Nir Y, Chen B, Schnyer R, Manber R. A randomized controlled pilot study of acupuncture for postmenopausal hot flashes: effect on nocturnal hot flashes and sleep quality. *Fertil Steril.* 2006;86(3):700-710.
135. Vincent A, Burton DL, Mandrekar JN, et al. Acupuncture for hot flashes: a randomized, sham-controlled clinical study. *Menopause.* 2007;14(1):45-52.
136. Michlewitz H. Benign vulvar disorders. In: Carlson KJ, Eisenstat SA, Frigoletto FD Jr, Schiff I, eds. *Primary Care of Women.* New York: Mosby; 1995:226-229.
137. Davis SR. Sexual health consequences of premature ovarian failure. *Menopause.* 2008;15(1):5-6.
138. Osphena [package insert]. Florham Park, NJ: Shionogi; 2013.
139. Management of symptomatic vulvovaginal atrophy: 2013 position statement of The North American Menopause Society. *Menopause.* 2013;20(9):888-902.
140. Stika CS. Atrophic vaginitis. *Dermatol Ther.* 2010;23(5):514-522.
141. Palacios S. Managing urogenital atrophy. *Maturitas.* 2009;63(4):315-318.
142. Lee YK, Chung HH, Kim JW, Park NH, Song YS, Kang SB. Vaginal pH-balanced gel for the control of atrophic vaginitis among breast cancer survivors: a randomized controlled trial. *Obstet Gynecol.* 2011;117(4):922-927.
143. Bygedman M, Swahn ML. Replens versus dienoestrol cream in the symptomatic treatment of vaginal atrophy in postmenopausal women. *Maturitas.* 1996;23(3):259-263.
144. Nachtigal LE. Comparative study: Replens versus local estrogen in menopausal women. *Fertil Steril.* 1994;61(1):178-180.
145. Estrace [package insert]. Rockaway, NJ: Warner Chilcott; 2011.
146. Premarin vaginal cream [package insert]. Philadelphia, PA: Wyeth Pharmaceuticals; 2012.
147. Estragyn vaginal cream [product monograph]. Concord, Ontario, Canada: Triton Pharma; 2010.
148. Estring [package insert]. New York: Pharmacia & Upjohn Co; 2008.
149. Femring [package insert]. Rockaway, NJ: Warner Chilcott; 2005.
150. Vagifem [package insert]. Princeton, NJ: Novo Nordisk; 2012.
151. Bachmann G, Bouchard C, Hoppe D, et al. Efficacy and safety of low-dose regimens of conjugated estrogens cream administered vaginally. *Menopause.* 2009;16(4):719-727.
152. Suckling J, Lethaby A, Kennedy R. Local oestrogen for vaginal atrophy in postmenopausal women. *Cochrane Database Syst Rev.* 2006;(4):CD001500.
153. Portman DJ, Bachmann GA, Simon JA; Ospemifene Study Group. Ospemifene, a novel selective estrogen receptor modulator for treating dyspareunia associated with postmenopausal vulvar and vaginal atrophy. *Menopause.* 2013;20(6):623-630.

Chapter 3

154. Bachmann GA, Komi JO; Ospemifene Study Group. Ospemifene effectively treats vulvovaginal atrophy in postmenopausal women: results from a pivotal phase 3 study. *Menopause.* 2010;17(3):480-486.
155. Simon J, Portman D, Mabey RG Jr; Ospemifene Study Group. Long-term safety of ospemifene (52-week extension) in the treatment of vulvar and vaginal atrophy in hysterectomized postmenopausal women. *Maturitas.* 2014;77(3):274-281.
156. Soe LH, Wurz GT, Kao CJ, DeGregorio MW. Ospemifene for the treatment of dyspareunia associated with vulvar and vaginal atrophy: potential benefits in bone and breast. *Int J Women's Health.* 2013;5:605-611.
157. Labrie F, Archer D, Bouchard C, et al. Effect of intravaginal dehydroepiandrosterone (Prasterone) on libido and sexual dysfunction in postmenopausal women. *Menopause.* 2009;16(5):923-931.
158. Labrie F, Archer D, Bouchard C, et al. Serum steroid levels during 12-week intravaginal dehydroepiandrosterone administration. *Menopause.* 2009;16(5):897-906.
159. Panjari M, Bell RJ, Jane F, Adams J, Morrow C, Davis SR. The safety of 52 weeks of oral DHEA therapy for postmenopausal women. *Maturitas.* 2009;63(3):240-245.
160. Raz R, Gennesin Y, Wasser J, et al. Recurrent urinary tract infections in postmenopausal women. *Clin Infect Dis.* 2000;30(1):152-156.
161. McMurdo ME, Argo I, Phillips G, Daly F, Davey P. Cranberry or trimethoprim for the prevention of recurrent urinary tract infections? A randomized controlled trial in older women. *J Antimicrob Chemother.* 2009;63(2):389-395.
162. Wang CH, Fang CC, Chen NC, et al. Cranberry-containing products for prevention of urinary tract infections in susceptible populations: a systematic review and meta-analysis of randomized controlled trials. *Arch Intern Med.* 2012;172(13):988-996.
163. Lüthje P, Brauner H, Ramos NL, et al. Estrogen supports urothelial defense mechanisms. *Sci Transl Med.* 2013;5(190):190ra80.
164. Perrotta C, Aznar M, Mejia R, Albert X, Ng CW. Oestrogens for preventing recurrent urinary tract infection in postmenopausal women. *Cochrane Database Syst Rev.* 2008;(2):CD005131.
165. ACOG Committee on Gynecologic Practice. ACOG Committee Opinion: Number 345, October 2006: vulvodynia. *Obstet Gynecol.* 2006;108(4):1049-1052.
166. Gunter J. Vulvodynia: new thoughts on a devastating condition. *Obstet Gynecol Surv.* 2007;62(12):812-819.
167. Reed BD, Harlow SD, Sen A, Edwards RM, Chen D, Haefner HK. Relationship between vulvodynia and chronic comorbid pain conditions. *Obstet Gynecol.* 2012;120(1):145-51.
168. Scheinfeld N. The role of gabapentin in treating disease with cutaneous manifestations and pain. *Int J Dermatol.* 2003;42(6):491-495.
169. ACOG Practice Bulletin No. 93: diagnosis and management of vulvar skin disorders. *Obstet Gynecol.* 2008;111(5):1243-1253.
170. Farage MA, Miller KW, Ledger WJ. Determining the cause of vulvovaginal symptoms. *Obstet Gynecol Surv.* 2008;63(7):445-464.
171. Pappas PG, Kauffman CA, Andes D, et al; Infectious Diseases Society of America. Clinical practice guidelines for the management of candidiasis: 2009 update by the Infectious Diseases Society of America. *Clin Infect Dis.* 2009;48(5):503-535.
172. Amsel R, Totten PA, Spiegel CA, Chen KC, Eschenbach D, Holmes KK. Nonspecific vaginitis. Diagnostic criteria and microbial and epidemiologic associations. *Am J Med.* 1983;74(1):14-22.
173. Sobel JD, Ferris D, Schwebka J, et al. Suppressive antibacterial therapy with 0.75% metronidazole vaginal gel to prevent recurrent bacterial vaginosis. *Am J Obstet Gynecol.* 2006;194(5):1283-1289.
174. Olsson A, Selva-Nayagam P, Oehler M. Postmenopausal vulvar disease. *Menopause Int.* 2008;14(4):169-172.
175. Jones RW, Scurry J, Neill S, MacLean AB. Guidelines for the follow up of women with vulvar lichen sclerosus in specialist clinics. *Am J Obstet Gynecol.* 2008;198(5):496.e1-496.e3.
176. Hannestad YS, Rortveit G, Sandvik H Hunskaar S; Norwegian EPINCONT study. Epidemiology of Incontinence in the County of Nord-Trøndelag. A community-based epidemiological survey of female urinary incontinence: the Norwegian EPINCONT study. Epidemiology of Incontinence in the County of Nord-Trøndelag. *J Clin Epidemiol.* 2000;53(11):1150-1157.
177. Hunskaar S, Arnold EP, Burgio K, Diokno AC, Herzog AR, Mallett VT. Epidemiology and natural history of urinary incontinence. *Int Urogynecol J Pelvic Floor Dysfunct.* 2000;11(5):301-319.
178. Waetjen LE, Feng WY, Ye J, et al; Study of Women's Health Across the Nation. Factors associated with worsening and improving urinary incontinence across the menopausal transition. *Obstet Gynecol.* 2008;111(3):667-677.
179. Waetjen LE, Ye J, Feng WY, et al; Study of Women's Health Across the Nation. Association between menopausal transition and the development of urinary incontinence. *Obstet Gynecol.* 2009;114(5):989-998.
180. Grodstein F, Lifford K, Resnick NM, Curhan GC. Postmenopausal hormone therapy and risk of developing urinary incontinence. *Obstet Gynecol.* 2004;103(2):254-260.
181. Waetjen LE, Johnson WO, Xing G, Feng WY, Greendale GA, Gold EB; Study of Women's Health Across the Nation. Serum estradiol levels are not associated with urinary incontinence in midlife women transitioning through menopause. *Menopause.* 2011;18(12):1283-1290.
182. Gopal M, Sammel MD, Arya LA, Freeman EW, Lin H, Gracia C. Association of change in estradiol to lower urinary tract symptoms during the menopausal transition. *Obstet Gynecol.* 2008;112(5):1045-1052.
183. Grady D, Brown JS, Vittinghoff E, Applegate W, Varner E, Snyder T; HERS Research Group. Postmenopausal hormones and incontinence: the Heart and Estrogen/Progestin Replacement Study. *Obstet Gynecol.* 2001;97(1):116-120.
184. Hendrix SL, Cochrane BB, Nygaard IE, et al. Effects of estrogen with and without progestin on urinary incontinence. *JAMA.* 2005;293(8):935-948.
185. Melville JL, Fan MY, Rau H, Nygaard IE, Katon WJ. Major depression and urinary incontinence in women: temporal associations in an epidemiologic sample. *Am J Obstet Gynecol.* 2009;201(5):490.e1-490.e7.
186. Danforth KN, Townsend MK, Lifford K, Curhan GC, Resnick NM, Grodstein F. Risk factors for urinary incontinence among middle-aged women. *Am J Obstet Gynecol.* 2006;194(2):339-345.
187. Sampselle CM, Harlow SD, Skurnick J, Brubaker L, Bondarenko I. Urinary incontinence predictors and life impact in ethnically diverse perimenopausal women. *Obstet Gynecol.* 2002;100(6):1230-1238.
188. Hägglund D, Walker-Engström ML, Larsson G, Leppert J. Quality of life and seeking help in women with urinary incontinence. *Acta Obstet Gynecol Scand.* 2001;80(11):1051-1055.
189. Moore EE, Jackson SL, Boyko EJ, Scholes D, Fihn SD. Urinary incontinence and urinary tract infection: temporal relationships in postmenopausal women. *Obstet Gynecol.* 2008;111(2 pt 1):317-323.
190. Holroyd-Leduc JM, Straus S. Management of urinary incontinence in women: scientific review. *JAMA.* 2004;291(8):986-995.
191. Shamliyan TA, Kane RL, Wyman J, Wilt TJ. Systematic review: randomized controlled trials of nonsurgical treatments for urinary incontinence in women. *Ann Intern Med.* 2008;148(6):459-473. Erratum in: *Ann Intern Med.* 2011;155(11):796.
192. Subak LL, Wing RW, West DS, et al; PRIDE Investigators. Weight loss to treat urinary incontinence in overweight and obese women. *N Engl J Med.* 2009;360(5):481-490.
193. Mariappan P, Alhasso A, Ballantyne Z, Grant A, N'Dow J. Duloxetine, a serotonin and noradrenaline reuptake inhibitor (SNRI) for the treatment of stress urinary incontinence: a systematic review. *Eur Urol.* 2007;51(1):67-74.
194. Cody JD, Richardson K, Moehrer B, Hextall A, Glazener CM. Oestrogen therapy for urinary incontinence in post-menopausal women. *Cochrane Database Syst Rev.* 2009;(4):CD001405. Update in: *Cochrane Database Syst Rev.* 2012;10:CD001405.
195. Dmochowski RR, Blaivas JM, Gormley EA, et al; Female Stress Urinary Incontinence Update Panel of the American Urological Association Education and Research, Inc, Whetter LE. Update of AUA guideline on the surgical management of female stress urinary incontinence. *J Urol.* 2010;183(5):1906-1914.
196. Burgio KL, Goode PS, Locher JL, et al. Behavioral training with and without biofeedback in the treatment of urge incontinence in older women: a randomized controlled trial. *JAMA.* 2002;288(18):2293-2299.
197. Latini JM, Alipour M, Kreder KJ Jr. Efficacy of sacral neuromodulation for symptomatic treatment of refractory urinary urge incontinence. *Urology.* 2006;67(3):550-554.
198. Visco AG, Brubaker L, Richter HE, et al; Pelvic Floor Disorders Network. Anticholinergic therapy vs. onabotulinumtoxina for urgency urinary incontinence. *N Engl J Med.* 2012;367(19):1803-1813.
199. Irwin DE, Milsom I, Hunskaar S, et al. Population-based survey of urinary incontinence, overactive bladder, and other lower urinary tract symptoms in five countries: results of the EPIC study. *Eur Urol.* 2006;50(6):1306-1315.

200. Tyagi S, Thomas CA, Hayashi Y, Chancellor MB. The overactive bladder: epidemiology and morbidity. *Urol Clin North Am.* 2006;33(4):433-438.

201. Brubaker L. Urinary urgency and frequency: what should a clinician do? *Obstet Gynecol.* 2005;105(3):661-667.

202. Association of Reproductive Health Professionals. *Screening, Treatment, and Management of IC/PBS.* Published May 2008. www.arhp.org/publications-and-resources/clinical-proceedings/screening-treatment-and-management-of-ICPBS. Accessed May 15, 2014.

203. Chapple CR, Kullar V, Gabriel Z, Muston D, Bitoun CE, Weinstein D. The effects of antimuscarinic treatment in overactive bladder: an update of a systematic review and meta-analysis. *Eur Urol.* 2008;54(3):543-562.

204. Nelken RS, Ozel BZ, Leegant AR, Felix JC, Mishell DR Jr. Randomized trial of estradiol vaginal ring versus oxybutynin for the treatment of overactive bladder. *Menopause.* 2011;18(9):962-966.

205. Campbell JD, Gries KS, Watanabe JH, Ravelo A, Dmochowski RR, Sullivan SD. Treatment success for overactive bladder with urinary urge incontinence refractory to oral antimuscarinics: a review of published evidence. *BMC Urol.* 2009;9:18.

206. Burgio KL. Update on behavioral and physical therapies for incontinence and overactive bladder: the role of pelvic floor muscle training. *Curr Urol Rep.* 2013;14(5):457-464.

207. Emmons SL, Otto L. Acupuncture for overactive bladder: a randomized controlled trial. *Obstet Gynecol.* 2005;106(1):138-143.

208. Cardozo L, Lose G, McClish D, Versi E. A systematic review of the effects of estrogens for symptoms suggestive of overactive bladder. *Acta Obstet Gynecol Scand.* 2004;83(10):892-897.

209. Costilla VC, Foxx-Orenstein AE, Mayer AP, Office-based management of fecal incontinence. *Gastroenterol Hepatol (N Y).* 2013;9(7):423-433.

210. Mowatt G, Glazener C, Jarrett M. Sacral nerve stimulation for fecal incontinence and constipation in adults: a short version Cochrane review. *Neurourol Urodyn.* 2008;27(3):155-161.

211. Shifren JL, Monz BU, Russo PA, Segreti A, Johannes CB. Sexual problems and distress in United States women: prevalence and correlates. *Obstet Gynecol.* 2008;112(5):970-978.

212. Lindau ST, Schumm LP, Laumann EO, Levinson W, O'Muircheartaigh CA, Waite LJ. A study of sexuality and health among older adults in the United States. *N Engl J Med.* 2007;357(8):762-774.

213. American Psychiatric Association. *Diagnostic and Statistical Manual of Mental Disorders (DSM-5).* 5th ed. Washington, DC: American Psychiatric Association; 2013.

214. Davison SL, Bell R, Donath S, Montalto JG, Davis SR. Androgen levels in adult females: changes with age, menopause, and oophorectomy. *J Clin Endocrinol Metab.* 2005;90(7):3847-3853.

215. Masters WH, Johnson VE. *Human Sexual Response.* Boston: Little, Brown and Co; 1966.

216. Basson R. Recent advances in women's sexual function and dysfunction. *Menopause.* 2004;11(6 pt 2):714-725.

217. Avis NE, Stellato R, Crawford S, Johannes C, Longcope C. Is there an association between menopause status and sexual functioning? *Menopause.* 2000;7(5):297-309.

218. Dennerstein L, Lehert P, Burger H, Guthrie J. Sexuality. *Am J Med.* 2005;118(suppl 12B):59-63.

219. Davis SR, Davison SL, Donath S, Bell RJ. Circulating androgen levels and self-reported sexual function in women. *JAMA.* 2005;294(1):91-96.

220. Basson R. Clinical practice. Sexual desire and arousal disorders in women. *N Engl J Med.* 2006;354(14):1497-1506.

221. Menopause Health Questionnaire. North American Menopause Society Web site. www.menopause.org/docs/default-document-library/questionnaire.pdf?sfvrsn=0. Published July 2005. Accessed May 15, 2014.

222. Utian WH, MacLean DB, Symonds T, Symons J, Somayaji V, Sisson M. A methodology study to validate a structured diagnostic method used to diagnose female sexual dysfunction and its subtypes in postmenopausal women. *J Sex Marital Ther.* 2005;31(4):271-283.

223. Watts RJ. Sexual functioning, health beliefs, and compliance with high blood pressure medications. *Nurs Res.* 1982;31(5):278-283.

224. Rosen R, Brown C, Heiman J, et al. The Female Sexual Function Index (FSFI): a multidimensional self-report instrument for the assessment of female sexual function. *J Sex Marital Ther.* 2000;26(2):191-208.

225. Meston CM, Derogatis LR. Validated instruments for assessing female sexual function. *J Sex Marital Ther.* 2002;28(suppl 1):155-164.

226. Rosen RC, Taylor JF, Leiblum SR, Bachmann GA. Prevalence of sexual dysfunction in women: results of a survey study of 329 women in an outpatient gynecological clinic. *J Sex Marital Ther.* 1993;19(3):171-188.

227. Marwick C. Survey says patients expect little physician help on sex. *JAMA.* 1999;281(23):2173-2174.

228. Sarwer D, Durlak J. A field trial of the effectiveness of behavioral treatment for sexual dysfunctions. *J Sex Marital Ther.* 1997;23(2):87-97.

229. Dhikav V, Karmarkar G, Gupta R, et al. Yoga in female sexual functions. *J Sex Med.* 2010;7(2 pt 2):964-970.

230. Shifren JL, Desindes S, McIlwain M, Doros G, Mazer NA. A randomized, open label, crossover study comparing the effects of oral versus transdermal estrogen therapy on serum androgens, thyroid hormones, and adrenal hormones in naturally menopausal women. *Menopause.* 2007;14(6):985-994.

231. Segraves RT, Clayton A, Croft H, Wolf A, Warnock J. Bupropion sustained release for the treatment of hypoactive sexual desire disorder in premenopausal women. *J Clin Psychopharmacol.* 2004;24(3):339-342.

232. Safarinejad MR, Hosseini SY, Asgari MA, Dadkhah F, Taghva A. A randomized, double-blind, placebo-controlled study of the efficacy and safety of bupropion for treating hypoactive sexual desire disorder in ovulating women. *BJU Int.* 2010;106(6):832-839.

233. Nurnberg HG, Hensley PL, Heiman JR, Croft HA, Debattista C, Paine S. Sildenafil treatment of women with antidepressant-associated sexual dysfunction: a randomized controlled trial. *JAMA.* 2008;300(4):395-404.

234. Basson R, McInnes R, Smith M, Hodgson G, Koppiker N. Efficacy and safety of sildenafil citrate in women with sexual dysfunction associated with female sexual arousal disorder. *J Womens Health Gend Based Med.* 2002;11(4):367-377.

235. Billups KL, Berman L, Berman J, Metz ME, Glennon ME, Goldstein I. A new non-pharmacological vacuum therapy for female sexual dysfunction. *J Sex Marital Ther.* 2001;27(5):435-441.

236. *2007 Women and Sleep. Sleep in America Polls.* National Sleep Foundation Web site. www.sleepfoundation.org/article/sleep-america-polls/2007-women-and-sleep. Accessed May 15, 2014.

237. Kravitz HM, Ganz PA, Bromberger J, Powell LH, Sutton-Tyrrell K, Meyer PM. Sleep difficulty in women at midlife: a community survey of sleep and the menopausal transition. *Menopause.* 2003;10(1):19-28.

238. Chasens ER, Twerski SR, Yang K, Umlauf MG. Sleepiness and health in midlife women: results of the National Sleep Foundation's 2007 Sleep in America poll. *Behav Sleep Med.* 2010;8(3):157-171.

239. Shaver J, Giblin E, Lentz M, Lee K. Sleep patterns and stability in perimenopausal women. *Sleep.* 1988;11(6):556-561.

240. Young T, Rabago D, Zgierska A, Austin D, Laurel F. Objective and subjective sleep quality in premenopausal, perimenopausal, and postmenopausal women in the Wisconsin Sleep Cohort Study. *Sleep.* 2003;26(6):667-672.

241. Freedman RR, Roehrs TA. Lack of sleep disturbance from menopausal hot flashes. *Fertil Steril.* 2004;82(1):138-144.

242. Joffe H, Crawford S, Economou N, et al. A gonadotropin-releasing hormone agonist model demonstrates that nocturnal hot flashes interrupt objective sleep. *Sleep.* 2013;36(12):1977-1985.

243. Freedman RR, Kruger ML, Wasson SL. Heart rate variability in menopausal hot flashes during sleep. *Menopause.* 2011;18(8):897-900.

244. de Zambotti M, Colrain IM, Sassoon SA, Nicholas CL, Trinder J, Baker FC. Vagal withdrawal during hot flashes occurring in undisturbed sleep. *Menopause.* 2013;20(11):1147-1153.

245. Freedman RR, Roehrs TA. Sleep disturbance in menopause. *Menopause.* 2007;14(5):826-829.

246. Parry BL. Sleep disturbances at menopause are related to sleep disorders and anxiety symptoms. *Menopause.* 2007;14(5):812-814.

247. Dancey DR, Hanly PJ, Soong C, Lee B, Hoffstein V. Impact of menopause on the prevalence and severity of sleep apnea. *Chest.* 2001;120(1):151-155.

248. Collop NA, Adkins D, Phillips BA. Gender differences in sleep and sleep-disordered breathing. *Clin Chest Med.* 2004;25(2):257-268.

249. Resta O, Caratozzolo G, Pannacciulli N, et al. Gender, age and menopause effects on the prevalence and the characteristics of obstructive sleep apnea in obesity. *Eur J Clin Invest.* 2003;33(12):1084-1089.

250. Harvey AG. Sleep hygiene and sleep-onset insomnia. *J Nerv Ment Dis.* 2000;188(1):53-55.

251. Landolt HP, Werth E, Borbély AA, Dijk DJ. Caffeine intake (200 mg) in the morning affects human sleep and EEG power spectra at night. *Brain Res.* 1995;675(1-2):67-74.

252. Afonso RF, Hachul H, Kozasa EH, et al. Yoga decreases insomnia in postmenopausal women: a randomized clinical trial. *Menopause.* 2012;19(2):186-193.

101

Chapter 3

253. Hachul H, Garcia TK, Maciel AL, Yagihara F, Tufik S, Bittencourt L. Acupuncture improves sleep in postmenopause in a randomized, double-blind, placebo-controlled study. *Climacteric.* 2013;16(1):36-40.
254. Siebern AT, Manber R. Insomnia and its effective non-pharmacologic treatment. *Med Clin North Am.* 2010;94(3):581-591.
255. Hainer BL, Matheson EM. Approach to acute headaches in adults. *Am Fam Physician.* 2013;87(10):682-687.
256. Stovner LJ, Hagen K, Jensen R, et al. The global burden of headache: a documentation of headache prevalence and disability worldwide. *Cephalalgia.* 2007;27(3):193-210.
257. Headache Classification Committee of the International Headache Society (IHS). The International Classification of Headache Disorders, 3rd edition (beta version). *Cephalalgia.* 2013;33(9):629-808.
258. Ravishankar K. The art of history-taking in a headache patient. *Ann Indian Acad Neurol.* 2012;15(suppl 1): S7-S14.
259. Loder EW. Headache in the primary care setting. In: Loder EW, Martin VT, eds. *Headache: A Guide for the Primary Care Physician.* Philadelphia, PA: American College of Physicians; 2004:1-10.
260. Chasman D, Schürks M, Anttila V, et al. Genome-wide association study reveals three susceptibility loci for common migraine in the general population. *Nature Genetics.* 2011;43(7):695-698.
261. Chowdhury D. Tension type headache. *Ann Indian Acad Neurol.* 2012;15(suppl 1): S83-S88.
262. Bezov D, Ashina S, Jensen R, Bendtsen L. Pain perception in tension-type headaches. *Headache.* 2011;51(2):262-271.
263. Spierings EL, Ranke AH, Honkoop PC. Precipitating and aggravating factors of migraine versus tension-type headache. *Headache.* 2001;41(6):554-558.
264. Matharu MS, Cohen AS, Frackowiak RS, Goadsby PJ. Posterior hypothalamic activation in paroxysmal hemicrania. *Ann Neurol.* 2006;59(3):535-545.
265. Cohen AS. Short-acting unilateral neuralgiform headache attacks with conjunctival injection and tearing. *Cephalalgia.* 2007;27(7):824-832.
266. Burstein R, Collins B, Jakubowski M. Defeating migraine pain with triptans: a race against the development of cutaneous allodynia. *Ann Neurol.* 2004;55(1):19-26.
267. MacGregor EA. Migraine headache in perimenopausal and menopausal women. *Curr Pain Headache Rep.* 2009;13(5):399-403.
268. Martin VT, Behbehani M. Ovarian hormones and migraine headache: understanding mechanisms and pathogenesis—part 2. *Headache.* 2006;46(3):365-386.
269. MacGregor EA. Estrogen replacement and migraine. *Maturitas.* 2009;63(1):51-55.
270. Tepper SJ. Tailoring management strategies for the patient with menstrual migraine: focus on prevention and treatment. *Headache.* 2006;46(suppl 2): S61-S68.
271. Pringsheim T, Davenport WJ, Dodi D. Acute treatment and prevention of menstrually related migraine headache: evidence-based review. *Neurology.* 2008;70(17):1555-1563.
272. Maizels M, Blumenfeld A, Burchette R. A combination of riboflavin, magnesium, and feverfew for migraine prophylaxis: a randomized trial. *Headache.* 2004;44(9):885-890.
273. Lipton RB, Göbel H, Einhäupl KM, Wilks K, Mauskop A. Petasites hybridus root (butterbur) is an effective preventive treatment for migraine. *Neurology.* 2004;63(12):2240-2244.
274. Bousser MG, Welch KM. Relation between migraine and stroke. *Lancet Neurol.* 2005;4(9):533-542.
275. Shuster LT, Faubion SS, Sood R, Casey PM. Hormonal manipulation strategies in the management of menstrual migraine and other hormonally related headaches. *Curr Neurol Neurosci Rep.* 2011;11(2):131-138.
276. Kurth T, Kase CS, Schürks M, Tzourio C, Buring JE. Migraine and risk of haemorrhagic stroke in women: prospective cohort study. *BMJ.* 2010;341:c3659.
277. Kurth T. The association of migraine with ischemic stroke. *Curr Neurol Neurosci Rep.* 2010;10(2):133-139.
278. Mancia G, Rosei EA, Ambrosioni E, et al; MIRACLES Study Group. Hypertension and migraine comorbidity: prevalence and risk of cerebrovascular events: evidence from a large, multicenter, cross-sectional survey in Italy (MIRACLES study). *J Hypertens.* 2011;29(2):309-318.
279. World Health Organization. Reproductive Health and Research. *Medical Eligibility for Contraceptive Use.* 3rd ed. Geneva: World Health Organization; 2004. http://whqlibdoc.who.int/publications/2004/9241562668.pdf. Accessed May 15, 2014.
280. Kurth T, Gaziano JM, Cook NR, Logroscino G, Diener HC, Buring JE. Migraine and risk of cardiovascular disease in women. *JAMA.* 2006;296(3):283-291. Erratum in: *JAMA.* 2006;296(3):1 p following 291; *JAMA.* 2006;296(6):654.
281. Young WB. Blocking the greater occipital nerve: utility in headache management. *Curr Pain Headache Rep.* 2010;14(5):404-408.
282. Linde K, Allais G, Brinkhaus B, Manheimer E, Vickers A, White AR. Acupuncture for migraine prophylaxis. *Cochrane Database Syst Rev.* 2009;(1):CD001218.
283. Moloney MF, Strickland OL, DeRossett SE, Melby MK, Dietrich AS. The experiences of midlife women with migraines. *J Nurs Scholarsh.* 2006;38(3):278-285.
284. Sullivan Mitchell E, Fugate Woods N. Midlife women's attributions about perceived memory changes: observations from the Seattle Midlife Women's Health Study. *J Womens Health Gend Based Med.* 2001;10(4):351-362.
285. Henderson VW. Menopause, cognitive ageing and dementia: practice implications. *Menopause Int.* 2009;15(1):41-44.
286. Maki PM, Drogos LL, Rubin LH, Banuvar S, Shulman LP, Geller SE. Objective hot flashes are negatively related to verbal memory performance in midlife women. *Menopause.* 2008;15(5):848-856.
287. Weber MT, Maki PM, McDermott MP. Cognition and mood in perimenopause: a systematic review and meta-analysis. *J Steroid Biochem Mol Biol.* 2014;142C:90-98.
288. Greendale GA, Huang MH, Wight RG, et al. Effects of the menopause transition and hormone use on cognitive performance in midlife women. *Neurology.* 2009;72(21):1850-1857.
289. Greendale GA, Wight RG, Huang MH, et al. Menopause-associated symptoms and cognitive performance: results from the study of women's health across the nation. *Am J Epidemiol.* 2010;171(11):1214-1224.
290. Henderson VW, Popat RA. Effects of endogenous and exogenous estrogen exposures in midlife and late-life women on episodic memory and executive functions. *Neuroscience.* 2011;191:129-138.
291. Henderson VW, Sherwin BB. Surgical versus natural menopause: cognitive issues. *Menopause.* 2007;14(3 pt 2):572-579.
292. Avis NE, Stellato R, Crawford S, et al. Is there a menopausal syndrome? Menopausal status and symptoms across racial/ethnic groups. *Soc Sci Med.* 2001;52(3):345-356.
293. Phillips SM, Sherwin BB. Effects of estrogen on memory function in surgically menopausal women. *Psychoneuroendocrinology.* 1992;17(5): 485-495.
294. Reitz C, Brayne C, Mayeux R. Epidemiology of Alzheimer disease. *Nat Rev Neurol.* 2011;7(3):137-152.
295. Gauthier S, Reisberg B, Zaudig M, et al; International Psychogeriatric Association Expert Conference on Mild Cognitive Impairment. Mild cognitive impairment. *Lancet.* 2006;367(9518):1262-1270.
296. Williams JW, Plassman BL, Burke J, Holsinger T, Benjamin S. *Preventing Alzheimer's Disease and Cognitive Decline.* Evidence Report/Technology Assessment No. 193. AHRQ Publication No. 10-E005. Rockville, MD: Agency for Healthcare Research and Quality; 2010.
297. Sofi F, Valecchi D, Bacci D, et al. Physical activity and risk of cognitive decline: a meta-analysis of prospective studies. *J Intern Med.* 2011;269(1):107-117.
298. Kang JH, Cook N, Manson J, Buring JE, Grodstein F. A randomized trial of vitamin E supplementation and cognitive function in women. *Arch Intern Med.* 2006;166(22):2462-2468.
299. Malouf R, Grimley Evans J. Folic acid with or without vitamin B12 for the prevention and treatment of healthy elderly and demented people. *Cochrane Database Syst Rev.* 2008;(4):CD004514. Update of: *Cochrane Database Syst Rev.* 2003;(4):CD004514.
300. DeKosky ST, Williamson JD, Fitzpatrick AL, et al. Ginkgo biloba for prevention of dementia: a randomized controlled trial. *JAMA.* 2008;300(19):2253-2262.
301. Snitz BE, O'Meara ES, Carlson MC, et al; Ginkgo Evaluation of Memory (GEM) Study Investigators. Ginkgo biloba for preventing cognitive decline in older adults: a randomized trial. *JAMA.* 2009;302(24):2663-2670.
302. Vellas B, Coley N, Ousset PJ, et al; GuidAge Study Group. Long-term use of standardised Ginkgo biloba extract for the prevention of Alzheimer's disease (GuidAge): a randomised placebo-controlled trial. *Lancet Neurol.* 2012;11(10):851-859.
303. Grimley Evans J, Malouf R, Huppert FAH, van Niekerk JK. Dehydroepiandrosterone (DHEA) supplementation for cognitive function in healthy elderly people. *Cochrane Database Syst Rev.* 2006;4:CD006221.

304. Henderson VW, St John JA, Hodis HN, et al; WISH Research Group. Long-term soy isoflavone supplementation and cognition in women: a randomized, controlled trial. *Neurology.* 2012;78(23):1841-1848.
305. Sydenham E, Dangour AD, Lim WS. Omega 3 fatty acid for the prevention of cognitive decline and dementia. *Cochrane Database Syst Rev.* 2012;6:CD005379.
306. McGuinness B, Todd S, Passmore P, Bullock R. Blood pressure lowering in patients without prior cerebrovascular disease for prevention of cognitive impairment and dementia. *Cochrane Database Syst Rev.* 2009;(4):CD004034.
307. Henderson VW. Alzheimer's disease: review of hormone therapy trials and implications for treatment and prevention after menopause. *J Steroid Biochem Mol Biol.* 2014;142C:99-106.
308. Shumaker SA, Legault C, Rapp SR, et al, WHIMS Investigators. Estrogen plus progestin and the incidence of dementia and mild cognitive impairment in postmenopausal women: the Women's Health Initiative Memory Study: a randomized controlled trial. *JAMA.* 2003;289(20):2651-2662.
309. Shumaker SA, Legault C, Kuller L, et al; Women's Health Initiative Memory Study. Conjugated equine estrogens and incidence of probable dementia and mild cognitive impairment in postmenopausal women: Women's Health Initiative Memory Study. *JAMA.* 2004;291(24):2947-2985.
310. Moyer VA; US Preventive Services Task Force. Menopausal hormone therapy for the primary prevention of chronic conditions: US Preventive Services Task Force recommendation statement. *Ann Intern Med.* 2013;158(1):47-54.
311. Marjoribanks J, Farquhar C, Roberts H, Lethaby A. Long term hormone therapy for perimenopausal and postmenopausal women. *Cochrane Database Syst Rev.* 2012;7:CD004143.
312. Henderson VW, Benke KS, Green RC, Cupples LA, Farrer LA; Mirage Study Group. Postmenopausal hormone therapy and Alzheimer's disease risk: interaction with age. *J Neurol Neurosurg Psychiatry.* 2005;76(1):103-105.
313. Henderson VW, Espeland MA, Hogan PE, et al. Prior use of hormone therapy and incident Alzheimer's disease in the Women's Health Initiative Memory Study [abstract]. *Neurology.* 2007;68(suppl 1):A205.
314. Shao H, Breitner JC, Whitmer RA, et al; Cache County Investigators. Hormone therapy and Alzheimer disease dementia: new findings from the Cache County study. *Neurology.* 2012;79(18):1846-1852.
315. Whitmer RA, Quesenberry CP, Zhou J, Yaffe K. Timing of hormone therapy and dementia: the critical window theory revisited. *Ann Neurol.* 2011;69(1):163-169.
316. Resnick SM, Maki PM, Rapp SR, et al; Women's Health Initiative Study of Cognitive Aging Investigators. Effects of combination estrogen plus progestin hormone treatment on cognition and affect. *J Clin Endocrinol Metab.* 2006;91(5):1802-1810.
317. Resnick SM, Espeland MA, An Y, et al; Women's Health Initiative Study of Cognitive Aging Investigators. Effects of conjugated equine estrogens on cognition and affect in postmenopausal women with prior hysterectomy. *J Clin Endocrinol Metab.* 2009;94(11):4152-4161.
318. Asthana S, Gleason CE, Wharton W, et al. The Kronos Early Estrogen Prevention Study: results of the Cognitive and Affective Sub-Study (KEEPS Cog) [abstract]. *Menopause.* 2012;19(12):1365.
319. Espeland MA, Shumaker SA, Leng I, et al; WHIMSY Study Group. Long-term effects on cognitive function of postmenopausal hormone therapy prescribed to women aged 50 to 55 years. *JAMA Intern Med.* 2013;173(15):1429-1436.
320. Phung TK, Waltoft BL, Laursen TM, et al. Hysterectomy, oophorectomy and risk of dementia: a nationwide historical cohort study. *Dement Geriatr Cogn Disord.* 2010;30(1):43-50.
321. Rocca WA, Bower JH, Maraganore DM, et al. Increased risk of cognitive impairment or dementia in women who underwent oophorectomy before menopause. *Neurology.* 2007;69(11):1074-1083.
322. Kritz-Silverstein D, Barrett-Connor E. Hysterectomy, oophorectomy, and cognitive function in older women. *J Am Geriatr Soc.* 2002;50(1):55-61.
323. Rossouw JE, Prentice RL, Manson JE, et al. Postmenopausal hormone therapy and risk of cardiovascular disease by age and years since menopause. *JAMA.* 2007;297(13):1465-1477. Erratum in: *JAMA.* 2008;299(12):1426.
324. Grodstein F, Manson JE, Stampfer MJ, Rexrode K. Postmenopausal hormone therapy and stroke: role of time since menopause and age at initiation of hormone therapy. *Arch Intern Med.* 2008;168(8):861-866.
325. Henderson VW, Lobo RA. Hormone therapy and the risk of stroke: perspectives 10 years after the Women's Health Initiative trials. *Climacteric.* 2012;15(3):229-234.
326. Renoux C, Dell'aniello S, Garbe E, Suissa S. Transdermal and oral hormone replacement therapy and the risk of stroke: a nested case-control study. *BMJ.* 2010;340:c2519.
327. Farina N, Isaac MG, Clark AR, Rusted J, Tabet N. Vitamin E for Alzheimer's dementia and mild cognitive impairment. *Cochrane Database Syst Rev.* 2012;11:CD002854.
328. Jaturapatporn D, Isaac MG, McCleery J, Tabet N. Aspirin, steroidal and non-steroidal anti-inflammatory drugs for the treatment of Alzheimer's disease. *Cochrane Database Syst Rev.* 2012;2:CD006378.
329. McGuinness B, O'Hare J, Craig D, Bullock R, Malouf R, Passmore P. Statins for the treatment of dementia. *Cochrane Database Syst Rev.* 2010;(8):CD007514.
330. Mazereeuw G, Lanctôt KL, Chau SA, Swardfager W, Herrmann N. Effects of ω-3 fatty acids on cognitive performance: a meta-analysis. *Neurobiol Aging.* 2012;33(7):1482.e.17-e.29.
331. Bond M, Rogers G, Peters J, et al. The effectiveness and cost-effectiveness of donepezil, galantamine, rivastigmine and memantine for the treatment of Alzheimer's disease (review of Technology Appraisal No. 111): a systematic review and economic model. *Health Technol Assess.* 2012;16(21):1-470.
332. Bromberger JT, Matthews KA, Schott LL, et al. Depressive symptoms during the menopausal transition: the Study of Women's Health Across the Nation (SWAN). *J Affect Disord.* 2007;103(1-3):267-272.
333. Cohen LS, Soares CN, Vitonis AF, Otto MW, Harlow BL. Risk for new onset of depression during the menopause transition. *Arch Gen Psychiatry.* 2006;63(4):385-390.
334. Freeman EW, Sammel MD, Lin H, Nelson DB. Associations of hormones and menopausal status do women with depressed mood in women with no history of depression. *Arch Gen Psychiatry.* 2006;63(4):375-382.
335. Rapkin AJ, Mikacich JA, Moatakef-Imani B, Rasgon N. The clinical nature and formal diagnosis of premenstrual, postpartum, and perimenopausal affective disorders. *Curr Psychiatry Rep.* 2002;4(6):419-428.
336. Payne JL, Palmer JT, Joffe H. A reproductive subtype of depression: conceptualizing models and moving toward etiology. *Harv Rev Psychiatry.* 2009;17(2):72-86.
337. Rocca WA, Grossardt BR, Geda YE, et al. Long-term risk of depressive and anxiety symptoms after early bilateral oophorectomy. *Menopause.* 2008;15(6):1050-1059.
338. Gibson CJ, Joffe H, Bromberger JT, et al. Mood symptoms after natural menopause and hysterectomy with and without bilateral oophorectomy among women in midlife. *Obstet Gynecol.* 2012;119(5):935-941.
339. Utian WH, Boggs PP. The North American Menopause Society 1998 Menopause Survey. Part I: postmenopausal women's perceptions about menopause and midlife. *Menopause.* 1999;6(2):122-128.
340. Schmidt PJ, Murphy JH, Haq N, Rubinow DR, Danaceau MA. Stressful life events, personal losses, and perimenopause-related depression. *Arch Womens Ment Health.* 2004;7(1):19-26.
341. Bailey JW, Cohen LS. Prevalence of mood and anxiety disorders in women who seek treatment for premenstrual syndrome. *J Womens Health Gend Based Med.* 1999;8(9):1181-1184.
342. Freeman EW, Sammel MD, Liu L, Gracia CR, Nelson DB, Hollander L. Hormones and menopausal status as predictors of depression in women in transition to menopause. *Arch Gen Psychiatry.* 2004;61(1):62-70.
343. Gibbs Z, Lee S, Kulkarni J. What factors determine whether a woman becomes depressed during the perimenopause? *Arch Womens Ment Health.* 2012;15(5):323-332.
344. Wassertheil-Smoller S, Shumaker S, Ockene J, et al. Depression and cardiovascular sequelae in postmenopausal women: The Women's Health Initiative (WHI). *Arch Intern Med.* 2004;164(3):289-298.
345. Yaffe K, Blackwell T, Gore R, Sands L, Reus V, Browner WS. Depressive symptoms and cognitive decline in nondemented elderly women: a prospective study. *Arch Gen Psychiatry.* 1999;56(5):425-430.
346. Landau C, Milan FB. Assessment and treatment of depression during the menopause: a preliminary report. *Menopause.* 1996;3(4):201-207.
347. Joffe H, Groninger H, Soares CN, Nonacs R, Cohen LS. An open trial of mirtazapine in menopausal women with depression unresponsive to estrogen replacement therapy. *J Womens Health Gend Based Med.* 2001;10(10):999-1004. Erratum in: *J Womens Health Gend Based Med.* 2003;12(1):92.
348. Altshuler LL, Cohen LS, Moline ML, et al. Treatment of depression in women: a summary of the expert consensus guidelines. *J Psychiatr Pract.* 2001;7(3):185-208.
349. Maki PM, Freeman EW, Greendale GA, et al. Summary of the National Institute on Aging-sponsored conference on depressive symptoms and cognitive complaints in the menopausal transition. *Menopause.* 2010;17(4):815-822.

350. Campbell S, Whitehead M. Oestrogen therapy and the menopausal syndrome. *Clin Obstet Gynaecol.* 1977;4(1):31-47.
351. Joffe H, Hall JE, Soares CN, et al. Vasomotor symptoms are associated with depression in perimenopausal women seeking primary care. *Menopause.* 2002;9(6):392-398.
352. Avis NE, Brambilla D, McKinlay SM, Vass K. A longitudinal analysis of the association between menopause and depression: results from the Massachusetts Women's Health Study. *Ann Epidemiol.* 1994;4(3):214-220.
353. Freeman EW, Sammel MD, Lin H. Temporal associations of hot flashes and depression in the transition to menopause. *Menopause.* 2009;16(4):728-734.
354. Green SM, Haber E, McCabe RE, Soares CN. Cognitive-behavioral group treatment for menopausal symptoms: a pilot study. *Arch Womens Ment Health.* 2013;16(4):325-332.
355. Siebern AT, Suh S, Nowakowski S. Non-pharmacological treatment of insomnia. *Neurotherapeutics.* 2012;9(4):717-727.
356. Steiner M, Romano SJ, Babcock S, et al. The efficacy of fluoxetine in improving physical symptoms associated with premenstrual dysphoric disorder. *BJOG.* 2001;108(5):462-468.
357. Cohen LS, Soares CN, Yonkers KA, Bellew KM, Bridges IM, Steiner M. Paroxetine controlled release for premenstrual dysphoric disorder: a double-blind, placebo-controlled trial. *Psychosom Med.* 2004;66(5):707-713.
358. Yonkers KA, Halbreich U, Freeman E, et al. Symptomatic improvement of premenstrual dysphoric disorder with sertraline treatment. A randomized controlled trial. Sertraline Premenstrual Dysphoric Collaborative Study Group. *JAMA.* 1997;278(12):983-988.
359. Pearlstein TB, Bachmann GA, Zacur HA, Yonkers KA. Treatment of premenstrual dysphoric disorder with a new drospirenone-containing oral contraceptive formulation. *Contraception.* 2005;72(6):414-421.
360. Joffe H, Soares CN, Petrillo LF, et al. Treatment of depression and menopause-related symptoms with the serotonin-norepinephrine reuptake inhibitor duloxetine. *J Clin Psychiatry.* 2007;68(6):943-950.
361. Soares CN, Poitras JR, Prouty J, Alexander AB, Shifren JL, Cohen LS. Efficacy of citalopram as a monotherapy or as an adjunctive treatment to estrogen therapy for perimenopausal and postmenopausal women with depression and vasomotor symptoms. *J Clin Psychiatry.* 2003;64(4):473-479.
362. Soares CN, Arsenio H, Joffe H, et al. Escitalopram versus ethinyl estradiol and norethindrone acetate for symptomatic peri- and postmenopausal women: impact on depression, vasomotor symptoms, sleep, and quality of life. *Menopause.* 2006;13(5):780-786.
363. Diem SJ, Ruppert K, Cauley JA, et al. Rates of bone loss among women initiating antidepressant medication use in midlife. *J Clin Endocrinol Metab.* 2013;98(11):4355-4363.
364. Soares CN, Almeida OP, Joffe H, Cohen LS. Efficacy of estradiol for the treatment of depressive disorders in perimenopausal women: a double-blind, randomized, placebo-controlled trial. *Arch Gen Psychiatry.* 2001;58(6):529-534.
365. Schmidt PJ, Nieman L, Danaceau MA, et al. Estrogen replacement in perimenopause-related depression: a preliminary report. *Am J Obstet Gynecol.* 2000;183(2):414-420.
366. Cohen LS, Soares CN, Poitras JR, Prouty J, Alexander AB, Shifren JL. Short-term use of estradiol for depression in perimenopausal and postmenopausal women: a preliminary report. *Am J Psychiatry.* 2003;160(8):1519-1522.
367. Hlatky MA, Boothroyd D, Vittinghoff E, Sharp P, Whooley MA; Heart and Estrogen/Progestin Replacement Study (HERS) Research Group. Quality-of-life and depressive symptoms in postmenopausal women after receiving hormone therapy: results from the Heart and Estrogen/Progestin Replacement Study (HERS) trial. *JAMA.* 2002;287(5):591-597.
368. Morrison MF, Kallan MJ, Ten Have T, Katz I, Tweedy K, Battistini M. Lack of efficacy of estradiol for depression in postmenopausal women: a randomized, controlled trial. *Biol Psychiatry.* 2004;55(4):406-412.
369. Satterwhite CL, Torrone E, Meites E, et al. Sexually transmitted infections among US women and men: prevalence and incidence estimates, 2008. *Sex Transm Dis.* 2013;40(3):187-193.
370. Workowski KA, Berman S; Centers for Disease Control and Prevention (CDC). Sexually transmitted diseases treatment guidelines, 2010. *MMWR Recomm Rep.* 2010;59(RR-12):1-110. Erratum in: *MMWR Recomm Rep.* 2011;60(1):18.
371. Brooks JT, Buchacz K, Gebo KA, Mermin J. HIV infection and older Americans: the public health perspective. *Am J Public Health.* 2012;102(8):1516-1526.
372. Lindau ST, Leitsch SA, Lundberg KL, Jerome J. Older women's attitudes, behavior, and communication about sex and HIV: a community-based study. *J Womens Health.* 2006;15(6):747-753.
373. Piper JM, Shain RN, Korte JE, Holden AE. Behavioral interventions for prevention of sexually transmitted diseases in women: a physician's perspective. *Obstet Gynecol Clin North Am.* 2003;30(4):659-669.
374. Holmes KK, Levine R, Weaver M. Effectiveness of condoms in preventing sexually transmitted infections. *Bull World Health Organ.* 2004;82(6):454-461.
375. Shepard CW, Simard EP, Finelli AE, Fiore AE, Bell BP. Hepatitis B virus infection: epidemiology and vaccination. *Epidemiol Rev.* 2006;28:112-125.
376. Centers for Disease Control and Prevention. *Expedited Partner Therapy in the Management of Sexually Transmitted Diseases.* Atlanta, GA: US Dept of Health and Human Services; 2006.
377. Centers for Disease Control and Prevention. Recommendations for the laboratory-based detection of Chlamydia trachomatis and Neisseria gonorrhoeae—2014. *MMWR Recomm Rep.* 2014;639(RR-2):1-19.
378. Mark KE, Wald A, Magaret AS, et al. Rapidly cleared episodes of herpes simplex virus reactivation in immunocompetent adults. *J Infect Dis.* 2008;198(8):1141-1149.
379. Centers for Disease Control and Prevention. *Self-Study STD Modules for Clinicians: Genital Herpes Simplex Virus (HSV) Infection.* CDC Web site. Updated March 2014. www2a.cdc.gov/stdtraining/self-study/herpes/hsv_self_study_clinical.html. Accessed May 13, 2014.
380. Centers for Disease Control and Prevention (CDC). Update to CDC's sexually transmitted diseases treatment guidelines, 2006: fluoroquinolones no longer recommended for treatment of gonococcal infections. *MMWR Morb Mortal Wkly Rep.* 2007;56(14):332-336.
381. Weinbaum CM, Mast EE, Ward JW. Recommendations for identification and public health management of persons with chronic hepatitis B virus infection. *Hepatology.* 2009;49(5 suppl):S35-S44.
382. Mast EE, Weinbaum CM, Fiore AE, et al; Advisory Committee on Immunization Practices (ACIP) Centers for Disease Control and Prevention (CDC). A comprehensive immunization strategy to eliminate transmission of hepatitis B virus infection in the United States: recommendations of the Advisory Committee on Immunization Practices (ACIP) part II: immunization of adults. *MMWR Recomm Rep.* 2006;55(RR-16):1-33. Erratum in: *MMWR Morb Wkly Rep.* 2007;56(42):1114.
383. Mast EE, Margolis HS, Fiore AE; Advisory Committee on Immunization Practices (ACIP). A comprehensive immunization strategy to eliminate transmission of hepatitis B virus infection in the United States: recommendations of the Advisory Committee on Immunization Practices (ACIP) part I: immunization of infants, children, and adolescents. *MMWR Recomm Rep.* 2005;54(RR-16):1-31.
384. Smith BD, Morgan RL, Beckett GA, et al; Centers for Disease Control and Prevention. Recommendations for the identification of chronic hepatitis C virus infection among persons born during 1945-1965. *MMWR Recomm Rep.* 2012;61(RR-4):1-32. Erratum in: *MMWR Recomm Rep.* 2012;61(43):886.
385. Mahmood T, Yang PC. Western blot: technique, theory, and trouble shooting. *N Am J Med Sci.* 2012;4(9):429-434.
386. Hammer SM, Eron JJ Jr, Reiss P, et al; International AIDS Society-USA. Antiretroviral treatment of adult HIV infection: 2008 recommendations of the International AIDS Society-USA panel. *JAMA.* 2008;300(5):555-570.
387. Hartel D, Lo Y, Bauer C, et al. Attitudes toward menopause in HIV-infected and at-risk women. *Clin Interv Aging.* 2008;3(3):561-566.
388. Kanapathipillai R, Hickey M, Giles M. Human immunodeficiency virus and menopause. *Menopause.* 2013;20(9):983-990.
389. Gravitt PE, Rositch AF, Silver MI, et al. A cohort effect of the sexual revolution may be masking an increase in human papillomavirus detection at menopause in the United States. *J Infect Dis.* 2013;207(2:272-280.
390. Rositch AF, Burke AE, Viscidi RP, Silver MI, Chang K, Gravitt PE. Contributions of recent and past sexual partnerships on incident human papillomavirus detection: acquisition and reactivation in older women. *Cancer Res.* 2012;72(23):6183-6190.
391. Walboomers JM, Jacobs MW, Manos MM, et al. Human papilloma virus is a necessary cause of invasive cervical cancer worldwide. *J Pathol.* 1999;189(1):12-19.
392. Howlader N, Noone AM, Krapcho M, et al, eds. *SEER Cancer Statistics Review, 1975-2010: Cancer of the Corpus and Uterus, NOS (Invasive).* Bethesda, MD: National Cancer Institute; 2012. http://seer.cancer.gov/csr/1975_2010/results_merged/sect_07_corpus_uteri.pdf. Accessed May 15, 2014.

393. Saslow D, Solomon D, Lawson HW, et al; American Cancer Society; American Society for Colposcopy and Cervical Pathology; American Society for Clinical Pathology. American Cancer Society, American Society for Colposcopy and Cervical Pathology, and American Society for Clinical Pathology screening guidelines for the prevention and early detection of cervical cancer. *Am J Clin Pathol*. 2012;137(4):516-542.
394. Muzny CA, Schwebke JR. The clinical spectrum of Trichomonas vaginalis infection and challenges to management. *Sex Transm Infect*. 2013;89(6):423-425.

Chapter 4

Disease Risk

Clinicians who care for midlife women should be aware of risk factors for common diseases including cardiovascular disease, diabetes mellitus, osteoporosis, and cancers and know the strategies to lower these risks and treat these diseases.

Cardiovascular health

Cardiovascular disease (CVD) is the leading killer of women worldwide. More women die from CVD than from all cancers, tuberculosis, HIV/AIDS, and malaria combined.[1] In 2009, a total of 401,495 US women died from heart disease, accounting for more than half of all deaths.[2] Although rates of CVD in the United States are lowering because of significant advancements in prevention, diagnosis, and treatment, 1 in 3 women will die of heart disease regardless of race or ethnicity, and more women will die of CVD than men.

Heart disease awareness in women is increasing, yet only 52% of women identify heart disease as the leading cause of death in women, and a significant disconnect still remains in black and Hispanic women aged 25 to 34 years, with only 30% of them aware.[3]

Cardiovascular disease is an inclusive term used to describe many conditions:
- Arrhythmias
- Atherosclerosis
- Congenital cardiovascular defect
- Heart failure (HF)
- Coronary heart disease (CHD)
  - Myocardial infarction (MI)
  - Angina pectoris
  - Microvascular coronary dysfunction
- Hypertension
- Stroke and transient ischemic attack (TIA)
- Valvular heart disease
- Peripheral arterial disease
- Aortic disease
- Arterial and venous thrombosis and pulmonary embolism

Proper function of the myocardium depends on a positive balance of oxygen and nutrient supply and demand. Angina is most often associated with the narrowing or dysfunction of coronary arteries, caused by the formation of atherosclerotic plaques in the epicardial coronary arteries or abnormal vasomotor function of microvasculature in the heart. Chronic narrowing of the lumen of the coronary artery is most commonly associated with a continuous process of plaque formation, disruption, reorganization, and reformation that begins early in life and may lead to stable angina or even sudden death. Genetic, metabolic, behavioral, and environmental factors can all contribute to the process. Myocardial infarction usually occurs when a previously narrowed artery suddenly becomes completely occluded with a thrombus and less commonly because of microvascular dysfunction or coronary dissection, which is relatively more prevalent in women.[4]

Diseased peripheral blood vessels can lead to conditions such as stroke, TIA, and hypertension. In addition, peripheral vascular disease can result in difficulty walking and, if severe, amputation of the affected limb.

Palpitations

During menopausal vasomotor episodes, the heart rate can increase 7 to 15 beats per minute. Some women may interpret the perceived increase as palpitations. Although most are benign, the differential diagnosis for palpitations can be extensive and includes cardiac disorders, anemia, medication or caffeine use, and thyroid and anxiety disorders. Although it is unlikely that palpitations associated with vasomotor symptoms in perimenopausal and postmenopausal women are related to serious cardiac abnormalities, caution should be exercised if syncope or presyncope is reported. A stress test should be conducted if symptoms are accompanied by exercise intolerance, shortness of breath, or chest pain. Women with a high risk of CHD or with a strong family history of early cardiac death (ie, first-degree male relatives <50 y or female relatives <60 y) should also be assessed. Framingham Risk, Reynolds Risk,

CHAPTER 4

and the American College of Cardiology (ACC)/American Heart Association (AHA) global risk scores are useful for assessment of cardiovascular risk. Although each of these tools can overestimate risk, they are widely used, however known to be imperfect predictors of CHD or CVD risk.

Menopause and risk of cardiovascular disease
Most CVD in women occurs during the menopause period or after age 55. This has contributed to the idea that menopause results in an increased risk for CVD. However, the Atherosclerosis Risk in Communities surveillance study (1984-2004) from the National Heart, Lung, and Blood Institute shows no acceleration of absolute CVD rates after menopause. Further, menopause does not modulate the relation between blood pressure (BP) and CVD independent of age.[5] In fact, increasing systolic BP confers a higher CVD risk in premenopausal women compared with the same increase in systolic BP in postmenopausal women. Menopause does, however, appear to result in an accelerated increase in low-density lipoprotein cholesterol (LDL-C) and total cholesterol during the year immediately after the final menstrual period, whereas other risk factors (glycated hemoglobin A_{1c} [Hb A_{1c}] and BP) appear to maintain their usual trajectories during this transition period.[5,6] Carotid atherosclerosis has been shown to be more prevalent during menopause.[7] Metabolic syndrome also is more prevalent during these years.

Sex-specific initiatives and intervention
The results of the Women's Health Initiative (WHI) randomized, controlled trials (RCTs) demonstrate that hormone therapy (HT) is not cardioprotective for CHD in an older group of women (mean age, 63 y) and that estrogen therapy (ET) and estrogen-progestogen therapy (EPT) may even increase the risk for thrombosis and stroke in this population. Subsequent WHI analyses stratified by age at HT initiation demonstrate that the risk of CVD decreases when it is started in younger women and closer to the time of menopause.[8]

The Kronos Early Estrogen Prevention Study (KEEPS) was the first double-blind, placebo-controlled trial designed to address the question of whether HT is cardioprotective when given soon after menopause rather than later. Over 4 years, 727 women within 3 years of menopause were randomized to oral or transdermal estrogen with cyclic progesterone to assess the progression of atherosclerosis. Results showed a similar rate of progression for all treatment groups over the study period as measured by carotid intimal medial thickness and coronary calcium score. Although the study demonstrated no harmful progression of atherosclerosis, there was no evidence of a cardioprotective benefit.

There *does* seem to be a relationship between premature menopause and increased incidence of CVD morbidity and mortality. Menopause before age 35 has been associated with a 2- to 3-fold increased risk of MI. The Nurses' Health Study found an overall significant association between younger age at menopause and higher risk of CVD among women who experienced natural menopause and never used HT.[9] An increased risk was observed among current smokers and not among participants who never smoked.[10] Conversely, other data suggest that processes that increase the risk for CVD may be a determinant of early menopause rather than the presumed reverse scenario. One study reported that for each 1% increase in premenopausal Framingham Risk Score, there was an associated 1.8-year decrease in menopausal age.[11]

Low-density lipoprotein cholesterol and very-low-density lipoprotein cholesterol (VLDL-C) increase in women at menopause, and there is enhanced oxidation of LDL-C postmenopause. There also is an increase in non-high-density lipoprotein cholesterol (HDL-C; total cholesterol minus HDL-C), a variable that includes apolipoprotein B atherogenic triglyceride metabolized particles and VLDL-C. Non-HDL-C is an excellent marker for increased risk when it is elevated. In a cross-sectional analysis of 9,309 women who had never used HT, the increases in total cholesterol, LDL-C, and triglycerides from premenopause to postmenopause were 3% to 4% after adjusting for covariates such as smoking and age.[12] Adverse LDL-C changes and changes in apolipoprotein B levels occur independently of age during the menopause transition.[6]

The Women's Healthy Lifestyle Project, however, found that the menopause-related rise in LDL-C can be reduced through a lifestyle intervention program that focuses on 2 factors: decreasing saturated fat and cholesterol intake and preventing excess weight gain through increased physical exercise and reduced caloric and fat intake.[13]

The direct vascular effects of menopause-related hormone changes may be important. Estrogen and progesterone receptors are present in vascular tissues, including coronary arteries. Coagulation balance may also play a role in the hormone-vascular interaction during menopause changes. Certain fibrinolytic factors (eg, antithrombin III and plasminogen) increase, along with some procoagulation factors (eg, factor VII and fibrinogen). After menopause, blood flow in all vascular beds decreases, prostacyclin decreases, endothelin levels increase, and vasoconstriction occurs in response to acetylcholine challenges. Circulating plasma levels of nitric oxide increase, and levels of angiotensin-converting enzyme (ACE) decrease.[14]

Women who are healthy and not obese experience a decrease in carbohydrate tolerance as insulin resistance increases in postmenopause, which is aggravated in women who are obese.[15] Stress reactivity is exaggerated in postmenopausal women compared with younger women.[16] However, the role of diminished estrogen in these effects is not yet clear.

Risk factors
Major risk factors associated with CVD in women include age, cigarette smoking, hypertension, diabetes mellitus (DM),

abnormal plasma lipids, family history of premature CVD, poor exercise capacity on the treadmill test or abnormal heart rate recovery after stopping exercise, and evidence of subclinical atherosclerosis (eg, abnormal carotid intima-media thickness, coronary calcification). Minor risk factors include sedentary lifestyle and poor diet. Whether obesity and the metabolic syndrome are independent CVD risk factors or simply represent a convenient clustering of risk is unclear.[17-20] It remains controversial whether a decline in estrogen levels is an independent risk factor through either direct or indirect mechanisms.

The 2011 AHA guidelines on CVD prevention in women stratify risk by using these definitions[3]:

- *High risk (1 or more):* Established CHD; cerebrovascular disease; peripheral arterial disease; abdominal aortic aneurysm; end-stage or chronic kidney disease; DM; or a 10-year predicted CVD risk of 10% or more.

- *At risk (1 or more):* Cigarette smoking; systolic BP 120 mm Hg or higher; diastolic BP 80 mm Hg or higher or treated hypertension; total cholesterol 200 mg/dL or more; HDL-C less than 50 mg/dL or treated dyslipidemia; obesity, particularly central adiposity; poor diet; physical inactivity; family history of premature CVD in first-degree relatives (men <55 y or women <65 y); metabolic syndrome; evidence of advanced subclinical atherosclerosis (eg, coronary calcification, carotid plaque, or intimal medial thickness); poor exercise capacity on treadmill test or abnormal heart rate recovery after stopping exercise; systemic autoimmune collagen-vascular disease (eg, lupus or rheumatoid arthritis [RA]); or history of preeclampsia, gestational diabetes, or pregnancy-induced hypertension.

- *Ideal cardiovascular health (all of these):* Total cholesterol less than 200 mg/dL (untreated); BP less than 120/80 mm Hg (untreated); fasting blood glucose less than 100 mg/dL (untreated); body mass index (BMI) less than 25 kg/m^2; no smoking; moderate-intensity physical activity 150 minutes per week or more, vigorous intensity 75 minutes per week or more, or a combination; and healthy diet.

The greater the risk, the more aggressive should be the prevention strategy. American Heart Association guidelines note that a Framingham Risk Score of more than 10% could be used to identify a woman at high risk, but less than 10% is not sufficient to assure low risk. The guidelines focus on the lifetime risk for CVD and emphasize that at age 50, even 1 single risk factor increases lifetime risk for women.[3,21]

The AHA guidelines also highlight the cardiovascular and metabolic changes that occur during pregnancy, such as preeclampsia and gestational diabetes, as CVD risk factors. This unique time of increased cardiac output and circulating blood volume provides a natural stress test for cardiovascular health. In a meta-analysis of 8 studies, women with preeclampsia were found to have a 1.65- to 3.61-fold increased risk in ischemic heart disease later in life.[22]

Screening for risk factors
Developing a standardized procedure for evaluating and managing women at risk for CVD is important.

The 2013 ACC/AHA guidelines on the assessment of cardiovascular risk includes a gender- and ethnicity-based prediction risk assessment for heart attack and stroke.[23] The risk assessment tool is a formula based on age, sex, race, cholesterol, BP, DM, and smoking status and will provide a short-term (10 y) as well as a lifetime risk of developing heart disease and stroke for persons aged 40 to 79 years. Risk factors include age, total cholesterol, HDL-C, systolic BP,

---

The metabolic syndrome

The metabolic syndrome includes a cluster of signs and is closely associated with a generalized metabolic disorder of central obesity, hypertension, and insulin resistance. Criteria for diagnosing the metabolic syndrome are not universally accepted. Many healthcare clinicians, particularly in North America, use criteria proposed in the third report of the National Cholesterol Education Program Expert Panel on Detection, Evaluation, and Treatment of High Blood Cholesterol in Adults (Adult Treatment Panel III, or ATP III).

For women, ATP III defines the metabolic syndrome as the presence of 3 or more of the following factors (note that the mmol/L value for HDL-C is from Canadian guidelines, not directly converted from mg/dL):

- Central obesity (≥35-in or 88-cm waist measurement; 31.5 in South Asian women)
- Elevated serum triglycerides ≥150 mg/dL (1.70 mmol/L)
- Low serum HDL-C <50 mg/dL (1.3 mmol/L)
- Elevated blood pressure (≥130/85 mm Hg)
- Fasting plasma glucose level ≥100 mg/dL (5.6 mmol/L)

ATP III did not find conclusive evidence to recommend routine measurement of insulin resistance, prothrombotic state, or proinflammatory state. However, universal waist measurements using the National Health and Nutrition Examination Survey method is recommended.

Underlying causes of this syndrome are overweight/obesity, physical inactivity, and genetic factors. Women with the metabolic syndrome are at increased risk of cardiovascular heart disease, stroke, peripheral vascular disease, type 2 diabetes mellitus, and subclinical atherosclerosis.

ongoing treatment for hypertension, black race, and active cigarette smoking. The pooled risk equation estimates are more robust for atherosclerotic CVD prediction because of the inclusion of black populations and stroke. Low-density lipoprotein cholesterol remains the primary target of therapy.

The Framingham Risk Score has been validated in Canada and is also recommended by the Canadian Cardiovascular Society.[19] The Reynolds Risk Score was developed to better estimate risk in patients in the intermediate-risk category.[24] High-sensitivity C-reactive protein (hsCRP) is used as a screening and monitoring tool.[25,26] Oral estrogen is associated with elevated hsCRP, which can limit its use for monitoring.[27]

Hypertension. It is important to identify and manage hypertension. Hypertension is strongly related to the risk of cardiovascular, cerebrovascular, and renal diseases. Treatment and control of hypertension in the United States has contributed substantially to the reduction in stroke and heart disease mortality during the past 30 years, especially in women. If a woman has hypertension, the odds of having the other components of the metabolic syndrome are very high. High BP often develops as a late progressive metabolic syndrome.

Hypertension is defined by the Eighth Joint National Committee on Prevention, Detection, Evaluation, and Treatment of High Blood Pressure (JNC 8) as BP higher than 140 mm Hg systolic or 90 mm Hg diastolic in adults aged younger than 60 years and higher than 150 mm Hg systolic or 90 mm Hg diastolic in adults aged 60 years or older.[28] The JNC 8 guidelines define normal BP as less than 120 mg Hg systolic and 80 mm Hg diastolic (Table 1). In addition, JNC 8 revised prior recommendations for patients with diabetes and chronic kidney disease aged younger than 60 years to be treated if BP is higher than 140 mm Hg systolic or 90 mm Hg diastolic. Previous guidelines had recommended treatment in this group if BP was higher than 130/80 mm Hg.

Table 1. Eighth Joint National Committee Blood Pressure Recommendations

Patient subgroup	Target SBP, mm Hg	Target DBP, mm Hg
≥60 y	<150	<90
<60 y	<140	<90
>18 y with chronic kidney disease	<140	<90
>18 y with DM	<140	<90

Abbreviations: DBP, diastolic blood pressure; DM, diabetes mellitus; SBP, systolic blood pressure.
James PA, et al.[28]

Similarly, a 2006 AHA scientific statement on dietary approaches to prevent and treat hypertension calls for initial dietary intervention before pharmacotherapy in uncomplicated stage 1 hypertension levels established by JNC 8.[29]

Hypertension management does not require specialty consultation. Evaluation includes history, physical examination, and laboratory testing (urinalysis, checking for albuminuria, complete blood cell count, and blood chemistry, including electrolytes, creatinine, fasting glucose, and fasting lipids). An electrocardiogram should be performed initially to assess associated risks, target organ damage, and to assist in identifying potential secondary causes (including sleep apnea). More extensive testing for secondary causes may be needed, depending on initial screening results.

Dyslipidemia. Elevated serum cholesterol levels, particularly elevated LDL-C, are a clearly established major risk factor for CVD. The 2013 ACC/AHA guidelines on the treatment of cholesterol have diverged from National Cholesterol Education Program Expert Panel (ATP III) guidelines that targeted a specific cholesterol number. The updated guidelines now recommend moderate- or high-intensity statin therapy for 4 specific patient types: 1) those with CVD; 2) those with LDL-C of 190 mg/dL or higher; 3) patients aged 40 to 75 years with type 1 or type 2 DM and LDL-C between 70 mg/dL and 189 mg/dL; and 4) patients aged 40 to 75 years with LDL-C between 70 mg/dL and 189 mg/dL and 10-year risk of CVD (using their new risk calculator) of 7.5%.[30] As evidenced in clinical trials, high-intensity statin therapy should lower LDL-C by more than 50%, and moderate-intensity statin therapy should lower LDL-C by 30% to 50%.(Table 2).

The 10-year CVD risk calculator takes into account age, sex, race, cholesterol, BP, DM, and smoking status and estimates the future risk of MI and stroke. If a clinician remains uncertain about statin use on the basis of these calculations, additional parameters such as family history of premature CVD, hsCRP, coronary artery calcium score, and/or ankle-brachial index may be considered. These tests should include a measurement of total cholesterol, LDL-C, HDL-C, and triglycerides. Lipoprotein concentrations are better predictors of CVD before and after pharmacologic intervention.[31,32]

Fasting is not mandatory for screening, although knowing a patient's fasting status is helpful for interpretation of the results. Total cholesterol and HDL-C are not sensitive to fasting, so even if the patient did not fast, her lipid panel results are clinically useful. Fasting triglycerides should be lower than 150 mg/dL (1.7 mmol/L), and non-HDL-C should be no more than 30 mg/dL (0.8 mmol/L) higher than LDL-C targets.

Lifestyle modification. Women with modifiable CVD risk factors should be urged to initiate lifestyle changes to decrease overall risk.[3] American Heart Association guidelines for the prevention of CVD in women define lifestyle interventions as tobacco cessation, physical activity, dietary intake, weight maintenance and reduction, cardiac rehabilitation after a recent acute coronary event, and omega-3 fatty acids to lower triglycerides. The 2013 ACC/AHA guidelines on lifestyle management to reduce cardiovascular risk were published with the intent of evaluating diet, nutritional intake, and physical activity.[33] The key recommendations include eating a diet consistent with the Mediterranean diet based on fruits, vegetables, and lean meats and restricting saturated and trans fats, sugar, and sodium. The guidelines also recommend engaging in moderate to vigorous physical activity 40 minutes per session 3 to 4 times per week. These lifestyle interventions are important, not only because of their potential to reduce clinical CVD but also because heart-healthy lifestyles may prevent the development of major risk factors. Such prevention may minimize the need for more intensive future interventions and revascularization.[34,35]

Cigarette smoking. Use of tobacco is the single most important preventable risk factor for CVD in women. A woman who smokes is 2 to 6 times more likely to have a heart attack than a woman who does not smoke. The effect of smoking on risk of fatal CVD is dose related (ie, heavier smokers have a greater relative risk). However, if a woman stops smoking—no matter for how long or how much she has smoked—her risk of heart disease drops rapidly. The AHA guidelines for smoking cessation include counseling at each encounter, nicotine replacement, and other pharmacotherapy as indicated, in conjunction with a behavioral program or formal smoking cessation program.[3] Women should also avoid environmental (ie, secondhand) smoke. Although oral contraceptive (OC) use does not appreciably increase CVD risk in nonsmokers, use of OCs synergistically increases CVD risk, especially MI, in women who do smoke.[36] Studies have shown an increased risk of MI with the number of cigarettes smoked per day. Oral contraceptives are therefore not recommended for women aged 35 years or older who smoke.[37]

Physical activity. Middle-aged women who exercise regularly have lower weight, BP, and plasma glucose levels, as well as more favorable lipid profiles, than sedentary women. Regular physical activity, particularly aerobic exercise, promotes cardiovascular health. Adoption of a regular aerobic exercise program reduces the risk of coronary events in women. The AHA recommends that women accumulate at least 150 minutes per week of moderate-intensity exercise (eg, brisk walking), 75 minutes per week of vigorous exercise, or a combination equal to both aerobic activities. The guidelines also recommend that the aerobic activity should be performed in at least 10-minute increments, spread throughout the week.[3] Resistance training for 20 minutes,

Table 2. Statin Therapy Outcomes in Clinical Trials

Statin intensity	Treatment, mg per day	Outcome
Low	Simvastatin 10 Pravastatin 10-20 Lovastatin 20 Fluvastatin 20-40 Pitavastatin 1	Daily dose lowers LDL-C by <30%, on average
Moderate	Atorvastatin 10-20 Rosuvastatin 5-10 Simvastatin 20-40[a] Pravastatin 40 Lovastatin 40 Fluvastatin XL 80 Fluvastatin 40 (bid) Pitavastatin 2-4	Daily dose lowers LDL-C by approximately 30% to <50%, on average
High	Atorvastatin 40-80[b] Rosuvastatin 20-40	Daily dose lowers LDL-C by approximately ≥50%, on average

Individual responses to statin therapy varied in clinical trials and should be expected to vary in clinical practice. There may be a biologic basis for less-than-average response.
Abbreviation: LDL-C, low-density lipoprotein cholesterol.
a. Although simvastatin 80 mg was evaluated in clinical trials, initiation or titration to 80 mg is not recommended by FDA because of increased risk of myopathy, including rhabdomyolysis.
b. Evidence is from 1 clinical trial only. Down-titrate if patient unable to tolerate 80 mg.
Adapted from Stone NJ, et al.[30]

2 to 3 times a week on nonconsecutive days, also helps to reduce insulin resistance and facilitates weight loss.[38]

Dietary intake. American Heart Association guidelines suggest a heart-healthy nutrition strategy that includes intake of a variety of fruits and vegetables (≥4.5 cups/d) and wholegrain and high-fiber foods. A modified Mediterranean diet is the most practical way to implement a heart-healthy diet to reduce cardiometabolic risk and should include fish, especially oily fish, at least twice a week.[3] Intake of saturated fat (<7% of total energy) and cholesterol (<150 mg/d) should be limited, avoiding trans fatty acids. Sodium intake should be limited to less than 1.5 g per day (approximately one-third teaspoon salt). As an adjunct to diet, omega-3 fatty acid supplementation may be considered in women with severe hypertriglyceridemia. Several nonpharmacologic, nutritional strategies are available to reduce dyslipidemia.[39]

Additional nutrition-related approaches include

- *Antioxidants.* Epidemiologic studies have shown a lc incidence of heart disease in those who eat more grains and fruits and vegetables high in antio

To date, however, no large RCTs have established any benefit of taking antioxidant vitamin supplements such as vitamin C, vitamin E, beta-carotene, lycopene, or folic acid. Some studies suggest that supplements may cause harm. The AHA guidelines indicate that antioxidant vitamin supplements should not be used for primary or secondary prevention of CVD.[3]

- *B vitamins*. Supplements of the B vitamins folate, B[6], and B[12] will lower homocysteine levels, although multiple studies have failed to demonstrate benefit of folic acid with or without B vitamins for CVD prevention. Folic acid supplementation should not be used for the primary or secondary prevention of CVD.[3,40]

- *Vitamin D*. There are a growing number of studies suggesting an association between low vitamin D and heart health; however, prospective data analyzing CVD and vitamin D, although not designed or powered to specifically answer this question, have not shown a benefit, and the results of at least 1 study suggest potential cardiovascular harm in those receiving vitamin D supplementation.[41] In several meta-analyses, vitamin D deficiency has been associated with increased BP, higher risk of heart attacks, and early death.[42,43] The Multi-Ethnic Study of Atherosclerosis, however, found that such association varies by race and ethnicity and was not associated with greater risk in blacks or Hispanics.[44] These findings suggest that there are likely biologic variations in the metabolism of vitamin D. There are no formal recommendations for vitamin D supplementation and heart disease.

- *Plant sterols and stanols*. Naturally occurring plant sterols and stanols may help to reduce the risk of CVD by lowering blood cholesterol levels.[45] These compounds chemically resemble cholesterol and inhibit cholesterol absorption in the small intestine and have been incorporated into low-fat foods, including bread, cereals, dressings, low-fat milk and yogurt, and fruit juice.[46] Food products, such as spreads, containing stanols and sterols are available, as well as soft gel dietary supplements. The AHA in its diet and lifestyle recommendations advocates consumption of plant sterols and stanols from a variety of foods and beverages, similar to cholesterol-lowering medication, to maintain LDL-C reductions.[47] The AHA also noted that maximal effects are achieved at intakes of about 2 g per day. This is consistent with the ATP III evidence statement that daily intakes of 2 to 3 g per day will reduce LDL-C by 6% to 15%.[17,48] Patients on statin therapy may achieve further reductions in their blood cholesterol levels when consuming a diet with plant sterols and stanols. These compounds are even more effective than doubling the statin dose, which usually produces an additional lowering of LDL-C levels by only 5% to 7%. One review suggests long-term use of plant sterols or stanols resulted in a 20% reduction in the incidence of CHD.[49] Incorporating plant sterols or stanols into a healthy diet in older adults can help prevent aging-associated diseases.[50]

- *Soy isoflavones*. Although not mentioned specifically in the AHA guidelines, an AHA science advisory panel reviewed the use of soy and isoflavones and their effect on cardiovascular health in 22 RCTs.[47,51] The effect of isolated soy protein with isoflavones showed minimal LDL-C reductions, in the range of 3%. No significant effects on HDL-C, triglycerides, lipoprotein(a), or BP were evident. Further review of 19 studies of soy isoflavones showed no effect on LDL-C and other lipid risk factors. Use of isoflavone supplements in food or pills was not recommended. The review does note, however, that soy products may be beneficial to health as a replacement for animal protein because of their high content of polyunsaturated fats, fiber, vitamins, and minerals and their low content of saturated fat. Flavonoids in foods such as soy, as well as fruits and nuts, may be beneficial. A large RCT demonstrated efficacy of Mediterranean-style nutrition that included supplemental daily tree nuts or virgin olive oil for prevention of CVD in women and men with risk factors.[52] Although food appears to be beneficial, the effect of over-the-counter supplements on disease prevention and potential contraindications for aging women must be further determined.[53]

- *Alcohol consumption*. The AHA guidelines encourage limiting alcohol consumption to no more than 1 drink per day (a drink being equal to a 12-oz bottle of beer, a 5-oz glass of wine, or 1.5 oz of 80-proof spirit).[3] Some evidence suggests that light to moderate use of alcohol lowers CVD mortality among women aged older than 50 years who are at greater risk for CHD; however, higher levels (>7 drinks per week) may increase risk of hypertension, stroke, and ischemic heart disease.

Weight maintenance and reduction. Maintaining an ideal body weight has been estimated to reduce the overall risk of CVD by 35% to 55%. Central obesity (ie, apple shape) is more dangerous than subcutaneous obesity for heart health.[54] The AHA recommends weight maintenance or reduction through an appropriate balance of physical activity, caloric intake, and formal behavioral programs, when indicated, to maintain or achieve a BMI between 18.5 kg/m^2 and 24.9 kg/m^2 and a waist circumference of less than 35 inches (88 cm; 31.5 in for South Asian women).[3]

For women who need to lose weight or sustain weight loss, the AHA guidelines recommend a minimum of 60 to 90 minutes of moderate-intensity exercise on most and preferably all days of the week. A combined approach of exercise and diet is superior to diet only. Three 10-minute exercise sessions have been shown to be as least as effective as one 30-minute session. A reasonable goal is losing 10% of body weight over a 6-month period.

Psychosocial factors. Although RCTs have failed to demonstrate CVD reduction, postmenopausal women should be evaluated for depression and treated appropriately for quality-of-life (QOL) and mental health considerations.

Aspirin. The benefit of aspirin use in women and men with established CVD remains unchallenged, and the use of daily low-dose aspirin (81 mg) to prevent recurrence of MI, stroke, and TIA has become common practice. Dozens of studies have shown that aspirin impairs platelet function and reduces vascular inflammation.

A meta-analysis of pooled data from 5 trials examining the effects of aspirin for the primary prevention of cardiovascular events over periods of 4 to 7 years showed that daily or every-other-day aspirin therapy reduced the risk for CHD by 28%, with no significant effects on mortality and stroke. Most participants were men aged older than 50 years.[55]

Aspirin 100 mg every other day for primary prevention in women was evaluated in the Women's Health Study, which demonstrated reductions in stroke of 17%, including up to a 24% reduction in the risk of ischemic stroke, with a nonsignificant increase in the risk of hemorrhagic stroke and reduction in MI in those aged older than 65 years.[56] There was a significant 40% increase in gastrointestinal (GI) bleeding.

A meta-analysis reviewed aspirin for primary prevention of cardiovascular events in men and women.[57] The conclusion was that for women and for men, the risk of cardiovascular events was decreased because of a reduction in ischemic stroke in women and MI in men. Aspirin did increase the risk of bleeding to a similar effect in men and women.

One systematic review evaluated the dosing of aspirin for CVD prevention.[58] Clinical data do not support doses of aspirin greater than 75 mg to 81 mg per day. Higher doses, which may be commonly prescribed, have not been found to be more effective at preventing CVD events but are associated with increased risks of GI bleeding.

The AHA guidelines recommend that women at high risk for CVD take aspirin (75-325 mg/d) unless contraindicated.[3] If a woman at high risk is intolerant of aspirin therapy, clopidogrel should be substituted. Additionally, the guidelines recommend that for at-risk or healthy women aged 65 years or older, aspirin therapy (81 mg/d or 100 mg every other day) can be considered if BP is controlled and the benefit for ischemic stroke and MI prevention is likely to outweigh the risk of GI bleeding and hemorrhagic stroke. For women aged younger than 65 years, the same doses should be used when the benefit of ischemic stroke prevention is likely to outweigh the adverse events (AEs) of therapy.

Aspirin use has been shown to significantly increase the rate of upper GI bleeding and is contraindicated for those who have an allergy to aspirin, a tendency for bleeding, recent GI bleeding, or clinically active hepatic disease. Even enteric-coated or buffered aspirin may damage the intestinal lining. However, studies have shown that patients who regularly take aspirin (and other anti-inflammatory drugs) have unusually low rates of digestive tract cancers. Data are not clear regarding an adverse association with cancers of the pancreas, prostate, and breast.

Pharmacologic interventions

For women with higher risks for CVD, prescription therapies may be necessary. Recommendations for primary prevention based on the ACC/AHA guidelines focus on reducing risks through management of lipids (with a statin), hypertension, and DM.[28,33] If diet and exercise modifications for 6 weeks fail to obtain the desired levels for BP and cholesterol, appropriate pharmacologic intervention is recommended.

Dyslipidemia. Dyslipidemia can cause atherosclerosis and lead to ischemic heart disease, stroke, TIA, and MI. More than one-third of women have dyslipidemia. It is estimated that a 25% reduction in LDL-C can reduce heart disease risk by 50%. Reducing cholesterol to a normal range is a therapeutic goal.

Triglycerides appear to be a more significant predictor of CVD risk in women than in men. Attention should therefore be focused on the potential higher risk associated with women who have elevated triglyceride levels. The risk for CVD is elevated in women who have levels of triglycerides of 128 mg/dL (1.4 mmol/L) or greater along with increased waist circumference of 35 inches (88 cm) or greater.[54] Clinical trials to date have failed to demonstrate benefit of combination therapy (statin plus niacin, statin with fibrate) that addresses HDL-C and triglycerides for CVD reduction. Guidelines do not support HDL-C or triglycerides as pharmacologic treatment targets; further work is needed specifically in women.

Guidelines for the management of dyslipidemia focus on LDL-C as the target of therapy.[17] Updated cholesterol guidelines based on available clinical trial evidence recommend using optimized doses of potent statins rather than targeting LDL-C levels as evidence-based treatment goals.[21] The National Lipid Association and the International Atherosclerosis Association disagree and recommend continuing to optimize levels of LDL-C and non-HDL-C, based on all the evidence. Drug therapy for lowering LDL-C in women at high or moderate risk should be aimed toward achieving a 30% to 40% reduction in LDL-C. Benefits of LDL-C-lowering therapy apply to older women who are at greater absolute risk of stroke (Table 3).[17]

The protective role of lipid-lowering therapy in women, especially with the 3-hydroxy-3-methylglutaryl-coenzyme A reductase inhibitors (ie, statins), is well established by numerous RCTs, noting consistent reductions in CVD risk ranging

Table 3. Lipid-Lowering Guidelines for Women at High or Moderate Risk for Cardiovascular Disease

Levels of lipids and lipoproteins recommended by the American Heart Association through lifestyle approaches:

- LDL-C <100 mg/dL (2.6 mmol/L).
- HDL-C >50 mg/dL (1.3 mmol/L).
- Triglycerides <150 mg/dL (1.7 mmol/L).
- Non-HDL-C (total cholesterol minus HDL-C) <130 mg/dL (3.3 mmol/L).

If a woman is at high risk or has hypercholesterolemia:

- LDL-C-lowering drug therapy should be used simultaneously with lifestyle therapy in high-risk women to achieve an LDL-C <100 mg/dL (2.6 mmol/L). This is also indicated in women with other atherosclerotic CVD or diabetes mellitus or if 10-year risk >20%.
- LDL-C <70 mg/dL in very high-risk women with CHD is reasonable and may require an LDL-lowering drug combination.

For at-risk women:

- If there are multiple risk factors, LDL-C-lowering drug therapy should be used if LDL-C is ≥130 mg/dL (3.3 mmol/L) with lifestyle therapy, even if the 10-year absolute risk is 10% to 20%.
- LDL-C–lowering therapy should be used if LDL-C level is ≥160 mg/dL (4.1 mmol/L) with lifestyle therapy and multiple risk factors even if the 10-year absolute risk is <10%.
- LDL-C–lowering therapy should be used if LDL-C is ≥190 mg/dL (4.9 mmol/L), regardless of the presence or absence of other risk factors or CVD on lifestyle therapy.
- For women >60 years with an estimated CHD risk >10% and hsCRP >2 mg/dL, statin therapy may be considered after lifestyle modification and no acute inflammation present to account for hsCRP.

For low HDL-C or elevated non-HDL-C in high-risk women:

- Niacin or fibrate therapy should be used if HDL-C is low (<50 mg/dL) or non-HDL-C is elevated (>130 mg/dL) after LDL-C goal is reached.

Abbreviations: CHD, coronary heart disease; HDL-C, high-density lipoprotein cholesterol; hsCRP, high-sensitivity C-reactive protein; LDL-C, low-density lipoprotein cholesterol.
National Cholesterol Education Program (NCEP) Expert Panel on Detection, Evaluation, and Treatment of High Blood Cholesterol in Adults (Adult Treatment Panel III).[17]

from 11% to 54%.[59] Although the representation of women in most trials is relatively low (averaging <20% of the population), a positive trend for benefit was consistent across all trials. The protective effect of statins based on these trials appeared equivalent to or greater than that observed for men. Women taking statin therapy should be monitored for LDL-C AEs (and other potential drug AEs). Intensive lipid lowering can reverse atherosclerotic changes and prevent CVD events.[60]

Hypertension. Hypertension is more prevalent than dyslipidemia in women of all ages. On their own, long-term systolic and diastolic BP levels correlate with mortality from ischemic heart disease. This correlation is stronger than previously thought and slightly stronger in women than in men. Throughout middle age, differences of 20 mm Hg systolic BP and 10 mm Hg diastolic BP in women are associated with a 2-fold difference in ischemic heart disease mortality. Systolic BP predicts ischemic heart disease mortality more accurately than does diastolic BP.

American Heart Association guidelines recommend aiming for an optimal BP of less than 120/80 mm Hg through lifestyle approaches such as weight control, increased physical activity, alcohol moderation, sodium restriction, and increased dietary fruit, vegetables, and low-fat dairy. If BP is 140/90 mm Hg or higher, pharmacotherapy is indicated. For patients with DM or chronic kidney disease, pharmacotherapy is indicated if BP is 130/80 mm Hg or higher. A wide variety of antihypertensive agents, including diuretics, can be prescribed. The guidelines recommend including thiazide diuretics as part of the BP management plan for most women unless contraindicated or if there are compelling indications for other agents in specific vascular diseases. Initial treatment of women at high risk with acute coronary syndrome or MI should be with beta-blockers, ACE inhibitors, or angiotensin II receptor blockers (ARBs), with the addition of other drugs such as thiazides as needed to achieve BP goals. It is important to note that ACE inhibitors are contraindicated in pregnancy and should be used with caution in young women with the potential to become pregnant.

Diabetes mellitus. A potent independent risk factor for CVD morbidity and mortality in women is DM. Normal fasting plasma glucose is lower than 100 mg/dL. Diabetes mellitus is diagnosed in patients with fasting blood glucose higher than 126 mg/dL (7.0 mmol/L); an Hb A$_{1C}$ of 6.5% or more; a 2-hour value in an oral glucose tolerance test of 200 mg/dL or more; or a random plasma glucose of 200 mg/dL or more in the presence of symptoms. Diabetes mellitus accelerates atherosclerosis and increases the risk of ischemic heart disease in women. It is often associated with obesity, hypertension, and dyslipidemia, which act synergistically to raise CVD risk. Programs aimed at reducing this risk in women with DM focus on controlling plasma glucose and insulin levels, controlling cholesterol, reducing obesity, and promoting exercise.

Although a randomized trial demonstrated that physical activity and weight loss reduced progression to DM in patients with the metabolic syndrome, a randomized lifestyle trial failed to demonstrate CVD benefit in patients with DM despite improved physical activity and weight loss.[61,62] The AHA recommends lifestyle and pharmacotherapy to achieve an Hb A[1c] level less than 7%, if this can be accomplished without significant hypoglycemia.[3] Testing Hb A[1C] has become an additional diagnostic screening test, according to the American Diabetes Association (ADA) Workgroup statement from the International Expert Committee.[63]

Hormone therapy. Initiation of HT by women aged 50 to 59 years or by those within 10 years of menopause to treat typical menopause symptoms (eg, vasomotor, vaginal) does not seem to increase the risk of CVD events.[64] Although post hoc analyses suggest that initiation of ET in early postmenopause may reduce cardiovascular risk, the one trial testing this hypothesis to date was negative.[65-67]

Three primary cardiovascular outcomes have been studied in relation to HT: CHD, stroke, and venous thromboembolism (VTE). Hormone therapy is not recommended for cardiovascular protection in women of any age.

- *Coronary heart disease.* Most observational and preclinical studies support the potential benefits of systemic HT in reducing the risk of CHD. Most RCTs do not.[68] However, the characteristics of women participating in observational studies are different from those of women enrolled in RCTs, which may influence baseline cardiovascular risk and the HT effects.[69]

   Data indicate that the disparity in findings between observational studies and RCTs may be related in part to the timing of initiation of HT in relation to age and proximity to menopause. Most women studied in observational studies of CHD risk were aged younger than 55 years at the time HT was initiated and within 2 to 3 years of menopause, whereas the women enrolled in the cardiovascular RCTs were on average aged 63 to 64 years and were more than 10 years beyond menopause.[69,70] A secondary analysis of WHI data found a significant reduction in the composite endpoint of MI, coronary artery revascularization, and coronary death in women who were randomized to ET when aged 50 to 59 years.[70]

   Observational studies show that long-term HT is associated with less accumulation of coronary artery calcium, which is strongly correlated with atheromatous plaque burden and future risk of clinical cardiovascular events.[71] In an ancillary substudy of younger women (<60 y) in the WHI-ET trial, after an average of 7 years of treatment, women who had been randomized to ET had lower levels of exit coronary artery calcium than those randomized to placebo.[72,73] Conversely, the KEEPS trial failed to demonstrate a benefit in coronary artery calcium with HT initiated early in menopause, suggesting again that the observational and post hoc analyses may be misleading.[67]

- *Stroke.* Results of observational studies of the risk of stroke with HT have been inconsistent. Several studies (including the Nurses' Health Study, the largest prospective study of HT and stroke) indicated an increased risk of ischemic stroke consistent with the findings from the WHI,[74] whereas other studies showed no effect on stroke risk. The WHI-ET and -EPT trials demonstrated an increased risk of ischemic stroke and no effect on risk of hemorrhagic stroke.[75] There were 8 additional strokes per 10,000 women per year of EPT and 11 additional strokes per 10,000 women per year of ET when the entire cohort was analyzed. In analyses that combined results from the WHI-ET and -EPT trials, HT in younger women (50-59 y) at study entry had no significant effect on risk of stroke (relative risk [RR], 1.13; 95% confidence interval [CI], 0.73-1.76).[69] In the Framingham Heart Study, natural menopause at 42 years or younger was associated with elevated risk of ischemic stroke.[10]

   With few women in younger age groups in the WHI trials, the confidence intervals have been wide, meaning that there was not enough statistical power to reach a conclusion. In the Nurses' Health Study, in women aged 50 to 59 years, the relative risk of stroke for current EPT users tended to be elevated (RR, 1.34; 95% CI, 0.84-2.13) and was significantly increased for current users of ET (RR, 1.58; 95% CI, 1.06-2.37).[74] Lower doses of estrogen (eg, 0.3 mg conjugated estrogens [CE]) were not associated with an increased risk in the Nurses' Health Study, although this was based on the relatively few women who were taking lower doses.

   In women randomized in the WHI within 5 years of menopause, there were 3 additional strokes per 10,000 women per year of EPT, which is not statistically significant. The excess risk of stroke in this age group observed in the WHI studies would fall into the rare risk category. Stroke risk was not significantly increased in the Heart and Estrogen/Progestin Replacement Study (HERS).[76] The Women's International Study of Long Duration Oestrogen After Menopause found no excess of stroke in EPT users compared with women on placebo in 1 year.[77]

   No studies indicate that postmenopausal HT is effective for reducing the risk of a recurrent stroke among women with established CVD or for prevention of a first stroke, and it may increase the rate of first strokes, particularly in women initiating HT later than age 60. Although stroke was not increased in the group aged 50 to 59 years in the combined analysis of the WHI, it was almost doubled in the ET group with fewer than 10 years since menopause.[78] This apparent contradiction in the data is hard to explain but may be because of relatively few events and the difficulty in accurately timing onset of menopause in the ET group.

- *Venous thromboembolism.* Data from observational studies and from randomized trials demonstrate an increased risk of VTE with oral HT. In the WHI trials, there were 18 additional VTEs per 10,000 women per year of EPT and 7 additional VTEs per 10,000 women per year of ET when the entire cohort was analyzed.[79,80] Risk for VTE in randomized trials emerges soon after HT is initiated (ie, during the first 1-2 y), but the magnitude of the excess risk seems to decrease somewhat over time. In the WHI trials, the absolute excess VTE risk associated with either EPT or ET was lower in women who started HT before age 60 than in older women who initiated HT after age 60.[81,82] There were 7 additional VTEs per 10,000 women per year of EPT and 4 additional VTEs per 10,000 women per year of ET in women aged 50 to 59 years who were randomized to HT. These risks fall into the rare risk category.

The baseline risk of VTE also increases relative to BMI. For women who are obese (BMI >30), the baseline risk was almost 3-fold greater. At any BMI, the risk of VTE doubled with HT and returned to baseline soon after discontinuation.

Growing evidence suggests that women with a prior history of VTE or women who possess factor V Leiden are at increased risk with HT use.[83] Limited observational study data suggest lower risks of VTE with transdermal than with oral ET, but there are no comparative trial data.[84] Lower doses of oral ET may also confer less VTE risk than higher doses, but again no comparative trial data are available to confirm this assumption.

Treatment

Postmenopausal women with established CVD have a high risk for recurrent ischemic heart disease events and cardiovascular mortality. Therapies that result in even a small reduction in CVD risk can have a major effect on public health. In postmenopausal women with preexisting CVD, dietary and pharmacologic management of hypertension, dyslipidemia, and DM should be initiated where appropriate, according to established guidelines from leading US and Canadian organizations, including the AHA, the ACC, the National Lipid Association, and the International Atherosclerosis Association.

Aspirin. When used for secondary prevention of ischemic heart disease, an overview of randomized trials from the Antithrombotic Trialists' Collaboration found that aspirin (75-162 mg/d) was beneficial in women.[85] Among patients with an acute coronary syndrome, aspirin should be part of preventive management for women and men.

Statins. Statin therapy is recommended to lower LDL-C, based on increased CVD risk, and can be considered in women if hsCRP levels are more than 2 mg/dL after lifestyle modification and no inflammatory process is present.

Beta-blockers. Beta-blocker agents should be considered in all women after MI, acute coronary syndrome, or left ventricular dysfunction with or without HF symptoms, unless contraindicated.

Angiotensin-converting enzyme inhibitors/Angiotensin II receptor blockers. ACE inhibitors should be used (unless contraindicated) in women after MI and in those with clinical evidence of HF, a left ventricular ejection fraction (LVEF) of 40% or less, or DM. In women after MI and in those with clinical evidence of HF or an LVEF of 40% or less, or those with DM who are intolerant of ACE inhibitors, ARBs should be used instead.

Aldosterone blockade. Aldosterone blockade should be used after MI in women who do not have significant renal dysfunction or hyperkalemia, who are already receiving therapeutic doses of an ACE inhibitor and beta-blocker, and have an LVEF of 40% or less with symptomatic HF.

Hormone therapy. Several observational, secondary prevention studies had suggested that HT use could lower the risk of mortality and future cardiac events. However, on the basis of clinical trials that have found no effect of HT on clinical or anatomic progression of CVD, HT is not recommended by the North American Menopause Society (NAMS), the AHA, or other US or Canadian organizations for the secondary prevention of CVD. For women with CVD, it would be prudent to emphasize cardiovascular risk reduction with established evidence-based treatments.

Diabetes mellitus

Diabetes mellitus (DM) refers to a complex group of diseases that affect the processing of glucose. *Prediabetes* may be diagnosed when blood glucose levels are higher than normal but lower than that required for a diagnosis of DM. Prediabetes puts patients at risk for developing type 2 DM within 10 years.

Type 1 DM, often called *insulin-dependent diabetes mellitus* and formerly called *juvenile diabetes*, is a chronic condition in which the beta cells of the pancreas produce too little or no insulin. Type 1 DM is usually diagnosed in children, teenagers, and young adults.

Type 2 DM is the most common type of DM; about 90% to 95% of people with DM have type 2.[86] Type 2 DM was formerly referred to as *adult-onset diabetes*, but it can be diagnosed at any age, even during childhood. Type 2 DM occurs when a patient's body either resists the effects of insulin or does not produce enough insulin to maintain a normal glucose level.

The first stage of type 2 DM is usually insulin resistance, a condition linked to excess weight in which the body's cells do not use insulin efficiently. At first, the pancreas produces extra insulin, but over time, it loses the ability to do so, causing a rise in glucose levels.[87]

Screening
Screening for type 2 DM can be accomplished through the HbA[1c] test, a fasting plasma glucose test, or the oral glucose tolerance test (Figure).[87,88] The ADA recommends repeating a DM screening test every 3 years in people aged older than 45 years with no risk factors.[87]

The goal of glucose screening is to identify those who have or who are at high risk of developing type 2 DM. Screening should be considered for all women starting at age 45 and is strongly recommended if women are overweight (BMI >25 kg/m² to <30 kg/m²) or obese (BMI ≥30 kg/m²). Screening should also be considered in women who are overweight at any age with 1 or more additional risk factors[87]:

- Physical inactivity
- Having a first-degree relative with DM
- Being part of a high-risk ethnic population (black, Hispanic, North American Indian, Asian American, Pacific Islander)
- Having delivered a baby weighing more than 9 lb (4 kg) or having been diagnosed with gestational diabetes
- Hypertension (BP ≥140/90 mm Hg) or on therapy for hypertension
- High-density lipoprotein cholesterol level less than 35 mg/dL (0.9 mmol/L) or a triglyceride level more than 250 mg/dL (6.4 mmol/L)
- Polycystic ovary syndrome
- Prediabetes—an Hb A[1c] level of 5.7% to 6.4%; a fasting plasma glucose test result of 100 mg/dL to 125 mg/dL, indicating impaired fasting glucose; or a 2-hour oral glucose tolerance test result of 140 mg/dL to 199 mg/dL, indicating impaired glucose tolerance
- Acanthosis nigricans, a condition associated with insulin resistance and characterized by a dark, velvety rash around the neck or armpits
- History of CVD

The US Preventive Services Task Force (USPSTF) 2008 clinical guidelines are more conservative, recommending screening for DM in asymptomatic adults only if BP is greater than 135/80 mm Hg.[89]

Epidemiology
In the United States, 12% of people aged 35 to 64 years have DM; the incidence jumps to 28% after age 65.[90] Nearly 11% of all women aged older than 20 years have DM.[86] As women age, they are more likely to develop type 2 DM. Type 2 DM remains undiagnosed in approximately one-third of women with the disease and is more prevalent in nonwhite women.[91] Compared with non-Hispanic whites, the risk of DM diagnosis in Asians, Hispanics/Latinos, and non-Hispanic blacks is 18%, 66%, and 77%, respectively.[87] Diabetes mellitus is a significant health issue in Canada, where about 2.4 million adult Canadians—6.8% of the population—were diagnosed with DM in 2009.[92] This represented a 70% increase in the prevalence of DM since the publication of the 1998 Canadian Diabetes Association clinical practice guidelines.

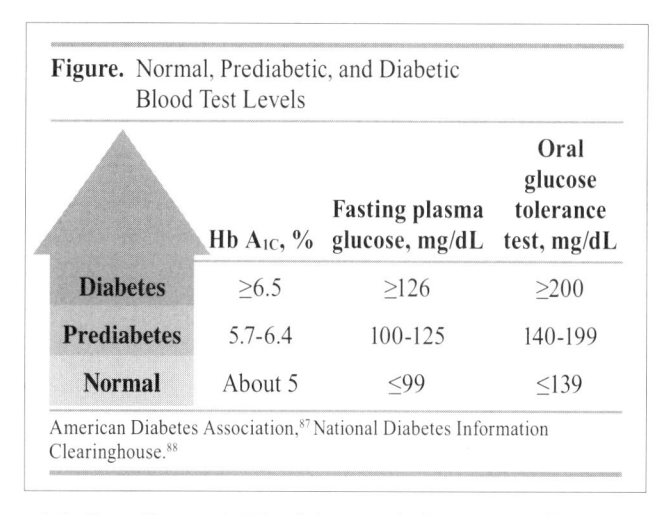

Worldwide, DM cases are expected to double between 2000 and 2030.[91] In the United States, it is estimated that for girls born in the year 2000, more than 1 in every 3 will develop DM in their lifetimes.[93]

Figure. Normal, Prediabetic, and Diabetic Blood Test Levels

	Hb A[1C], %	Fasting plasma glucose, mg/dL	Oral glucose tolerance test, mg/dL
Diabetes	≥6.5	≥126	≥200
Prediabetes	5.7-6.4	100-125	140-199
Normal	About 5	≤99	≤139

American Diabetes Association,[87] National Diabetes Information Clearinghouse.[88]

Menopausal risk factors
Adiposity. Women typically gain weight as they age; excess weight is associated with the development of type 2 DM. However, in studies that have controlled for age, menopause does not appear to influence weight gain significantly.[94,95] Body composition change is another driver of DM risk. Central fat accumulation appears to confer higher risk of type 2 DM compared with other types of tissue gain. Muscle loss likely worsens insulin resistance by reducing a type of tissue (muscle) that engages in insulin-mediated glucose uptake.

Menopause is widely thought to play a significant role in body composition change, with loss of estradiol seen as increasing central fat accumulation.[96,97] Cross-sectional and longitudinal data from the Study of Women Across the Nation (SWAN) corroborates an association between the menopause transition and increases in central adiposity and general fat mass in women.[98,99] A SWAN investigation on the temporal relationship between sex steroids and waist circumference found that the relationship between estradiol and waist circumference appeared reciprocal.[100] Higher estradiol levels appeared to contribute to a smaller waist circumference during the early menopause transition, whereas a higher waist circumference contributed to a higher estradiol level in the later menopause transition.

Ovarian hormones. Endogenous sex steroids may affect glucose metabolism, but this effect appears more pronounced in premenopausal women rather than postmenopausal women. In healthy premenopausal women, endogenous estradiol and progesterone levels during menstrual cycling are positively associated with worse insulin resistance.[101] Consistent with these findings, higher follicle-stimulating hormone levels (a surrogate of low sex steroid levels) are associated with better insulin sensitivity.

The hormonal changes associated with menopause appear to have less of an effect on glucose metabolism. In SWAN, glucose metabolism indices (glucose levels, insulin levels, insulin resistance) worsened as women aged. However, neither natural nor surgical menopause transitions appeared to worsen glucose metabolism in an age-independent way.[6,102] Other studies corroborate that menopause may not significantly worsen glucose metabolism, especially if aging, weight gain, and body composition change are taken into account.[103]

Complications

The excess glucose that results from type 2 DM deposits in the small vessels of the kidneys, eyes, and nerves, leading to the microvascular complications of nephropathy, retinopathy, and neuropathy, respectively. Evidence supports the conclusion that nephropathy and retinopathy can be prevented or delayed by optimizing glucose and BP control. This type of self-care is crucial; retinopathy is the number 1 cause of new cases of blindness in adults aged 20 to 74 years, and diabetic nephropathy is the leading cause of end-stage renal disease.[87] Urine albumin excretion should be checked annually in all patients with type 2 DM, starting at diagnosis. Serum creatinine should be measured annually to estimate glomerular filtration rate and to stage the level of chronic kidney disease, if present.[100] A dilated eye exam should be performed in all women diagnosed with DM.[87] The exam should be repeated annually if retinopathy is observed. Less frequent exams (every 2-3 y) may be considered in some patients who have one or more normal eye examinations.

Cardiovascular disease risk

Type 2 DM is considered equivalent to preexisting CHD because the risk of a future CHD event is so high.[101] Women with type 2 DM may have an even higher risk of a CHD event than women with known CHD but without DM. Prospective studies and meta-analyses reported an alarming, more than 300% increased risk of CHD mortality in women with DM compared with women with known CHD.[104] A later and larger meta-analysis, however, suggests a much smaller increased risk in women with DM compared with women without DM with known CHD (hazard ratio [HR], 1.28; 95% CI, 0.75-2.22).[105] No matter the exact hazard estimate, these data suggest that among women, targeting those with DM may be an especially important way of ameliorating heart disease burden.

Risk reduction recommendations

Glucose management. The Action to Control Cardiovascular Risk in Diabetes (ACCORD) study tested the hypothesis that controlling glucose to achieve an Hb A$_{1C}$ below 6% (similar to that of a healthy person without DM) versus a more standard target (7%-7.9%) would prevent CVD events.[106] The more aggressive strategy did reduce nonfatal MIs over 5 years, but this occurred at the expense of worse overall 5-year mortality. Thus, the conclusion of the study was that aggressive glucose lowering below an Hb A$_{1c}$ target of 7% should not be recommended. However, the participants in the ACCORD study had DM for an average of 10 years before the study's baseline examination, and debate surrounds the generalizability of this finding to younger, healthier patients with DM and those more recently diagnosed. Thus, the optimal glucose target for most midlife women with DM is debatable. The ADA sets an Hb A$_{1C}$ of 7% as a reasonable goal in nonpregnant adults, with acknowledgement that more stringent goals may be indicated for select patients, such as those with short durations of DM and long life expectancy, as long as hypoglycemia can be avoided.[87] In addition, the ADA recommends a preprandial capillary glucose level of between 70 mg/dL and 130 mg/dL (3.9-7.2 mmol/L) and a peak postprandial glucose level of less than 180 mg/dL (10 mmol/L). The American Association of Clinical Endocrinologists (AACE) guidelines propose that the Hb A$_{1c}$ should in fact be less than 6.5%, with preprandial glucose lower than 110 mg/dL (6.0 mmol/L) and postprandial glucose lower than 140 mg/dL (7.7 mmol/L).[107]

Lifestyle modification. Women at high risk for developing DM can improve their glucose metabolism, thereby delaying and sometimes preventing the onset of type 2 DM. Among a cohort of adults at high risk for DM, the Diabetes Prevention Program Research Group determined that a lifestyle intervention that included 150 minutes of exercise per week and eating less fat and fewer calories (with the goal of reducing weight by 7%) decreased the risk of type 2 DM in women by 57%.[108] Similarly, women with DM can improve glucose metabolism with this type of lifestyle intervention.

Among adults with DM, the Look AHEAD Research Group determined that an intensive lifestyle intervention (with a goal of 7% sustained weight loss) caused a remission of type 2 DM in more than 10% of the women studied.[109] This rate was 4 times greater (10.4% vs 2.5%) than in women receiving only an educational intervention. However, this intensive lifestyle intervention did not lead to a reduction in CVD events.[62]

Adult women should avoid excess alcohol and stop smoking. Women should have no more than 1 alcoholic drink per day, and women with DM should take extra precautions to prevent hypoglycemia, because excessive alcohol use is associated with hyperglycemia and hypoglycemia.[87] Smoking should be avoided; smokers with type 2 DM have an increased risk of microvascular diabetic complications, macrovascular events, and premature death.

Metformin therapy. The ADA recommends that metformin therapy be considered for the prevention of type 2 DM, especially for those women with an impaired DM screening test and a BMI greater than 35, those aged younger than 60 years, and those with a history of gestational DM.[87] Metformin therapy is the preferred initial pharmacologic intervention for type 2 DM.

Statin therapy. Per the 2013 ACC/AHA guidelines on the treatment of blood cholesterol to reduce atherosclerotic cardiovascular risk in adults, all women with DM aged between 40 and 75 years should be treated with statin therapy.[30] This was based on Class A evidence that statin therapy reduces macrovascular disease and mortality in persons with DM. Per the guidelines, measurement of LDL-C can be performed under the auspices of global CVD risk assessment to guide the aggressiveness of the statin regimen. These recommendations are significantly changed from previous CVD prevention recommendations that emphasized the need to achieve specific LDL-C thresholds (such as LDL-C <100 mg/dL). Checking a baseline alanine aminotransferase before initiating a statin (>3 times the upper limit of normal was considered a potential contraindication to therapy) was recommended, whereas checking a baseline creatinine phosphokinase was not.

The US Food and Drug Administration (FDA) has expanded its prescribing information on the use of statins to include reports of a small increased risk of raised blood sugar and the development of type 2 DM with their use.[110] The cardiovascular benefits of statins outweigh the risks, says FDA, but healthcare professionals prescribing them should monitor blood sugar levels after instituting statin therapy.

Blood pressure management. Blood pressure control is important because higher BP increases the risk of vascular complications.[87] In women with DM and BP higher than 120/80 mmHg, lifestyle modification should be encouraged. Antihypertensive therapy is indicated for BP 140/80 mmHg or higher in women with DM and should include agents with proven benefits against CVD events such as ACE inhibitors, angiotensin receptor blockers, beta-blockers, diuretics, and calcium-channel blockers. These drugs have been shown to delay the progression of nephropathy in patients with DM with hypertension and microalbuminuria (>300 mg/24 h).[103]

Aspirin therapy. In 2009, the USPSTF updated their recommendations regarding aspirin for the primary prevention of cardiovascular events.[111] They recommended aspirin use in women aged 55 to 79 years but did not specifically single out women with DM. In 2010, the ADA, the AHA, and the ACC outlined recommendations for aspirin therapy specifically for patients with DM, and the ADA reiterated many of these recommendations in their 2013 statement on the standard of medical care in DM.[102,112] In these statements, aspirin therapy was recommended in doses of 75 mg to 162 mg per day in persons with increased cardiovascular risk (10-y risk >10%) and no increased risk for bleeding. This risk cut point was estimated to include most women with DM aged older than 60 years with 1 other major risk factor for CHD (such as family history of CVD, hypertension, smoking, dyslipidemia, or albuminuria). Aspirin therapy was explicitly *not* recommended for low-risk women, including women with DM aged younger than 60 years with no other major CVD risk factors. The 2011 AHA Effectiveness-Based Guidelines for the Prevention of Cardiovascular Disease in Women were vaguer in their recommendations for women with DM, stating that aspirin therapy (75-325 mg/d) is a reasonable recommendation for women with DM unless it is contraindicated.[34]

Hormone therapy's effect on glucose metabolism and incident diabetes

The data on the effects of HT on glucose metabolism are inconsistent. Although there is some suggestion that HT (estrogen alone) may reduce the incidence of DM in postmenopausal women, it is possible that there is publication bias because incident DM is variably defined in clinical trials and is typically a secondary clinical endpoint. The Postmenopausal Estrogen/Progestin Intervention (PEPI) trial was a 3-year randomized trial of HT's effects on cardiovascular risk factors, including glucose metabolism, in 788 healthy postmenopausal women.[113] The PEPI trial found that ET (conjugated equine estrogens [CEE]) and EPT (medroxyprogesterone acetate [MPA] or micronized progesterone) decreased fasting blood glucose slightly compared with placebo but significantly increased post-challenge glucose concentrations in healthy women.

In a 2004 report from the WHI, an EPT (CEE plus MPA) trial that included 15,641 postmenopausal women, the incidence of self-reported type 2 DM was lower in women randomized to EPT compared with those receiving placebo (3.5% vs 4.2%, respectively; HR, 0.79; 95% CI, 0.67-0.93) after 5.6 years of follow-up.[114] A 2013 WHI report that included 8.2 years of "intervention phase" follow-up reported a very similar hazard ratio (HR, 0.81; 95% CI, 0.70-0.94), supporting a lower incidence of self-reported DM in those randomized to EPT.[8] In age-stratified analyses from the 2004 report, incidence of DM was lowest in women aged 50 to 59 years and 60 to 69 years (HR, 0.80; 95% CI, 0.61-1.05, and HR, 0.58; 95% CI, 0.45-0.74, respectively) and higher in women aged 70 to 79 years (HR, 1.46; 95% CI, 1.02-2.09).[114] In the subset of women who underwent biomarker analyses during the trial, it appeared that women who received EPT had a lowering of glucose and insulin as well as a decrease in insulin resistance.

In the WHI-ET (CEE) trial that included 10,739 post-menopausal women with hysterectomy, the incidence of self-reported type 2 DM was lower in women randomized to ET compared with those receiving placebo, although the difference was not significant (8.3% vs 9.3%, respectively; HR, 0.88; 95% CI, 0.77-1.01).[115] In age-stratified analyses, the results were similar. The 2013 report from the WHI that included a 6.6-year intervention phase follow-up reported a very similar hazard ratio, albeit one that became statistically significant because of the inclusion of more events as a result of longer follow-up (HR, 0.86; 95% CI, 0.76-0.98).[8] This finding supports a lower incidence of self-reported DM in those randomized to ET.

However, after approximately 13 years of extended follow-up of both these WHI trials, the reduction in incident DM with HT dissipated completely.[8] In age-stratified analysis, no statistically significant reduction in DM was found in any age group with either form of HT. In fact, in women aged 70 to 79 years, an increased risk of incident DM was observed in the women randomized to EPT (HR, 1.32; 95% CI, 1.06-1.32).

In HERS, a study that included 2,763 women with known CHD, the incidence of type 2 DM was lower at follow-up in those randomized to EPT (CEE plus MPA) compared with those receiving placebo (6.2% vs 9.5%, respectively; HR, 0.65; 95% CI, 0.48-0.89).[116] Researchers noted in their conclusions that the observed reduction in type 2 DM did not outweigh the 3-fold increased risk of VTE nor the increased risk of secondary coronary events observed with EPT compared with placebo.[116-118]

Based on evidence from these 4 trials (PEPI, WHI-ET, WHI-EPT, and HERS), NAMS concluded that there is inadequate evidence to recommend HT for the sole or primary indication of the prevention of type 2 DM in perimenopausal or postmenopausal women.[65]

Hormone therapy and its effect on vascular complications in diabetes mellitus

One of the main goals of DM management is to minimize the vascular morbidities associated with the disease. Researchers from the Wisconsin Epidemiologic Study of Diabetic Retinopathy concluded that use of OCs or HT among women with type 1 or type 2 DM did not seem to worsen diabetic retinopathy nor increase the incidence of macular edema.[119] More evidence regarding the effect of HT on microvascular complications (retinopathy, nephropathy, and neuropathy) is needed.

Cardiovascular disease, the number 1 cause of death in women, is more common in women with DM than women without DM. Consensus exists that HT carries a relative contraindication in women with known CVD; menopause guidelines suggest that the best candidate for HT for vasomotor symptom control is a woman currently in the menopause transition or only recently transitioned through menopause and who has low risk of CVD, including CHD, stroke, and VTE. Cardiovascular disease risk is on a continuum, and determining where women with type 2 DM fall on the CVD risk spectrum is a clinical challenge for those working to provide personalized care for midlife women with DM and menopause symptoms.

Some guidance on the general safety of HT in women with DM may be gleaned from guidelines on the use of contraceptives in women with DM. The 2010 US Centers for Disease Control and Prevention (CDC) guidelines on contraceptive choice advise against the use of combined oral contraception in women with known ischemic heart disease, stroke, or hypertensive vascular disease as an "unacceptable health risk."[37] Hypertension of more than 160 systolic and/or 100 diastolic is also in this "unacceptable health risk" category. Diabetes mellitus with microvascular complications (retinopathy, nephropathy, or neuropathy) or DM for 20 or more years is considered slightly less risky, with a recommendation between "theoretical or proven risks usually outweigh the benefit" and "unacceptable health risk" for combined hormonal contraceptives. Progestin-only pills, implants, and intrauterine devices (IUDs) are available as less-risky options.

The 2006 guidelines (reaffirmed in 2008) from the American Congress of Obstetricians and Gynecologists (ACOG) are more cautious, stating that combined hormone contraceptives should be limited to women with DM who are nonsmokers, aged younger than 35 years, and without hypertension, nephropathy, retinopathy, or other vascular disease.[120]

Some research on the relationship between HT, impaired glucose metabolism, and/or self-reported DM and CVD risk is available from the WHI.[121] Researchers reported that high glucose, high insulin, or treated DM at the baseline WHI exam put women at higher risk of CHD events but that this increased risk appeared to add to the risk rather than potentiate it when HT was given.

Researchers conducted a nested case-control study of women with CHD events over the first 4 years of the WHI (cases) and matched controls.[122] They investigated whether baseline metabolic syndrome (or its components) increased the risk of CHD in women receiving HT. They reported that among 164 cases and controls with a fasting glucose of 100 mg/dL or higher at the baseline exam, women receiving EPT were 2.5 times more likely to develop CHD compared with those receiving placebo (odds ratio [OR], 2.46; 95% CI, 1.15-5.24). This contrasted the findings in 273 cases and controls with normal baseline glucose. In these women, EPT did not appear to confer an increased risk of CHD (OR, 0.95; 95% CI, 0.51-1.77). Among 97 cases and controls with a fasting glucose of 100 mg/dL or higher at baseline exam in the ET trial, women receiving ET did not appear more likely to develop CHD compared with those receiving placebo (OR, 0.85; 95% CI, 0.28-2.54). These hazards were calculated after adjusting for multiple confounders, including age and other CHD risk factors. Taken together, these data reveal that EPT may exacerbate CHD risk in women with abnormal glucose metabolism, but ET may not. This suggests a potential interactive effect between EPT use and abnormal glucose metabolism that worsens CHD risk.

Osteoporosis

Osteoporosis—the most common bone disorder affecting humans—becomes a significant health threat for aging postmenopausal women by increasing their risk of fracture. It is the most common cause of morbidity in the menopausal woman. Osteoporotic fractures are associated with substantial morbidity and mortality in postmenopausal women, especially women aged older than 65 years.[123]

Osteoporosis is a silent skeletal disorder characterized by compromised bone strength, predisposing a person to an increased risk of fracture.[124] Bone strength (and hence, fracture risk) reflects the integration of 2 main features: bone quantity and bone quality, whereby bone mineral density (BMD) is the most commonly measured estimate of bone quantity. Peak bone mass is achieved by a woman's third decade of life.[125] The process of bone loss begins at that time and accelerates at menopause. By age 80, many women have lost, on average, approximately 30% of their peak bone mass.[126] However, low bone density is not always the result of bone loss. A woman who does not achieve an adequate peak bone mass as a young adult may have low bone density without substantial bone loss as she ages.

To standardize values from different bone densitometry tests, results are reported as either a Z-score or a T-score, both expressed as standard deviation (SD) units.

- A T-score is useful to express BMD in a postmenopausal population and is calculated by comparing current BMD to the mean peak BMD of a normal, young-adult female population and expressed in SD units. The reference database is white women.

- For premenopausal women, use of Z-scores is the preferred manner of expressing BMD. A Z-score is based on the difference between the person's BMD and the mean BMD of a reference population of the same sex, age, and ethnicity and also is expressed in SD units.

NAMS supports the World Health Organization (WHO) and the International Society for Clinical Densitometry definitions of osteoporosis in a postmenopausal woman or in a man aged older than 50 years as a BMD T-score of −2.5 or less at the total hip, femoral neck, or lumbar spine (at least 2 vertebral levels measured in the posterior-anterior projection and not the lateral projection; Table 4).[127]

In addition to diagnosis through densitometry, osteoporosis can be diagnosed clinically, regardless of the T-score. The presence of a fragility fracture constitutes a clinical diagnosis of osteoporosis, even in those with a normal T- or Z-score.

Osteoporosis has no warning symptoms. Often, the first indication of the disease is a fracture. Nearly all nonvertebral

Table 4. Definitions of Bone Mineral Density Based on Dual-Energy X-Ray Absorptiometry Score

Normal	T-score ≥ −1.0
Low bone mass (osteopenia)	T-score between −1.0 and −2.5
Osteoporosis	T-score ≤ −2.5

Kanis JA.[127]

fractures are caused by a fall; vertebral fractures, however, often occur without a fall, need not necessarily be painful, and frequently are not diagnosed at the time of occurrence. It is estimated that only one-third of vertebral fractures are painful. Marked height loss over the years may be a sign of underlying vertebral compression fractures, even without significant associated back pain. Wrist or other fractures may occur at a younger age than vertebral or hip fractures and may also be early clinical expressions of osteoporosis.[128]

Osteoporosis is categorized as either primary, secondary, or idiopathic. Primary osteoporosis is usually caused by bone loss that occurs with aging. Secondary osteoporosis is caused at least in part by other diseases (eg, malabsorption) or medications (eg, glucocorticoids) that adversely affect skeletal health. Idiopathic osteoporosis is characterized by low bone density and fractures in young adults without known cause.

The primary clinical goal of osteoporosis management is to reduce fracture risk. This may be accomplished by slowing or stopping bone loss, increasing bone mass, improving bone architecture, maintaining or increasing bone strength, and minimizing factors that contribute to falls. Management strategies include general preventive health measures and pharmacologic interventions.

Prevalence

The National Osteoporosis Foundation (NOF) estimates derived from the National Health and Nutrition Examination Survey III (NHANES III) indicate that 9.9 million US people have osteoporosis and 43 million have low bone density.[129] In addition, about 34 million people have low bone mass. Most cases of osteoporosis occur in postmenopausal women; the prevalence of the disorder as defined by low BMD increases with age. The prevalence of osteoporosis rises from 19% in women aged 65 to 74 years to more than 50% in women aged 85 years and older.[130]

In the United States, the rates of osteoporosis and fracture vary with ethnicity. In one large study of postmenopausal women from 5 ethnic groups (whites, blacks, Asians, Hispanics, and American Indians), blacks had the highest BMD, whereas Asians had the lowest; differences in weight explained the variability among whites, Asians, and Hispanics but not blacks.[131] After adjusting for weight, BMD, and other covariates, whites and Hispanics had the highest risk for osteoporotic fracture, followed by American Indians, Asians, and blacks.[132]

The rate of hip fractures in women is decreasing. Canadian data on hip fractures are reliably collected from hospital discharges. One analysis showed declining age-adjusted hip fracture incidence (decreases of 31.8% in women and 25% in men) over the 21 years of the study.[133] Data obtained in the United States report similar declines in hip fracture rate among women, with no clear explanation for this trend, which appears to extend beyond the United States and Canada.[134,135] The absolute number of fractures will likely increase, however, because of population growth.

Morbidity and mortality
Hip fractures, which occur on average at age 82, elicit a particularly devastating toll, resulting in higher cost, disability, and mortality than all other osteoporotic fracture types combined. Hip fractures cause up to a 25% increase in mortality within 1 year of the incident. Approximately 25% of women require long-term care after a hip fracture, and 50% will have some long-term loss of mobility.

Osteoporotic fractures take a psychological toll as well. Hip and vertebral fractures and the resultant pain, loss of mobility, changed body image, and loss of independence can have a strong negative effect on self-esteem and mood.

Pathophysiology
Bone remodeling is a coupled process of bone resorption followed by bone formation. At the cellular level, osteoclasts promote bone resorption by stimulating the production of acid and enzymes that dissolve bone mineral and proteins. Osteoblasts promote bone formation by creating a protein matrix consisting primarily of collagen that is soon calcified, resulting in mineralized bone.

In normal bone remodeling, bone resorption is balanced by bone formation. Bone loss occurs when there is an imbalance between bone resorption and bone formation, resulting in a decrease in bone mass and an increase in the risk of fracture.

Menopause is associated with a few years of rapid bone loss attributed to lower circulating levels of 17β-estradiol, related primarily to the loss of estrogen-mediated inhibition of bone resorption without a fully compensatory increase in bone formation.[130] However, there is only a weak association between serum estradiol levels and rates of bone turnover in postmenopausal women.

Clinical risk factors
In determining risk factors, it is important to distinguish between risk factors for osteoporosis as defined by BMD and risk factors for osteoporotic fracture. For BMD-defined osteoporosis, major risk factors in postmenopausal women are advanced age, genetics, lifestyle factors (eg, low calcium and vitamin D intake, smoking), thinness, and menopause status.

Clinical risk factors can be used to assess fracture risk or to help make the decision as to which postmenopausal women should be screened with dual-energy x-ray absorptiometry (DXA) before age 65. Such risk factors increase the likelihood of fracture 1.5- to 3-fold over that seen in unaffected persons. Women with multiple risk factors are at greater risk of fracture if they have a lower BMD. The use of BMD T-scores to assess fracture risk can be markedly improved by combining BMD with information about other risk factors, particularly the woman's age and fracture history.

WHO conducted a meta-analysis of the relationship of clinical risk factors and fracture using global epidemiology data.[136] Ten risk factors were identified (Table 5). These risk factors were then used to create a platform called FRAX to calculate the 10-year risk of major osteoporotic fracture (hip, shoulder, wrist, and clinical spine).[137] It has been adapted for use in 53 countries and is accessible in 28 languages (www.shef.ac.uk/FRAX/). FRAX can be used without BMD.

Bone mineral density and fracture risk. Bone mineral density is an important determinant of fracture risk, especially in women aged 65 years and older.[138,139] In general, lower BMD is associated with a higher risk of fracture.

Age. Age is one of the strongest risk factors for fracture, particularly hip fracture. In general, the risk of osteoporotic fracture doubles every 7 or 8 years after age 50. The median age for hip fracture is 82 years. The median age for vertebral fracture is thought to occur in a woman's 70s.[140] Based on BMD alone, it would be expected that the hip fracture risk would increase 4-fold between ages 55 and 85.[141]

Fracture history. It is well established from many cohort, case-control, and cross-sectional studies that a prior osteoporotic fracture increases the risk of future fractures. A prior forearm fracture is associated with a 2-fold increase in subsequent risk of fracture. In 2 analyses of studies, a perimenopausal or postmenopausal woman who has had a fracture has approximately a 2-fold increased risk of sustaining another fracture; adjustment for BMD did not significantly affect the risk.[142,143]

Genetics. The greatest influence on a woman's peak bone mass (the maximal BMD gained during the skeletal development and maturation phase) is heredity. Studies have suggested that up to 80% of the variability in peak BMD might be attributable to genetic factors.[130] Daughters of women who have osteoporotic fractures have lower BMD than would be expected for their age.[144,145] First-degree relatives (mother, sister) of women with osteoporosis also tend to have lower BMD than those with no family history of osteoporosis.[146] Inasmuch as patient recall of parental hip fracture is higher than of any fracture, parental hip fracture was chosen as a clinical risk factor in FRAX (Table 5).[136]

Body mass index and thinness. Being thin—often cited as a BMI less than 21 kg/m^2—is a risk factor for low BMD.[147,148] Thinness has also been associated with increased fracture risk, especially in older women.[149] Low BMI is a well-documented risk factor for future fracture, whereas high BMI may be protective.[127] In FRAX, BMI is used when BMD is not available.

Lifestyle factors

Several lifestyle factors are associated with BMD and fracture. These include thinness, nutrition, exercise, fall risk, cigarette smoking, and alcohol consumption.

Nutrition. A balanced diet is important for bone development and maintenance as well as for general health. In the specific context of the prevention and management of osteoporosis, a discussion of nutrition appropriately focuses on calcium and vitamin D, magnesium, isoflavones, and protein.

- *Calcium.* Expert opinion recommends that postmenopausal women obtain 1,200 mg of calcium per day.[129]

- *Vitamin D.* The NOF guidelines recommend that postmenopausal women obtain 800 IU to 1,000 IU of vitamin D per day.[129] Vitamin D status is assessed by measurement of its major circulating metabolite, 25-hydroxy vitamin D or 25-(OH) D, with the minimum desirable 30 ng/mL.[150,151] Many patients require supplements of vitamin D (2,000 IU daily or more) to achieve this level.

- *Magnesium.* The recommended daily allowance for magnesium is 320 mg per day in women aged 31 years and older.[152] Data supporting a role for magnesium supplementation in the prevention or treatment of postmenopausal osteoporosis, however, are inconclusive.[153-155]

Exercise. Weight-bearing and strength-training exercises are beneficial to bone development and maintenance.[156-158] Even mild forms of exercise that improve agility and balance can benefit the skeleton. Among women aged 75 years and older, muscle strengthening and balance exercises have been shown to reduce the risk of falls and fall-related injuries by 75%.[159]

Fall risk. Falls are the precipitating factor in nearly 90% of all appendicular fractures, including hip fracture.[160] In the United States and Canada, approximately one-third of women aged older than 60 years falls at least once a year.[161,162] The incidence of falls increases with age, rising to a 50% annual rate in people aged older than 80 years. Poor vision, hearing, and balance and muscle weakness become critical determinants of fall risk, hence fracture risk, in older patients. Implementing relatively inexpensive measures to eliminate safety hazards in the home may also reduce this risk (Table 6). Effective fall prevention interventions in the elderly include home safety evaluation for high-risk or visually impaired patients, withdrawal of psychoactive medications, cataract surgery, exercise interventions (such as tai chi), and vitamin D repletion in those with low vitamin D levels.[163,164] A Cochrane review found the overall evidence inconclusive regarding the efficacy of hip protectors in reducing hip fractures, although poor adherence is a key problem contributing to the continuing uncertainty on their effectiveness.[165]

Cigarette smoking. Compared with nonsmokers, women smokers tend to lose bone more rapidly, have lower bone mass, and reach menopause 2 years earlier, on average.[166-168] In addition, some data show that postmenopausal women who are current smokers have significantly higher fracture rates than nonsmokers.[169]

Alcohol consumption. Data suggest an association between moderate alcohol intake and increased BMD in postmenopausal women.[170-171] Nevertheless, this observation must be tempered by the increased risk of falling and osteoporotic fracture associated with alcohol consumption. The level of alcohol consumption associated with an increased risk of falls is more than 7 units a week, as established by the Framingham Heart Study.[172]

Menopause status

The increased rate of bone resorption immediately after menopause clearly indicates a hormonal influence on bone density in women. The most likely explanation for this increased resorption is the drop in ovarian estrogen production that accompanies menopause.

Table 5. Risk Factors for Osteoporotic Fracture Used in FRAX

- Age (FRAX is calibrated for ages 40-90 y)
- Sex
- Weight
- Height
- Femoral neck BMD
- Prior fragility fracture
- Parental history of hip fracture
- Current tobacco smoking
- Long-term use of glucocorticoids (≥5 mg/d of prednisone for ≥3 months, ever)
- Rheumatoid arthritis
- Other causes of secondary osteoporosis
- Alcohol intake of 3 or more units daily

Body mass index is automatically computed from height and weight.
Abbreviation: BMD, bone mineral density.
Silverman SL.[136]

Chapter 4

Table 6. Recommendations for Fall Prevention at Patient Home

Lighting
- Provide ample lighting
- Have easy-to-locate light switches for rooms and stairs
- Use night lights to illuminate pathways from bedroom to bathroom and kitchen
- Provide light on all stairways

Obstructions
- Remove clutter, low-lying objects
- Remove raised door sills to ensure smooth transition

Floors and carpets
- Provide nonskid rugs on slippery floors
- Repair/Replace worn, buckled, or curled carpet
- Use nonskid floor wax

Furniture
- Arrange furniture to ensure clear pathways
- Remove or avoid low chairs and armless chairs
- Adjust bed height if too high or low

Storage
- Install shelves and cupboards at accessible height
- Keep frequently used items at waist height

Bathroom
- Install grab bars in tub, shower, near toilet
- Use chair in shower and tub
- Install nonskid strips/decals in tub/shower
- Elevate low toilet seat or install safety frame

Stairways and halls
- Install handrails on both sides of stairs
- Remove or tape down throw rugs and runners
- Repair loose and broken steps
- Install nonskid treads on steps

Bone loss begins to accelerate approximately 2 to 3 years before the last menses; this acceleration ends 3 to 4 years after menopause. For an interval of a few years around menopause, women lose 1% to 2% of bone annually. Afterward, bone loss slows to about 0.5% to 1.0% per year.[173,174] A prospective, longitudinal study of white women reported BMD losses during this 5- to 7-year interval of 10.5% for the spine, 5.3% for the femoral neck, and 7.7% for the total body.[173] Although some of the decline can be attributed to age-related factors, lower estrogen levels were implicated as the cause for approximately two-thirds of the bone loss. Lower estrogen levels have also been significantly associated with increased fracture risk in older women (mean age, 75 y).[175]

Women experiencing menopause at or before age 40—either spontaneously or induced (eg, through bilateral oophorectomy, chemotherapy, or pelvic radiation therapy)—are at greater risk of low BMD than other women of the same age who have not reached menopause.[176] However, by age 70, when fractures are more likely to occur, these women have the same risk for low BMD or fracture as women who reached menopause at the average age.[177,178]

Causes of secondary osteoporosis. Various medications, disease states, and genetic disorders are associated with bone loss (Table 7).[179]

Evaluation

All postmenopausal women should be assessed for risk factors associated with osteoporosis and fracture. This assessment requires a history, physical examination, and any necessary diagnostic tests. The goals of this evaluation are to assess fracture risk, to rule out causes of secondary osteoporosis, to identify modifiable risk factors, and to determine appropriate candidates for pharmacologic therapy.

History and physical examination. The medical history and physical examination should solicit clinical risk factors for osteoporosis and fracture and also evaluate for causes of secondary osteoporosis and fragility fracture (Tables 5 and 7). Risk factors must be accurately collected, often with the aid of a simple questionnaire. Risk factors may help identify contributing causes of osteoporosis and are essential in the determination of FRAX. This tool, used with guidelines for treatment thresholds, is very helpful in identifying candidates for pharmacotherapy. Osteoporosis can be diagnosed by bone density testing in postmenopausal women aged older than 50 years. A fragility fracture may also indicate a clinical diagnosis of osteoporosis.

Height loss greater than 1.5 in (3.8 cm) increases the likelihood that a vertebral fracture is present.[123] Weight should also be recorded to identify those women with low BMI and to be aware of weight changes, which may interfere with the interpretation of changes in BMD over time. The evaluation should include eliciting symptoms of acute or chronic back pain, which may indicate the presence of vertebral fractures.

Because back pain, height loss, and kyphosis can occur without osteoporosis, and because two-thirds of vertebral fractures are asymptomatic,[180,181] vertebral fractures must be confirmed by lateral spine radiographs or vertebral fracture assessment—imaging of the spine using DXA equipment at the time of BMD testing.[182,183]

After menopause, a woman's risk for falls should be assessed. Clinical factors related to an increased risk of falls include

Table 7. Major Causes of Secondary Osteoporosis

Medications
- Aromatase inhibitors
- Cytotoxic agents
- Excessive thyroxine doses
- GnRH agonists or analogs
- Heparin for >3 mo
- Immunosuppressants (eg, cyclosporine)
- IM medroxyprogesterone
- Long-term use of certain anticonvulsants (eg, phenytoin, barbiturates, carbamazepine)
- Oral or IM use of glucocorticoids for >3 mo
- Excess vitamin A (>5,000 IU/d retinol)
- PPIs
- SSRIs
- Thiazolidinediones

Genetic disorders
- Hemochromatosis
- Hypophosphatasia
- Osteogenesis imperfecta
- Thalassemia
- Homocystinuria
- Ehlers-Danlos syndrome
- Marfan syndrome
- Glycogen storage diseases
- Gaucher disease
- Porphyria

Disorders of calcium balance
- Hypercalciuria
- Vitamin D deficiency

Endocrinopathies
- Cushing syndrome
- Gonadal insufficiency (primary and secondary)
- Hyperthyroidism
- Hyperparathyroidism
- Type 1 DM
- Type 2 DM

Gastrointestinal diseases
- Billroth I gastroenterostomy
- Chronic liver disease (eg, primary biliary cirrhosis)
- Malabsorption syndromes (eg, celiac disease)
- Total gastrectomy
- IBD

Other disorders and conditions
- Ankylosing spondylitis
- Chronic renal disease
- Lymphoma and leukemia
- Multiple myeloma
- MS
- Nutritional disorders (eg, anorexia nervosa)
- RA
- Sarcoidosis
- Systemic mastocytosis
- COPD
- Organ transplantation
- Sickle cell disease
- HIV
- Immobilization

Abbreviations: COPD, chronic obstructive pulmonary disease; DM, diabetes mellitus; GnRH, gonadotropin-releasing hormone; HIV, human immunodeficiency virus; IBD inflammatory bowel disease; IM, intramuscular; MS, multiple sclerosis; PPI, proton pump inhibitors; RA, rheumatoid arthritis; SSRIs, selective serotonin-reuptake inhibitors.
Watts NB, et al.[179]

- A history of falls, fainting, or loss of consciousness
- Muscle weakness
- Dizziness, coordination, or balance problems
- Difficulty standing or walking
- Arthritis of the lower extremities
- Neuropathy of the lower extremities
- Impaired vision and/or hearing

Bone mineral density measurement. Bone mineral density testing of the hip (femoral neck, total hip), spine (at least 2 vertebral bodies), or radius (one-third radius site) is required for a densitometric diagnosis of osteoporosis. A clinical diagnosis of osteoporosis can be made if fragility fractures are present, regardless of BMD.

The NOF guidelines recommend BMD testing for all women aged 65 years and older, which is in agreement with the 2011 USPSTF recommendations for postmenopausal women.[129,184] Testing should be done sooner in women with clinical risk factors for fracture such as low body weight, history of prior fracture, family history of osteoporosis, smoking, excessive alcohol intake, or long-term use of high-risk medications such as glucocorticoids.

Bone-testing options. Fracture risk can be estimated by a variety of technologies at numerous skeletal sites. Bone mineral density measured by DXA is the only diagnostic technology by which measurements are made at the hip and spine and sometimes at the one-third radius. These are also important sites of osteoporotic fracture.[185]

When BMD testing is indicated, measuring the total hip, femoral neck, and posterior-anterior lumbar spine and using the lowest of the 3 T-scores is recommended for diagnosis.[123] In some patients, degenerative changes or other artifacts at the spine site make measurements unreliable. In such cases, the distal one-third radius should be measured and used for diagnosis.

Follow-up bone mineral density testing. In most cases, repeat DXA testing in untreated postmenopausal women is not needed until 2 to 5 years have passed. Postmenopausal women, after substantial BMD losses in early postmenopause, generally lose about 0.5 T-score units in BMD every 5 years.[149,186]

For women receiving osteoporosis therapy, BMD monitoring may not provide clinically useful information after 1 to 2 years of treatment.[123] At that point, a BMD indicating significant loss should prompt a reevaluation for secondary causes of osteoporosis after adherence to therapy has been confirmed. If the BMD demonstrates either an improvement or stability (no statistically significant loss), further testing is not indicated unless a change in health status warrants repeat testing.

Bone turnover markers. Biochemical markers of bone turnover can be measured in serum or urine. They can indicate either osteoclastic bone resorption or osteoblast functioning. Bone turnover markers cannot diagnose osteoporosis and have varying ability to predict fracture risk when studied in groups of patients in clinical trials.[187,188] They also have varying value in predicting individual patient response to therapy. Nevertheless, these tests may show a patient's response to therapy earlier than BMD changes, sometimes within 2 to 3 months compared with the 1 to 2 years required with BMD.[189,190]

Tests for potential contributing factors. Low BMD in postmenopausal women is most often the result of low peak bone mass, postmenopausal declines in bone density (related to estrogen deficiency), or both. There are, however, important factors that contribute to bone loss that should be identified clinically and through appropriate laboratory testing (Table 8). Potential contributing factors are found in about 30% of postmenopausal women with osteoporosis, and it is critical to identify and address these in order to avoid further bone loss on therapy.[191,192]

Initial laboratory testing should include a complete blood count, complete metabolic panel (including creatinine, calcium, phosphorus, alkaline phosphatase, and liver function tests), 25-OH D to evaluate for vitamin D deficiency, thyroid-stimulating hormone (TSH) level, and a 24-hour urine calcium, sodium, and creatinine assay to check for calcium malabsorption or hypercalciuria. This work-up identifies about 90% of occult disorders at a reasonable cost.[193] The presence of laboratory abnormalities on this initial work-up may suggest certain etiologies and guide further testing in selected patients.

Pharmacologic interventions

A management strategy focused on lifestyle approaches may be all that is needed for postmenopausal women who are at low risk for osteoporotic fracture. Adding osteoporosis drug therapy in these populations is recommended:

- All postmenopausal women who have had an osteoporotic vertebral or hip fracture

- All postmenopausal women who have BMD values consistent with osteoporosis (T-scores −2.5 or worse) at the lumbar spine, femoral neck, or total hip region

- All postmenopausal women who have T-scores from −1.0 to −2.5 and a 10-year risk, based on the FRAX calculator, of major osteoporotic fracture (spine, hip, shoulder, or wrist) of at least 20% or of hip fracture of at least 3%

Several pharmacologic options are available for osteoporosis therapy (Table 9). The antiresorptive agents include bisphosphonates, the estrogen agonist/antagonist raloxifene, estrogen, the estrogen agonist/antagonist bazedoxifene (BZA) combined with CE, calcitonin, and the monoclonal antibody against RANK-ligand, denosumab. Teriparatide, recombinant human parathyroid hormone, is the only approved anabolic agent for the treatment of postmenopausal osteoporosis. No studies have prospectively compared these therapies for antifracture efficacy.

With the exception of estrogen, the effects of therapies on fracture have been demonstrated only in patients with either the clinical or BMD diagnosis of osteoporosis. The absolute reduction in fracture risk is greatest in patients at high risk of fracture.

Adherence to therapy is poor. In studies of 6 months to 1 year, adherence rates for prescription drugs ranged from below 25% to 81%, depending on the therapy.[194-196] Factors associated with nonadherence include advancing age, AEs, being unsure about BMD test results, patient health beliefs, and inadequate patient education.[197-199] Perhaps the most important follow-up measure for clinicians is to encourage adherence to the treatment plan and to identify barriers to nonadherence. Providing clear information

Table 8. Routine Laboratory Tests for Osteoporosis Evaluation

Test	Diagnostic result	Possible cause of secondary osteoporosis
CBC	Anemia	Multiple myeloma
Serum calcium	Elevated	Hyperparathyroidism
	Low	Vitamin D deficiency, GI malabsorption
Serum phosphate	Elevated	Renal failure
	Low	Hyperparathyroidism
Serum 25-hydroxyvitamin D	Low	Undersupplementation, GI malabsorption, celiac disease
Serum albumin	Used to interpret serum calcium, nutritional deficiencies	
Serum alkaline phosphatase	Elevated	Vitamin D deficiency, GI malabsorption, hyperparathyroidism, Paget disease of bone, liver/biliary disease
Urinary calcium excretion	Elevated	Renal calcium leak, multiple myeloma, metastatic cancer involving bone, hyperparathyroidism, hyperthyroidism
	Low	GI malabsorption, inadequate intake of calcium, vitamin D
TSH turnover)	Low	Hyperthyroidism (causes excess bone
Serum protein electrophoresis	Monoclonal band	Multiple myeloma
Tissue transglutaminase (gluten enteropathy) with normal IgA total	Elevated	Predictive of celiac disease antibody
Creatinine	Elevated	Renal osteodystrophy, possible contraindication to bisphosphonates

Abbreviations: CBC, complete blood count; GI, gastrointestinal; IgA, immunoglobulin A; TSH, thyroid-stimulating hormone.

to women regarding their risk for fracture and the purpose of osteoporosis therapy may be the optimal way to improve adherence.

Antiresorptive agents. Antiresorptive agents are pharmacologic options that inhibit osteoclast-mediated bone resorption.

Bisphosphonates. This class of drugs works by inhibiting the activity of osteoclasts and shortening their life spans, thereby reducing bone resorption.[200] The most common AE of oral bisphosphonate therapy is esophageal and gastric irritation, particularly affecting patients who dose inappropriately. Clinical trials have demonstrated that bisphosphonates significantly increase BMD at the spine and hip in a dose-dependent manner in younger and older postmenopausal women. In women with osteoporosis, bisphosphonates have reduced the risk of vertebral fractures by 40% to 70% and reduced the incidence of nonvertebral fracture, including hip fracture, by about half this amount.[186,201]

Most of the bisphosphonates approved for osteoporosis therapy in the United States (alendronate, ibandronate, and risedronate) and in Canada (alendronate, etidronate, and risedronate) are available in oral formulations for daily and intermittent (weekly or monthly) dosing regimens. Ibandronate and zoledronic acid are available as intravenous (IV) formulations.

Oral bisphosphonates are not well absorbed (<1% of an oral dose is absorbed, and absorption is completely blocked if taken with calcium or food), so these must be taken first

Chapter 4

Table 9. Bone-Specific Prescription Drugs Approved for Postmenopausal Osteoporosis

Composition	Product	Form	Indication	Dosage
Bisphosphonates				
Alendronate	Fosamax	Oral tablet, solution[a]	Treatment	70 mg/wk
	Various generics	Oral tablet	Prevention	5 mg/d or 35 mg/wk
			Treatment	10 mg/d or 70 mg/wk
Alendronate + cholecalciferfol (vitamin D$_3$)	Fosamax Plus D[a] Fosavance[b]	Single tablet	Treatment	70 mg + 2,800 IU /wk 70 mg + 5,600 IU/wk[a]
Risedronate	Actonel	Oral tablet	Prevention + treatment	5 mg/d; 35 mg/wk; 150 mg/mo
	Atelvia	Oral tablet (delayed release)	Treatment	35 mg/wk
Risedronate + calcium carbonate	Actonel with calcium	Packet of oral tablets (not combined therapies) with 4-wk supply	Prevention + treatment	35 mg/wk (day 1) + 1,250 mg calcium for no-risedronate days (days 2-7 of 7-d cycle)
Ibandronate	Boniva[a]	Oral tablet IV injection	Prevention Treatment	150 mg/mo 3 mg q 3 mo
Etidronate	Didrocal[b]	Oral tablet (packaged with calcium carbonate)	Prevention + treatment	400 mg/d for 14 d q 3 mo, with calcium taken between cycles
Zoledronic acid	Reclast[a]	IV infusion	Prevention Treatment	5 mg/2 y 5 mg/y
	Aclasta[b]	IV infusion	Treatment	5 mg/y
Estrogen agonist/antagonist				
Raloxifene	Evista	Oral tablet	Prevention + treatment	60 mg/d
Calcitonin				
Calcitonin-salmon	Fortical[a]	Nasal spray	Treatment (>5 y postmenopause)	200 IU/d
	Miacalcin	Nasal spray	Treatment (>5 y postmenopause)	200 IU/d
		SC or IM injection[a]	Treatment (>5 y postmenopause)	100 IU every other day
Parathyroid hormone				
Teriparatide (recombinant human PTH 1-34)	Forteo	SC injection	Treatment (high fracture risk)	20 µg/d
RANK ligand inhibitor				
Denosumab	Prolia	SC injection	Treatment	60 g q 6 mo

Unless noted, products are available in the United States and in Canada.
Abbreviations: IM, intramuscular; IV, intravenous; SC, subcutaneous.
a. Available in the United States but not Canada.
b. Available in Canada but not the United States.

thing in the morning on an empty stomach. Food, drink, and medications (including supplements) must be avoided for 30 minutes (alendronate and risedronate) to 60 minutes (ibandronate) after dosing; etidronate labeling recommends waiting 2 hours. Calcium and vitamin D must be continued but not taken at the same time as the bisphosphonate. There is a specially formulated version of weekly risedronate that may be taken with food, immediately after breakfast.

Several AEs are associated with the different dosings of bisphosphonates:

- Oral bisphosphonates may cause upper GI disorders such as dysphagia, esophagitis, and esophageal ulcers and are contraindicated in patients with esophageal abnormalities that delay esophageal emptying or in those who are unable to stand or sit upright for at least 30 to 60 minutes after ingestion.

- All bisphosphonates carry precautions on hypocalcemia and renal impairment. Serum calcium and serum creatinine should be measured in all patients before beginning osteoporosis therapy. Revised labeling for zoledronic acid states that it is contraindicated in patients with creatinine clearance less than 35 mL per minute or with acute renal impairment.

- A transient flu-like illness, often called an acute-phase reaction, occurs infrequently with large doses of oral or IV bisphosphonates; symptoms are usually mild, resolve on their own, and are usually limited to the first dose.

- Jaw lesions (known as osteonecrosis of the jaw [ONJ]), usually after dental extraction, have been observed with bisphosphonate use, most often in patients treated with large IV doses for cancer-related bone diseases.[201-203] There are no data to suggest that dental surgery is contraindicated in patients on bisphosphonate therapy. Routine dental care is recommended for all patients.

- FDA has warned of a possible risk of a rare type of thigh bone (subtrochanteric femur) fracture with bisphosphonates approved for osteoporosis.[204,205] These fractures had been described in patients who have not received any treatment for osteoporosis. Along with the increased femoral fracture risk warning, labeling now also recommends reassessing the need for continued therapy at 5 years.

The long-term safety concerns of bisphosphonate therapy are not supported by evidence from RCTs. Trials of more than 5 years' duration with zoledronic acid (6 y), risedronate (7 y), and alendronate (10 y) have demonstrated persistent but not progressive reduction of bone turnover without evidence of unexpected AEs or abnormal bone histomorphometry.[206-211] In a retrospective review of the Health Outcomes and Reduced Incidence with Zoledronic Acid Once Yearly (HORIZON) trial with IV zoledronic acid, one case of ONJ was reported in the treatment group and another in the placebo group.[212] A total of 12 fractures in 10 women were classified as subtrochanteric in secondary analyses of the Fracture Intervention Trial (FIT), the FIT Long-term Extension trial, and the HORIZON Pivotal Fracture trial, indicating that the risk of such fractures with use of bisphosphonates was very low, even in women treated for up to 10 years.[213]

Discontinuation studies have yielded variable results, depending on which bisphosphonate is being considered. Zoledronic acid has the highest binding avidity of the oral bisphosphonates to hydroxyapatite in osteoclasts, followed by alendronate, ibandronate, and then risedronate. In the 3-year extension of the zoledronate HORIZON Pivotal Fracture Trial, BMD dropped slightly in the placebo group compared with the treatment group but remained above pretreatment levels at the end of 6 years.[211] After discontinuation of alendronate after 5 years of therapy, BMD remained stable or decreased slowly while bone turnover markers remained below baseline values for up to 5 years.[207,208,214] Such studies excluded women at highest risk for fracture. Discontinuation of risedronate therapy after 2 years in young postmenopausal women (mean age, 51-52 y) was shown to result in significant bone loss at the spine and the hip during the first year after treatment is stopped.[215] No data are available regarding discontinuation of etidronate or ibandronate therapy. Data from clinical trials suggest that the risk of vertebral fractures is reduced beyond 3 to 5 years of therapy and that continuing treatment for 10 years seems to be a better choice for high-risk patients. For lower-risk patients, it is reasonable to consider a "drug holiday" at 3 to 5 years, because bisphosphonates accumulate in bone with some persistent antifracture efficacy after therapy is stopped.[216] There is considerable controversy regarding the optimal duration of therapy and the length of the holiday, both of which should be based on individual assessments of risk and benefit. If a drug holiday is advised, reassessment of risk should occur sooner for drugs with lower skeletal affinity, with a suggestion to reassess after 1 year for risedronate, 1 to 2 years for alendronate, and 2 to 3 years for zoledronic acid.[216,217]

Estrogen agonists/antagonists. These nonsteroidal agents of various chemical structures act as estrogen agonists and/or antagonists. Raloxifene 60 mg per day is approved for the prevention and treatment of osteoporosis. No other estrogen agonist/antagonist is approved for osteoporosis therapy, although several are in clinical development. Raloxifene has beneficial effects on BMD, in reducing osteoporotic vertebral fractures but not hip or nonvertebral fractures, and decreasing bone turnover, as assessed by biochemical marker as seen in the Multiple Outcomes of Raloxifene Evaluation (MORE) trial.[218,219] In addition to its effects on bone, raloxifene has been associated with a reduced risk of invasive breast cancer in postmenopausal women with osteoporosis.

Chapter 4

Estrogen. Systemic estrogen products—ET for women without a uterus (Table 10) and EPT for women with a uterus (Table 11)—are government approved in the United States and Canada for prevention, but not treatment, of postmenopausal osteoporosis.[220-226]

- *Bone mineral density.* The beneficial effects of systemic oral or transdermal ET or EPT at standard doses on BMD preservation are well established.[227] Effects of lower-than-standard doses of ET or EPT on BMD have been investigated.[222-226] Significant BMD improvements have also been noted with systemic estrogen doses delivered via a vaginal ring.[228] A dose-dependent response on bone density is seen with ET, and BMD losses occur rapidly when therapy is discontinued.

- *Fracture.* Evidence from RCTs and observational studies indicate that standard doses of ET or EPT (including 0.625 mg/d CE or the equivalent) reduce fracture risk in postmenopausal women.[229-233] Lower doses have not been examined with regard to fracture efficacy.

- *Discontinuation of therapy.* The benefits of HT on bone mass dissipate quickly after treatment is discontinued. Studies have shown a BMD loss of 3% to 6% during the first year after cessation of systemic ET or EPT.[214,234-236] Data also indicate that the fracture risk reduction with ET or EPT does not persist after therapy is discontinued.[232]

Bazedoxifene/Conjugated estrogens. Bazedoxifene combined with conjugated estrogens (BZA/CE) is a tissue-selective estrogen complex that has prevented bone loss and decreased bone turnover without stimulating the endometrium in healthy postmenopausal women with normal or low BMD.[237,238] A 2-year trial involving 3,397 postmenopausal women with a BMD score between −1.0 SD and −2.5 SD tested multiple doses of BZA/CE and found that all doses resulted in significantly higher BMD scores in the treatment group compared with the placebo group. Similarly, bone turnover markers were significantly decreased in the BZA/CE group compared with placebo.[238] Bazedoxifene 20 mg combined with CE 0.45 mg has been government approved for prevention of osteoporosis in postmenopausal women and for treatment of moderate to severe vasomotor symptoms.

Calcitonin. Salmon calcitonin is government approved for treatment of osteoporosis in women 5 years beyond their age of menopause when other treatments are not suitable. It is available in the United States as a nasal spray and an intramuscular or subcutaneous injection. Calcitonin is an inhibitor of bone resorption. In clinical use, however, the reduction in bone turnover with calcitonin is much less than with other antiresorptive agents. In 2012, the European Medicines Agency's Committee for Medicinal Products for Human Use did a review of data on calcitonin and found an increased risk of cancer in general with its use. On the basis of this review and the overall risk-benefit

Table 10. Estrogen-Only Prescription Drugs Approved for the Prevention of Postmenopausal Osteoporosis

Composition	Product	Form	Dosage
Conjugated estrogens	Premarin	Oral tablet	0.3, 0.45,[a] 0.645, 0.9, 1.25 mg/d
Estropipate	Ogen	Oral tablet	0.625 (0.75 estropipate, calculated as sodium estrone sulfate sodium estrone sulfate 0.625), 1.25 (1.5), 2.5 (3.0) mg/d (approved only for treatment in Canada)
17β-estradiol	Alora[a]	Matrix patch	0.025, 0.05, 0.075, 0.1 mg (twice/wk)
	Climara	Matrix patch	0.025,[a] 0.0375, 0.05, 0.075, 0.1 mg (once/wk) (0.025 dose not approved in Canada)
	Estrace	Oral tablet	0.5, 1.0, 2.0 mg/d
	Menostar[a]	Matrix patch	0.014 mg (once/wk)
	Vivelle[a]	Matrix patch	0.025,[a] 0.0375,[a] 0.05, 0.075,[a] 0.1[a] mg (twice/wk)
	Vivelle-Dot[a] Estradot[b]	Matrix patch	0.025, 0.0375, 0.05, 0.075, 0.1 mg (twice/wk)
	Estraderm	Reservoir patch	0.05, 0.1 mg (twice/wk)

Unless noted, products are available in the United States and in Canada.
a. Available in the United States but not Canada.
b. Available in Canada but not the United States.

Table 11. Combination Drugs Approved for the Prevention of Postmenopausal Osteoporosis (Intact Uterus)

Composition	Product	Form	Dosage
Conjugated estrogens (E) + medroxyprogesterone acetate (P) (continuous-cyclic)	Premphase[a]	Oral	0.625 mg E + 5.0 mg P/d (2 tablets: E for days 1-14 followed by E+P on days 15-28)
Conjugated estrogens (E) + medroxyprogesterone acetate (P) (continuous-combined)	Prempro[a]	Oral	0.3 or 0.45 mg E + 1.5 mg P/d (1 tablet) 0.625 mg E + 2.5 mg or 5.0 mg P (1 tablet)
Ethinyl estradiol (E) + norethindrone acetate (P)	femhrt[a] femHRT[b]	Oral	2.5 µg E + 0.5 mg P/d (1 tablet) 5 µg E + 1 mg P/d (1 tablet)
17β-estradiol (E) + norethindrone acetate (P)	Activella[a]	Oral	0.5 mg E + 0.1 mg P/d (1 tablet) 1 mg E + 0.5 mg P/d (1 tablet)
17β-estradiol (E) + norgestimate (P) (intermittent-combined)	Prefest[a]	Oral	1 mg E + 0.09 mg P (2 tablets: E for 3 d followed by E+P for 3 d, repeated continuously)
17β-estradiol (E) + levonorgestrel (P) (continuous-combined)	Climara Pro[a]	Patch	0.045 mg E + 0.015 mg P (22 cm^2 patch, once/wk)
Bazedoxifene (BZA) + conjugated estrogens (E)	Duavee[a]	Oral	20 mg BZA + 0.45 mg E (1 tablet)

a. Available in the United States but not Canada.
b. Available in Canada but not the United States.

profile, the agency withdrew salmon calcitonin for treatment of osteoporosis from the European market.[239] Canada withdrew 3 nasal spray salmon calcitonin products from its market in 2013.[240] FDA sent a notification to US healthcare professionals of the increased cancer risk.

Denosumab. Denosumab is a fully human monoclonal antibody to receptor activator of nuclear factor-B ligand (RANKL), a member of the tumor necrosis factor superfamily expressed on the surface of osteoblasts. RANKL binding to its receptor RANK on the surface of osteoclast precursors promotes the proliferation and differentiation of osteoclasts. By blocking the interaction between RANKL and RANK, denosumab inhibits bone resorption by osteoclasts. In postmenopausal women with low bone mass, denosumab increased BMD in various skeletal sites similar to or slightly more than did alendronate 70 mg per week.[241] In women with osteoporosis, denosumab reduced the incidence of vertebral fractures by 68%, hip fracture by 40%, and nonvertebral fractures by 20% compared with placebo.[242]

Bone mineral density of the lumbar spine and total hip regions increased with denosumab therapy compared with placebo by 9.2% and 6.0%, respectively. Denosumab was also generally safe and well tolerated after 8 years of exposure in a phase 2 clinical trial.[243] Skin reactions (including infections) occurred more commonly with treatment than with placebo. Other AEs include low calcium levels, infections, jaw bone problems, and atypical femur fractures. A detailed analysis examining the incidence and types of infections with denosumab revealed that serious AEs of infections (skin, GI, ear, urinary, and cardiac valvular infections) were numerically higher in the denosumab group, but the number of events was small, and the differences between groups were not statistically significant.[244]

Tibolone. Tibolone is approved in many countries, but not the United States or Canada, for the prevention of osteoporosis. In the Long-Term Intervention on Fractures With Tibolone study, tibolone reduced the risk of vertebral and nonvertebral fracture, breast cancer, and possibly colon cancer but increased the risk of stroke in older postmenopausal women with osteoporosis.[245]

Anabolic agents. Pharmacologic options such as parathyroid hormone directly stimulate osteoblastic bone formation.

Parathyroid hormone. Parathyroid hormone and its analogs, given by subcutaneous injection once daily, are anabolic agents that directly stimulate osteoblastic bone formation, resulting in substantial increases in trabecular bone density and connectivity in women with postmenopausal osteoporosis. Teriparatide (recombinant human parathyroid hormone 1-34) is approved in the United States and in Canada for the treatment of osteoporosis in postmenopausal women who are at high risk for fracture. Drug-related AEs include muscle cramps, transient hypercalcemia, nausea, and dizziness. There are anecdotal reports that teriparatide may be beneficial in the treatment of ONJ and atypical femoral fracture, but it is not approved for these indications.[246,247]

Strontium ranelate. Oral strontium ranelate is approved for the prevention and treatment of osteoporosis in many countries outside of North America. However, in 2014, the European Medicines Agency further restricted its use to patients who cannot use any of the other osteoporosis medications. Safety concerns include cardiovascular risk (such as an increase in thromboembolism and MI) and a concern for Stevens-Johnson syndrome. This drug is unusual in that it increases deposition of new bone by osteoblasts and reduces the resorption of bone by osteoclasts. Dosing involves dissolving 2 g of strontium ranelate in water and drinking it before bedtime. Other strontium salts are available as supplements, but no studies are available evaluating their effectiveness and safety.

Combining therapies. Combining potent antiresorptive agents results in small additional increments in bone density. In postmenopausal women (mean age, 61-62 y) who have low bone mass, BMD improvements in the spine and hip with combined alendronate and ET were significantly greater (8.3%) than results for either agent alone (6.0%).[248] However, fracture data are unavailable for these combinations, and combining antiresorptive agents is not generally recommended.

Combining an anabolic agent such as teriparatide with an antiresorptive agent has been considered. Significant increases in BMD occurred in a clinical trial when teriparatide was added to ongoing ET.[249] A study comparing the effects of adding versus switching to teriparatide in postmenopausal women who had received at least 18 months of alendronate or raloxifene showed that greater bone turnover increases were achieved by switching to teriparatide, whereas greater BMD increases were achieved by adding teriparatide.[250] Combination therapy with teriparatide and denosumab appears to increase BMD to a greater extent than either therapy alone.[251] Based on available data, recommendations cannot be made for or against combining antiresorptive and anabolic drugs. Given the absence of fracture and long-term follow-up data and the additional cost and AEs of taking 2 agents, it seems reasonable to switch to rather than add teriparatide in patients who have received antiresorptive therapy but require additional therapy for osteoporosis. There are no data to suggest that discontinuing long-term bisphosphonates requires a latent period before starting teriparatide. An antiresorptive agent, preferably a bisphosphonate or RANKL inhibitor, should be used to preserve or increase gains in BMD acquired with teriparatide therapy after it is discontinued.

Promising therapies. Several new drugs have demonstrated fracture efficacy in published trials for the treatment or prevention of osteoporosis or both. Some are now available outside of North America, and others are in clinical development.

Parathyroid hormone 1-84. The full-length parathyroid hormone, parathyroid hormone 1-84, is available in Europe. In an randomized trial of 2,532 women with postmenopausal osteoporosis, parathyroid hormone 1-84 administered as a daily subcutaneous injection in a 100-μg dose increased BMD in the lumbar spine by 6.9% and in the total hip region by 2.1% compared with placebo.[252] The proposed indication for this drug appears to be hypoparathyroidism.

Cathepsin-K inhibitors (ie, odanacatib) inhibit matrix dissolution, decrease bone resorption, and improve BMD in postmenopausal women.[253,254]

Sclerostin antibody inhibitors (ie, romosozumab) have also been shown to improve BMD in postmenopausal women by binding to sclerostin and increasing bone formation.[255]

There are also promising trials assessing the safety and efficacy of different formulations of recombinant parathyroid hormone, including a transdermal patch and a once-daily oral treatment.[256,257] In addition, parathyroid hormone-related protein (1-36) and synthetic parathyroid hormone-related protein analogs have shown promise as novel skeletal anabolic agents.[258,259]

Gallbladder disease

The incidence of gallstones in the US population has been estimated to be at 8% to 10%.[260] NHANES III estimates 6.3 million men and 14.2 million women in the United States have gallbladder disease and that it occurs 2 times more frequently in women than in men. American Indians have the highest rate of gallstones because of the increased cholesterol in their bile; almost 65% of American Indian women have gallstones. Mexican Americans comprise the next highest group.

A woman's risk of gallstones increases with obesity, parity, and hormone use. They occur more commonly during rapid weight loss, such as with low-calorie diets or bariatric surgery, because extra cholesterol is secreted into bile. Ovarian hormones, whether OCs or menopausal HT, increase biliary cholesterol saturation, a prerequisite for cholesterol gallstone formation. Warning signs include abdominal pain lasting more than 5 hours, nausea and vomiting, fever or chills, jaundice, tea-colored urine, and light-colored stools, which may signify serious infection or inflammation of the gallbladder, liver, or pancreas.

A review of the epidemiologic literature, which included the Nurses' Health Study and 2 clinical trials, PEPI and HERS, concluded that HT increases risk of gallbladder disease and cholecystectomy.[261] Furthermore, HERS found that HT use among postmenopausal women (average age, 68 y) with known coronary disease resulted in a marginally significant increase in the risk of biliary tract surgery—

1 additional woman undergoing surgery for every 185 women treated with CE 0.625 mg/MPA 2.5 mg.

In the WHI, with an average participant age of 63 years, treatment with ET or EPT increased the risk of cholecystitis and cholelithiasis. Risk increased with duration of use. Attributable risk in the ET arm of the WHI was 15.5 per 1,000 per 5 years of use, with similar risks seen with EPT.[262,263]

Overall risk of gallbladder disease from WHI and HERS for EPT revealed an increase after 5.6 years of use, with an absolute risk increase of 27 cases per 1,000 woman-years (95% CI, 21 to 34), whereas ET after 7 years showed an increase in absolute risk of 45 cases per 1,000 woman-years (95% CI, 36 to 57).[8,261]

In the Million Women Study, current estrogen users were 64% more likely (95% CI, 1.58-1.69) to experience gallbladder disease than never users (RR, 1.6).[264] Oral estrogen use raised risk more than did transdermal estrogen use (RR, 1.7 vs 1.2). One RCT compared the effect of transdermal and oral estrogens on gallstone formation and focused on biliary markers of gallstone formation, an intermediate outcome, compared with clinical gallstone formation.[265] The study found that both estrogen formulations altered bile comparably in ways that would be expected to form gallstones.

One review of the literature postulated that estrogen increases the risk of developing cholesterol gallstones by increasing the hepatic secretion of biliary cholesterol, which, in turn, leads to an increase in cholesterol saturation of bile.[266] A small, nonrandomized study suggested that the degree of elevation of circulating estrone levels manifested during oral, but not transdermal, ET may predict the level of lithogenic bile during oral ET use.[267] Minimal data are available regarding gallbladder cancer and estrogen use, with no cases reported in the WHI.[262]

A large prospective cohort study designed to examine hormonal and environmental factors that affect diseases in women included data on 70,928 women who were followed for a mean of 11.5 years (total follow-up period, 819,889 person-years); 45,984 (64.8%) participants reported ever using menopausal HT.[268] There were 2,819 incident cholecystectomies performed during the study period, with data on HT available for 2,608 participants. Adjustments were made for BMI, parity, hypercholesterolemia, DM, and level of education. Compared with never use of HT, any use was associated with an adjusted HR for cholecystectomy of 1.10 (95% CI, 1.01-1.20). The increase in risk was associated only with oral unopposed estrogens (adjusted HR, 1.16; 95% CI, 1.06-1.27), which was significantly greater than with transdermal estrogens (P=.03) or with oral preparations that combined estrogen with a progestogen (P=.03). Oral CE alone was associated with a significantly higher risk than oral CE plus a progestogen (P=.01). Over 5 years, about 1 cholecystectomy in excess would be expected in every 150 women using oral ET without progestogens compared with women not using ET.

Hormone therapy should be administered with caution to postmenopausal women who have gallstones or a history of gallbladder disease. Gallbladder-related risks should be discussed.

Arthritis and arthralgia

There are more than 100 types of arthritis, many of which affect women at midlife and beyond. The term *arthritis* refers to diseases of the joints and is generally classified into *noninflammatory* forms, those for which inflammation and immunologic sources are not thought to be central to the disease process, and *inflammatory*, in which autoimmune or inflammatory processes cause the disease. Musculoskeletal syndromes that cause pain around the joints but do not actually harm the joints themselves are referred to as *arthralgias*.

Osteoarthritis

Osteoarthritis, or degenerative joint disease, is overwhelmingly the most common form of joint disease and is the most important noninflammatory arthritis. It is predominantly a disease of aging, and hence its prevalence is growing dramatically as the population ages; virtually everyone will have evidence of some structural joint degeneration by age 70, although only a minority will have symptoms of osteoarthritis. Typically, weight-bearing joints are affected, including the knees, hips, and feet, as well as the cervical and lumbosacral spine. In addition, several small joints of the hand are often involved. Although simplistic, it is useful to think of osteoarthritis in these joints as a "wearing out."

Aside from aging, important risk factors for the development of osteoarthritis include obesity, significant joint injury, and overuse. Especially important are major knee injuries during recreational sports; for example, torn cruciate ligaments confer a greater than 50% risk of subsequent osteoarthritis development.[269] Certain patterns of osteoarthritis such as so-called nodal or *generalized* osteoarthritis, in which the distal joints of the fingers may be affected, may predominate in women.

One variant of this condition, erosive osteoarthritis, is of particular significance because it affects predominantly women aged in their mid-40s and beyond. There is a major hereditary component to erosive osteoarthritis; many affected women will have a first-degree relative with the condition. The small joints of the fingers, particularly the proximal interphalangeal (midfinger) and distal interphalangeal (fingertip) joints, are the targets of involvement. Initially, these joints may be inflamed with redness, warmth, and pain mimicking other forms of arthritis, but over months and years the inflammation resolves, leaving a typical gnarled, knobby joint that is most often relatively pain free. To date, there is no convincing explanation as to why women are targeted by erosive osteoarthritis, although genetics may play a role.

Chapter 4

The first carpometacarpal joint (at the base of the thumb) is another frequent area of osteoarthritis involvement and can be exceptionally disabling. Perhaps because of better mechanics, primary osteoarthritis rarely affects the wrists, elbows, ankles, or shoulders, and when found in these joints, look for other causes of symptoms such as rotator cuff tear or history of trauma. Osteoarthritis, for the most part, has a low-grade inflammatory component, which may be related to exacerbating pain and fostering disease progression. However, osteoarthritis is not considered a systemic inflammatory process, therefore involvement of organs outside of the musculoskeletal system is not expected nor are systemic symptoms such as malaise.

Physical findings typically include joint tenderness, limitation of motion, and crepitus. Joint swelling may be present, but significant warmth and redness should prompt concern about the diagnosis. Chondrocalcinosis (deposition of calcium pyrophosphate dihydrate) is frequently found on radiographs of the osteoarthritis joint, particularly in the knee and wrist. Release of these crystals into the joint space may cause an intense inflammatory response. This is always a prime consideration in an older woman with acute joint pain and swelling in the knees or wrists.

Management of osteoarthritis. To date, there is no means of either preventing or curing osteoarthritis. Management as recommended by experts in the field may provide significant therapeutic benefit.[270] Maintaining ideal weight has been shown to delay and reduce the severity of degeneration of the lumbar spine and weight-bearing joints. Because osteoarthritis is driven by aberrant biomechanics, a variety of modalities to improve the way we load joints can be beneficial[271]; for example, exercise to strengthen periarticular muscles and improve posture has been shown to provide pain relief. Physical therapy can be useful for getting patients started on appropriate exercise, for aerobic conditioning and balance, and for strengthening. Applications of heat or cold and splinting of affected joints can be useful for slowing exacerbation. Often, however, medication is necessary to control symptoms.

Nonprescription therapy. Acetaminophen, in doses up to 2 g per day (1 double-strength pill 4 times/d) is often recommended as first-line treatment for relatively minor osteoarthritis pain, but it is most useful for short-term painful flares of osteoarthritis rather than chronic ongoing pain. Nonsteroidal anti-inflammatory drugs (NSAIDS) such as ibuprofen or naproxen are available over the counter and can be effective in low doses.

Prescription therapy. Nonsteroidal anti-inflammatory drugs are often prescribed for osteoarthritis pain and have been demonstrated in several controlled studies to be effective. Adverse effects of these drugs, which often limit their use, include fluid retention, secondary hypertension, and decreases in renal function. Serious cardiovascular events may also be increased in frequency. The most common AE of NSAIDs as a group is GI irritation and bleeding, which can be life threatening; thus, in middle-aged and elderly patients, additional medications to protect the stomach lining are often prescribed with the NSAIDs.

Alternatively, cyclooxygenase-2 selective inhibitors may be safer for the GI tract than conventional NSAIDs; only celecoxib is available in the United States. Topical NSAIDs such as diclofenac are available and may be effective for osteoarthritis involving superficial joints such as the knees or the knuckles. Other alternatives include the pure analgesics such as tramadol, and under certain circumstances, opiates can provide substantial pain relief. There has been great interest in a possible neuropathic component of osteoarthritis pain, and duloxetine, a neuroactive medicine, has been approved by FDA for use in osteoarthritis.

Systemic steroids are rarely, if ever, indicated for treatment of pure osteoarthritis, but intra-articular injection of a long-acting corticosteroid agent such as triamcinolone or methylprednisolone can be effective for alleviating symptoms. Intra-articular hyaluronans given as a series of injections may provide fairly long-term relief for selected patients with osteoarthritis of the knee.

Complementary and alternative approaches. The majority of osteoarthritis patients have tried a variety of complementary strategies for pain relief. These include nutriceuticals as well as acupuncture and various Eastern exercise regimens. Although glucosamine remains very popular, it has been demonstrated to have little incremental value beyond that of placebo.[272,273] Nonetheless, the placebo effect in osteoarthritis pain is quite potent, and in controlled trials involving placebos, the placebo treatments themselves consistently provide substantial relief. Thus, for agents or approaches that have low toxicity, there may be great value appreciated by many persons.

Joint replacement. Finally, joint replacement remains the option of choice for those patients in whom joint pain affects daily activity and even sleep.

Rheumatoid arthritis

Rheumatoid arthritis is considered the archetypal *inflammatory* arthritis. It occurs 3 times as often in women as men; peak age of onset is between ages 35 and 55, commonly affecting perimenopausal and postmenopausal women. The etiology of RA remains an enigma. There is a somewhat higher incidence of disease in first-degree relatives, but in most cases overt hereditary factors are absent. Rheumatoid arthritis often goes into remission during pregnancy, but a direct connection to hormone levels has not yet been defined.

Rheumatoid arthritis typically affects multiple peripheral joints in a symmetric pattern producing the classic findings of inflammation, pain, swelling, heat, and erythema. Patients complain of prolonged morning stiffness and generalized symptoms of fatigue and low-grade fever. At times, vasculitis and involvement of lungs, eyes, and other organs emphasize the systemic nature of the disease. Laboratory studies reveal elevated acute-phase reactants such as the sedimentation rate or CRP; rheumatoid factor is commonly found in patients with RA, but it is also present in patients with other connective tissue diseases, with liver function abnormalities, and with aging per se. Antibodies to cyclic citrullinated peptide antibody tend to be more specific for RA than rheumatoid factor, but many patients without RA may also be positive.

Rheumatoid inflammation, over time, leads to the growth of pannus, a destructive immune/inflammatory tissue within affected joints. The release of damaging enzymes and cytokines by infiltrating lymphocytes and macrophages leads to loss of cartilage and bony erosion. Joint limitation, instability, and functional impairment are the end result.

Management of rheumatoid arthritis. Enormous advances in the treatment of RA have made it possible to prevent this progression and make early diagnosis and aggressive treatment vital.[274] Although NSAIDs and low-dose corticosteroids can provide symptomatic improvement, disease-modifying antirheumatic drugs such as low-dose methotrexate and leflunomide have been proven to prevent cartilage and bone damage as well as control clinical manifestations. Modern biologic agents have become available; these tend to be composed of large complex proteins that are generated by biotechnology methods and include the tumor necrosis factor-α inhibiting agents as well as inhibitors of interleukins and of other aspects of the immune response. These agents have transformed the treatment of RA, and it is rare to see the advanced joint deformities that were so common 30 years ago.

Gout and pseudogout

The crystal deposition diseases represent a category of inflammatory arthritis whereby crystals precipitated in the joint capsule induce an immune response that results in joint swelling and acute pain; fever may accompany these attacks, which may be confused with an infectious source. The 2 common forms of this disease, gout and pseudogout, each occur in middle-aged and aging women.[275]

Gout. Gout is caused by excessively high serum uric acid levels and by the subsequent precipitation of monosodium urate crystals in the joints and other tissues. Although it is predominant in men during early life, it has significant prevalence among postmenopausal women. In that demographic, it is commonly associated with hypertension, diuretic use, and kidney disease, as well as with the metabolic syndrome and obesity. Acute gouty attacks are thought to be related to the inflammatory response elicited by the precipitation of the monosodium urate crystals in the synovial fluid of joints and may occur spontaneously or be triggered by any changes in health status, such as minor trauma or acute infections, or by alcohol ingestion. In addition, dose alterations of medications that influence serum uric acid levels, such as diuretics and aspirin, can trigger gouty attacks.

The diagnosis of acute gout is confirmed by detecting monosodium urate crystals in synovial fluid obtained from an involved joint, typically using polarizing microscopy. Classically, acute gout involves the base of the great toe, but any joint can be involved, and often multiple joints are affected simultaneously. These episodes are characterized by abrupt onset of severe pain, redness, and swelling of the involved joints. The pain is sufficiently severe that often patients do not tolerate even the weight of a bed sheet on involved toes. Chronic gout can lead to deposition of crystals in tissues other than the joints; when this happens, the resulting masses are called tophi and may be present in the skin or in any other tissue.

Management of gout. Acute attacks may be aborted if treated early with colchicine or with high doses of NSAIDs, if tolerated. After an attack is fully established, treatment with NSAIDs is effective, although many gout patients cannot tolerate this class of medication because of renal, cardiac, or GI concerns. In those patients, either intra-articular or systemic corticosteroid treatment is highly effective; typically oral prednisone or prednisolone is employed. In rare cases when corticosteroids are insufficient, inhibition of interleukin-1 with monoclonal antibodies has been shown to be useful. Chronic gout that is complicated by tophi or by frequent disabling attacks should be treated with long-term medication using agents that lower the serum uric acid level; these include allopurinol, febuxistat, uricosuric agents, and pharmaceutical uricase, the enzyme that degrades uric acid. With normalization of serum uric acid concentrations, tophi will resorb over time.

Pseudogout. Calcium pyrophosphate dihydrate deposition is a common feature of aging joints and may be detected by radiography as *chondrocalcinosis*. Occasionally, these crystals trigger an inflammatory response similar to that seen in gout and may cause a syndrome that is clinically indistinguishable from true gout, *pseudogout*. The diagnosis can only be made definitively by detecting calcium pyrophosphate dihydrate crystals by microscopy. Pseudogout occurs most commonly among middle-aged and elderly patients with evidence of some degenerative changes in the affected joints. Like gout, it may occur spontaneously or be triggered by trauma or changes in systemic medical conditions. Unlike gout, it most commonly involves the large joints such as the knees; nonetheless, any joint may be affected by acute pseudogout.

Management of pseudogout. Acute pseudogout attacks are managed in a manner similar to gout. High-dose NSAIDs are effective, if tolerated. In cases where NSAIDs are not practical, intra-articular or systemic corticosteroids are effective. Unlike gout, there are no effective strategies that result in crystal resorption. For patients with frequent attacks, prophylactic use of colchicine has been tried, as have long-term NSAIDs.

Arthralgias

The sensation of pain around one or more joints is exceptionally common and usually is self-limited and does not bring a patient into contact with a physician. Perhaps the commonest cause of acute arthralgias is viral infection. Infection with parvovirus B19, the agent of the childhood exanthema erythema infectiosum, may be the etiology in a significant percentage of patients presenting with recent-onset arthralgia or arthritis. Rash may be minor or absent in adults with parvovirus infection, but arthralgias and even frank arthritis involving peripheral joints occur frequently and may mimic early RA. Viral serologies confirm the diagnosis. Other viral sources, including common cold viruses as well as uncommon viruses, may cause arthralgias but usually in association with unambiguous viral syndromes, and the arthralgias are typically self-limited and resolve with treatment of the acute viral syndrome.

Arthralgias and arthritis are often seen in the prodrome of hepatitis B infection. In this stage, a significant immune response is being mounted against the virus, leading to large-scale production of circulating immune complexes. Deposition of these complexes within the synovium produces an intense response with severe polyarthralgias and frank arthritis. Rash (frequently urticarial) and fever are often observed in association with the joint symptoms. This systemic serum sickness-type prodrome resolves as the hepatitis becomes more obvious.

Fibromyalgia syndrome. Among the most common sources of chronic arthralgia and myalgia in adult women is fibromyalgia, or *myofascial pain syndrome*. The cause of this condition is not yet understood, but it appears to be noninflammatory and to involve heightened pain sensitivity. Pain tends to be primarily axial, with diffuse aching in the neck, shoulders, back, and pelvis. There is no joint swelling or synovitis, and muscle strength is normal. The key finding is the presence of characteristic tender points, although patients with fibromyalgia tend to display heightened pain sensitivity diffusely as well. Arthralgias and myalgias in these patients are typically accompanied by other subjective symptoms of poor sleep, chronic fatigue, headache, and irritable bowel and bladder. It is likely that there is a common pathogenesis to these manifestations.

Treatment of fibromyalgia is often unsatisfying. Patient education and institution of an aerobic conditioning program can be helpful. Minor analgesics and anti-inflammatory medications such as ibuprofen can also provide modest relief. Interestingly, opiates have been found to be ineffective in the treatment of this form of pain. Consistent with the concept that the pain of fibromyalgia is related to neurologic mechanisms, the medications that have been approved by FDA for treatment of fibromyalgia are each neuroactive drugs—pregabalin, duloxetine, and milnacipran—although a variety of other medications have been found to be effective and are commonly employed, especially the tricyclic antidepressants as well as the later-generation antidepressants.

Thyroid disease

Thyroid disorders are common in women, increasing in prevalence with age. In a subset of more than 3,000 multiethnic women aged 42 to 52 years participating in SWAN, approximately 1 in 10 women had evidence of thyroid dysfunction—a TSH level outside of the normal range (two-thirds were higher than normal, and one-third was below normal).[276] In NHANES III, the percentage of women with evidence of thyroid antibodies, a harbinger of autoimmune thyroid dysfunction, increased from 15.8% in 40- to 49-year-olds to 26.5% in those aged older than 80 years.[277] Symptoms of thyroid dysfunction (altered menstrual cycle length, change in amount of bleeding, sleep disruption, fatigue, mood swings, forgetfulness, heat intolerance, palpitations) can be confused with symptoms common to the menopause transition.

The primary function of the thyroid is to regulate metabolism. Thyroid hormone is synthesized when the thyroid gland extracts iodine from the circulation, combines it with the amino acid tyrosine, and converts it to the thyroid hormones triiodothyronine (T_3) and thyroxine (T_4). The thyroid gland stores thyroid hormone until it is released into the bloodstream. Most thyroid hormones circulate bound to proteins. Thyroid hormones affect the liver, muscle, heart, bone, and central nervous system. Thyroid-stimulating hormone secreted by the pituitary gland reflects circulating thyroid hormone concentration and, via a negative feedback loop, regulates thyroid hormone release.

Screening

Recommendations for screening for thyroid disease vary. The American Thyroid Association (ATA) recommends screening all adults beginning at age 35 and every 5 years thereafter, whereas the USPSTF concluded that the evidence is insufficient to recommend for or against routine screening for thyroid disease in adults.[278,279] The Canadian Task Force on the Periodic Health Examination recommends maintaining a high index of clinical suspicion for nonspecific symptoms consistent with hypothyroidism when examining perimenopausal and postmenopausal women.[280] The AACE recommends screening older patients (age not specified), especially women; the American College of Physicians suggests that women aged 50 years and older with an incidental finding suggestive of symptomatic thyroid disease should be evaluated.[281] Other than the ATA recommendations, intervals for screening are not specified.

Hypothyroidism

Hypothyroidism, most often caused by Hashimoto thyroiditis, is the most common thyroid disorder in women,

DISEASE RISK

occurring 7 times more often in women than men, with an increased incidence in midlife.[282] A woman with hypothyroidism may complain of fatigue, dry skin, leg cramps, and heavier, longer menstrual cycles. The risk of hypothyroidism increases if a woman has a family history of thyroid disorders, experienced postpartum thyroiditis, received radioactive iodine treatment for Graves disease or multinodular goiter, or reports a history of type 2 DM, polycystic ovarian syndrome, or other endocrine/autoimmune disorders.

The serum TSH determination is the gold standard to detect hypothyroidism.[283] The normal range is defined as 0.4 mIU/L to 4.5 mIU/L, although some experts propose reducing the upper limit of normal. If the TSH level is elevated, free T_4 and antithyroperoxidase antibodies should be measured; a low free T_4 value confirms the diagnosis of overt hypothyroidism. A high TSH value with elevated free T_4 may be suggestive of a rare TSH-producing pituitary adenoma but more likely may confirm that a patient may have taken extra thyroid hormone before her appointment. If the patient has symptoms of hypothyroidism, low free T_4 and low TSH, the possibility of central hypothyroidism arises, and an evaluation of the pituitary and hypothalamus is indicated.[284] Slight elevations in TSH with normal free T_4, especially in older persons, could be consistent with subclinical hypothyroidism, often reported to increase with age. The presence of antithyroperoxidase antibodies in patients with subclinical hypothyroidism predicts progression to overt hypothyroidism.[281] Alternatively, the increased incidence of TSH elevation might simply represent a normal manifestation of the aging hypothalamic pituitary-thyroid axis.[285] Age-stratified norms have yet to be formally established.[281]

Patients with overt hypothyroidism merit replacement T_4 therapy.[281] The usual replacement dose of synthetic T_4 (levothyroxine) averages 1.6 μg per kg of body weight per day. Therapy should be initiated at 50 μg to 100 μg per day. In patients aged older than 50 years without CHD, start at the lower dose. Among patients with known CHD, the starting dose is 12.5 μg to 25 μg per day. Titrate at 6- to 8-week intervals by 12.5 μg to 25 μg, depending on the TSH levels. Titrate more gingerly in an older patient or one who may be at substantial risk for CHD. In treated patients, the target for TSH is within the normal range.

Once the replacement dose is established, monitor TSH values every 6 to 12 months. If the patient changes thyroid hormone preparations (eg, insurance or pharmacy change), recheck the TSH after 6 to 8 weeks. Because concurrent administration of T_4 with food, vitamins, calcium, and iron may significantly interfere with absorption, patients should take T_4 separately. Compliance may be enhanced by recommending that T_4 be taken with water 30 to 60 minutes before breakfast; alternatively, some patients prefer taking T_4 3 to 4 hours after the last meal of the day.

Role of estrogen therapy. If the patient receiving thyroid hormone starts oral ET, monitor TSH levels 6 to 8 weeks later. Anticipate that the dose of T_4 may need to be increased. Oral (but not transdermal) estrogens increase thyroid-binding globulin, which in turn reduces the free T_4 values; androgen therapy manifests the opposite effect.[286,287] A normally functioning thyroid gland compensates by increasing thyroid hormone production to maintain free T_4, but a hypothyroid gland with compromised thyroid reserve cannot. Conversely, when HT is discontinued, monitor thyroid function again 6 to 8 weeks later. The dose of T_4 may need to be reduced. Case reports suggest that an increase in the dose of T_4 might be necessary when raloxifene or soy supplements are initiated in hypothyroid women.

Subclinical hypothyroidism. A healthy, asymptomatic woman with no history or signs of thyroid disease with an elevated TSH level in the presence of normal thyroid hormone concentrations might qualify for a diagnosis of *subclinical hypothyroidism*. The prevalence of subclinical hypothyroidism is between 4% and 8.5%, increasing to 15% in elderly populations.[288] Before making the diagnosis, repeat the TSH test after 3 to 6 months to confirm. Up to 60% of cases will regress to euthyroidism over 5 years, whereas 1% to 5% of cases per year, perhaps more in those with positive thyroperoxidase antibodies, will become frankly hypothyroid.[282]

Some, but not all, observational studies link subclinical hypothyroidism with an increased risk for CHD, HF, and mortality.[283] These events may depend on the age of the patient as well as the relative degree of thyroid failure. In one analysis, even persons whose TSH level was on the high side of the normal range had subtle increases in BP and lipid levels.[288] Paradoxically, cardiovascular events and mortality appear to be increased more often in persons aged younger than 65 to 70 years with subclinical hypothyroidism rather than in the elderly.[281,282,285,289,290] In a nested case-cohort design in the WHI observational study, subclinical hypothyroidism was not associated with increased risk of MI. Hazard ratios for MI by age showed an elevation in risk in women aged 50 to 64 years compared with older women with subclinical hypothyroidism, although the CIs were wide, and the differences were not statistically significant.[291] In an evaluation from the 55,000-participant Thyroid Studies Collaboration, subclinical hypothyroidism was associated with a 2-fold increase in CHD events and mortality but only if the TSH level was higher than 10 mIU/L.[292]

Whether a midlife woman with subclinical hypothyroidism should be treated is a hotly debated topic and one on which the experts do not necessarily agree. In the absence of clinical trial evidence substantiating improved clinical outcomes, recommendations for replacement therapy are largely based on observational studies and expert opinion.[281-283,288] In an analysis from the UK General Practitioner Research Database, treatment of subclinical hypothyroidism in patients with TSH levels of 5 mIU/L to 10 mIU/L was associated with fewer CHD events in younger patients (40-70 y), but similar benefit was not seen for persons aged older than 70 years.[293]

In AACE/ATA guidelines, an individualized approach to treatment is recommended.[281] Treatment should be considered for patients whose TSH level falls between the upper limit of normal and 10 mIU/L and who have symptoms of hypothyroidism (dry skin, cold sensitivity, fatigue, muscle cramps, voice changes, constipation), positive thyroperoxidase antibodies, or evidence of atherosclerotic CVD, HF, or associated risk factors. Treatment is also recommended for patients with TSH levels more than 10 mIU/L.[281-283] Patients with subclinical hypothyroidism do not necessarily require full replacement doses; treatment with 25 μg to 75 μg of T$_4$ daily usually suffices in normalizing thyroid status and might reduce the likelihood of overtreating and inducing subclinical hyperthyroidism.[281,288]

Hyperthyroidism
Symptoms of hyperthyroidism—anxiety, palpitations, lighter and less frequent menses, and heat intolerance—also mimic the menopause transition. Hyperthyroidism occurs less frequently than hypothyroidism.[294] The most common etiologies include Graves disease, toxic multinodular goiter, and solitary hyperfunctioning adenoma.

The initial diagnostic test of choice for hyperthyroidism remains the TSH level. If the TSH value is suppressed, free T$_4$ should be measured to assess the degree of thyroid hormone excess. If free T$_4$ is normal, total T$_3$ should also be measured and, if elevated, might point to the presence of an autonomously functioning thyroid nodule. When free T$_4$ level is above the normal range, a radioactive iodine uptake scan can distinguish the cause of thyroid hormone excess and define thyroid anatomy.

Markedly increased uptake in a homogenous distribution is consistent with Graves disease, whereas a heterogeneous distribution is consistent with multinodular goiter. A solitary "hot" nodule may be responsible for hyperthyroidism, especially if the T$_3$ is elevated. A lack of uptake points to the diagnosis of thyroiditis, either Hashimoto autoimmune thyroiditis or glandular destruction caused by a viral infection.

Management of hyperthyroidism. Most women who have hyperthyroidism should be referred to an endocrinologist for consultation. The diagnosis should be confirmed, and the patient begun on therapy with long-term monitoring. Initial therapy often includes beta-blockers for symptomatic relief and, if the diagnosis is Graves disease or multinodular goiter, concurrent antithyroid drugs (methimazole). Radioactive iodine thyroid ablation is the most definitive nonsurgical therapy for Graves disease and toxic multinodular goiter, but it is used less often for treatment of Graves disease because it can result in permanent thyroid destruction and the requirement of lifelong thyroid hormone replacement.[295]

Subclinical hyperthyroidism. If the TSH level falls below the normal range in the presence of normal thyroid hormone levels, the patient might meet criteria for the diagnosis of *subclinical hyperthyroidism*. Concerns with subclinical hyperthyroidism include increased osteoporosis risk and fracture, atrial fibrillation, HF, and possibly increased CHD and CHD mortality, especially in patients of advanced age.[282,296]

Subclinical hyperthyroidism occurs in less than 2% of the population, with the mild form being more common.[282] Suppressed TSH can be related to severe nonthyroidal illness, as well as to advanced age and to black race, because of changes in the hypothalamic-pituitary set point. It is therefore reasonable to monitor an asymptomatic, healthy woman over 3 to 6 months to document persistence of these findings. If the TSH remains below the normal range with normal thyroid hormone concentrations, particularly if suppressed to less than 0.1 mIU/L, the specific thyroid disorder should be determined. The most common cause of subclinical hyperthyroidism is toxic multinodular goiter, followed by Graves disease and solitary autonomous nodules.[294]

The 2011 AACE/ATA guidelines recommend treatments similar to those for overt hyperthyroidism if the TSH level is persistently less than 0.1 mIU/L in persons aged 65 years and older, in postmenopausal women not taking estrogen or bisphosphonates (and therefore at risk of accelerated bone loss), and in persons aged younger than 65 years with heart disease, osteoporosis, or persistent hyperthyroid symptoms.[294] Treatment can also be considered if TSH values fall between 0.1 mIU/L and 0.4 mIU/L in persons aged older than 65 years and in those aged 65 years and younger with heart disease, who are postmenopausal, or with hyperthyroid symptoms. With treatment, hypothyroidism may result, and ultimately, thyroid replacement therapy could be required.

Bone effects. In the Study of Osteoporotic Fractures, use of thyroid hormone itself did not increase risk of fracture if the TSH level was maintained in the normal range.[297] However, in women aged older than 65 years, suppressed TSH levels (<0.1 mIU/L), either as a result of excess endogenous thyroid hormone production or exogenous thyroid hormone use, were associated with a 3-fold increase in hip fractures and a 4-fold increase in vertebral fractures. As assessed by TSH measurements, approximately 20% of patients receiving T$_4$ therapy may be overtreated.[298] Bone mineral density should be measured, preferably at a cortical site such as the hip, in women with a long history of T$_4$ therapy; doses used in the past were often higher than what is now recommended.[299]

Thyroid nodules
A thyroid nodule is a discrete lesion within the thyroid gland that is radiologically distinct from the surrounding thyroid parenchyma.[300] Thyroid nodules are palpable in about 5% of women. Ultrasound examination of asymptomatic patients suggests that thyroid nodules occur in as many as 19% to

67% of the US population. Most of the nodules are benign, but 5% to 15% harbor thyroid cancers. Thyroid cancer is diagnosed in women 3 times more often than in men, with peak incidence occurring between ages 40 and 50 years. The risk of thyroid cancer increases with age, a history of radiation exposure, a family history of thyroid cancer, rapid growth of the nodule, and hoarseness.

The ATA updated its guidelines for evaluation and management of thyroid nodules and thyroid cancers in 2009; the AACE, along with Mexican and European experts, updated its recommendations in 2010.[300,301] If a thyroid nodule is detected on physical examination, the TSH level should be measured. If the TSH level is low, a radionucleotide thyroid scan should be obtained to determine the functional status of the nodule. Hyperfunctioning hot nodules are rarely malignant; therapy for hyperthyroidism should be considered. Although the ATA recommended in 2009 that aspiration of a hot nodule is not required,[300] a 2013 review reported an estimated 3.1% prevalence of malignancy in hyperfunctioning thyroid nodules.[302] Depending on the clinical situation, a lower threshold for aspirating autonomously functioning nodules might be prudent.

If the TSH value is normal or elevated in a patient with a thyroid nodule, the next step is a diagnostic thyroid ultrasound to define the anatomy of the gland, accurately measure the diameter of the nodule(s), and ascertain clinical features of the nodule(s), all important parameters for management decisions. If ultrasound confirms the presence of a nodule, the patient should be referred to an endocrinologist for fine-needle aspiration.

Management. The cytology of the cellular aspirate, in conjunction with the medical history, clinical findings, and ultrasound characteristics, will dictate further management. Most benign nodules can be monitored with serial annual ultrasounds, and depending on whether the nodule has grown, a repeat fine-needle aspiration may be indicated.

Epilepsy

Epilepsy is a chronic neurologic disorder that is characterized by recurrent seizures. The prevalence of epilepsy is about 1% in the general population. It increases to 3% in the elderly aged older than 75 years, likely as a result of the increased incidence of stroke and Alzheimer disease.[303]

In most women with epilepsy, seizures do not occur randomly. Instead, in more than 50% of cases, they tend to cluster. Seizure clusters, in turn, may occur with temporal rhythmicity in a significant proportion of women (35%) and men (29%).[304]

Role of ovarian hormones
In women, the temporal rhythmicity of seizure clusters may align with that of the menstrual cycle, in which case it is known as catamenial epilepsy. This catamenial predilection is attributable to the neuroactive properties of reproductive hormones and the cyclic variation of their serum levels.[304]

Estrogen generally has neuroexcitatory (glutamatergic) properties that can promote seizure occurrence. Progesterone, in contrast, has reduced metabolites, such as allopregnanolone, that have potent antiseizure (GABAergic) effects.[305] Midcycle elevations in estrogen and premenstrual withdrawal of progesterone are triggers for seizures in about one-third of women with epilepsy.[304]

Statistical evidence supports the concept of catamenial epilepsy and the existence of at least 3 distinct patterns of seizure exacerbation in relation to the menstrual cycle: 1) perimenstrual, 2) preovulatory patterns in women with ovulatory cycles, and 3) entire luteal-phase and perimenstrual-phase pattern in women with anovulatory or inadequate luteal phase cycles.[304] Inadequate luteal-phase cycles are more common among women with epilepsy than in the general population. This may result from epilepsy-related disruption of pulsatile gonadotropin secretion, ovulation, and luteal progesterone production.[306,307]

Menopause occurs a few years earlier in women with epilepsy than in the general population, especially in women with a high lifetime seizure frequency and with polytherapy using enzyme-inducing antiepileptic drugs.[308,309]

Perimenopause is sometimes associated with increased seizure frequency, which is more pronounced in women who have shown previous evidence of hormonal sensitivity in the form of catamenial seizure exacerbation.[310] Perimenopausal seizure exacerbation may relate to unopposed estrogen effects that accompany the greater frequency of anovulatory cycles during this transition.

Role of hormone therapy
Progesterone therapy may benefit some women with catamenial epilepsy. Two open-label trials have shown that cyclic, oral progesterone supplementation at physiologic-range levels during the luteal phase of each cycle may be associated with substantially and significantly lower seizure frequencies than optimal antiepileptic drug therapy alone. In contrast, oral progestogens alone, administered cyclically or continuously, have not proven to be an effective therapy.

A National Institutes of Health (NIH)-sponsored randomized, double-blind, multicenter investigation has shown that adjunctive cyclic natural progesterone supplement is not superior to placebo overall in the treatment of women with epilepsy but did show a clinically important and statistically significantly greater responder rate in patients who demonstrated perimenstrual seizure exacerbation in the baseline phase ($P=.0372$).[311] The responder rate correlated significantly with the level of catameniality for women treated with progesterone but not placebo.

The effects of menopausal HT on epilepsy have not been rigorously assessed, although estrogen has demonstrated epileptogenic effects in women with epilepsy who do not

CHAPTER 4

have an intact uterus. A small, randomized, double-blind, placebo-controlled multicenter NIH investigation did show that treatment of postmenopausal women with epilepsy using EPT was associated with a significant increase in the frequency of the most severe seizure type during the 3-month treatment phase compared with the 3-month baseline phase.[312] The increase in seizure frequency correlated with the dosage of EPT.

Antiepileptic drug interaction effects with HT have not been established, but they may be similar to the effects on OCs.[313] Enzyme-inducing antiepileptic drugs can make OCs less effective, reducing steroid concentrations in OC users by up to 50%.[314] These include drugs that induce cytochrome P450 isoenzyme 3A4 such that there is accelerated hepatic metabolism of hormone preparations resulting in a decrease in biologically active sex steroids in serum (carbamazepine, oxcarbazepine, phenobarbital, phenytoin, primidone, topiramate). Antiepileptic medications that do not seem to interfere, or interfere minimally, with the effectiveness of OCs include gabapentin, lamotrigine, levetiracetam, tiagabine, and the infrequently used felbamate. However, lamotrigine and (somewhat less so) valproate levels drop markedly, from as much as 20% to more than 50%, on the active OCs and recover within days on the inactive tablets.[313,315] A comparable effect of HT needs to be considered but data are limited.

Management issues
In addition to the relationship between hormones and epilepsy, there are additional important issues for the menopause practitioner to consider. There is a decline in antiepileptic drug clearance and decrease in albumin levels with maturity that can affect antiepileptic drug use in the aging population. Therefore, mature patients with epilepsy need to be monitored carefully for increasing drug levels that could lead to toxicity.[316,317]

It also is important for the menopause practitioner to realize that antiepileptic drug therapy results in a significant increase in the risk of osteoporosis and fracture.[318,319] Enzyme-inducing antiepileptic drugs induce the hydrolase enzymes in the hepatic microsomal system to accelerate the conversion of vitamin D sterols to inactive polar metabolites. They also reduce levels of 1,25-dihydroxycholecalciferol, the vitamin D metabolite needed for transport of calcium from the intestine into the bloodstream and for bone formation. The precise magnitude of osteoporosis risk, however, is difficult to establish because of the frequent coexistence of other risk factors, such as lack of ambulation, falls, and inadequate sunlight exposure. The use of vitamin D and calcium supplements, as well as bone absorption inhibitors, may be particularly important in women with epilepsy, especially those who take or have taken enzyme-inducing antiepileptic drugs.[303,318-320]

Some studies have found that the antiseizure medication gabapentin is effective in managing mild hot flashes. Incorporating gabapentin into an existing epilepsy treatment regime should involve the neurologist who is managing the epilepsy.

Asthma

The relation between sex hormones and asthma is complex. Before puberty, boys are more likely to be diagnosed with asthma than are girls, at least in part because of biologic factors.[321] After puberty, the prevalence of asthma and of severe asthma becomes higher in women. Asthma exacerbations are more likely to occur during the premenstrual or preovulatory phase of the menstrual cycle or both.[321,322] Sharp decreases in serum estradiol levels may be associated with an increased risk of asthma flares. Women also have more frequent and longer hospital admissions than men from complications of asthma throughout the rest of the life span.[323,324]

Data are conflicting regarding the relationship of asthma and menopause. Large observational studies have shown that pulmonary symptoms, including wheezing, are more prevalent after menopause, including surgical menopause.[325,326] A systematic review and meta-analysis of studies, however, found no association between asthma incidence and either the menopause transition or postmenopausal status.[327]

When it occurs, postmenopausal-onset asthma may be particularly severe.[328] Forced expiratory volume in one second is usually decreased, and the forced vital capacity is reduced. This trend exists even in women who have never smoked.[325] The association between menopause and respiratory changes is stronger in lean women than in heavier women.

Several large observational studies have shown an association between the increased risk of asthma and current use of HT, either with ET but not EPT or with ET and also EPT.[327,329,330] This association may be more prominent in lean women.[326]

Several small interventional trials performed in the early 2000s demonstrated neutral or beneficial effects from HT on the airways. A prospective, crossover study of women with asthma (N=20) who were at least 2 years postmenopausal found that neither discontinuing nor reinitiating HT had any effect on objective measures of airway function.[331] However, women with corticosteroid-dependent asthma, those aged older than 70 years, and smokers were not included in the study. The researchers concluded that until data to the contrary are available, HT should not be withheld from postmenopausal women because of concerns about detrimental effects on asthma.

A nonrandomized study of asthmatic (n=55) and healthy (n=20) postmenopausal women aged 48 to 60 years measuring endocrine and spirometric parameters before and after 6 months of transdermal 17β-estradiol and cyclic oral MPA treatment concluded that EPT use in postmenopausal women with asthma had a favorable influence on the course of asthma.[332] Estrogen-progestogen therapy was found to reduce daily use of glucocorticoids and frequency of asthma exacerbations. It may relax the bronchial smooth muscle and may be associated with higher forced expiratory volume in 1 second.

Adequately sized RCTs are needed to evaluate the effects of ET and EPT on the course of asthma to help resolve the contradictions in the literature between the findings in large observational and small interventional studies.

Cancer

Cancer continues to be the first and second leading causes of death for US and Canadian women, respectively.[333,334] In 2013, approximately 805,500 US women will be diagnosed with cancer, and 273,431 will die from their disease.[335] During the same time period, 91,400 Canadian women will be diagnosed with cancer, and 36,100 will die from their disease.[336] Estimated 2013 cancer statistics indicate that although breast cancer affects more women, a greater number continue to die of lung cancer (Table 12).[336-338]

There are specific modifiable and nonmodifiable risk factors for cancer in general:

- *Age* is a key risk factor. The incidence of cancer increases with age. Approximately 77% of all cancers are diagnosed in persons aged 55 years and older.[336] Following approved age-related guidelines for cancer prevention and screening is critical in the care of our patients, particularly postmenopausal women.

- *Obesity* places women at higher risk for several specific types of malignancies. In a prospectively studied population of more than 900,000 US adults (404,576 men and 495,477 women), increased body weight alone was associated with increased mortality for all cancers combined.[339] The metabolic dysregulation associated with obesity is often manifested in metabolic syndrome, an established risk factor for many cancers. Cancer risk and progression, within the proinflammatory environment of the obese state, may be enhanced by a variety of mechanisms, including cross talk among macrophages, adipocytes, and epithelial cells that occurs via obesity-associated hormones, cytokines, and other mediators.[340]

- *Socioeconomic status* in the United States and Canada has been linked to cancer care. A review of Canadian literature demonstrates that income has the most consistent effect on access to cancer screening.[341]

- *Race* alone alters various cancer incidence and mortality rates, as has been shown in multiple studies. In the United States, blacks develop cancer at a much higher rate than any other racial or ethnic group.[342]

- *Alcohol consumption* is a major contributor to cancer mortality and years of potential life lost. Higher consumption increases risk, and there is no safe threshold with respect to cancer risk.[343]

- *Exercise* has been shown in population-wide studies to decrease cancer incidence. The amount and intensity of exercise required to measure a survival benefit appear to vary by primary tumor type.[344]

- *Specific nutritional* considerations play a role in several types of cancers, but nutrition as it relates to obesity is of utmost importance.

- *A family history* of breast or ovarian cancer is common in women diagnosed with these cancers. For women with a family history of breast cancer, the lifetime risk of breast cancer is twice as high as that of the general population.[345] However, less than 10% of all breast cancers and less than 15% of ovarian cancers are associated with known inherited genetic mutations such as *BRCA1* and *BRCA2*, suggesting that environmental factors or genetic variation play a role.[346,347] Women with Lynch syndrome are at increased risk of colon, endometrial, and ovarian cancer.[348]

Breast Cancer

Breast cancer is the most common cancer diagnosed in US women.[349] Many of the known breast cancer risk factors,

Table 12. Estimated New Cancer Cases and Cancer Deaths in Women, 2013

	United States		Canada	
Site	Estimated new cases	Estimated deaths	Estimated new cases	Estimated deaths
Breast	232,340	39,620	23,855	5,018
Lung	110,110	72,220	12,156	9,494
Colon	52,390	24,530	10,602	4,188
Endometrium	49,560	8,190	5,575	902
Thyroid	45,310	1,040	4,387	NA
Skin (melanoma)	31,630	3,200	2,742	397
Pancreas	22,480	18,980	2,376	2,166
Ovary	22,240	14,030	2,650	1,697
Kidney	24,720	4,900	2,285	650
Bladder	17,960	4,390	2,010	614
Cervix	12,340	4,030	1,462	361
Vulva	4,700	990	NA	NA
Vagina	2,890	840	NA	NA
TOTAL	805,500	273,431	91,400	36,100

Canadian Cancer Society's Advisory Committee on Cancer Statistics,[336] Centers for Disease Control and Prevention,[333] American Cancer Society.[335]

such as race, age, family history, early menarche, and late menopause, are not modifiable. Modifiable factors, which increase the risk of developing breast cancer, include postmenopausal obesity, menopausal HT, alcohol consumption, and physical inactivity. Screening remains important, but the appropriate time interval is still under debate. For many women, breast cancer is their primary health concern. Breast cancer is the second major cause of cancer mortality in US and Canadian women.[350,351]

Incidence. The incidence of breast cancer in the United States has been rising since the early 1930s.[352] A significant decline in breast cancer incidence occurred in 2003 and 2004 and then leveled off through 2006.[352-355] A US woman's lifetime risk of developing breast cancer is approximately 1 in 8.

Nearly one-half of all breast cancer cases occur in women aged 65 years and older. Less than 10% of breast cancers occur in US women aged younger than 40 years, and approximately 15% occur in women aged younger than 50 years. Estimates are that by age 50, 2% of US women will have developed breast cancer. By age 60, between 4% and 5% will have the disease; by age 70, approximately 7%; and by age 80, between 9% and 10%.[356] Contralateral breast cancer in women with a personal history of breast cancer is estimated to occur at a rate of 0.5% to 1% per year after the initial diagnosis.

Among US racial and cultural groups, white, non-Hispanic women have the highest incidence of breast cancer, although black women have the highest mortality from the disease, possibly related to later stages of diagnosis, more ER-negative tumors, and more aggressive tumors.[350,353,357] The 5-year survival rate for blacks is 71% versus 86% for whites.

Although the incidence of breast cancer has increased, mortality rates have decreased, perhaps because of earlier intervention.[350] Smaller, less-advanced tumors that would have been missed without mammography can now be detected. According to US statistics, if breast cancer is detected while it is still localized, the 5-year survival rate is 99%, up from 72% in the 1940s. For regional metastases, however, the rate is 84%. For distant metastases, the rate is 24%. Survival at 10 years is also stage dependent.[358]

The Canadian Cancer Society estimates the lifetime risk of breast cancer in Canadian women to be 1 in 9, with a corresponding mortality of 1 in 28.[351] In Canada, the 5-year survival rate is 86%. After 3 decades of small annual increases, breast cancer incidence in women has leveled off since 1993, and the mortality rate has declined to the lowest rate since 1950. These trends are attributed to screening programs and improved treatments.

Risk factors. Medical research has identified several potential cancer-causing genes, including *BRCA1* (linked to breast and ovarian cancers) and *BRCA2* (linked to breast cancer and postmenopausal ovarian cancer).[359] Although the genes have been identified, more research is needed to target which women to test, how to protect them from discrimination based on genetic findings, and what to do if the test results are positive.

Data regarding the importance of a positive family history as a risk factor for breast cancer are not conclusive. Most breast cancers occur in women without a positive family history.

The National Cancer Institute has developed a breast cancer risk assessment tool, based on the Gail model (Table 13).[360] It assesses the 5-year risk based on 5 primary factors: a woman's age, age at first live birth, age at menarche, previous breast biopsy results, and personal or family (first-degree relatives) history of cancer. The Gail model works best in postmenopausal women with ER-positive cancers. A model with fewer variables (age, breast cancer in first-degree relatives, and previous breast biopsy) seems to offer similar results for predicting risk of ER-positive breast cancer in postmenopausal women.[361]

Mammographic breast density and circulating sex steroid hormones have been associated with an increased risk for breast cancer in premenopausal and postmenopausal women.[362-366] A prospective study within the Nurse's Health Study consisting of a subcohort of 253 postmenopausal women with no cancer history who were not taking HT on entry to the study but were diagnosed to have breast cancer within 10 years of joining the study were compared with 520 age-matched controls.[365] All the women, including controls, had baseline mammograms and blood drawn for circulating estradiol and testosterone levels. The study reported that breast density and increased circulating levels of estradiol and testosterone were strongly and independently associated with breast cancer risk. Adding breast density to quantitative models can improve discriminatory accuracy. However, sex steroid hormone assays should not be included in risk assessment because they lack standardization and are quite variable in the clinical setting.

Role of hormone therapy. Hormone therapy may stimulate the growth of benign breast masses.[367] Most studies show an association between HT and breast cancer risk,[75,368-372] and many studies report a greater increase in breast cancer risk with EPT than with ET.[363,371,373]

Some data link greater occurrence of lobular breast cancers with progestogen use.[363,374-376] One observational study suggested that the type of progestogen administered with the estrogen was important inasmuch as there was no increase in breast cancer incidence noted with EPT with the use of estrogen plus progestogen (RR, 1.00) or estrogen plus dydrogesterone (RR, 1.16) versus estrogen plus other progestogens (RR, 1.69).[377] A report of a cohort of women in the Nurses' Health Study also suggested an increased risk with estrogen plus testosterone compared with estrogen alone.[365]

DISEASE RISK

Epidemiologic data suggest an association between the timing of menopause and breast cancer risk. The data have shown that early menopause is associated with decreased risk, and delayed menopause is associated with an increased risk. A trial examining the "gap" hypothesis of breast cancer found that women who started HT less than 5 years from menopause were more likely to be diagnosed with breast cancer than those who started treatment more than 5 years afterward.[378]

Based on the results from large randomized and observational trials, breast cancer risk is increased with use of EPT beyond 3 to 5 years (Table 14).[65] In the WHI, 8 additional invasive cancers per 10,000 person-years occurred in the group receiving EPT.[75] There was no increase in breast cancer risk in ET users versus placebo after 7.1 years of use and a decrease in breast cancer risk in a 10.7-year follow-up.[379] There are limited observational studies suggesting that using ET for more than 15 years may increase the risk of breast cancer. Lower doses of HT have not been tested in long-term trials.[356]

It is recommended that all women have a breast examination and mammogram before beginning HT if they have not had one in the past 12 months and at regular intervals thereafter.

Role of oral contraceptives. The use of OCs and risk of breast cancer has been reported in 2 population-based, case-control studies, the Cancer and Steroid Hormone Study and the Women's Contraceptive and Reproductive Experiences Study.[380] Both studies provided strong evidence that OCs do not increase a woman's risk of developing breast cancer. An update of the Cancer and Steroid Hormone Study demonstrated no difference in breast cancer or overall mortality for OC users compared with nonusers on the basis of duration of OC use, time since first use, time since last use, and age at first use. There was no association identified for survival based on specific pill formulations. It should be noted that WHO does not recommend OC use in women known to have breast cancer.[1] Results of OC breast cancer studies vary and are influenced by current-use or ever-use analyses. Studies that focus on current use of OCs tend to report an increased risk of breast cancer that dissipates 5 to 10 years after discontinuation.[381]

Women with a history of breast cancer. The number of women surviving breast cancer has increased because of earlier detection through widespread application of mammographic screening and the efficacy of adjuvant systemic therapies. For women in remission, breast cancer recurrence is a possibility.

During perimenopause or postmenopause, if breast cancer survivors need relief from menopause-related symptoms, primarily vasomotor and genitourinary symptoms, therapeutic choices must be weighed for their potential to cause breast cancer recurrence.

Table 13. Established Epidemiologic Risk Factors for Breast Cancer

- Personal history of breast, endometrial, ovarian, or (possibly) colon carcinoma
- History of breast cancer in a mother, sister, or daughter, especially while premenopausal
- History of breast cancer in a father or any male relative
- Menarche before age 12
- Late menopause (after age 55)
- Nulliparity or having a first child after age 30
- Obesity after menopause (≥20 kg [44 lb] weight gain)
- Alcohol consumption (>2 drinks/d)
- Lack of exercise (<4 h/wk)
- Low levels of vitamin D
- Diet low in vegetables and fruits
- Exposure to chest wall or nodal radiation (eg, for lymphoma or thymoma)
- Long-term use (>5 y) of estrogen-progestogen therapy

National Cancer Institute.[360]

- *Systemic hormone therapy use in women with a history of breast cancer.* Systemic HT use is generally contraindicated in women with a history of breast cancer. The rationale is that avoiding hormones will reduce the risk of recurrence and of new contralateral tumors. Also, systemic HT increases mammographic density and could potentially decrease surveillance effectiveness for new breast cancer. A breast cancer survivor experiencing debilitating menopause-related symptoms such as hot flashes and night sweats without relief from nonhormonal alternatives may elect HT after consultation with her oncologist and a thorough discussion of her individual risks and benefits.

A number of studies, mostly uncontrolled, have evaluated the effects of HT in women with a history of breast cancer.[382,383] Most, but not all, enrolled women 10 or more years after the initial breast cancer diagnosis and reported no deleterious effects on tumor recurrence. One RCT was stopped early because of a significant increase in breast cancer among women randomized to HT.[384]

A history of breast cancer is generally considered an absolute contraindication for HT use. In certain situations,

Chapter 4

Table 14. North American Menopause Society Position on Breast Cancer Risk Associated With Hormone Therapy

- Breast cancer risk is increased with EPT use beyond 3-5 years. Progestogen seems to contribute substantially to that adverse effect. EPT, and to a lesser extent ET, increase breast cell proliferation, breast pain, and mammographic density.
- EPT may impede the diagnostic interpretation of mammograms.
- The effects of HT on risk for breast cancer in symptomatic perimenopausal women have not been established in clinical trials. The findings from trials in different populations (eg, the WHI) should, therefore, be extrapolated with caution. There is, however, no evidence that symptomatic women differ from asymptomatic women in cancer outcomes.

Abbreviations: EPT, estrogen-progestogen therapy; ET, estrogen-only therapy; HT, hormone therapy; WHI, Women's Health Initiative.
North American Menopause Society.[65]

---

the therapeutic benefits of HT may outweigh its risks in women with or at high risk for breast cancer. The decision must be made with the woman's full awareness that therapy may promote more rapid tumor growth. Caution is recommended in all cases, inasmuch as there are no specific data from clinical trials regarding particular stages or histologic types of the disease to provide guidance regarding women at highest risk. Alternatives always should be tried first.

- *Cognitive dysfunction.* Women who reach menopause as a result of adjuvant therapy for breast cancer often report complaints of difficulty with thinking and memory.[385] These complaints could be the result of a direct neurotoxic effect of chemotherapy. Additional studies are needed to further define these effects. Similarly, little is known about the potential effects of tamoxifen on cognitive decline with aging.

- *Weight gain.* After breast cancer, weight gain may be precipitated by adjuvant chemotherapy, decreased exercise during treatment, or increased food intake related to depression. Overweight and obesity are important health concerns for postmenopausal breast cancer survivors (as they are for all postmenopausal women) because they increase the risk for CVD and DM. In some studies, weight gain has been associated with an increased risk of breast cancer recurrence, possibly because of higher levels of endogenous estrogen. Obesity has been statistically associated with an increased risk for second primary contralateral breast cancers.[386]

Women with benign breast disease. Women with premalignant breast disease are at increased risk for breast cancer.[387,388] Compared with women with nonproliferative benign histology, those with proliferative, nonmalignant breast disease have an increased risk for developing breast cancer (RR, 3.6 and 1.8, respectively, with and without atypical hyperplasia). Hormone therapy use has not been found to affect these risks. Women at risk for breast cancer because of family history can be referred for evaluation of genetic testing for *BRCA1* and *BRCA2*.[389-393] Ductal lavage is sometimes performed as a diagnostic modality for high-risk women.

Screening. The value of monthly self-examination in detecting breast disease of significance is controversial. Women should be encouraged to report any changes in their breasts to a clinician for evaluation. Clinical breast examinations plus mammography are recommended for breast assessment/screening. The overall sensitivity of mammography is approximately 79% but less in younger women because of increased breast density.[394] Mammogram specificity is 67%.

Clinical examination. A clinical breast examination should be performed annually (close to the scheduled mammogram). The best time for a breast examination or mammogram is immediately after menses or EPT-induced uterine bleeding. From a practical perspective, however, most clinicians do not order mammography on a timed basis.

These physical signs and symptoms should be investigated by mammography:
- Breast lump, thickening, swelling, distortion, or tenderness
- Skin irritation or dimpling
- Nipple pain, scaliness, or retraction

Mammography. Mammography is a screening tool and does not provide a specific diagnosis. The false-negative rate for screening mammography is approximately 10% to 15%. Recommendations differ on frequency of mammograms in perimenopausal and postmenopausal women (Table 15).[351,395-398]

Mammography sensitivity depends on a number of factors, including the size of the lesion, the woman's age, current use of any HT, and the extent of follow-up. The appearance of breast tissue on a mammogram changes according to its composition. Fat is radiolucent and appears dark on a mammogram, whereas stromal and epithelial tissues have greater optical density and appear light.

Increased breast density is a risk factor for breast cancer. Factors associated with a reduction in breast density include increasing age, menopause, an elevated BMI, pregnancy at an early age, and tamoxifen treatment. Factors associated with an increase in breast density include an older age at first birth and postmenopausal use of ET or EPT. Women with breast implants and those aged older than 40 years with fibrocystic changes have denser breasts, but they are not necessarily at greater risk for breast cancer.

The mammographic appearance of the breasts becomes increasingly radiolucent after menopause in response to decreased estrogen and progesterone levels. For example, 76% of women aged 75 to 79 years and not using HT have radiolucent breasts compared with 38% of women aged 25 to 29 years.

Digital mammography is similar to regular mammography. Images are digitized and can be stored on film.[399] This detection technology may improve the sensitivity of mammography in women with dense breasts, although clinical trials are needed to confirm this.

Ultrasound and ductal lavage. Ultrasound is being used more frequently to evaluate focal asymmetric densities and any palpable masses of the breast.[400] Ductal lavage is an approved, minimally invasive technique in which a small flexible catheter is inserted into a periareolar duct to collect cells for examination.[401]

Magnetic resonance imaging. Prospective trials from Europe support the use of magnetic resonance imaging (MRI) in the routine evaluation of women of reproductive age who have an inherited susceptibility to breast cancer.[402]

American Cancer Society (ACS) guidelines for women at increased risk for breast cancer suggest use of MRI as an adjunct to mammography.[402] Magnetic resonance imaging is more sensitive but less specific (more false positives) in identifying mammographically occult disease in this targeted population, identified as women who have at least 1 of these conditions:

- *BRCA1* or *BRCA2* mutation
- First-degree relative (parent, sibling, child) with a *BRCA1* or *BRCA2* mutation, even if they have yet to be tested themselves
- Lifetime risk of breast cancer at 20% to 25% or greater, based on 1 of several accepted risk-assessment tools that look at family history and other factors
- Radiation to the chest when aged between 10 and 30 years
- Li-Fraumeni syndrome, Cowden syndrome, or Bannayan-Riley-Ruvalcaba syndrome or one of these syndromes in a first-degree relative

It should be noted that all studies to date have reported that the specificity for MRI in detecting breast cancer is significantly lower than that of mammography.[403] This may be acceptable to women at very high risk for breast cancer, such as women with an inherited predisposition to develop breast cancer.[404,405] Magnetic resonance imaging for women at low risk for breast cancer is inappropriate inasmuch as the technique will lead to an excessive number of recalls and biopsies for benign disease.

Lifestyle modification. All women should be assisted in modifying unhealthy lifestyle habits, some with a significant effect on breast cancer risk.

Recreational physical activity. Physical activity seems to reduce the risk of breast cancer, but more research is needed to determine the level of activity necessary.[366,406] A lifetime of physical activity may be the key. A report from the California Teachers Study evaluated recreational physical

---

Table 15. Recommendations for Mammograms in Perimenopausal and Postmenopausal Women

- *American Cancer Society*: Annual mammograms for all women beginning at age 40 in the absence of unusual findings.

- *Canadian Cancer Society*: Mammogram every 2 years for women aged between 50 and 69 years, with more frequent mammograms or more detailed testing when abnormalities are found. Women aged 70 years and older should talk to their doctors about the need for screening mammograms.

- *National Cancer Institute*: Screening mammograms every 1 to 2 years at age 40 and older.

- *National Comprehensive Cancer Network*: Screening annual mammogram for women at normal risk aged 40 years and older. An annual breast exam is also recommended.

- *US Preventive Services Task Force*: Screening mammography, with or without clinical breast examination, every 2 years for women aged 50 to 74 years. The decision to start biennial screening mammography when younger than age 50 should be an individualized one, taking into account the patient's values regarding specific benefits and harm. Insufficient evidence exists to assess the additional benefits and harm to screening mammograms in women aged 75 years and older. Recommends against teaching breast self-examinations because evidence suggests that it does not reduce breast cancer mortality. The recommendations are applicable for women who do not have an increased risk of breast cancer on the basis of an inherited genetic mutation or a history of chest radiation.

Public Health Agency of Canada[351]; American Cancer Society[395]; National Cancer Institute[396]; Bevers TB, et al[397]; US Preventive Services Task Force.[398]

activity in 3,539 breast cancer survivors.[407] Women reporting moderate to high levels of long-term physical activity had a significantly lower risk of dying from breast cancer than those with low physical activity levels. This finding was true regardless of their tumor's ER status or their cancer stage, but it was limited to women who were overweight.

Diet. Diet also affects breast cancer risk.[366,406,408,409] Consumption of well-done meats and exposure to heterocyclic amines (or other compounds) formed during high-temperature cooking may increase breast cancer risk. The evidence linking dietary fat intake to breast cancer risk has been conflicting. In the Women's Intervention Nutrition Study of 2,400 women with early stage, resected breast cancer, relapse-free and overall survivals were significantly improved in women on a low-fat diet compared with controls.[408] No improvement in survival was seen in ER-positive patients with breast cancer on the low-fat diet. The benefits accrued in patients whose cancers were ER-negative and progesterone-negative. Even after a diagnosis of breast cancer, it is important to use dietary discretion and recommend a low-fat diet. The role of isoflavones on breast cancer risk is being explored but with mixed results.

Alcohol consumption has been associated with breast cancer in many studies, although there is some evidence that excess risk from alcohol consumption may be reduced by adequate folate intake.[366,406,410] A report from the Million Women Study showed a significant increased risk for breast cancer associated with "low" alcohol ingestion (3-6 drinks/wk) and "moderate" alcohol ingestion (7-14 drinks/wk).[411] The trends were similar for those who drank wine exclusively. A long-term follow-up of the Nurses' Health Study found the highest risk of breast cancer to be in postmenopausal women who consumed alcohol and used HT (RR, 1.99; 95% CI, 1.42-2.79).[412]

A meta-analysis of 63 observational studies found a protective relationship between sufficient vitamin D status and lower risk of cancer.[413] However, use of higher doses has been associated with invasive breast cancers.[414]

Weight management. Managing one's weight is also important. One report found that avoiding adult weight gain may contribute to the prevention of breast cancer after menopause, particularly among women who do not use HT.[415] A positive association between adiposity and breast cancer risk has been documented.[366,416] Breast cancer risk may be influenced by the local breast conversion of circulating androgens via aromatization to estrogen.[417]

Pharmacologic interventions. Various prescription options are available. Selective ER modulators (SERMs), also known as estrogen agonists/antagonists, have now moved into the clinical realm for the primary reduction of breast cancer risk.

- *Tamoxifen*, the first clinically significant SERM, was noted in the 1960s to prevent the initiation and promotion of rat mammary carcinogenesis. It was subsequently shown to decrease the incidence of contralateral breast cancer in postmenopausal women with ER-positive breast cancers.[366] However, tamoxifen stimulated the growth of endometrial cancer.

  The National Surgical Adjuvant Breast and Bowel Project P-1 trial demonstrated that tamoxifen (20 mg/d) reduced the risk of breast cancer by 50% in women at high risk for breast cancer whose Gail model scores were 1.6 or higher.[418] Two European trials support the long-term chemopreventive effect of tamoxifen on breast cancer reduction once it is discontinued, supporting the value of tamoxifen in the long-term prevention of estrogen-dependent breast cancer.[419,420]

  Tamoxifen was approved in the United States in 1999 for reduction of breast cancer incidence in high-risk women and in 2000 for reduction of risk of invasive cancer and in situ ductal carcinoma. Tamoxifen provides significant net benefit to all high-risk premenopausal women (with no increased risk of uterine malignancy or clotting) and substantial net benefit to postmenopausal women whose Gail scores are more than 3.0% in 5 years, who have atypical ductal or lobular hyperplasia, and women with lobular carcinoma in situ.[421] In 2002, labeling was revised to include a black box warning for uterine malignancies, stroke, and pulmonary embolism. Use of the drug has been limited because reports indicate that many high-risk women have been unwilling to accept the potential risks of therapy. Generic tamoxifen is available in the United States and Canada.

  In Canada and the United States, tamoxifen is indicated for the adjuvant treatment of early breast cancer in women with ER-positive tumors and for the treatment of women with hormone-responsive breast cancer that is locally advanced or metastatic. Tamoxifen does not have an indication for the prevention of breast cancer in high-risk Canadian women. Although tamoxifen requires metabolism to its active form by CYP2D6, measurement of this enzyme is not required in women taking tamoxifen for either treatment of breast cancer or for primary breast cancer risk reduction.[422]

- *Raloxifene*, another clinically effective SERM, is government approved in the United States for the prevention and treatment of osteoporosis and in Canada for the treatment of osteoporosis. The MORE trial and its extension through 8 years, the Continuing Outcomes Relative to Evista trial, found that raloxifene significantly reduces the incidence of postmenopausal breast cancer compared with placebo in osteoporotic women.[423-426]

  The results of National Surgical Adjuvant Breast and Bowel Project Study of Tamoxifen and Raloxifene

P-2 trial revealed that raloxifene is equivalent to tamoxifen in reducing the incidence of invasive breast cancer in postmenopausal women at high risk for the disease.[427-429] Raloxifene reduced the risk of developing noninvasive breast cancer as well as tamoxifen.[430] The risk of clotting events was 30% lower in women taking raloxifene compared with those taking tamoxifen. Compared with women who received tamoxifen therapy, women who received raloxifene therapy had a 45% lower incidence of uterine cancer; lower risks of endometrial hyperplasia, leiomyomas, and endometrial polyps; and fewer procedures performed to evaluate the uterus. Women receiving tamoxifen therapy had more hot flashes, vaginal discharge, and vaginal bleeding compared with women taking raloxifene.[431] There was no placebo control arm in the National Surgical Adjuvant Breast and Bowel Project Study of Tamoxifen and Raloxifene P-2 trial. In the Raloxifene Use for the Heart trial, a 44% reduction in breast cancer was seen.[432]

In mid-2007, raloxifene was approved by the US government to reduce invasive breast cancer risk in postmenopausal women who had osteoporosis and in postmenopausal women at high risk for breast cancer (raloxifene has not been approved for this indication in Canada). It is not approved to treat existing breast cancer, reduce the risk of recurrent breast cancer, or reduce the risk of all forms of breast cancer.[433] A black box warning in the raloxifene labeling emphasizes that the drug is contraindicated in women with an active or past history of VTE and that women at risk for stroke should use raloxifene only after evaluating the risk-benefit ratio.[434] Expert panels in Europe and in the United States have recommended the use of tamoxifen or raloxifene in high-risk, postmenopausal women for the reduction of breast cancer risk.[435-437] There are millions of US and Canadian women who would derive significant net benefit from the use of SERMs for the reduction of their risk of breast cancer.[438]

Meta-analysis of the prospective, randomized trials of SERMs to reduce the risk of breast cancer included more than 83,000 randomly assigned participants with more than 300,000 woman-years of follow-up (median follow-up, 65 mo).[439] Overall, there was a 38% reduction in breast cancer incidence (42 women would need to be treated to prevent 1 breast cancer in the first 10 y of follow-up). The reduction was larger in the first 5 years of follow-up than in years 5 through 10. Thromboembolic events were increased with all SERMs. There was also a reduction of 34% in vertebral fractures and a small effect for nonvertebral fractures. For all SERMs, the incidence of invasive ER-positive breast cancer decreased during treatment and for at least 5 years after completion. Similar to other preventive interventions, careful consideration of risks and benefits is needed to identify women who are most likely to benefit from these drugs.

- *Aromatase inhibitors.* Aromatase inhibitors (AIs) are being evaluated as chemoprevention for women at high risk for breast cancer. These agents (anastrozole, letrozole, exemestane) lower the amount of estrogen produced outside the ovaries by inhibiting the enzyme aromatase from converting androgen into estrogen. With less estrogen in the bloodstream reaching ERs, there is less cancer cell growth. Aromatase inhibitors have been shown to be superior to tamoxifen in clinical trials for reducing contralateral breast cancer in postmenopausal women with ER-positive breast cancer.[440-443]

In the National Cancer Institute of Canada MAP 3 study, 4,560 women with a median Gail risk score of 2.3% were randomly assigned to either exemestane or placebo.[444] At a median follow-up of 35 months, there was a 65% relative reduction in the annual incidence of invasive breast cancer. The annual incidence of invasive plus noninvasive (ductal carcinoma in situ) breast cancers was 0.35% on exemestane and 0.77% on placebo. Adverse events occurred in 88% of the exemestane group and 85% of the placebo group, with no significant differences between the 2 groups in terms of skeletal fractures, cardiovascular events, other cancers, or treatment-related deaths. Minimal QOL differences were observed.

Patients treated with AIs may be more likely to experience worsening of osteoporosis, bone fractures, arthralgia, low-grade hypercholesterolemia, and cardiovascular events other than ischemia and cardiac failure, although these events are uncommon. Zoledronic acid 4 mg intravenously every 6 months has been shown to be effective in preventing osteoporosis when initiated with an AI in premenopausal and postmenopausal patients with breast cancer.[445,446]

In selecting a therapy for the primary prevention of breast cancer, raloxifene would be the optimal therapy for postmenopausal women who have or do not have osteoporosis.[435-437]

For women with *BRCA1* and *BRCA2* gene mutations, risk-reducing bilateral salpingo-oophorectomy (the prophylactic removal of both ovaries and fallopian tubes) has been associated with a significant reduction (up to 53%) in their risk for breast cancer and ovarian cancer.[393,447,448] It has been reported that 68% of American and 54% of Canadian women have undergone this operation on learning that they carry a mutation in one of these genes.[392] A case-control study of 472 postmenopausal women with *BRCA1* gene mutations, half of whom had been diagnosed with breast cancer, showed a significant reduction in breast cancer among women who had used ET and no increased risk for breast cancer in the group receiving EPT.[449] However, until more studies are conducted, the results of the Hormonal Replacement Therapy After Breast Cancer Diagnosis study that showed a clinically significant increased risk of a new cancer event in survivors who used HT should influence treatment decisions for these patients.[384]

Because many breast cancer risk factors are nonmodifiable, and some risks are unknown, early detection remains the best strategy.

Endometrial Cancer

Endometrial cancer is the fourth most common cancer among women after breast, lung, and colorectal cancer, and it is the most common gynecologic malignancy in North America. More than 47,000 new cases of endometrial cancer are diagnosed, and about 8,000 women die from it annually in the United States.[335] This cancer is uncommon in women younger than 45 years of age. Although endometrial cancer occurs more frequently in white women, mortality rates are higher in black women, 3.9 per 100,000 versus 7.1 per 100,000, respectively.[450] The etiology of the racial and ethnic disparities is multifactorial.

Most uterine cancers arise from endometrial glands. Approximately 2% of uterine cancers are sarcomas.[451] Endometrial cancers are classified into type 1 and type 2 on the basis of their etiologic and histologic grade (Table 16).[452-459]

Type 1 tumors consist of endometrioid tumors grade 1 or 2, comprising 80% of endometrial cancers.

The precursor of type 1 endometrial cancer is endometrial hyperplasia—20% to 60% of endometrial biopsy specimens interpreted as atypical endometrial hyperplasia are associated with an invasive endometrial cancer at the time of hysterectomy.[454,460,461] It is classified according to the severity of glandular crowding and the presence of nuclear atypia.[462] WHO and ACOG categorize hyperplasia as simple hyperplasia, complex hyperplasia, simple atypical hyperplasia, or complex atypical hyperplasia. A study among women with nonatypical endometrial hyperplasia showed only a moderate increase in risk of endometrial cancer, from 1.2% to 4.6%, over 19 years.[463] In contrast, among women with atypical endometrial hyperplasia, the risk of endometrial cancer increased from 8.2% to 27.5% over 19 years.

Type 2 papillary serous and clear cell carcinomas are more aggressive malignancies, which arise in atrophic endometrium and spread intraperitoneally, similar to ovarian epithelial tumors (Table 17).[464]

Women with type 2 are more likely to be older at diagnosis, of nonwhite race, and have a history of additional primary tumors. They are less likely to be obese and have a significantly worse prognosis compared with type 1 patients.[465]

Risk factors and pathophysiology of endometrial cancer. Epidemiologic and experimental studies have identified factors associated with endometrial cancer (Table 18). These factors can prospectively identify some women at risk of developing type 1 endometrial cancer. Type 2 endometrial cancers often develop in normoestrogenic, nonobese women who may have a family history of endometrial cancer.

Hyperestrogenic endometrial milieu. Type 1 endometrial cancer is associated with exposure to estrogen. Mitogenic stimuli in the endometrium are associated with the ER-α.[466] Estrogen stimulates endometrial cell proliferation, inhibits apoptosis, and promotes angiogenesis.[467,468] Type 2 endometrial cancers are not affected by the ER pathways and are unrelated to hyperestrogenism. Endometrial hyperestrogenic milieu and excessive activation of the ER-α pathway have been associated with

- A history of hyperestrogenism before menopause (early menarche, nulliparity, anovulation, infertility, late menopause).[469-471]

- Unopposed exogenous estrogen use after menopause, regardless of the route of administration, which can result in endometrial hyperplasia, atypical hyperplasia, or eventually type 1 endometrial cancer. The effect is dose and duration dependent. When used for more than 3 years, unopposed estrogen treatment is associated with a 5-fold increased risk of endometrial cancer; if used for 10 years, the risk increases 10-fold, and the increased risk can persist for several years after discontinuing estrogen.[472] The risk of endometrial cancer is lower in women in whom estrogen treatment is opposed by the concurrent use of a progestin and in women with decreased estrogen levels.[473,474]

- Use of estrogen agonists/antagonists. In the uterus, raloxifene and tamoxifen impart estrogenic effects that involve stimulation of ER-α.[475] Tamoxifen is associated with the development of endometrial polyps, endometrial hyperplasia, and endometrial cancer.[418,476] Raloxifene has only mild uterine proestrogenic effects, and in postmenopausal women its use is associated with a lower risk of type 1 endometrial cancer compared with tamoxifen or estrogen users.[477-479]

- In situ production of estrogen.[480]

- Polymorphic variations in the ER-α-1 gene, which are associated with endometrial cancer risk.[481-483]

Estrogen-like effects. These effects bypass the ER mechanism.

- Hyperinsulinemia and type 2 DM. Although the effect is mediated in part by obesity, the mechanism involves activation of signaling cascades downstream of the ER (eg, the insulin-like growth factor).[484-488]

- Aberrant activity of intracellular pathways (eg, tumor protein 53, human epidermal growth factor receptor 2, and others).[489-497]

Defective control of estrogen endometrial effects. The endometrial effects of estrogen are physiologically controlled

DISEASE RISK

Table 16. Endometrial Cancer Types

Characteristic	Type 1	Type 2
Percentage of cases	80	20
Main histologic features	Endometrioid	Papillary serous or clear cell
Common tissue background	Endometrial hyperplasia	Atrophic endometrium
Usual precursor	Atypical complex hyperplasia	Endometrial intraepithelial carcinoma
Hyperestrogenism	+	–
Menopause status	Early	Late
Grade (at diagnosis)	Usually low	Usually high
Confined to uterus	>70% of cases	<40% of cases
Extramural spread	<25% of cases	>60% of cases
5-year survival rate	>85%	<50%

Bokhman JV[452]; Creasman WT, et al[453]; Levine RL, et al[454]; Emons G, et al[455]; Clement PB, et al[456]; Amant F, et al[457]; Hamilton CA, et al[458]; Leslie WD, et al.[459]

by progesterone and by the action of proapoptotic pathways. Attenuated control of estrogen endometrial effects can be associated with endometrial cancer by

- History of low progestinic activity (nulliparity, anovulatory cycles, polycystic ovary syndrome, infertility).[498]

- Defective activity of proapoptotic pathways such as the $P2X_7$ mechanism and mitochondrial DNA polymorphism.[499-500]

Obesity. A BMI greater than 25 kg/m² doubles a woman's risk of endometrial cancer; a BMI above 30 kg/m² triples the risk.[501-505] In the United States and other developed countries, obesity has become an epidemic that can pose an increasing endometrial cancer risk for women. Over the past 4 decades, the incidence of endometrial cancer has increased in the United States (mainly in black women) and in other developed countries (eg, the United Kingdom).[335,506,507] Between 1987 and 2012, the number of US women newly diagnosed with endometrial cancer increased from 35,000 to 47,000; the number of deaths rose from 2,900 to 8,000.[335,508]

Obesity increases the risk of endometrial cancer by a number of mechanisms. In premenopausal women, obesity causes insulin resistance, ovarian androgen excess, anovulation, and chronic progesterone deficiency.[456,509] Obesity is associated with excess white adipose tissue, which can metabolize and store steroid hormones. Adipose tissue is a primary source of extragonadal estrogens via aromatase-induced conversion of androgens. In postmenopausal women, peripheral conversion of androgens to estrogens is enhanced in peripheral fat stores, leading to increased blood concentrations of estrogens and an increased risk of endometrial cancer.[510]

Diabetes mellitus. Diabetes mellitus increases the risk of endometrial cancer via factors related to hyperinsulinemia and obesity.[484,485,487,488] Mechanisms related to hyperinsulinemia involve, in part, an increase in free estrogen levels via decreased sex hormone-binding globulin, effects on the insulin-growth factor system, and increased levels of insulin-growth factor-1 and of insulin-growth factor-binding protein-1.[487,511-513]

Physical inactivity and sedentary lifestyle. A sedentary lifestyle has been correlated with increased endometrial cancer risk.[514] In contrast, studies found an inverse, independent association between physical activity and risk for

Table 17. Routes of Endometrial Cancer Metastases

- Contiguous extension (associated with grade 3 disease and lymphovascular invasion)

- Hematogenous dissemination (associated with myometrial invasion)

- Lymphatic embolization (associated with cervical and lymph node invasion)

- Exfoliation with intraperitoneal spread (observed in advanced stages of the disease)

Mariani A, et al.[464]

Chapter 4

Table 18. Endometrial Cancer Risk Factors

- Age (>50 y)
- Hyperestrogenic endometrial milieu
  - History of hyperestrogenism (early menarche, nulliparity, unovulatory cycles, infertility, late menopause)
  - Unopposed estrogen use
  - Long-term SERM use
  - Defective estrogen metabolization
- Polymorphic variations in the estrogen receptor-α-1 gene
- Estrogen-like effect
  - Hyperinsulinemia and activation of insulin-growth-factor-1 pathways
  - Aberrant activation of intracellular pathways
- Defective control of estrogen endometrial effects
  - History of hypoprogesteronism (nulliparity, unovulatory cycles, PCOS)
  - Defective activity of proapoptotic pathways
- Obesity and high caloric intake
- Physical inactivity and sedentary lifestyle
- Diabetes mellitus
- Genetic factors and familial traits
  - Hereditary nonpolyposis colorectal cancer syndrome (Lynch II)
  - Familial predisposition for endometrial cancer
  - Familial breast cancer or endometrial cancer

Abbreviations: PCOS, polycystic ovary syndrome; SERM, selective estrogen-receptor modulator.

endometrial cancer after adjusting for BMI and other risk factors.[514-517]

Genetic factors and familial traits. Multiple gene complexes have been found to be associated with endometrial cancer. About 10% of cases of endometrial cancer have a familial-hereditary basis.[518] Three genetic models have been suggested in the development of endometrial cancer: hereditary nonpolyposis colorectal cancer syndrome (Lynch II), familial endometrial cancer alone (both of which are inherited in an autosomal dominant fashion),[519] and familial breast cancer or endometrial cancer.

Hereditary nonpolyposis colorectal cancer is a disorder with high penetrance (80%-85%) and is characterized by early age at onset (<45 y) and by neoplastic lesions in a variety of tissues (colorectal, endometrial, gastric, ureteral, ovarian, skin cancers). As reported in a population-based study, a history of endometrial cancer in a first-degree relative increases its risk by nearly 3-fold after adjusting for age, obesity, and number of relatives.[520] Endometrial cancer and breast cancer share some of the same reproductive and hormonal risk factors, such as nulliparity and exposure to unopposed estrogen. Earlier reports suggested a link between these 2 cancers,[521] but the familial association between breast cancer and endometrial cancer is uncertain.

Alcohol consumption. A prospective-questionnaire, multiethnic, cohort study on the effect of alcohol intake on endometrial cancer risk in postmenopausal women showed that alcohol consumption of 2 drinks per day was associated with a relative risk of 2.01, but there was no increased risk associated with fewer than 2 drinks per day.[522]

Cigarette smoking. The risks of endometrial hyperplasia with atypia and of endometrial cancer appear to be lower in cigarette smokers, possibly through the antiestrogenic effects of nicotine on estrogen production and metabolism.[502,523,524]

Antioxidants. No association was found in the Nurses' Health Study between endometrial cancer risk (or reduced risk) and the intake of vitamins A, C, or E or carotenoids from foods or supplements.[525]

Diagnosis and staging of endometrial cancer. Diagnosis usually results from evaluation of a woman's report of abnormal uterine bleeding (AUB). In postmenopausal women, AUB is associated with endometrial cancer in 1% to 14% of patients and with endometrial hyperplasia, endometrial polyps, or other pathology of the endometrium in 20% to 40% of patients.[526] However, in about 50% to 70% of patients, no organic cause of bleeding is found, and the postmenopausal AUB is often attributed to endometrial or vaginal atrophy. Nevertheless, any postmenopausal bleeding warrants an initial evaluation for endometrial cancer.

Although dilation and curettage of the uterus was standard evaluation in the past, less-invasive methods (eg, blind endometrial biopsy using a suction piston biopsy instrument) can be used initially in an office setup without anesthesia. This is only a stopping point if it is positive for cancer or atypical hyperplasia. When pathology occupies less than 50% of the uterine surface once blind biopsy is not sensitive enough, even in cases of known carcinoma,[527] alternative approaches to evaluate AUB involve office hysteroscopy or transvaginal solography and saline infusion sonohysterography where indicated.

In 2009, the Féderation Internationale de Gynécologie et d'Obstétrique (FIGO) published a revised staging system for endometrial cancer based on surgical findings that better predicts patients' stage-dependent prognosis (Table 19).[528]

- Exclusive endometrial glandular involvement is considered stage I, regardless of tumor grade (because there were no significant differences in 5-year survival rates based on tumor grade).

DISEASE RISK

- Pelvic and para-aortic lymph node involvement are considered separately (because the involvement of para-aortic lymph nodes carries a worse prognosis).

- Positive cytology should be noted separately, but it has been excluded as a factor in the new surgical staging.

A key point of the revised FIGO staging system is that every patient with endometrial cancer should undergo surgery as part of staging and management planning.

Treatment of precursor lesions. The use of office-based diagnostic techniques results in earlier diagnosis of endometrial hyperplasia.

Hyperplasia without atypia, either simple or complex, has a low likelihood (<5%) of progressing to carcinoma; however, women with risk factors for developing endometrial cancer should be treated with a progestin (eg, MPA or megestrol acetate), administered either in a cyclic or in a continuous fashion.[529,530] Treatment with a progestin-releasing IUD has a higher regression rate and a lower relapse rate than oral progestogen therapy.[531] Perimenopausal women with oligo-ovulatory or anovulatory cycles can be prescribed OCs if there is no contraindication. In patients at high risk for developing endometrial cancer, follow-up endometrial evaluation is recommended every 3 to 6 months until regression to normal endometrium occurs. If abnormal vaginal bleeding recurs, endometrial evaluation should be performed more often.[532] Hysterectomy may be considered in postmenopausal women at risk for developing endometrial cancer who have hyperplasia without atypia.

Hysterectomy and bilateral adnexal removal is the recommended treatment for women with atypical hyperplasia because atypical hyperplasia is the immediate precursor to endometrial cancer. Women with atypical hyperplasia have an estimated 30% risk of developing invasive carcinoma, and about one-third of women with histologic finding of atypical hyperplasia in their dilation-and-curettage specimen already have invasive carcinoma in their hysterectomy specimen.[463,533] Conservative treatment with high-dose progestogen therapy may be implemented in compliant younger patients seeking to preserve fertility or in poor surgical candidates, but it requires meticulous follow-up. Conservative treatment in such cases carries a 30% chance of recurrence, and those women should be carefully followed and advised to undergo surgical treatment after their last pregnancy.[534] Atypical hyperplasia can regress after treatment with progestogens in 60% to 95% of patients, but close follow-up is indicated.[529,532,535]

Treatment of invasive endometrial cancer. Standard therapy for endometrial cancer is surgery, including hysterectomy and removal of adnexal structures, as well as surgical staging, including pelvic and para-aortic lymph node sampling in patients considered at risk for extra-uterine disease.[457,536] The surgical findings will determine disease staging and prognosis and serve as the guide for further lymph node dissection and adjuvant therapy.

Routine pelvic/para-aortic lymphadenectomy as part of the surgical treatment of endometrial cancer remains controversial.[537-545] Proponents suggest that pelvic and para-aortic lymph node dissection could be used as a diagnostic tool to determine the need for and extent of postoperative treatment, as a staging tool to define the extent of disease spread, and as a therapeutic modality.[540,546-549] Data tend to support use of lymphadenectomy to prolong survival in advanced-stage endometrial carcinoma and in poorly differentiated stage I carcinoma.[538,541]

Postoperative adjuvant treatment options depend on surgical staging and pelvic and para-aortic lymph node assessment. Recurrences usually occur in patients with high-grade tumors or with deep myometrial invasion and usually involve the vaginal apex.[550] Vaginal brachytherapy and/or external pelvic radiotherapy, or both, may be used postoperatively in such patients.[457,536] External pelvic radiotherapy improves local control of the disease but it does not substantially increase survival.[550-553] The PORTEC-2A RCT of adjuvant external teletherapy versus vaginal brachytherapy showed no significant differences with respect to vaginal recurrence rates, the occurrence of distant metastases, disease-free survival, or overall survival.[554] However, women who had received only vaginal brachytherapy had significantly fewer AEs and reported a better QOL.[555]

Systemic chemotherapy trials reported that the most active agents for chemotherapy-naive patients are platinum agents,

Table 19. 2009 FIGO Staging System for Endometrial Cancer

IA	Tumor confined to the uterus; <50% myometrial invasion
IB	Tumor confined to the uterus; ≥50% myometrial invasion
II	Cervical stromal invasion but not beyond uterus
IIIA	Tumor invades serosa or adnexa
IIIB	Vaginal and/or parametrial involvement
IIIC1	Pelvic node involvement
IIIC2	Para-aortic involvement
IVA	Tumor invasion bladder and/or bowel mucosa
IVB	Distant metastases including abdominal metastases and/or inguinal lymph nodes

Abbreviation: FIGO, Féderation Internationale de Gynécologie et d'Obstétrique.
Creasman W, et al.[528]

taxanes, and anthracyclines, all producing response rates of 20% to 30%, and that HT with progestins can produce 20% response rates in properly selected patients.[508,556-559] Palliative external beam radiotherapy and/or intrauterine brachytherapy combined with HT or chemotherapy have been used to treat medically inoperable patients with liver and extra-abdominal metastases and improve disease-free and overall survival.[560-562]

Endometrial cancer and hormone therapy. Premenopausal patients with endometrial cancer undergoing hysterectomy and bilateral salpingo-oophorectomy may develop menopause symptoms and are at a greater risk of osteoporosis.[563] Estrogen therapy has been avoided because of the potential risk of cancer recurrence. One study reported that ET only minimally increased the risk.[564] In 2006, a randomized, double-blind, placebo-controlled trial was designed to determine whether ET increased rates of disease recurrence in women with stage I or II endometrial cancer, but it closed early because of a decline in accrual after the findings of the WHI were made public in 2002.[565] Although the study was insufficiently powered despite enrollment of more than 1,200 patients, it showed a very low risk of recurrent disease in the cohort receiving ET.

Prescribing either ET or EPT for women after endometrial cancer remains controversial. In the absence of data from well-designed studies, the decision to recommend HT for women after endometrial cancer should be based on the severity of menopausal symptoms and prognostic indicators, including depth of invasion, degree of differentiation, and cell type. Moreover, careful counseling regarding perceived benefits and risks should be conducted to assist each woman in making an informed decision. The need for adding a progestogen is undetermined, although progestogen supplementation has not been found to affect the recurrence rate.[566]

Preventive measures. The ACS recommends that all women aged 40 years and older should have an annual pelvic examination. Although a pelvic examination may not uncover endometrial cancer, it is generally valuable for detecting adverse health conditions. Lifestyle modification (healthy diet and regular exercise) have been shown to reduce the risks of a number of medical conditions, including endometrial cancer, and prolong life, usually by controlling the health-related risks of obesity, DM, and hypertension.

Preventive considerations:

- Perimenopause can be a time of relative progesterone deficiency. Anovulatory cycles and intermittently high estrogen levels may lead to an estrogen-dominant hormone milieu. Use of a menstrual calendar may facilitate identification of anovulatory cycles, so that measures can be taken to provide adequate progestogen, including continuous or cyclic progestogen, low-dose hormone contraception, or a progestogen-containing intrauterine system, depending on the needs and preferences of the patient.

- After menopause, use of ET alone should be reserved for women who have undergone hysterectomy. If ET is used by a woman with a uterus despite this recommendation, women should undergo an endometrial evaluation at baseline and periodically thereafter. Endometrial evaluation should be performed after any episode of uterine bleeding; reevaluation is necessary when uterine bleeding is persistent.

- Women with a uterus using EPT after menopause should undergo endometrial evaluation if irregular uterine bleeding persists for more than 6 months after beginning therapy or sooner if there are other risk factors such as obesity, DM, or family history of endometrial cancer. The use of progestogen reduces the risks of endometrial hyperplasia and endometrial cancer induced by ET to the level found in women not taking hormones.[220,567,568] In the WHI, postmenopausal women taking oral CE 0.625 mg per day plus MPA 2.5 mg per day did not experience a significant increase in endometrial cancer, and no appreciable differences were found in the distribution of tumor histology, stage, or grade compared with women assigned to placebo.[569] However, women taking EPT required significantly more endometrial biopsies for uterine bleeding than women taking placebo.

- When an oral progestogen used in a cyclic regimen combined with a standard estrogen dose (eg, 0.625 mg CE, 1 mg oral estradiol, or 0.05 mg transdermal estradiol), the minimum effective dose for endometrial protection is 5 mg MPA per day (or equivalent) for 12 to 14 days each month. With oral micronized progesterone, the dose is 200 mg per day for 12 to 14 days each month. Progestin-containing IUDs or vaginal suppositories or gels offer another possibility for endometrial protection, but long-term efficacy data are lacking regarding their protection against endometrial cancer, and they are not FDA approved for this purpose. Continuous-combined EPT dose schedules, in which a smaller amount of progestogen is taken daily along with estrogen, usually result in amenorrhea over time. However, some women (particularly those who are recently postmenopausal) may have uterine spotting and bleeding during the first year or so of this regimen. With continuous-combined EPT, the minimum effective dose of oral progestogen for endometrial protection against standard doses of estrogen is 2.5 mg per day of MPA (or equivalent) or 100 mg per day of oral micronized progesterone. The continuous-combined regimen is the most popular regimen in the United States.

- Other alternatives to reduce HT-induced uterine bleeding include dosing progestogen less frequently, but these dosing regimens are not recommended with standard doses of estrogen and may require uterine evaluation periodically to monitor for endometrial proliferation changes.

Women using these regimens should be encouraged to report any uterine bleeding that occurs at unusual times.

Cervical Cancer

In North America, cervical cancer rates have fallen more than 50% and death rates from cervical cancer by nearly 70% over the past 30 years because of the widespread use of the Papanicolaou (Pap) test.[570] Mortality rates are still concerning, however. Cervical cancer is a slow-growing cancer caused by the high-risk strains of the human papillomavirus (HPV), an extremely common sexually transmitted infection in women. As screening with the Pap test has become more prevalent, preinvasive lesions are detected more frequently.

Incidence. The ACS estimates that in 2013 about 12,360 new cases of invasive cervical cancer will have been diagnosed, and about 4,020 women will have died from it.[570] In 2010, the CDC found that 11,818 US women were diagnosed with cervical cancer, and 3,939 women died from it.[337] Most cases of cervical cancer are found in women aged younger than 50 years; however, nearly 20% of women with cervical cancer are diagnosed when they are aged older than 65 years. In Canada, 2013 estimates are that 1,450 Canadian women were diagnosed with cervical cancer, and 380 women had died from it.[571]

The 1-year survival rate for cervical cancer is 89%, with an overall 5-year survival rate of 70%.[572] When detected at an early stage, the 5-year survival rate improves to 92%. Survival with preinvasive lesions is nearly 100%. However, many women who develop invasive cervical cancer have never had a Pap test. Black women are more likely than white women to be diagnosed with and die from cervical cancer. Hispanic/Latina women, however, have the highest cervical cancer incidence rate. White women living in Appalachia suffer a disproportionately higher risk for developing cervical cancer compared with other white women.[573] Incident rates are higher in black women, and they are more likely to have cancers detected at a later stage.

Cervical cancer rates reflect unequal access to healthcare.[574] The National Cancer Institute recommends using culturally sensitive trained healthcare professionals, particularly women of the same race or ethnicity, and removing cultural and economic barriers to ensure equality of cervical cancer preventive measures and care.

Risk factors. Several risk factors for cervical cancer have been identified (Table 20).[572] Virtually all cervical cancers are related to infection by the sexually transmitted, high-risk (oncogenic) types of HPV. An HPV infection may be identified by benign growths in the genital area (genital warts) in men and women, but many infections, especially those of the cervix, lack obvious signs. One study of HPV infection in US women aged 15 to 59 years suggested that 24.9 million women in this age range have prevalent HPV infections.[575] There was a statistically significant trend for increasing HPV prevalence with each year of age from 14 to 24 years ($P<.001$), followed by a significant gradual decline in HPV prevalence through 59 years ($P=.06$). Multivariate analysis demonstrated that being a single woman aged younger than 25 years and having a large number of recent or lifetime sex partners were factors independently associated with HPV infection.

Oral contraceptives may be associated with a higher risk of cervical cancer. One review of literature found that the risk of cervical cancer was doubled in women who took OCs longer than 5 years, but the risk returned to normal 10 years after they were stopped.[576]

Women taking combined HT in the WHI had a significantly higher annual incidence of new abnormalities (179 per 10,000 person-years) than those in the placebo arm (130 per 10,000 person-years), and sexually active unmarried women had a higher incidence (20 per 10,000 person-years) than either unmarried women who were not sexually active (11 per 10,000 person-years) or married women (5 per 10,000 person-years).[577]

No epidemiologic studies have linked HT with squamous cell cancers of the cervix, but one small epidemiologic study demonstrated a statistically increased risk for cervical cancer among users of unopposed ET.[578] In the same study, women using a progestogen had no statistically increased risk for the development of adenocarcinoma of the cervix. In the WHI, women using EPT had no significant increase in cervical cancer compared with those using placebo.[569]

Symptoms. Symptoms of cervical cancer include abnormal bleeding and spotting as well as abnormal vaginal discharge. These symptoms do not necessarily indicate that the cancer is at an advanced stage. Prompt medical evaluation is necessary when these symptoms occur.

Screening. A pelvic examination and Pap test are key elements of a comprehensive physical examination for women aged older than 40 years. However, approximately one-half of US women diagnosed with cervical cancer have never had a Pap test. In addition, many women stop having pelvic examinations and Pap tests when they reach menopause. Most deaths from cervical cancer could be prevented through routine Pap tests and safer sex practices.

Pap tests are especially important in women with risk factors—those who smoke cigarettes, do not use condoms, have had HPV detected in their Pap test, have had genital warts, or have HIV/AIDS.

Advanced tests and methods have been developed that increase the accuracy of the Pap test analysis. A computer-based evaluation technique is available in which a computer screens and identifies the most abnormal cells to be reviewed. Liquid-based, thin-layer cytology Pap testing is a technique in which cells are washed into a fluid, allowing abnormal cells to be more easily detected by reducing preparation variables and decreasing ambiguous atypical cells. These techniques may improve Pap test accuracy in

Chapter 4

> **Table 20.** Risk Factors for Cervical Cancer
>
> - Human papillomavirus
> - Sexual intercourse at an early age
> - Multiple sexual partners
> - Sexual partners who have had multiple partners
> - HIV/AIDS
> - Smoking
>
> American Cancer Society.[572]

the detection of precancerous changes by as much as 30%, but there is no "best" method.[579] Liquid-based Pap tests also can be used to detect HPV and other viruses.

An annual pelvic examination is recommended for all perimenopausal and postmenopausal women. Because cervical cancer is slow growing, considerable uncertainty surrounds the issue of the optimal cervical cancer screening interval.

Joint recommendations of the ACS, the American Society for Colposcopy and Cervical Pathology, and the American Society for Clinical Pathology say that women aged 30 years and older who have had 3 consecutive negative cervical cytology test results may be screened with cytology and HPV testing ("co-testing") every 5 years (preferred) or cytology alone every 3 years (acceptable).[580,581] More frequent screenings are recommended for women with HIV, immunosuppression, exposure to diethylstilbestrol in utero, or previously treated for cervical intraepithelial neoplasia (CIN) 2, CIN 3, or cervical cancer. Women vaccinated against HPV should follow the same screening guidelines as unvaccinated women (Table 21).[580,581]

ACOG recommends that routine cervical cytology testing be discontinued in women (regardless of age) who have had a total hysterectomy with removal of the cervix for noncancerous reasons, as long as there is no history of high-grade CIN. Women who have had a hysterectomy with removal of the cervix for benign disease rarely have important abnormalities found on Pap testing. ACOG recommends against screening in women who have had a hysterectomy with removal of the cervix and who do not have a history of a high-grade precancerous lesion (ie, CIN 2 or 3) or cervical cancer.

ACOG recommends stopping cervical cancer screening at age 65 in women who have had 3 or more negative cytology results in a row and no abnormal test results in the past 10 years or are not otherwise at high risk for cervical cancer.

The USPSTF recommendations are similar—screening for women aged 21 to 65 years with cytology every 3 years, or for women who want to lengthen the time between screenings, screening with a combination of cytology and HPV testing every 5 years.[582] It recommends against screening with HPV testing, alone or in combination with cytology, in women aged younger than 30 years. It also recommends against screening in women aged younger than 21 years but also recommends against screening in women aged older than 65 years who have had adequate prior screening and are not otherwise at high risk.

Lifestyle modification. Smoking cessation, changes in sexual behavior, and use of condoms may reduce the risks for cervical cancer.

Prevention. The single most important clinical development in gynecologic oncology has been the introduction of vaccines to prevent cervical cancer.[583] Two different HPV vaccines have been government approved for use in the United States and Canada. Gardasil protects against HPV types 6, 11, 16, and 18. Cervarix protects against HPV types 16 and 18. More HPV vaccines are being developed and tested.[584,585] Worldwide, approximately 70% of invasive cervical cancers are caused by HPV types 16 and 18.[570] Additionally, about 500,000 cases of precancerous lesions (CIN 2 and 3) are diagnosed annually in the United States. Approximately 50% to 60% of CIN 2 and CIN 3 are attributable to HPV 16 and 18.

The ACS has developed recommendations for the use of the vaccines.[572] Research has shown that since 2006, when the HPV vaccine was introduced, vaccine-type HPV prevalence dropped 56% among girls aged between 14 and 19 years.[586]

The vaccines are not licensed for women aged older than 26 years nor are they being recommended for older women. One longitudinal study concluded that the vaccine would be of low value in the older age group because of lower infection and progression rates.[587] ACOG says that the vaccine could be considered for off-label use in older women on a case-by-case basis.[588]

Even if a woman has been vaccinated against HPV 16 and 18, she still is at risk for cervical cancer caused by other high oncogenic risk HPV types. Immediate HPV genotype-specific testing for HPV 16 alone or HPV 16 and 18 can be used as an adjunct in women with negative Pap test results but who have tested positive for HPV by an assay testing for 13 or 14 high-risk types. Women who test positive for HPV 16 or HPV 16 and 18 should be referred directly for colposcopy. Women with negative results for HPV 16 or HPV 16 and 18 should be co-tested in 12 months.[580] Pap test screening remains important for all women, even those who have been immunized against HPV 16 and 18.

Ovarian Cancer

Cancer of the ovaries causes more deaths than any other cancer of the reproductive system, primarily because it is usually detected at an advanced stage.

Incidence and significance. In 2013, there will be an expected 22,240 cases of ovarian cancer in the United States, with an estimated 14,030 deaths; ovarian cancer is the ninth most common cancer in women (3% of cancers)

Table 21. ACOG Cervical Cancer Screening Recommendations

- Screening should begin at age 21.

- Pap cytology screening is recommended every 3 years for women aged 21-29 years.

- For women aged 30-65 years, co-testing with cervical cytology screening and HPV testing is preferred and should be performed every 5 years. Screening with cytology alone every 3 years is acceptable.

- Liquid-based and conventional methods of Pap cytology are acceptable for screening.

- In women who have had a total hysterectomy and have never had CIN 2 or higher, routine cytology screening and HPV testing should be discontinued and not restarted for any reason.

- Women who have a history of cervical cancer, have HIV infection, are immunocompromised, or were exposed to diethylstilbestrol in utero should not follow routine screening guidelines.

- Screening by any modality should be discontinued in women older than 65 years with evidence of adequate negative prior screening results and no history of CIN 2 or higher.[a]

Abbreviations: ACOG, American Congress of Obstetricians and Gynecologists; CIN, cervical intraepithelial neoplasia; HPV, human papillomavirus.
a. Adequate negative prior screening results are defined as 3 consecutive negative cytology results or 2 consecutive negative co-test results within the previous 10 years, with the most recent test performed within the past 5 years.
Committee on Practice Bulletins—Gynecology,[580] Saslow D, et al.[581]

---

but the fifth most common cause of cancer death (5% of deaths for women) and remains the most lethal of gynecologic malignancies.[350]

The ovary is comprised of 3 cell types—germ, stromal, and epithelial—and cancer can arise in any one of them. Most ovarian cancers are epithelial. It is the deadliest type and occurs primarily in postmenopausal women.[350] The 5-year survival rate for invasive ovarian cancers diagnosed in the United States from 2003 to 2009 was 44.2%.[589] If ovarian cancer is stage I at diagnosis, nearly 92% of women survive at least 5 years; however, only 15% of cases diagnosed from 2003 to 2009 were detected at stage I.

Etiology. The underlying mechanism of epithelial ovarian cancer development is unclear. There are several different hypotheses, including inflammation, incessant ovulation, and gonadotropin or hormone exposure. There has been focused discussion on whether there are 2 pathways to ovarian cancer, with a low-grade pathway (eg, low-grade serous, endometrioid, mucinous subtypes) versus a high-grade pathway (eg, high-grade serous).[590] Risk factors and pathogenesis for each subtype would then be different, based on the cell type.

With regard to the high-grade serous cancers, emerging data implicate the fallopian tube as the site of origin.[591] Support for this theory originated from risk-reducing bilateral salpingo-oophorectomy in *BRCA* mutation carriers in which most occult ovarian cancers coexisted with tubal involvement or occult fallopian tube carcinoma in isolation. Other molecular studies that have replicated serous cancers by manipulation of fallopian tube cells in mouse models also lend further credence to this innovative theory and raise intriguing questions about early detection and prevention of ovarian cancer.[592] The jury is still out on the exact etiology of the various ovarian epithelial tumors, but they remain among the most deadly cancers because they are most often found in late stages and cure rates remain discouraging.

Risk factors. The risk of ovarian cancer increases with age and peaks during the eighth decade.[593] Women with a family or personal history of breast or ovarian cancer, including those with *BRCA1* and *BRCA2* gene mutations, are at the highest risk for the disease (Table 22).[594] Women who carry the *BRCA1* mutation and those with the *BRCA2* mutation carry a 39% and an 11% to 17% lifetime risk, respectively, of developing ovarian cancer by age 70 years.[589,595] An association has been found between the hereditary nonpolyposis colorectal cancer syndrome (Lynch syndrome) and ovarian cancer, with women having approximately a 10% lifetime risk of developing ovarian cancer.[596]

Numerous case-control epidemiologic studies have reported an association between genital-area talc exposure and ovarian cancer risk. However, associations with the extent or duration of talc use have generally not been observed, and this association remains controversial.[597-601] Endometriosis has also been consistently linked to a modestly increased 2-fold risk of ovarian cancer, but this association appears to be most significant for the low-grade and endometrioid subtypes rather than the high-grade serous types, supporting the theory that these arise through separate mechanisms.[602]

A history of pregnancy, breastfeeding, past use of OCs, or bilateral tubal ligation have been consistently associated in multiple studies with lower ovarian cancer risk.[603-606]

CHAPTER 4

Table 22. Risk Factors for Ovarian Cancer

Factor	Relative risk
BRCA 1 or *BRCA2* carrier	14-35
Relative with ovarian cancer	3-4
Lynch syndrome	3-4
Older age	3
Infertility	2-5
Nulligravidity	2-3
Endometriosis	2
Higher socioeconomic status	1.5-2
Early menarche or late menopause	1.5-2
Hysterectomy or bilateral tubal ligation	0.5-0.7
Oral contraceptive pill use	0.3-0.5

Ramus SJ, et al[594]; Chen S, et al[595]; Howlader N, et al[589]; South SA, et al[596]; Collaborative Group on Epidemiological Studies of Ovarian Cancer, et al[603]; Jordan SJ, et al[604]; Kjaer SK, et al[605]; Purdie DM, et al.[606]

Progressive risk reductions are observed with an increasing number of full-term births, months of breastfeeding, and use of OCs.

Role of hormone therapy. Published data on the role of HT and the risk of ovarian cancer are conflicting.[65] Older epidemiologic studies generally reported no association or a modest increase in risk, and only a few more studies have separately examined ET and EPT regimens. It is unclear whether HT increases risk, but if it does, it only increases it marginally, and the studies that demonstrated more risk were generally large, observational rather than RCTs. Because the incidence of ovarian cancer is low, it would take a very large RCT to demonstrate significant risk.

In the WHI, the only RCT to date to study ovarian cancer, postmenopausal women taking daily continuous-combined CE (0.625 mg) and MPA (2.5 mg) for an average follow-up of 5.6 years did not exhibit a statistically significant increase in ovarian cancer.[569] There were 20 cases of invasive ovarian cancer among EPT recipients (n=8,506) and 12 cases among those taking placebo (n=8,102). This translates to 42 cases per 100,000 per year for EPT users and 27 cases per 100,000 per year for the placebo group (HR, 1.58; 95% CI, 0.48-1.36). Data from the WHI-ET trial have not been published.

In a cohort of 44,241 postmenopausal women who participated in the Breast Cancer Detection Demonstration Project, use of unopposed ET, especially for more than 10 years, increased the risk of ovarian cancer.[607] The risk increased with duration of use; those who used ET for 10 to 19 years had a relative risk of 1.8, and those with 20 or more years had a relative risk of 3.2. Women who used combined EPT did not have a significantly increased risk of developing ovarian cancer.

In the Million Women Study, the relative risk of ovarian cancer among current users of EPT was 1.09 (95% CI, 0.91-1.30) for those using it fewer than 5 years and 1.17 (95% CI, 1.02-1.34) for those using it 5 years or longer.[608] A larger risk was observed among long-term current users of estrogen-alone therapy, with a relative risk of 0.89 (95% CI, 0.64-1.89) for those using it fewer than 5 years and 1.53 (95% CI, 1.27-1.84) for those using it 5 years or longer. No increase in risk was observed among past users of HT overall (RR, 0.98; 95% CI, 0.88-1.11), but data were not provided regarding risk associated with specific regimens (ET vs EPT) in former users.

In a subsequent large cohort study conducted in Denmark, current HT users were at increased risk of ovarian cancer overall (RR, 1.38; 95% CI, 1.26-1.51) and of epithelial ovarian cancer (RR, 1.44; 95% CI, 1.30-1.58); risk did not vary by type of HT.[609] Among former users of ET or EPT, relative risk declined with time, from 1.22 (95% CI, 1.02-1.46) within 2 years to 0.63 (95% CI, 0.41-0.96) more than 6 years after stopping.

A US case-control study of women diagnosed with ovarian cancer from 2002 to 2005 reported increased risk among current or recent users with 5 years or more of ET use (OR, 1.6 and 1.8; 95% CI, 1.1-2.5 and 0.8-3.7, respectively).[610] There was little evidence of increased risk among former ET users. There was also increased risk for current users of EPT (OR, 1.1; 95% CI, 0.8-1.5), but risk declined with increasing time since stopping in women who had discontinued use more than 3 years previously (OR, 0.5; 95% CI, 0.3-0.70).

Further data are needed to better characterize risks associated with different HT regimens. However, as is with many of the risks associated with therapy, discontinuation of HT results in declining risk.

Role of tamoxifen. Use of tamoxifen may result in the development of benign ovarian cysts, but an increase in ovarian cancer risk has not been found.[611]

Signs and symptoms. The most common sign of ovarian cancer is enlargement of the abdomen, caused by accumulation of fluid or a large ovarian mass. However, many women have bloating or weight gain in the abdominal area, making this sign nonspecific. In women aged older than 40 years, digestive disturbances (stomach discomfort, gas, distention) that persist and cannot be explained by any other cause indicate the need for a thorough evaluation for ovarian cancer, including a carefully performed pelvic examination and ultrasound. Abnormal uterine bleeding is rarely associated with ovarian cancer.

Ovarian cancer symptoms are often subtle. A study of 1,725 US and Canadian women who had been diagnosed with ovarian cancer revealed that most experienced symptoms for

3 to 6 months before the disease was identified.[612] A second study reported that the most common symptoms associated with ovarian cancer were bloating, increased abdominal size, fatigue, urinary tract symptoms, and pelvic or abdominal pain. These symptoms were more frequent and more severe in patients with ovarian cancer than in women presenting to a general health clinic.[422]

The Gynecologic Cancer Foundation, the Society of Gynecologic Oncology, and the ACS issued a consensus statement in 2007 recommending that women who have symptoms of abdominal bloating, abdominal or pelvic pain, early satiety, or urinary urgency or frequency that occurs almost daily for a few weeks see their healthcare professional, with the hope that prompt medical evaluation may lead to the early detection of ovarian cancer.[613] However, 1 study estimated that the use of these symptoms to trigger evaluation for ovarian cancer is likely to result in diagnosis of the disease in only 1 of 100 women in the general population with such symptoms.[614]

Screening. Given the abysmal mortality rates with advanced stage ovarian cancer, the Holy Grail in gynecologic oncology has always been the pursuit of an effective screening mechanism. Yet, in order to have an effective cancer screening test, the screening modality must be technically feasible, have acceptable detection rates, and positively affect the treatment and outcomes of the cancer in question. To date, there is not an accepted or recommended ovarian cancer screening regimen for normal-risk women, although several modalities, including transvaginal ultrasonography and cancer antigen-125 (CA-125) or other potential tumor markers (human epididymis protein 4, leptin, prolactin, osteoponin) tests have been in screening trials for years.

The Prostate, Lung, Colorectal and Ovarian Cancer Screening Trial was a randomized trial evaluating the efficacy of annual transvaginal ultrasound in combination with cancer antigen-125 tests in more than 74,000 US women.[615] Across 4 screening rounds, the predictive value of a positive screen was quite low (approximately 1%). The overall ratio of surgeries to screen-detected cancers was 19.5 to 1, and 72% of screen-detected cancers were advanced stage. In 2011, the mortality results of the Prostate, Lung, Colorectal and Ovarian Cancer Screening study were reported and showed no reduction in mortality and concluded that false-positive screens were associated with complications.[616] One other large screening trial in the United Kingdom (The UK Collaborative Trial of Ovarian Cancer Screening) has enrolled more than 200,000 women and is evaluating no screening versus CA-125 tests versus ultrasound. Survival data are expected in 2014.

Multiple other biomarkers (human epididymis protein 4, mesothelin, B7-H4, decoy receptor 3, spondin-2) with potential application to ovarian cancer have been evaluated, but none have proven superior to CA-125 tests and none are recommended for screening.

No screening mechanism has been proven effective for ovarian cancer screening, and no major group endorses testing for normal-risk women. The potential for harm (unnecessary testing and/or surgery for benign conditions) outweighs the potential benefits. The National Comprehensive Cancer Network does recommend consideration of screening (with ultrasound, physical exam, and CA-125 tests) for women at high risk because of hereditary syndromes such as hereditary breast and ovarian cancer or Lynch syndrome until definitive risk-reducing surgery is deemed appropriate.

Lifestyle modification. Ovarian cancer, like many other cancers, is more likely to develop in overweight women, although the association is not strong. Dietary discretion may be one approach to reduce risk. Increasing physical activity may further reduce risk, either through reduction in body weight or other mechanisms.[617] Breastfeeding also seems to reduce risk, perhaps by extending the time period for postpartum anovulation. Pregnant women should be encouraged to breastfeed postpartum, not only for the benefits to their child but also for the health benefit they might gain for reduced risk of ovarian cancer.

Pharmacologic interventions for risk reduction. It is now well recognized that factors suppressing ovulation—including pregnancy, postpartum breastfeeding, and OC use—are associated with a reduced incidence of ovarian cancer. The simplest pharmacologic intervention to suppress ovulation is the use of OCs. Numerous observational studies of ovarian cancer have consistently reported risk reductions in association with OC use. These findings have been summarized in a worldwide collaborative reanalysis of data from 45 epidemiologic studies that include 23,257 women with ovarian cancer and 87,303 controls.[603] Ever use of OCs was associated with about a 30% reduction in disease risk. Reduction in risk was greater the longer women had used OCs, with the overall risk declining by 20% for each 5 years of use. Risk reductions persisted for more than 30 years, although they were somewhat attenuated over time. After accounting for time since last use, risk reductions did not seem to vary substantially according to the calendar time that OCs had been used, despite declining estrogen dosages. Few data are yet available to assess whether nonoral types of estrogen-progestin contraceptives or progestin only applications may also reduce ovarian cancer risk.

Case-control studies have generally supported the finding that OC use also is effective in preventing ovarian cancer in women at highest risk for the disease—women who have inherited a mutation in the *BRCA1* or *BRCA2* genes. In one study, the strength of association of ovarian cancer risk for ever use and duration of use of OCs was similar in *BRCA1* mutation carriers and noncarriers.[618]

Surgical risk reduction. For women at highest risk for disease (*BRCA* or hereditary nonpolyposis colorectal cancer [Lynch syndrome] mutation carriers), a risk-reducing surgery

CHAPTER 4

with removal of the ovaries and fallopian tubes is recommended after completion of childbearing or when a woman is aged between 35 and 40 years. One of the largest studies on women with *BRCA* mutations demonstrated improved all-cause mortality, breast cancer-specific mortality, and ovarian cancer-specific mortality in women undergoing a bilateral salpingo-oophorectomy.[448] This study found an 80% reduction in ovarian cancer risk with prophylactic salpingo-oophorectomy. Given data about the fallopian tube as a potential source of serous ovarian cancer, there has been interest in prophylactic salpingectomy alone to improve QOL by reducing the AEs of oophorectomy.[619] There is an ongoing study in the United Kingdom looking at initial salpingectomy (followed by a later oophorectomy) in women who are mutation carriers to try and reduce the effect of early menopause. Given the growing body of evidence suggesting the fallopian tube as a source for the development of ovarian cancer, all patients undergoing surgery for benign disease should be counseled about the risks and benefits of salpingectomy with ovarian preservation at the time of surgery.

Lung Cancer
Between 2005 and 2009, lung cancer rates decreased 1.1% each year among women, from 57 to 54 cases per 100,000, according to the CDC.[620] It has been 50 years since the first report of the US Surgeon General linking cigarette smoking to lung cancer, and smoking prevalence has been decreasing because of increased tobacco control, increased tobacco prices, and more smoke-free laws.

Lung cancer occurs mainly in older people—2 out of 3 people diagnosed with lung cancer are aged 65 years or older.[621] The average age at diagnosis is 70 years. The ACS estimates that there will be 224,210 (108,210 women) new cases of lung cancer diagnosed and 159,260 lung cancer deaths (72,330 women) in the United States in 2014. It is by far the leading cause of cancer death in women and in men. In Canada, 12,200 women will be diagnosed with lung cancer, and 9,500 will die from it. About 1 in 15 Canadian women is expected to develop lung cancer during her lifetime, and 1 in 18 will die from it.[622]

Each year, more people die of lung cancer than of colon, breast, and prostate cancers combined. It is the second most common cancer among white and American Indian/Alaska Native women and the third most common cancer among black, Asian/Pacific Islander, and Hispanic women.[573]

Lung cancers are divided into 2 major categories: small cell lung cancer (SCLC), representing about 15% of lung cancers, and non-small cell lung cancer (NSCLC), which includes adenocarcinomas, squamous carcinomas, and large cell carcinomas.[621] More than 80% of all lung cancers are related to smoking, and almost all SCLCs, a very aggressive form of lung cancer, are associated with smoking.

Among men and women who smoke, women are more likely to have aggressive lung cancers, and although the cause of most lung cancers is thought to be cigarette smoking, other factors include exposure to asbestos, radon, environmental factors, and secondhand smoke. Among men and women who do not smoke, women are also more likely to get lung cancer. A genetic link has been found for NSCLC in women.[621] Smoking cessation has been shown to lower lung cancer incidence. Smoking remains the leading cause of preventable death and disease in the United States.

Preclinical evidence in animal studies suggests that NSCLC can have ERs and respond to estradiol with increased gene transcription and growth.[623] In humans, ERs and aromatase, the enzyme that synthesizes 17β-estradiol, have been found in NSCLC.[624] Higher estrogen levels have been correlated with higher mortality. In the WHI, post hoc analyses found a significant increase in lung cancer death in women randomized to HT related to effects on NSCLC: these cancers were more commonly poorly differentiated and were diagnosed at metastatic stage.[625] The hazard ratio for women receiving EPT exhibited a trend (not statistically significant) toward a higher incidence of NSCLC, with an absolute attributable risk of 1.8 per 1,000 women using EPT for 5 years.[263] No increase in lung cancer was observed for those aged 50 to 59 years. Associations have been found among ER, type of lung cancer, prognosis, and epidermal growth factor-receptor mutations.[623] However, large observational studies have shown protective effects of OCs and HT on lung cancer risk.[626-628]

A Cochrane review of HT showed that continuous-combined HT was associated with an increased risk of lung cancer death after 5.6 years of use plus 2.4 years of additional follow-up (absolute risk, 9/1,000; 95% CI, 6-13) but not with estrogen alone.[261]

A study of women with NSCLC found that among 485 women, median survival time was 80 months for women on HT and 37.5 months for women not receiving HT. Combined EPT was associated with a slightly higher median survival time (87.0 mo) than ET (83.0 mo).[629]

Studies on the effects of hormone use on lung cancer and lung cancer survival are limited, with inconsistent results. Additional research is needed to evaluate the significance of long-term use of HT on outcomes in lung cancer, including characterization of tumors for ERs and PRs. Research is focusing on differences in female physiology, including bronchial responsiveness, airway size, cytochrome P450, and differences in DNA repair.[630-632] Early limited studies have suggested that antiestrogen agents may improve lung cancer outcomes, which could have substantial implications for clinical practice.[633]

Colorectal Cancer
Colorectal cancer is the third most commonly diagnosed cancer and the second leading cause of cancer death in US men and women, with an estimated 142,820 new cases of colon and rectal cancer in 2013.[589] An estimated 24,530 women will die from this disease.[338] From 2005 to

2009, the incidence has declined by 4.1% per year in persons who are aged older than 50 years.[589] In women, the incidence ranges from 31.6 per 100,000 per year in Hispanics to 49.2 per 100,000 per year in blacks. The age-adjusted mortality rate for women is 13.9 per 100,000 per year. About 5% of Americans are expected to develop the disease within their lifetimes, and about half of those will die from it.

The most important reason for the decline in colorectal cancer is thought to be the removal of polyps at the first screening colonoscopy.[634] The lifetime risk of colorectal cancer is 5.20%, or 1 in 19. The median age at diagnosis is 69 years.[589] Of women aged between 50 and 70 years, 1.54% are expected to be diagnosed with cancer of the colon and rectum. These numbers are higher in black women. Expected survival rate depends on the stage of the cancer at diagnosis. The overall 5-year survival rate was 65% from 2003 to 2009.

Risk factors. Various modifiable and nonmodifiable risk factors for colorectal cancer have been identified (Table 23).[635-641]

One inherited form of colorectal cancer is known as hereditary nonpolyposis colorectal cancer, or Lynch syndrome.[642] It is caused by a germline mutation in a mismatch repair gene. It is characterized by an increased risk of colon cancer as well as cancers of the urinary tract, brain, skin, endometrium, ovary, stomach, small intestine, and hepatobiliary tract.

For patients with Lynch syndrome, lifetime risks for colorectal cancer are 52% to 82% (mean age at diagnosis, 44-61 y); 25% to 60% for endometrial cancer (mean age at diagnosis, 48-62 y); 6% to 13% for gastric cancer (mean age at diagnosis, 56 y); and 4% to 12% for ovarian cancer (mean age at diagnosis, 42.5 y; approximately 30% are diagnosed before age 40).[643] The risk for other Lynch syndrome-related cancers is lower, although substantially increased over general population rates.[644]

Another inherited condition is familial adenomatous polyposis, in which people develop hundreds to thousands of adenomatous polyps in the colon and rectum.[645] There is a 100% risk of developing cancer by age 40, with some patients developing cancer by age 20. This condition accounts for 1% of all colorectal cancers.

Dietary intake of vitamin D has not been shown to predict risk for colorectal cancer. In a large study evaluating blood levels of vitamin D, persons who had midlevel concentrations of serum vitamin D between 50.0 nmol/L and 75.0 nmol/L were compared with those with levels in the highest quintile; the latter had a 40% lower risk of developing colorectal cancer than those in the lowest quintile.[646] Dietary vitamin D was not associated with disease risk. Levels of 25-hydroxyvitamin D below 74.88 nmol/L (20 ng/mL) are associated with a 30% to 50% increased risk of incident colon, prostate, and breast cancer, along with higher mortality from these cancers, according to prospective and retrospective epidemiologic studies.[413] For instance, pooled data for 980 women showed that the highest vitamin D intake compared with the lowest correlated with a 50% lower risk of breast cancer.[647]

Screening. The goals of screening include, first, prevention and, second, early detection of cancer.[648] The primary screening tests for detecting colorectal cancer are fecal occult blood testing (FOBT), flexible sigmoidoscopy, colonoscopy, barium enema, and computed tomography colonoscopy, with colonoscopy being the gold standard.

Women at average risk of colorectal cancer should be screened with a colonoscopy every 10 years, beginning at age 50.[648]

- *Fecal occult blood testing.* The purpose of this test is to detect the presence of blood in the GI tract that is not visible to the naked eye.[649] The original guiaic test, which is still in use, is the least expensive test available for this purpose. It results in a change in dye color when hemoglobin is present. However, the positive predictive value for cancer with this test is approximately only 5% to 10%. Follow-up of a false-positive test can result in discomfort, cost, and occasional complications from unnecessary tests. A more advanced type of FOBT is achieved by using an immunochemical method. This method uses an antibody to the hemoglobin protein in order to detect the presence of blood in the stool. This is about 5 times more expensive than the guiaic-based test. It appears to be able to detect left-sided tumors better than right sided. The fecal immunochemical test is considered a cancer-detecting test and is recommended annually.[648] A stool DNA test can identify several markers for colon cancer, but this is about 10 times more expensive than the guiaic test and is not generally available. The USPSTF does not recommend use of this test for average-risk adults.[650]

- *Sigmoidoscopy* uses a flexible sigmoidoscope to examine the colon from the anus to the proximal descending colon. Its primary use is to detect left-sided cancers. Other findings may include internal hemorrhoids and polyps. If there is a polyp present, photographs of the lesion(s) are taken, and colonoscopy is indicated. Combining sigmoidoscopy with fecal occult blood testing increases the identification of cancer to 76% relative to colonoscopy. Air is introduced through the sigmoidoscope to distend the intestinal walls to enhance visualization of mucosal lesions. The risk of perforation is approximately 3.4 per 10,000 procedures, but the risk depends on the skill of the physician performing the procedure in addition to patient anatomy.[651-653]

- *Colonoscopy* is the examination of the large intestine with a flexible fiber optic colonoscope. Air introduced through the colonoscope distends the intestinal walls to enhance visualization. Colonoscopy evaluates polypoid

Chapter 4

Table 23. Risk Factors for Colorectal Cancer

Risks you cannot change

- Ethnicity
- Age (risk increases markedly after age 50)
- Family history of colorectal cancer
- Inherited syndromes such as familial adenomatous polyposis coli
- Personal history of inflammatory bowel disease

Risks you can change

- Type 2 diabetes mellitus
- Diet high in red meats and processed meats
- Physical inactivity
- Obesity
- Smoking
- Heavy alcohol use
- Low blood levels of vitamin D_3

American Cancer Society[635]; Mills KT, et al[636]; Nimptsch K, et al[637]; Doubeni CA, et al[638]; Bardou M, et al[639]; Cho EL, et al[640]; Zgaga L, et al.[641]

lesions that are beyond the reach of a sigmoidoscope. During colonoscopy, polyps are removed for histologic evaluation, and photographs of visualized lesions are taken. Colonoscopy is repeated at more frequent intervals when women have a prior history of polyps, colon cancer, or high-risk factors, such as family history or genetic predisposition.

Colonoscopy is considered the gold standard for screening because of its ability to visualize, sample, and remove lesions from the entire colon. Data from the largest study to date revealed an expected perforation rate of 0.082%, which is lower than previously thought.[654] Risk factors for perforation include increasing age, significant comorbidity, female sex, hospital setting, removal of polyps larger than 10 cm, and invasive interventions during the procedure. There is a higher perforation rate when nongastroenterologists perform the procedure, perhaps because of the lower volume and differences in training.[655,656]

Obstruction is a contraindication for colonoscopy. Colonoscopy combined with polypectomy has been shown to decrease morbidity and mortality from colorectal cancer. Data from the National Polyp study calculated an expected reduction in cancer to be 90%.[657] The observed decrease is thought to reflect the effect of the initial colonoscopy with polyp removal. For those patients who prefer not to have this procedure, annual FOBT can be done. The fecal immunochemical test is preferred but may not be available.

- *Barium enema* with air contrast increases the quality of x-rays of the rectum. The sensitivity of this procedure, however, is only 48% for polyps 1 cm and larger.[657] Most polyps that are not detected are in the proximal colon. Polyps also can be missed in the sigmoid and transverse colon because of redundancy. Inadequate colonic distention with air, poor bowel preparation, and the presence of diverticulitis may be factors contributing to the poor sensitivity.[658]

- *Computed tomography* can be used to examine the colon and reconstruct the images in a 3-dimensional format, so-called *virtual colonoscopy*.[659] This technique has not yet been approved as a screening tool by Medicare. It can be used as a follow-up examination when traditional colonoscopy could not be completed for technical reasons or when colonoscopy is contraindicated because of a medical reason such as anticoagulation or an inherited coagulation defect. Bowel preparation is still required. Radiologists may not identify lesions less than 5 mm. There is a perforation rate associated with this procedure, estimated to be 0.08%, secondary to insufflation with air for visualization of the mucosal wall.[660]

Alternative testing. Flexible sigmoidoscopy every 5 to 10 years in combination with annual FOBT is recommended. Computed tomography of the colon can be offered every 5 years but at present may not be reimbursed by insurance, and a bowel preparation is necessary as for routine colonoscopy.

Risk-specific testing. Screening for colorectal cancer should be done when a patient's family history is positive for colorectal cancer. Having a single first-degree relative diagnosed with colorectal cancer or advanced adenoma when aged older than 60 years results in the same recommendation for screening as an average-risk patient. When a patient has a single first-degree relative diagnosed with colorectal cancer or advanced adenoma when aged younger than 60 years or has 2 first-degree relatives with colorectal cancer or advanced adenoma at any age, the recommended screening is every 5 years starting at age 40 or 10 years younger than age at diagnosis of the youngest affected relative.

Familial adenomatous polyposis (>100 adenomas). Genetic counseling is recommended for women at risk of familial adenomatous polyposis based on family history. Given a 100% risk of colorectal cancer by age 40, an annual flexible sigmoidoscopy or colonoscopy is recommended until colectomy is deemed appropriate.

Hereditary nonpolyposis colorectal cancer. Patients who meet the Bethesda criteria should have genetic testing.[661] Those with positive testing should undergo colonoscopy

DISEASE RISK

every 2 years beginning at age 20 to 25 years until age 40, then annually thereafter.

Lifestyle modification. Colorectal cancer risk may be lowered by exercise and healthy lower fat intake. Populations with a fat intake significantly lower than the US population have one-third the risk of colorectal cancer. However, the WHI Dietary Modification Trial, a randomized trial involving 48,835 postmenopausal women, demonstrated that reducing fat ingestion and increasing intake of fruits, vegetables, and grains did not reduce the incidence of colorectal cancer.[662] In the trial, intervention-group participants reduced fat as a percentage of energy intake by 10.7% more than the control group at 1 year and most maintained this difference (8.1%) at 6 years. There was no evidence that this intervention reduced colorectal cancer incidence in subsequent years. Many women in the study were taking aspirin, HT, and calcium and vitamin D supplementation, which may have influenced the findings. These findings were consistent with those of the Polyp Prevention Trial, which showed no reduction in polyp formation in 2,079 participants followed for 4 years.[663] The results were also consistent with a pooled analysis of prospective cohort studies evaluating dietary fiber intake and the risk of colorectal cancer.[664]

Postpolypectomy guideline. In 1990, a different type of precancerous polyp, called a *serrated polyp*, was described.[665] This is a type of hyperplastic polyp that tends to be found in the right side of the colon, is more common in women, and has a shorter progression to cancer than the traditional tubular adenoma. The traditional tubular adenoma is more likely to be found in the left side of the colon, is more common in men, and has at least a 10-year interval progression to colon cancer. There are different mutations involved. The serrated polyps can be difficult to detect because they are usually flatter. Postpolypectomy guidelines now reflect this classification so that practitioners will see different recommendations after polyp removal than in the past.[666]

Prevention. There is some evidence that aspirin at least every other day may be chemoprotective against colon cancer in patients who have Lynch syndrome.[667,668] Patients with familial adenomatous polyposis have been taking sulindac and celcoxib to delay recurrence of adenomas in the rectum after subtotal colectomy and to delay development of adenomas in the upper and lower GI tract.

There is also some evidence that a daily folate supplement may be chemopreventive in a subset of patients with colon cancer[669]; however, there is no generally accepted recommendation for any of these supplements because there is no single strategy that is applicable to all of the different types of colon cancer.

A nitric oxide-modified form of aspirin may be chemoprotective for colorectal cancer.[670] The mechanism of action appears to be inhibition of cell growth by affecting intracellular cell signaling. However, this product is not yet ready for clinical use.

Randomized, controlled trials, including the WHI, have shown that EPT use is associated with decreased risk of colorectal cancer, with 6 fewer cases per 10,000 women over 1 year.[671] Overall, there was a 44% decrease in the risk for colorectal cancer in the EPT group. However, the colorectal tumors diagnosed in EPT users tended to have more lymph node involvement. One of the noted differences between the groups was that the women in the HT group had more vaginal bleeding than did women in the placebo group, which may have delayed their evaluation for colorectal cancer.[672] Data are insufficient at this time to support a global recommendation for EPT use to reduce the risk of colorectal cancer in postmenopausal women.

In the ET arm of the WHI, there were no statistically significant differences between the incidence of colorectal cancer in the estrogen users versus the placebo group; tumor grades, stages, and deaths were noted to be similar.

Halting screening. The age at which to stop screening should be individualized based on risk factors and symptoms. At present, asymptomatic women aged between 50 and 75 years should be screened regularly. Routine screening of asymptomatic persons aged between 75 and 85 years is not recommended; screening should be done in this population on an individual basis. Screening is not recommended in asymptomatic persons aged older than 85 years who have previously been adequately screened.[650]

Pancreatic Cancer
Pancreatic cancer is more common in men than in women, yet it is of particular interest to menopause practitioners because ERs are present in the exocrine pancreas from which 95% of pancreatic cancers arise. It is a highly lethal tumor that remains a therapeutic challenge, with low survival rates.[673]

Incidence. Pancreatic cancer is the fourth-leading cause of cancer death in US and Canadian women.[674] It is more likely to occur in postmenopausal than in premenopausal women.[589] It affects the black population more than any other race.[675] A prospective cohort study of 89,835 Canadian women who were followed for a mean of 16.4 years failed to show an association between pancreatic cancer risk and age at first live birth, parity, age at menarche, use of OCs, or use of HT.[676] Studies also have not shown a significant link between pancreatic cancer risk and reproductive factors.[677-680]

Pancreatic cancer is a rapidly progressive, fatal disease. For all stages combined, the 1-year survival rate is 26%; 5-year survival is 6%.[338] Average survival is 6 months or less from date of diagnosis.

Risk factors. Cigarette smoking (including smokeless tobacco) is the only well-established risk factor for pancreatic cancer, as well as a 70% increase risk of death.[338,681]

161

Chapter 4

Risk of pancreatic cancer seems to increase with age, high-fat diet, and, possibly, alcohol intake. Other studies suggest a causal role for type 2 DM, chronic pancreatitis, chronic inflammation, and obesity.[339,682-687] There are several hereditary cancer syndromes.[346,688]

After reading case reports and animal studies indicating an increased risk for pancreatitis with use of glucagon-like peptide-1-based therapies, researchers examined the pancreases of patients who had died of causes unrelated to pancreatic diseases.[689] They found that the pancreases of those patients who used sitagliptin or exenatide contained lesions and cancerous lesions compared with persons without DM or persons with DM who had not taken those medications.

Screening. There are no effective methods for the early detection of pancreatic cancer. Cancer of the pancreas is generally asymptomatic until advanced stages. Jaundice may be the first symptom if the cancer develops near the common bile duct. Other symptoms can include weight loss, upper abdominal and back pain, and glucose intolerance.[338] Pancreatic cancer frequently presents with lower extremity deep vein thrombosis, thrombophlebitis migrans, and pulmonary emboli.[690] Portal vein thrombosis in patients with pancreatic cancer is more frequently being recognized on routine computed tomography scans in the absence of symptoms. A patient presenting with manifestations of thromboembolic disease must be evaluated promptly for the possibility of pancreatic cancer.

Lifestyle modification. Cigarette smoking and dietary indiscretion should be avoided. Several studies have reported reduced survival in patients who have pancreatic cancer associated with high levels of tobacco use.

Although no relationship is seen with respect to reproductive factors, there is some evidence that estrogen exposure during menopause may be protective. The California Teachers Study cohort study followed 118,164 participants, of which 323 were diagnosed with invasive pancreatic cancer.[691] Current ET users at baseline had a lower risk of pancreatic cancer than never users (HR, 0.59). No increased risk of pancreatic cancer was associated with EPT.

Few studies have examined dietary patterns and pancreatic cancer risks. Researchers calculated Healthy Eating Index 2005 scores for 537,218 men and women in the NIH-American Association of Retired Persons Diet and Health Study to estimate the association between dietary guidelines and pancreatic cancer risk.[692] They calculated survey responses to food-frequency questionnaires to estimate hazard ratios for risk of pancreatic cancer and adherence to dietary guidelines. A reduced risk of pancreatic cancer (HR, 0.85) was observed between those who met the most dietary guidelines to those with the fewest. This was seen most dramatically in overweight men.

Dietary studies have also shown a relationship between increased selenium and nut intake and reduced risk of pancreatic cancer.[693,694]

The relationship between vitamin D and pancreatic cancer is controversial. An analysis of 2 large prospective cohort studies (the Nurses' Health Study and the Health Professionals Follow-up Study) observed a 41% lower risk for pancreatic cancer in participants consuming 600 IU or more per day of vitamin D compared with those consuming less than 150 IU per day, suggesting that increasing vitamin D consumption may serve as a primary prevention.[695] However, 1 prospective case-control study involving 29,133 male smokers reported a 3-fold increased risk of pancreatic cancer among those in the highest quintile of serum vitamin D level compared to these in the lowest quintile.[696]

Treatment interventions. No prescription therapies are known to reduce the risk of pancreatic cancer. Treatment of pancreatic cancer with surgery (including minimally invasive approaches), radiation, and chemotherapy may extend survival and relieve symptoms but is seldom curative.[338]

Skin Cancer

Skin cancer is by far the most common form of cancer in the United States. Nonmelanoma skin cancers are the most prevalent, with an estimated annual incidence of 3.5 million US cases in 2006. Melanoma, although less common, is responsible for most skin cancer deaths. The ACS anticipates more than 76,000 cases of melanoma in 2013.[335] Despite public health efforts to warn about this cancer and its association with sun exposure, the public tends to minimize the risk and seriousness of the disease.[697,698]

Melanoma. The most deadly form of skin cancer is melanoma. Its incidence has been increasing significantly for decades, with a rate of about 2.8% annually from 1981 to 2008.[699] Melanoma is a malignancy arising from melanocytes. Because most of these malignant cells maintain the ability to produce melanin, melanoma tumors are usually brown or black. Some melanomas do not contain pigment and are difficult to diagnose. The strongest predictor of long-term survival in melanoma is tumor thickness.[700] The 5-year survival rate for melanoma diagnosed at stage IA is 97%; the 10-year survival rate is about 95%. If diagnosed at stage IV, the 5-year survival rate is 15% to 20%; the 10-year survival rate is 10% to 15%.[701] Early detection of melanoma can therefore be lifesaving.

Melanoma is predominantly a cutaneous disease but may in rare instances occur primarily at other sites, including mucous membranes (vulva, vagina, perianal region, lip, throat, and esophagus) and the eye (uvea and conjunctiva). Melanomas in these sites have a worse prognosis than cutaneous melanomas.

Risk factors for melanoma include excessive exposure to ultraviolet radiation, specifically intense, intermittent sun exposure. Having severe sunburns during childhood greatly increases the risk for melanoma later in life. Although fair-skinned persons are at highest risk, those with darkly pigmented skin are not risk free. Additional risk factors include a family history of melanoma and multiple nevi or atypical nevi.

Nonmelanomas. The most common cancers of the skin are nonmelanomas, usually basal cell and squamous cell cancers. The cell of origin in nonmelanoma skin cancer is the keratinocyte. Because they metastasize less frequently, they are less worrisome than melanomas.

Benign tumors that develop from other types of skin cells include

- *Actinic keratoses*: Sun-induced growths that are sometimes burning and tender. These common skin lesions are considered "premalignant." Although they carry a potential for malignant progression, the frequency of this transformation is not well defined and likely very low.[702] Actinic keratoses are strongly associated with an increased risk of squamous cell cancer.

- *Seborrheic keratoses*: Benign tan, brown, or black raised spots with a waxy texture or rough surface.

- *Hemangiomas*: Benign blood vessel growths often called strawberry spots or port wine stains.

- *Warts*: Rough-surfaced benign growths caused by a virus.

- *Lipomas*: Soft growths of benign fat cells.

Cumulative exposure to sunlight is strongly associated with the risk of actinic keratoses and thus squamous cell cancer. Intermittent, intense episodes of burning seem to be more important in the development of basal cell skin cancer. Risk factors for photoaging and skin cancer include fair skin, difficulty tanning, ease of sunburning, sunburns before age 20, tanning bed use, and advancing age. Smoking is an independent risk factor for wrinkling, telangiectasia, and squamous cell cancer. Other risk factors for the development of nonmelanoma skin cancer include exposure to arsenic, tar and aromatic hydrocarbons, ionizing radiation, immunosuppression, and HPV infection. There are also several important hereditary cancer syndromes that include a number of skin cancers.[346,688]

Screening. All women, but particularly those who are fair skinned, should undergo total body skin examinations periodically for skin cancers and precursors to skin cancer. Although there are no definitive recommendations regarding the frequency of skin exams, people at increased risk require more frequent monitoring. This includes those who are immunosuppressed as well as those with significant sun exposure or numerous acquired or atypical nevi.

Moles should be evaluated for asymmetry, border irregularities, variability in color, diameter greater than 6 mm, or a sudden or progressive increase in size. The typical presenting sign of melanoma is any change in appearance of a mole or other dark pigmented growths or spots. Other signs and symptoms of melanoma include a change in appearance of a skin bump or nodule, spread of pigmentation beyond the border, scaliness, oozing, bleeding, change in sensation, itchiness, tenderness, or pain.

Basal cell carcinoma may present with a persistent, nonhealing sore on the skin; a reddish or irritated patch of skin; a shiny bump or nodule that may be mistaken for a mole; a pink, elevated growth; or a scar-like area on the skin.

Squamous cell tumors appear thick, rough, horny, and shallow on the skin. They may ulcerate, meaning that the epidermis above the cancer is not intact.

Lifestyle modification. It is well established that prolonged exposure to ultraviolet (UV) radiation is the major cause of photoaging and skin cancers. Shorter wavelength UVB radiation has long been targeted as the main cause of skin malignancy, whereas UVA was implicated in the changes of photoaging. It is now felt that UVA and UVB contribute to malignant transformation in the skin. These strategies can be employed to reduce the risk of developing skin cancer[702]:

- Avoid the sun during midday hours (10 AM to 2 PM).

- When in the sun, wear clothing (including broad-brimmed hats) and sunglasses to avoid excessive ultraviolet radiation.

- Apply adequate amounts of sunscreen to dry skin, 15 minutes before going outdoors, and reapply sunscreen every 2 hours or after swimming or sweating heavily. Use a sunscreen that is labeled as broad-spectrum (protecting against UVA and UVB) and water resistant, with a skin protection factor of at least 30. Self-tanning lotions containing dihydroxyacetone may be used to achieve a darker appearance.

- Avoid tanning salons because exposure to UVA radiation may induce photoaging and photoallergic responses. Tanning outdoors also should be avoided. Patients can be reminded that there is no such thing as a "healthy tan"—tanned skin means that skin is damaged.

- Do not smoke.

References

1. World Health Organization. *The World Health Report 2004: Changing History.* Geneva: World Health Organization; 2004.
2. Go AS, Mozaffarian D, Roger VL, et al; American Heart Association Statistics Committee and Stroke Statistics Subcommittee. Executive summary: heart disease and stroke statistics—2013 update: a report from the American Heart Association. *Circulation.* 2013;127(1):143-152.

3. Mosca L, Benjamin EJ, Berra K, et al; American Heart Association. Effectiveness-based guidelines for the prevention of cardiovascular disease in women—2011 update: a guideline from the American Heart Association. *J Am Coll Cardiol*. 2011;57(12):1404-1423. Erratum in: *J Am Coll Cardiol*. 2012;59(18):1663.
4. Shaw LJ, Bugiardini R, Merz CN. Women and ischemic heart disease: evolving knowledge. *J Am Coll Cardiol*. 2009;54(17):1561-1575.
5. Gierach GL, Johnson BD, Bairey Merz CN, et al; WISE Study Group. Hypertension, menopause, and coronary artery disease risk in the Women's Ischemia Syndrome Evaluation (WISE) Study. *J Am Coll Cardiol*. 2006;47(3 suppl):S50-S58.
6. Matthews KA, Crawford SL, Chae CU, et al. Are changes in cardiovascular disease risk factors in midlife women due to chronological aging or to the menopausal transition? *J Am Coll Cardiol*. 2009;54(25):2366-2373.
7. El Khoudary SR, Wildman RP, Matthews K, Thurston RC, Bromberger JT, Sutton-Tyrrell K. Progression rates of carotid intima-media thickness and adventitial diameter during the menopausal transition. *Menopause*. 2013;20(1):8-14.
8. Manson JE, Chlebowski RT, Stefanick ML, et al. Menopausal hormone therapy and health outcomes during the intervention and extended poststopping phases of the Women's Health Initiative randomized trials. *JAMA*. 2013;310(13):1353-1368.
9. Hu FB, Grodstein F, Hennekens CH, et al. Age at natural menopause and risk of cardiovascular disease. *Arch Intern Med*. 1999;159(10):1061-1066.
10. Murabito JM, Yang Q, Fox C, Wilson PW, Cupples LA. Heritability of age at natural menopause in the Framingham Heart Study. *J Clin Endocrinol Metab*. 2005;90(6):3427-3430.
11. Kok HS, van Asselt KM, van der Schouw YT, et al. Heart disease risk determines menopausal age rather than the reverse. *J Am Coll Cardiol*. 2006; 47(10):1976-1983.
12. de Aloysio D, Gambacciani M, Meschia M, et al. The effect of menopause on blood lipid and lipoprotein levels. The Icarus Study Group. *Atherosclerosis*. 1999;147(1):147-153.
13. Kuller LH, Simkin-Silverman LR, Wing RR, Meilahn EN, Ives DG. Women's Healthy Lifestyle Project: a randomized clinical trial: results at 54 months. *Circulation*. 2001;103(1):32-93.
14. Mendelsohn ME, Karas RH. Molecular and cellular basis of cardiovascular gender differences. *Science*. 2005;308(5728):1583-1587.
15. Feng Y, Hong X, Wilker E, et al. Effects of age at menarche, reproductive years, and menopause on metabolic risk factors for cardiovascular diseases. *Atherosclerosis*. 2008;196(2):590-597.
16. Lobo RA. Menopause and aging. In: Strauss JF III, Barbieri RL, eds. *Yen & Jaffe's Reproductive Endocrinology: Physiology, Pathophysiology, and Clinical Management*. 7th ed. Philadelphia: Saunders Elsevier; 2013:309-339.
17. National Cholesterol Education Program (NCEP) Expert Panel on Detection, Evaluation, and Treatment of High Blood Cholesterol in Adults (Adult Treatment Panel III). Third Report of the National Cholesterol Education Program (NCEP) Expert Panel on Detection, Evaluation, and Treatment of High Blood Cholesterol in Adults (Adult Treatment Panel III) final report. *Circulation*. 2002;106(25):3143-3421.
18. National Heart, Lung, and Blood Institute. *Risk Assessment Tool for Estimating Your 10-Year Risk of Having a Heart Attack*. National Institutes of Health Web site. http://cvdrisk.nhlbi.nih.gov/calculator.asp. Updated May 2013. Accessed May 21, 2014.
19. Genest J, Frohlich J, Fodor G, McPherson R; the Working Group on Hypercholesterolemia and Other Dyslipidemias. Recommendations for the management of dyslipidemia and the prevention of cardiovascular disease: 2003 update. Online only. October 28, 2003. www.cmaj.ca/content/suppl/2003/11/06/169.9.921.DC1/dysonline.pdf. Accessed May 21, 2014.
20. Kramer H, Cao G, Dugas L, Luke A, Cooper R, Durazo-Arvizu R. Increasing BMI and waist circumference and prevalence of obesity among adults with type 2 diabetes: the National Health and Nutrition Examination Surveys. *J Diabetes Complications*. 2010;24(6):368-374.
21. Grundy SM, Cleeman JI, Merz CN, et al; National Heart, Lung, and Blood Institute; American College of Cardiology Foundation; American Heart Association. Implications of recent clinical trials for the National Cholesterol Education Program Adult Treatment Panel III guidelines. *Circulation*. 2004;110(2):227-239. Erratum in: *Circulation*. 2004;110(6):763.
22. Bellamy L, Casas JP, Hingorani AD, Williams DJ. Pre-eclampsia and risk of cardiovascular disease and cancer in later life: systematic review and meta-analysis. *BMJ*. 2007;335(7627):974.
23. Goff DC Jr, Lloyd-Jones DM, Bennett G, et al. 2013 ACC/AHA Guideline on the Assessment of Cardiovascular Risk: a report of the American College of Cardiology/American Heart Association Task Force on Practice Guidelines. *Circulation*. 2014;129(25 suppl 2):S49-S73.
24. Ridker PM, Buring JE, Rifai N, Cook NR. Development and validation of improved algorithms for the assessment of global cardiovascular risk in women: the Reynolds Risk Score. *JAMA*. 2007;297(6):611-619. Erratum in: *JAMA*. 2007;297(13):1433.
25. Ridker PM, Wilson PW, Grundy SM. Should C-reactive protein be added to metabolic syndrome and to assessment of global cardiovascular risk? *Circulation*. 2004;109(23):2818-2825.
26. Ridker PM, Rifai N, Cook NR, Bradwin G, Buring JE. Non-HDL cholesterol, apolipoproteins A-I and B100, standard lipid measures, lipid ratios, and CRP as risk factors for cardiovascular disease in women. *JAMA*.2005;294(3):326-333.
27. Walsh BW, Paul S, Wild RA, et al. The effects of hormone replacement therapy and raloxifene on C-reactive protein and homocysteine in healthy postmenopausal women: a randomized, controlled trial. *J Clin Endocrinol Metab*. 2000;85(1):214-218.
28. James PA, Oparil S, Carter BL, et al. 2014 evidence-based guidelines for the management of high blood pressure in adults: report from the panel members appointed to the Eighth Joint National Committee (JNC 8). *JAMA*. 2014;311(5):507-520. Erratum in: *JAMA*. 2014;311(17):1809.
29. Appel LJ, Brands MW, Daniels SR, Karanja N, Elmer PJ, Sacks FM; American Heart Association. Dietary approaches to prevent and treat hypertension: a scientific statement from the American Heart Association. *Hypertension*. 2006;47(2):296-308.
30. Stone NJ, Robinson J, Lichtenstein AH, et al. 2013 ACC/AHA guideline on the treatment of blood cholesterol to reduce atherosclerotic cardiovascular risk in adults: a report of the American College of Cardiology/American Heart Association Task Force on Practice Guidelines. *Circulation*. 2014;129(25 suppl 2):S1-S45.
31. Dayspring TD, Pokrywka G. The impact of triglycerides on lipid and lipoprotein biology in women. *Gend Med*. 2010;7(3):189-205.
32. Harper CR, Jacobson TA. Using apolipoprotein B to manage dyslipidemic patients: time for a change? *Mayo Clin Proc*. 2010;85(5):440-445.
33. Eckel RH, Jakicic JM, Ard JD, et al. 2013 AHA/ACC guideline on lifestyle management to reduce cardiovascular risk: a report of the American College of Cardiology/American Heart Association Task Force on Practice Guidelines. *J Am Coll Cardiol*. 2014;63(25 pt B):2960-2984.
34. Mosca L, Linfante AH, Benjamin EJ, et al. National study of physician awareness and adherence to cardiovascular disease prevention guidelines. *Circulation*. 2005;111(4):499-510.
35. Mosca L, Merz NB, Blumenthal RS, et al. Opportunity for intervention to achieve American Heart Association guidelines for optimal lipid levels in high-risk women in a managed care setting. *Circulation*. 2005;111(4):488-493.
36. Chasan-Taber L, Stampfer MJ. Epidemiology of oral contraceptives and cardiovascular disease. *Ann Intern Med*. 1998;128(6):467-477.
37. Centers for Disease Control and Prevention (CDC). US medical eligibility criteria for contraceptive use, 2010. *MMWR Recomm Rep*. 2010;59(RR-4):1-86.
38. Segar ML, Eccles JS, Richardson CR. Type of physical activity goal influences participation in healthy midlife women. *Womens Health Issues*. 2008;18(4):281-291.
39. Houston MC, Fazio S, Chilton FH, et al. Nonpharmacologic treatment of dyslipidemia. *Prog Cardiovasc Dis*. 2009;52(2):61-94.
40. Bazzano LA, Reynolds K, Holder KN, He J. Effect of folic acid supplementation on risk of cardiovascular diseases: a meta-analysis of randomized controlled trials. *JAMA*. 2006;296(22):2720-2726. Erratum in: *JAMA*. 2007;297(9):952.
41. Inkovaara J, Gothoni G, Halttula R, Heikinheimo R, Tokola O. Calcium, vitamin D and anabolic steroid in treatment of aged bones: double-blind placebo-controlled long-term clinical trial. *Age Ageing*. 1983;12(2):124-130.
42. Brøndum-Jacobsen P, Benn M, Jensen GB, Nordestgaard BG. 25-hydroxyvitamin D levels and risk of ischemic heart disease, myocardial infarction, and early death: population-based study and meta-analyses of 18 and 17 studies. *Arterioscler Thromb Vasc Biol*. 2012;32(11):2794-2802.
43. Wang L, Song Y, Manson JE, et al. Circulating 25-hydroxy-vitamin D and risk of cardiovascular disease: a meta-analysis of prospective studies. *Circ Cardiovasc Qual Outcomes*. 2012;5(6):819-829.
44. Robinson-Cohen C, Hoofnagle AN, Ix JH, et al. Racial differences in the association of serum 25-hydroxyvitamin D concentration with coronary heart disease events. *JAMA*. 2013;310(2):179-188.

45. Katan MB, Grundy SM, Jones P, Law M, Miettinen T, Paoletti R; Stresa Workshop Participants. Efficacy and safety of plant stanols and sterols in the management of blood cholesterol levels. *Mayo Clin Proc*. 2003;78(8):965-978.
46. Devaraj S, Jialal I, Vega-López S. Plant sterol-fortified orange juice effectively lowers cholesterol levels in mildly hypercholesterolemic healthy individuals. *Arterioscler Thromb Vasc Biol*. 2004;24(3):e25-e28.
47. American Heart Association Nutrition Committee; Lichtenstein AH, Appel LJ, et al. Diet and lifestyle recommendations revision 2006: a scientific statement from the American Heart Association Nutrition Committee. *Circulation*. 2006;114(1):82-96. Erratum in: *Circulation*. 2006;114(1):e27; *Circulation*. 2006;114(23):e629.
48. Marangoni F, Poli A. Phytosterols and cardiovascular health. *Pharmacol Res*. 2010;61(3):193-199.
49. Clearfield M. Coronary heart disease risk reduction in postmenopausal women: the role of statin therapy and hormone replacement therapy. *Prev Cardiol*. 2004;7(3):131-136.
50. Rudkowska I. Plant sterols and stanols for healthy ageing. *Maturitas*. 2010;66(2):158-162.
51. Sacks FM, Lichtenstein A, Van Horn L, Harris W, Kris-Etherton P, Winston M; American Heart Association Nutrition Committee. Soy protein, isoflavones, and cardiovascular health: an American Heart Association Science Advisory for professionals from the Nutrition Committee. *Circulation*. 2006;113(7):1034-1044.
52. Estruch R, Ros E, Salas-Salvadó J, et al; PREDIMED Study Investigators. Primary prevention of cardiovascular disease with a Mediterranean diet. *N Engl J Med*. 2013;368(14):1279-1290.
53. Prasain JK, Carlson SH, Wyss JM. Flavonoids and age-related disease: risk, benefits and critical windows. *Maturitas*. 2010;66(2):163-171.
54. Tankó LB, Bagger YZ, Qin G, Alexandersen P, Larsen PJ, Christiansen C. Enlarged waist combined with elevated triglycerides is a strong predictor of accelerated atherogenesis and related cardiovascular mortality in postmenopausal women. *Circulation*. 2005;111(15):1883-1890.
55. Hayden M, Pignone M, Phillips C, Mulrow C. Aspirin for the primary prevention of cardiovascular events: a summary of the evidence for the US Preventive Services Task Force. *Ann Intern Med*. 2002;136(2):161-172.
56. Ridker PM, Cook NR, Lee IM, et al. A randomized trial of low-dose aspirin in the primary prevention of cardiovascular disease in women. *N Engl J Med*. 2005;352(13):1293-1304.
57. Berger JS, Roncaglioni MC, Avanzini F, Pangrazzi I, Tognoni G, Brown DL. Aspirin for the primary prevention of cardiovascular events in women and men: a sex-specific meta-analysis of randomized controlled trials. *JAMA*. 2006;295(3):306-313.
58. Campbell CL, Smyth S, Montalescot G, Steinhubl SR. Aspirin dose for the prevention of cardiovascular disease: a systematic review. *JAMA*. 2007;297(18):2018-2024.
59. Cholesterol Treatment Trialists' (CTT) Collaboration; Baigent C, Blackwell L, Emberson J, et al. Efficacy and safety of more intensive lowering of LDL cholesterol: a meta-analysis of data from 170,000 participants in 26 randomised trials. *Lancet*. 2010;376(9753):1670-1681.
60. Nissen SE, Tuzcu EM, Schoenhagen P, et al; Reversal of Atherosclerosis with Aggressive Lipid Lowering (REVERSAL) Investigators. Statin therapy, LDL cholesterol, C-reactive protein, and coronary artery disease. *N Engl J Med*. 2005;352(1):29-38.
61. Orchard TJ, Temprosa M, Goldberg R, et al; Diabetes Prevention Program Research Group. The effect of metformin and intensive lifestyle intervention on the metabolic syndrome: the Diabetes Prevention Program randomized trial. *Ann Intern Med*. 2005;142(8):611-619.
62. Look AHEAD Research Group; Wing RR, Bolin P, Brancati FL, et al. Cardiovascular effects of intensive lifestyle intervention in type 2 diabetes. *N Engl J Med*. 2013;369(2):145-154.
63. International Expert Committee. International Expert Committee report on the role of the A1C assay in the diagnosis of diabetes. *Diabetes Care*. 2009;32(7):1327-1334.
64. Rossouw JE, Prentice RL, Manson JE, et al. Postmenopausal hormone therapy and risk of cardiovascular disease by age and years since menopause. *JAMA*. 2007;297(13):1465-1477. Erratum in: *JAMA*. 2008;299(12):1426.
65. North American Menopause Society. The 2012 hormone therapy position statement of: The North American Menopause Society. *Menopause*. 2012;19(3):257-271.
66. Salpeter SR, Walsh JM, Greyber E, Salpeter EE. Brief report: coronary heart disease events associated with hormone therapy in younger and older women. A meta-analysis. *J Gen Intern Med*. 2006;21(4):363-366. Erratum in: *J Gen Intern Med*. 2008;23(10):1728.
67. Harman SM. Effects of oral conjugated estrogen or transdermal estradiol plus oral progesterone treatment on common carotid artery intima media thickness (CIMT) and coronary artery calcium (CAC) in menopausal women: initial results from the Kronos Early Estrogen Prevention Study (KEEPS) [abstract]. *Menopause*. 2012;19(12):1365.
68. Hodis HN, Mack WJ. Randomized controlled trials and the effects of postmenopausal hormone therapy on cardiovascular disease: facts, hypotheses and clinical perspective. In: Lobo RA, ed. *Treatment of the Postmenopausal Woman*. 3rd ed. San Diego, CA: Academic Press; 2007:529-564.
69. Prentice RL, Langer RD, Stefanick ML, et al; Women's Health Initiative Investigators. Combined analysis of Women's Health Initiative observational and clinical trial data on postmenopausal hormone treatment and cardiovascular disease. *Am J Epidemiol*. 2006;163(7):589-599.
70. Manson JE, Bassuk SS. Invited commentary: hormone therapy and risk of coronary heart disease why renew the focus on the early years of menopause? *Am J Epidemiol*. 2007;166(5):511-517.
71. Manson JE, Allison MA, Rossouw JE, et al; WHI and WHI-CACS Investigators. Estrogen therapy and coronary-artery calcification. *N Engl J Med*. 2007;356(25):2591-2602.
72. Allison MA, Manson JE, Langer RD, et al; Women's Health Initiative and Women's Health Initiative Coronary Artery Calcium Study Investigators. Oophorectomy, hormone therapy, and subclinical coronary artery disease in women with hysterectomy: the Women's Health Initiative coronary artery calcium study. *Menopause*. 2008;15(4 pt 1):639-647.
73. Allison MA, Manson JE. The complex interplay of vasomotor symptoms, hormone therapy, and cardiovascular risk. *Menopause*. 2009;16(4):619-620.
74. Grodstein F, Manson JE, Stampfer MJ, Rexrode K. Postmenopausal hormone therapy and stroke: role of time since menopause and age at initiation of hormone therapy. *Arch Intern Med*. 2008;168(8):861-866.
75. Rossouw JE, Anderson GL, Prentive RL, et al; Writing Group for the Women's Health Initiative Investigators. Risks and benefits of estrogen plus progestin in healthy postmenopausal women: principal results from the Women's Health Initiative randomized controlled trial. *JAMA*. 2002;288(3):321-333.
76. Grady D, Herrington D, Bittner V, et al; HERS Research Group. Cardiovascular disease outcomes during 6.8 years of hormone therapy: Heart and Estrogen/progestin Replacement Study follow-up (HERS II). *JAMA*. 2002; 288(1):49-57.
77. Vickers MR, MacLennan AH, Lawton B, et al; WISDOM group. Main morbidities recorded in the women's international study of long duration oestrogen after menopause (WISDOM): a randomised controlled trial of hormone replacement therapy in postmenopausal women. *BMJ*. 2007; 335(7613):239.
78. Hendrix SL, Wassertheil-Smoller S, Johnson KC, et al; WHI Investigators. Effects of conjugated equine estrogen on stroke in the Women's Health Initiative. *Circulation*. 2006;113(20):2425-2434.
79. Curb JD, Prentice RL, Bray PF, et al. Venous thrombosis and conjugated equine estrogen in women without a uterus. *Arch Intern Med*. 2006;166(7):772-780.
80. Cushman M, Kuller LH, Prentice R, et al; Women's Health Initiative Investigators. Estrogen plus progestin and risk of venous thrombosis. *JAMA*. 2004;292(13):1573-1580.
81. Canonico M, Oger E, Plu-Bureau G, et al; Estrogen and Thromboembolism Risk (ESTHER) Study Group. Hormone therapy and venous thromboembolism among postmenopausal women: impact of the route of estrogen administration and progestogens: the ESTHER Study. *Circulation*. 2007;115(7):840-845.
82. Canonico M, Plu-Bureau G, Lowe GD, Scarabin PY. Hormone replacement therapy and risk of venous thromboembolism in postmenopausal women: systematic review and meta-analysis. *BMJ*. 2008;336(7655):1227-1231.
83. Scarabin PY, Oger E, Plu-Bureau G; EStrogen and THromboEmbolism Risk Study Group. Differential association of oral and transdermal oestrogen-replacement therapy with venous thromboembolism risk. *Lancet*. 2003;362(9382):428-432.
84. Canonico M, Fournier A, Carcaillon L, et al. Postmenopausal hormone therapy and risk of idiopathic venous thromboembolism: results from the E3N cohort study. *Arterioscler Thromb Vasc Biol*. 2010;30(2):340-345.
85. Antithrombotic Trialists' Collaboration. Collaborative meta-analysis of randomised trials of antiplatelet therapy for prevention of death, myocardial infarction, and stroke in high risk patients. *BMJ*. 2002;324(7329):71-86. Erratum in: *BMJ*. 2002;324(7330):141.
86. National Diabetes Education Program. *The Facts About Diabetes: A Leading Cause of Death in the U.S*. Centers for Disease Control and Prevention Web site. http://ndep.nih.gov/diabetes-facts/. Updated January 2011. Accessed May 21, 2014.

CHAPTER 4

87. American Diabetes Association. Standards of medical care in diabetes—2013. *Diabetes Care.* 2013;36(suppl 1):S11-S66.
88. National Diabetes Information Clearinghouse (NDIC). *Diagnosis of Diabetes and Prediabetes.* US Dept of Health and Human Services, National Institute of Diabetes and Digestive and Kidney Diseases (NIDDK) Web site. http://diabetes.niddk.nih.gov/dm/pubs/diagnosis/index.aspx. Updated August 29, 2012. Accessed May 21, 2014.
89. US Preventive Services Task Force. Screening for type 2 diabetes mellitus in adults: US Preventive Services Task Force recommendation statement. *Ann Intern Med.* 2008;148(11):846-854. Erratum in: *Ann Intern Med.* 2008;149(2):147.
90. Cheng YJ, Imperatore G, Geiss LS, et al. Secular changes in the age-specific prevalence of diabetes among U.S. adults: 1988-2010. *Diabetes Care.* 2013; 36(9):2690-2696.
91. Cowie CC, Rust KF, Ford ES, et al. Full accounting of diabetes and pre-diabetes in the US population in 1988-1994 and 2005-2006. *Diabetes Care.* 2009;32(2):287-294. Erratum in: *Diabetes Care.* 2011;34(10):2338.
92. Canadian Task Force on Preventive Health Care; Pottie K, Jaramillo A, Lewin G, et al. Recommendations on screening for type 2 diabetes in adults. *CMAJ.* 2012;184(15):1687-1696. Erratum in: *CMAJ.* 2012;184(16):1815.
93. Narayan KM, Boyle JP, Thompson TJ, Sorensen SW, Williamson DF. Lifetime risk for diabetes mellitus in the United States. *JAMA.* 2003; 290(14):1884-1890.
94. Akahoshi M, Soda M, Nakashima E, et al. Effects of age at menopause on serum cholesterol, body mass index, and blood pressure. *Atherosclerosis.* 2001;156(1):157-163.
95. Crawford SL, Casey VA, Avis NE, McKinlay SM. A longitudinal study of weight and the menopause transition: results from the Massachusetts Women's Health Study. *Menopause.* 2000;7(2):96-104.
96. Ley CJ, Lees B, Stevenson JC. Sex- and menopause-associated changes in body-fat distribution. *Am J Clin Nutr.* 1992;55(5):950-954.
97. Carr M. The emergence of the metabolic syndrome with menopause. *J Clin Endocrinol Metab.* 2003;88(6):2404-2411.
98. Sowers M, Zheng H, Tomey K, et al. Changes in body composition in women over six years at midlife: ovarian and chronological aging. *J Clin Endocrinol Metab.* 2007;92(3):895-901.
99. Sternfeld B, Bhat AK, Wang H, Sharp T, Quesenberry CP Jr. Menopause, physical activity, and body composition/fat distribution in midlife women. *Med Sci Sports Exerc.* 2005;37(7):1195-1202.
100. Wildman RP, Tepper PG, Crawford S, et al. Do changes in sex steroid hormones precede or follow increases in body weight during the menopause transition? Results from the Study of Women's Health Across the Nation. *J Clin Endocrinol Metab.* 2012;97(9):E1695-E1704.
101. Yeung EH, Zhang C, Mumford SL, et al. Longitudinal study of insulin resistance and sex hormones over the menstrual cycle: the BioCycle Study. *J Clin Endocrinol Metab.* 2010;95(12):5435-5442.
102. Matthews KA, Gibson CJ, El Khoudary SR, Thurston RC. Changes in cardiovascular risk factors by hysterectomy status with and without oophorectomy: Study of Women's Health Across the Nation. *J Am Coll Cardiol.* 2013;62(3):191-200.
103. Soriguer F, Morcillo S, Hernando V, et al. Type 2 diabetes mellitus and other cardiovascular risk factors are no more common during menopause: longitudinal study. *Menopause.* 2009;16(4):817-821.
104. Huxley R, Barzi F, Woodward M. Excess risk of fatal coronary heart disease associated with diabetes in men and women: meta-analysis of 37 prospective cohort studies. *BMJ.* 2006;332(7533):73-78.
105. Lee C, Joseph L, Colosimo A, Dasgupta K. Mortality in diabetes compared with previous cardiovascular disease: a gender-specific meta-analysis. *Diabetes Metab.* 2012;38(5):420-427.
106. ACCORD Study Group; Gerstein HC, Miller ME, Genuth S, et al. Long-term effects of intensive glucose lowering on cardiovascular outcomes. *N Engl J Med.* 2011;364(9):818-828.
107. Rodbard HW, Blonde L, Braithwaite SS, et al; AACE Diabetes Mellitus Clinical Practice Guidelines Task Force. American Association of Clinical Endocrinologists medical guidelines for clinical practice for the management of diabetes mellitus. *Endocr Pract.* 2007;13(suppl 1):1-68. Erratum in: *Endocr Pract.* 2008;14(6):802-803.
108. Knowler WC, Barrett-Connor E, Fowler SE, et al; Diabetes Prevention Program Research Group. Reduction in the incidence of type 2 diabetes with lifestyle intervention or metformin. *N Engl J Med.* 2002;346(6):393-403.
109. Gregg EW, Chen H, Wagenknecht LE, et al; Look AHEAD Research Group. Association of an intensive lifestyle intervention with remission of type 2 diabetes. *JAMA.* 2012;308(23):2489-2496.
110. US Food and Drug Administration. FDA expands advice on statin risks. FDA Web page. www.fda.gov/forconsumers/consumerupdates/ucm293330.htm#3. Updated May 5, 2014. Accessed May 21, 2014.
111. US Preventive Services Task Force. Aspirin for the prevention of cardiovascular disease: U.S. Preventive Services Task Force recommendation statement. *Ann Intern Med.* 2009;150(6):396-404.
112. Pignone M, Alberts MJ, Colwell JA, et al. Aspirin for primary prevention of cardiovascular events in people with diabetes: a position statement of the American Diabetes Association, a scientific statement of the American Heart Association, and an expert consensus document of the American College of Cardiology Foundation. *Circulation.* 2010;121(24):2694-2701.
113. Espeland MA, Hogan PE, Fineberg SE, et al. Effect of postmenopausal hormone therapy on glucose and insulin concentrations. PEPI Investigators. Postmenopausal Estrogen/Progestin Interventions. *Diabetes Care.* 1998; 21(10):1589-1595.
114. Margolis KL, Bonds DE, Rodabough RJ, et al; Women's Health Initiative Investigators. Effect of oestrogen plus progestin on the incidence of diabetes in postmenopausal women: results from the Women's Health Initiative Hormone Trial. *Diabetologia.* 2004;47(7):1175-1187.
115. Bonds DE, Lasser N, Qi L, et al. The effect of conjugated equine oestrogen on diabetes incidence: the Women's Health Initiative randomised trial. *Diabetologia.* 2006;49(3):459-468.
116. Kanaya AM, Herrington D, Vittinghoff E, et al; Heart and Estrogen/progestin Replacement Study. Glycemic effects of postmenopausal hormone therapy: the Heart and Estrogen/progestin Replacement Study. A randomized, double-blind, placebo-controlled trial. *Ann Intern Med.* 2003;138(1):1-9.
117. Hulley S, Grady D, Bush T, et al. Randomized trial of estrogen plus progestin for secondary prevention of coronary heart disease in postmenopausal women. Heart and Estrogen/progestin Replacement Study (HERS) Research Group. *JAMA.* 1998;280(7):605-613.
118. Grady D, Wenger NK, Herrington D, et al. Postmenopausal hormone therapy increases risk for venous thromboembolic disease. The Heart and Estrogen/progestin Replacement Study. *Ann Intern Med.* 2000;132(9):689-696.
119. Klein BE, Klein R, Moss SE. Exogenous estrogen exposures and changes in diabetic retinopathy. The Wisconsin Epidemiologic Study of Diabetic Retinopathy. *Diabetes Care.* 1999;22(12):1984-1987.
120. ACOG Committee on Practice Bulletins-Gynecology. ACOG practice bulletin. No. 73: Use of hormonal contraception in women with coexisting medical conditions. *Obstet Gynecol.* 2006;107(6):1453-1472.
121. Rossouw JE, Cushman M, Greenland P, et al. Inflammatory, lipid, thrombotic, and genetic markers of coronary heart disease risk in the women's health initiative trials of hormone therapy. *Arch Intern Med.* 2008;168(20):2245-2253.
122. Wild RA, Wu C, Curb JD, et al. Coronary heart disease events in the Women's Health Initiative hormone trials: effect modification by metabolic syndrome: a nested case-control study within the Women's Health Initiative randomized clinical trials. *Menopause.* 2013;20(3):254-260.
123. Management of osteoporosis in postmenopausal women: 2010 position statement of The North American Menopause Society. *Menopause.* 2010; 17(1):25-54.
124. NIH Consensus Development Panel on Osteoporosis Prevention, Diagnosis, and Therapy. Osteoporosis prevention, diagnosis, and therapy. *JAMA.* 2001; 85(6):785-795.
125. Khosla S, Riggs BL. Pathophysiology of age-related bone loss and osteoporosis. *Endocrinol Metab Clin North Am.* 2005;34(4):1015-1030.
126. Looker AC, Wahner HW, Dunn WL, et al. Updated data on proximal femur bone mineral levels of US adults. *Osteoporos Int.* 1998;8(5):468-489.
127. Kanis JA on behalf of the World Health Organization Scientific Group. *Assessment of Osteoporosis at the Primary Health Care Level.* Technical Report. World Health Organization Collaborating Centre for Metabolic Bone Diseases. Sheffield, UK: University of Sheffield; 2008.
128. Eastell R. Forearm fracture. *Bone.* 1996;18(suppl 3):203S-207S.
129. National Osteoporosis Foundation. *Clinician's Guide to Prevention and Treatment of Osteoporosis.* Washington, DC: National Osteoporosis Foundation; 2014.
130. Brennan K, Chaudhuri G, Nathan L. Osteoporosis and falls. In: DiSaia PJ, Chaudhuri G, Guidice MD, Moore TR, Smith LH Jr, Porto M, eds. *Women's Health Review: A Clinical Update in Obstetrics-Gynecology.* Philadelphia, PA: Saunders; 2012:427-436.
131. Barrett-Connor E, Siris ES, Wehren LE, et al. Osteoporosis and fracture risk in women of different ethnic groups. *J Bone Miner Res.* 2005;20(2):185-194.
132. Wright NC, Saag KG, Curtis JR, et al. Recent trends in hip fracture rates by race/ethnicity among older US adults. *J Bone Miner Res.* 2012;27(11): 2325-2332.

133. Leslie WD, O'Donnell S, Jean S, et al; Osteoporosis Surveillance Expert Working Group. Trends in hip fracture rates in Canada. *JAMA.* 2009; 303(8):883-839.
134. Stevens JA, Rudd RA. The impact of decreasing US hip fracture rates on future hip fracture estimates. *Osteoporos Int.* 2013;24(10):2725-2728.
135. Amin S, Achenbach SJ, Atkinson EJ, Khosla S, Melton LJ 3rd. Trends in fracture incidence: a population-based study over 20 years. *J Bone Miner Res.* 2014;29(3):581-589.
136. Silverman SL. Selecting patients for osteoporosis therapy. *Curr Osteoporos Rep.* 2006;4(3):91-95.
137. McCloskey E, Kanis JA. FRAX updates 2012. *Curr Opin Rheumatol.* 2012;24(5):554-560.
138. Johnell O, Gullberg B, Kanis JA, et al. Risk factors for hip fracture in European women: the MEDOS Study. Mediterranean Osteoporosis Study. *J Bone Miner Res.* 1995;10(11):1802-1815.
139. Cummings SR, Black DM, Nevitt MC, et al. Bone density at various sites for prediction of hip fractures. The Study of Osteoporotic Fractures Research Group. *Lancet.* 1993;341(8837):72-75.
140. Jiang X, Westermann LB, Galleo GV, Demko J, Marakovits KA, Schnatz PF. Age as a predictor of osteoporotic fracture compared with current risk-prediction models. *Obstet Gynecol.* 2012;122(5):1040-1046.
141. Kanis JA, Johnell O, Oden A, Dawson A, De Laet C, Jonsson B. Ten-year probabilities of osteoporotic fractures according to bone mineral density and diagnostic thresholds. *Osteoporos Int.* 2001;12(12):989-995.
142. Klotzbuecher CM, Ross PD, Landsman PB, Abbott TA 3rd, Berger M. Patients with prior fractures have an increased risk of future fractures: a summary of the literature and statistical synthesis. *J Bone Miner Res.* 2000; 15(4):721-739.
143. Kanis JA, Johnell O, De Laet C, et al. A meta-analysis of previous fracture and fracture risk. *Bone.* 2004;35(2):375-382.
144. Bauer DC, Browner WS, Cauley JA, et al. Factors associated with appendicular bone mass in older women. The Study of Osteoporotic Fractures Research Group. *Ann Intern Med.* 1993;118(9):657-665.
145. Seeman E, Hopper JL, Bach LA, et al. Reduced bone mass in daughters of women with osteoporosis. *N Engl J Med.* 1989;320(9):554-558.
146. Evans RA, Marel GM, Lancaster EK, Kos S, Evans M, Wong SY. Bone mass is low in relatives of osteoporotic patients. *Ann Intern Med.* 1988;109(11): 870-873.
147. Cummings SR, Nevitt MC, Browner WS, et al. Risk factors for hip fracture in white women. Study of Osteoporotic Fractures Research Group. *N Engl J Med.* 1995;332(12):767-773.
148. Ensrud KE, Lipschutz RC, Cauley JA, et al. Body size and hip fracture risk in older women: a prospective study. Study of Osteoporotic Fractures Research Group. *Am J Med.* 1997;103(4):274-280.
149. van der Voort DJ, Geusens PP, Dinant GJ. Risk factors for osteoporosis related to their outcome: fractures. *Osteoporos Int.* 2001;12(8):630-638.
150. Holick MF, Binkley NC, Bischoff-Ferrari HA, et al; Endocrine Society. Evaluation, treatment, and prevention of vitamin D deficiency: an Endocrine Society clinical practice guideline. *J Clin Endocrinol Metab.* 2011;96(7):1911-1930. Erratum in: *J Clin Endocrinol Metab.* 2011;96(12):3908.
151. Holick MF, Binkley NC, Bischoff-Ferrari HA, et al. Guidelines for preventing and treating vitamin D deficiency and insufficiency revisited. *J Clin Endocrinol Metab.* 2012;97(4):1153-1158.
152. Standing Committee on the Scientific Evaluation of Dietary Reference Intakes. Food and Nutrition Board Institute of Medicine. *DRI Dietary Reference Intakes: Calcium, Phosphorus, Magnesium, Vitamin D, and Fluoride.* Washington, DC: National Academy Press; 1997.
153. Mutlu M, Argun M, Kilic E, Saraymen R, Yazar S. Magnesium, zinc and copper status in osteoporotic, osteopenic and normal post-menopausal women. *J Int Med Res.* 2007;35(5):692-695.
154. Nieves JW. Osteoporosis: the role of micronutrients. *Am J Clin Nutr.* 2005; 81(5):1232S-1239S.
155. Odabasi E, Turan M, Aydin A, Akay C, Kutlu M. Magnesium, zinc, copper, manganese, and selenium levels in postmenopausal women with osteoporosis. Can magnesium play a key role in osteoporosis? *Ann Acad Med Singapore.* 2008;37(7):564-567.
156. Lunt M, Masaryk P, Scheidt-Nave C, et al. The effects of lifestyle, dietary dairy intake on bone density and vertebral deformity prevalence: the EVOS study. *Osteoporos Int.* 2001;12(8):688-698.
157. Wilsgaard T, Emaus N, Ahmed LA. Lifestyle impact on lifetime bone loss in women and men: the Tromsø Study. *Am J Epidemiol.* 2009;169(7):877-886.
158. Dook JE, James C, Henderson NK, Price RI. Exercise and bone mineral density in mature female athletes. *Med Sci Sports Exerc.* 1997;29(3):291-296.
159. Robertson MC, Campbell AJ, Gardner MM, Devlin N. Preventing injuries in older people by preventing falls: a meta-analysis of individual-level data. *J Am Geriatr Soc.* 2002;50(5):905-911.
160. Cummings SR, Melton LJ. Epidemiology and outcomes of osteoporotic fractures. *Lancet.* 2002;359(9319):1761-1767.
161. Genant HK, Jergas M, Palermo L, et al. Comparison of semiquantitative visual and quantitative morphometric assessment of prevalent and incident vertebral fractures in osteoporosis. The Study of Osteoporotic Fractures Research Group. *J Bone Miner Res.* 1996;11(7):984-996.
162. O'Loughlin JL, Robitaille Y, Boivin JF, Suissa S. Incidence of and risk factors for falls and injurious falls among the community-dwelling elderly. *Am J Epidemiol.* 1993;137(3):342-354.
163. Gillespie LD, Robertson MC, Gillespie WJ, et al. Interventions for preventing falls in older people living in the community. *Cochrane Database Syst Rev.* 2012;9:CD007146.
164. Waldron N, Hill AM, Barker A. Falls prevention in older adults—assessment and management. *Aust Fam Physician.* 2012;41(12):930-935.
165. Gillespie WJ, Gillespie LD, Parker MJ. Hip protectors for preventing hip fractures in older people. *Cochrane Database Syst Rev.* 2010;(10):CD001255.
166. Slemenda CW, Hui SL, Longcope C, Johnston CC Jr. Cigarette smoking, obesity, and bone mass. *J Bone Miner Res.* 1989;4(5):737-741.
167. Kato I, Toniolo P, Akhmedkhanov A, et al. Prospective study of factors influencing the onset of natural menopause. *J Clin Epidemiol.* 1998;51(12):1271-1276.
168. Krall EA, Dawson-Hughes B. Smoking and bone loss among postmenopausal women. *J Bone Miner Res.* 1991;6(4):331-338.
169. Baron JA, Farahmand BY, Weiderpass E, et al. Cigarette smoking, alcohol consumption, and risk for hip fracture in women. *Arch Intern Med.* 2001; 161(7):983-988.
170. Tucker KL, Jugdaohsingh R, Powell JJ, et al. Effects of beer, wine, and liquor intakes on bone mineral density in older men and women. *Am J Clin Nutr.* 2009;89(4):1188-1196.
171. Felson DT, Zhang Y, Hannan MT, Kannel WB, Kiel DP. Alcohol intake and bone mineral density in elderly men and women. The Framingham Study. *Am J Epidemiol.* 1995;142(5):485-492.
172. Felson DT, Kiel DP, Anderson JJ, Kannel WB. Alcohol consumption and hip fractures: the Framingham Study. *Am J Epidemiol.* 1988;128(5):1102-1110.
173. Recker R, Lappe J, Davies K, Heaney R. Characterization of perimenopausal bone loss: a prospective study. *J Bone Miner Res.* 2000;15(10):1965-1973.
174. Pouillès JM, Trémollières F, Ribot C. Vertebral bone loss in perimenopause. Results of a 7-year longitudinal study [article in French]. *Presse Med.* 1996; 25(7):277-280.
175. Devine A, Dick IM, Dhaliwal SS, Naheed R, Beilby J, Prince RL. Prediction of incident osteoporotic fractures in elderly women using the free estradiol index. *Osteoporos Int.* 2005;16(2):216-221.
176. Pouillès JM, Trémollières F, Bonneu M, Ribot C. Influence of early age at menopause on vertebral bone mass. *J Bone Miner Res.* 1994;9(3):311-315.
177. Ohta H, Sugimoto I, Masuda A, et al. Decreased bone mineral density associated with early menopause progresses for at least ten years: cross-sectional comparisons between early and normal menopausal women. *Bone.* 1996;18(3):227-231.
178. Gerdhem P, Obrant KJ. Bone mineral density in old age: the influence of age at menarche and menopause. *J Bone Miner Metab.* 2004;22(4):372-375.
179. Watts NB, Bilezikian JP, Camacho PM, et al; AACE Osteoporosis Task Force. American Association of Clinical Endocrinologists Medical Guidelines for Clinical Practice for the diagnosis and treatment of postmenopausal osteoporosis. *Endocr Pract.* 2010;16(suppl 3):1-37.
180. Majumdar SR, Kim N, Colman I, et al. Incidental vertebral fractures discovered with chest radiography in the emergency department: prevalence, recognition, and osteoporosis management in a cohort of elderly patients. *Arch Intern Med.* 2005;165(8):905-909.
181. Schneider DL, von Mühlen D, Barrett-Connor E, Sartoris DJ. Kyphosis does not equal vertebral fractures: the Rancho Bernardo study. *J Rheumatol.* 2004;31(4):747-752.
182. Greenspan SL, von Stetten E, Emond SK, Jones L, Parker RA. Instant vertebral assessment: a noninvasive dual x-ray absorptiometry technique to avoid misclassification and clinical mismanagement of osteoporosis. *J Clin Densitom.* 2001;4(4):373-380.
183. Ferrar L, Jiang G, Barrington NA, Eastell R. Identification of vertebral deformities in women: comparison of radiological assessment and quantitative morphometry using morphometric radiography and morphometric x-ray absorptiometry. *J Bone Miner Res.* 2000;15(3):575-585.
184. US Preventive Services Task Force. Screening for osteoporosis: US preventive services task force recommendation statement. *Ann Intern Med.* 2011;154(5):356-364.

Chapter 4

185. Kanis JA, Borgstrom F, De Laet C, et al. Assessment of fracture risk. *Osteoporos Int.* 2005;16(6):581-589.
186. Knoke JD, Barrett-Connor E. Weight loss: a determinant of hip bone loss in older men and women. The Rancho Bernardo Study. *Am J Epidemiol.* 2003;158(12):1132-1138.
187. Schousboe JT, Bauer DC, Nyman JA, Kane RL, Melton LJ, Ensrud KE. Potential for bone turnover markers to cost-effectively identify and select post-menopausal osteopenic women at high risk of fracture for bisphosphonate therapy. *Osteoporos Int.* 2007;18(2):201-210.
188. Delmas PD, Munoz F, Black DM, et al; HORIZON-PFT Research Group. Effects of yearly zoledronic acid 5 mg on bone turnover markers and relation of PINP with fracture reduction in postmenopausal women with osteoporosis. *J Bone Miner Res.* 2009;24(9):1544-1551.
189. Marcus R, Holloway L, Wells B, et al. The relationship of biochemical markers of bone turnover to bone density changes in postmenopausal women: results from the Postmenopausal Estrogen/Progestin Interventions (PEPI) trial. *J Bone Miner Res.* 1999;14(9):1583-1595.
190. Miller PD, Baran DT, Bilezikian JT, et al. Practical clinical applications of biochemical markers of bone turnover: consensus of an expert panel. *J Clin Densitom.* 1999;2(3):323-342.
191. Cerdá Gabaroi D, Peris P, Monegal A, et al. Search for hidden secondary causes in postmenopausal women with osteoporosis. *Menopause.* 2010;17(1):135-139.
192. Hudec SM, Camacho PM. Secondary causes of osteoporosis. *Endocr Pract.* 2013;19(1):120-128.
193. Tannenbaum C, Clark J, Schwartzman K, et al. Yield of laboratory testing to identify secondary contributors to osteoporosis in otherwise healthy women. *J Clin Endocrinol Metab.* 2002;87(10):4431-4437.
194. McCombs JS, Thiebaud P, McLaughlin-Miley C, Shi J. Compliance with drug therapies for the treatment and prevention of osteoporosis. *Maturitas.* 2004;48(3):271-287.
195. Tosteson AN, Grove MR, Hammond CS, et al. Early discontinuation of treatment for osteoporosis. *Am J Med.* 2003;115(3):209-216.
196. Segal E, Tamir A, Ish-Shalom S. Compliance of osteoporotic patients with different treatment regimens. *Isr Med Assoc J.* 2003;5(12):859-862.
197. Penning-van Beest, FJ, Erkens, JA, Olson, M, Herings, RM. Determinants of non-compliance with bisphosphonates in women with postmenopausal osteoporosis. *Curr Med Res Opin.* 2008;24(5):1337-1344.
198. Papaioannou A, Kennedy CC, Dolovich L, Lau E, Adachi JD. Patient adherence to osteoporosis medications: problems, consequences and management strategies. *Drugs Aging.* 2007;24(1):37-55.
199. Gold DT, Silverman S. Review of adherence to medications for the treatment of osteoporosis. *Curr Osteoporos Rep.* 2006;4(1):21-27.
200. McClung M. Bisphosphonates. *Endocrinol Metab Clin North Am.* 2003;32(1):253-271.
201. Migliorati CA, Casiglia J, Epstein J, Jacobsen PL, Siegel MA, Woo SB. Managing the care of patients with bisphosphonate-associated osteonecrosis: an American Academy of Oral Medicine position paper. *J Am Dent Assoc.* 2005;136(12):1658-1668. Erratum in: *J Am Dent Assoc.* 2006;137(1):26.
202. Ruggiero SL, Mehrotra B, Rosenberg TJ, Engroff SL. Osteonecrosis of the jaws associated with the use of bisphosphonates: a review of 63 cases. *J Oral Maxillofac Surg.* 2004;62(5):527-534.
203. Khosla S, Burr D, Cauley J, et al; American Society for Bone and Mineral Research. Bisphosphonate-associated osteonecrosis of the jaw: report of a task force of the American Society for Bone and Mineral Research. *J Bone Miner Res.* 2007;22(10):1479-1491.
204. Dell RM, Adams AL, Greene DF, et al. Incidence of atypical nontraumatic diaphyseal fractures of the femur. *J Bone Miner Res.* 2012;27(12):2544-2550.
205. Shane E, Burr D, Abrahamsen B, et al. Atypical subtrochanteric and diaphyseal femoral fractures: second report of a task force of the American Society for Bone and Mineral Research. *J Bone Miner Res.* 2013;29(1):1-23.
206. McClung MR, Wasnich RD, Hosking DJ, et al; Early Postmenopausal Intervention Cohort Study. Prevention of postmenopausal bone loss: six-year results from the Early Postmenopausal Intervention Cohort Study. *J Clin Endocrinol Metab.* 2004;89(10):4879-4885.
207. Ensrud KE, Barrett-Connor EL, Schwartz A, et al; Fracture Intervention Trial Long-Term Extension Research Group. Randomized trial of effect of alendronate continuation versus discontinuation in women with low BMD: results from the Fracture Intervention Trial long-term extension. *J Bone Miner Res.* 2004;19(8):1259-1269.
208. Bone HG, Hosking D, Devogelaer JP, et al; Alendronate Phase III Osteoporosis Treatment Study Group. Ten years' experience with alendronate for osteoporosis in postmenopausal women. *N Engl J Med.* 2004;350(12):1189-1199.
209. Mellström DD, Sörensen OH, Goemaere S, Roux C, Johnson TD, Chines AA. Seven years of treatment with risedronate in women with postmenopausal osteoporosis. *Calcif Tissue Int.* 2004;75(6):462-468.
210. Black DM, Schwartz AV, Ensrud KE, et al; FLEX Research Group. Effects of continuing or stopping alendronate after 5 years of treatment: the Fracture Intervention Trial Long-term Extension (FLEX): a randomized trial. *JAMA.* 2006;296(24):2927-2938.
211. Black DM, Reid IR, Boonen S, et al. The effect of 3 versus 6 years of zoledronic acid treatment of osteoporosis: a randomized extension to the HORIZON-Pivotal Fracture Trial (PFT). *J Bone Miner Res.* 2012;27(2):243-254.
212. Grbic JT, Black DM, Lyles KW, et al. The incidence of osteonecrosis of the jaw in patients receiving 5 milligrams of zoledronic acid: data from the health outcomes and reduced incidence with zoledronic acid once yearly clinical trials program. *J Am Dent Assoc.* 2010;141(11):1365-1370.
213. Black DM, Kelly MP, Genant HK, et al; HORIZON Pivotal Fracture Trial Steering Committee. Bisphosphonates and fractures of the subtrochanteric or diaphyseal femur. *N Engl J Med.* 2010;362(19):1761-1771.
214. Wasnich RD, Bagger YZ, Hosking DJ, et al; Early Postmenopausal Intervention Cohort Study Group. Changes in bone density and turnover after alendronate or estrogen withdrawal. *Menopause.* 2004;11(6 pt 1):622-630.
215. Mortensen L, Charles P, Bekker PJ, Digennaro J, Johnston CC Jr. Risedronate increases bone mass in an early postmenopausal population: two years of treatment plus one year of follow-up. *J Clin Endocrinol Metab.* 1998;83(2):396-402.
216. Diab DL, Watts NB. Use of drug holidays in women taking bisphosphonates. *Menopause.* 2014;21(2):195-197.
217. Compston JE, Bilezikian JP. Bisphosphonate therapy for osteoporosis: the long and short of it. *J Bone Miner Res.* 2012;27(2):240-242.
218. Delmas PD, Bjarnason NH, Mitlak BH, et al. Effects of raloxifene on bone mineral density, serum cholesterol concentrations, and uterine endometrium in postmenopausal women. *N Engl J Med.* 1997;337(23):1641-1647.
219. Ettinger B, Black DM, Mitlack BH, et al. Reduction of vertebral fracture risk in postmenopausal women with osteoporosis treated with raloxifene: results from a 3-year randomized clinical trial. Multiple Outcomes of Raloxifene Evaluation (MORE) Investigators. *JAMA.* 1999;282(7):637-645.
220. Effects of hormone therapy on bone mineral density: results from the Postmenopausal Estrogen/Progestin Interventions (PEPI) trial. The Writing Group for the PEPI. *JAMA.* 1996;276(17):1389-1396.
221. Cauley JA, Robbins J, Chen Z, et al; Women's Health Initiative Investigators. Effects of estrogen plus progestin on risk of fracture and bone mineral density: the Women's Health Initiative randomized trial. *JAMA.* 2003;290(13):1729-1738.
222. Lindsay R, Gallagher JC, Kleerekoper M, Pickar JH. Effect of lower doses of conjugated equine estrogens with and without medroxyprogesterone acetate on bone in early postmenopausal women. *JAMA.* 2002;287(20):2668-2676.
223. Prestwood KM, Kenny AM, Kleppinger A, Kulldorff M. Ultralow-dose micronized 17beta-estradiol and bone density and bone metabolism in older women: a randomized controlled trial. *JAMA.* 2003;290(8):1042-1048.
224. Ettinger B, Ensrud KE, Wallace R, et al. Effects of ultralow-dose transdermal estradiol on bone mineral density: a randomized clinical trial. *Obstet Gynecol.* 2004;104(3):443-451.
225. Recker RR, Davies KM, Dowd RM, Heaney RP. The effect of low-dose continuous estrogen and progesterone therapy with calcium and vitamin D on bone in elderly women. A randomized, controlled trial. *Ann Intern Med.* 1999;130(11):897-904.
226. Weiss SR, Ellman H, Dolker M. A randomized controlled trial of four doses of transdermal estradiol for preventing postmenopausal bone loss. Transdermal Estradiol Investigator Group. *Obstet Gynecol.* 1999;94(3):330-336.
227. Wells G, Tugwell P, Shea B, et al; Osteoporosis Methodology Group and the Osteoporosis Research Advisory Group. Meta-analyses of therapies for postmenopausal osteoporosis. V. Meta-analysis of the efficacy of hormone replacement therapy in treating and preventing osteoporosis in postmenopausal women. *Endocr Rev.* 2002;23(4):529-539.
228. Al-Azzawi F, Lees B, Thompson J, Stevenson JC. Bone mineral density in postmenopausal women treated with a vaginal ring delivering systemic doses of estradiol acetate. *Menopause.* 2005;12(3):331-339.
229. Grady D, Rubin SM, Petitti DB, et al. Hormone therapy to prevent disease and prolong life in postmenopausal women. *Ann Intern Med.* 1992;117(12):1016-1037.
230. Torgerson DJ, Bell-Syer SE. Hormone replacement therapy and prevention of nonvertebral fractures: a meta-analysis of randomized trials. *JAMA.* 2001;285(22):2891-2897.

231. Siris ES, Miller PD, Barrett-Connor E, et al. Identification and fracture outcomes of undiagnosed low bone mineral density in postmenopausal women: results from the National Osteoporosis Risk Assessment. *JAMA.* 2001;286(22):2815-2822.
232. Banks E, Beral V, Reeves G, Balkwill A, Barnes I; Million Women Study Collaborators. Fracture incidence in relation to the pattern of use of hormone therapy in postmenopausal women. *JAMA.* 2004;291(18):2212-2220.
233. Anderson GL, Limacher M, Assaf AR, et al; Women's Health Initiative Steering Committee. Effects of conjugated equine estrogen in postmenopausal women with hysterectomy: the Women's Health Initiative randomized controlled trial. *JAMA.* 2004;291(14):1701-1712.
234. Gallagher JC, Rapuri PB, Haynatzki G, Detter JR. Effect of discontinuation of estrogen, calcitriol, and the combination of both on bone density and bone markers. *J Clin Endocrinol Metab.* 2002;87(11):4914-4923.
235. Greenspan SL, Emkey RD, Bone HG, et al. Significant differential effects of alendronate, estrogen, or combination therapy on the rate of bone loss after discontinuation of treatment of postmenopausal osteoporosis. A randomized, double-blind, placebo-controlled trial. *Ann Intern Med.* 2002;137(11):875-883.
236. Trémollieres FA, Pouilles JM, Ribot C. Withdrawal of hormone replacement therapy is associated with significant vertebral bone loss in postmenopausal women. *Osteoporos Int.* 2001;12(5):385-390.
237. Pinkerton JV, Harvey JA, Lindsay R, et al; SMART-5 Investigators. Effects of bazedoxifene/conjugated estrogens on the endometrium and bone: a randomized trial. *J Clin Endocrinol Metab.* 2014;99(2):E189-E198.
238. Lindsay R, Gallagher JC, Kagan R, Pickar JH, Constantine G. Efficacy of tissue-selective estrogen complex of bazedoxifene/conjugated estrogens for osteoporosis prevention in at-risk postmenopausal women. *Fertil Steril.* 2009;92(3):1045-1052.
239. European Medicines Agency. Calcitonin. European Medicines Agency Web site. www.ema.europa.eu/ema/index.jsp?curl=pages/medicines/human/referrals/Calcitonin/human_referral_000319.jsp&mid=WC0b01ac0580024e99. Accessed May 20, 2014.
240. Healthy Canadians. Synthetic calcitonin (salmon) nasal spray (NS)—market withdrawal of all products, effective October 1st, 2013—for health professionals. Healthy Canadians Web site. Published July 31, 2013. http://healthycanadians.gc.ca/recall-alert-rappel-avis/hc-sc/2013/34783a-eng.php. Accessed May 10, 2014.
241. McClung MR, Lewiecki EM, Cohen SB, et al; Bone Loss Study Group. Denosumab in postmenopausal women with low bone mineral density. *N Engl J Med.* 2006;354(8):821-831.
242. Cummings SR, San Martin J, McClung MR, et al; FREEDOM Trial. Denosumab for prevention of fractures in postmenopausal women with osteoporosis. *N Engl J Med.* 2009;361(8):756-765. Erratum in: *N Engl J Med.* 2009;361(19):1914.
243. McClung MR, Lewiecki EM, Geller ML, et al. Effect of denosumab on bone mineral density and biochemical markers of bone turnover: 8-year results of a phase 2 clinical trial. *Osteoporos Int.* 2013;24(1):227-235.
244. Watts NB, Roux C, Modlin JF, et al. Infections in postmenopausal women with osteoporosis treated with denosumab or placebo: coincidence or causal association? *Osteoporos Int.* 2012;23(1):327-337.
245. Cummings SR, Ettinger B, Delmas PD, et al; LIFT Trial Investigators. The effects of tibolone in older postmenopausal women. *N Engl J Med.* 2008;359(7):697-708.
246. Yoshiga D, Yamashita Y, Nakamichi I, et al. Weekly teriparatide injections successfully treated advanced bisphosphonate-related osteonecrosis of the jaws. *Osteoporos Int.* 2013;24(8):2365-2369.
247. Chiang CY, Zebaze RM, Ghasem-Zadeh A, Iuliano-Burns S, Hardidge A, Seeman E. Teriparatide improves bone quality and healing of atypical femoral fractures associated with bisphosphonate therapy. *Bone.* 2013;52(1):360-365.
248. Bone HG, Greenspan SL, McKeever C, et al. Alendronate and estrogen effect in postmenopausal women with low bone mineral density. Alendronate/Estrogen Study Group. *J Clin Endocrinol Metab.* 2000;85(2):720-726.
249. Lindsay R, Nieves J, Formica C, et al. Randomised controlled study of effect of parathyroid hormone on vertebral-bone mass and fracture incidence among postmenopausal women on oestrogen with osteoporosis. *Lancet.* 1997;350(9077):550-555.
250. Cosman F, Wermers RA, Recknor C, et al. Effects of teriparatide in postmenopausal women with osteoporosis on prior alendronate or raloxifene: differences between stopping and continuing the antiresorptive agent. *J Clin Endocrinol Metab.* 2009;94(10):3772-3780.
251. Tsai JN, Uihlein AV, Lee H, et al. Teriparatide and denosumab, alone or combined, in women with postmenopausal osteoporosis: the DATA study randomised trial. *Lancet.* 2013;382(9886):50-56.
252. Greenspan SL, Bone HG, Ettinger MP, et al; Treatment of Osteoporosis with Parathyroid Hormone Study Group. Effect of recombinant human parathyroid hormone (1-84) on vertebral fracture and bone mineral density in postmenopausal women with osteoporosis: a randomized trial. *Ann Intern Med.* 2007;146(5):326-339.
253. Langdahl B, Binkley N, Bone H, et al. Odanacatib in the treatment of postmenopausal women with low bone mineral density: five years of continued therapy in a phase 2 study. *J Bone Miner Res.* 2012;27(11):2251-2258.
254. Brixen K, Chapurlat R, Cheung AM, et al. Bone density, turnover, and estimated strength in postmenopausal women treated with odanacatib: a randomized trial. *J Clin Endocrinol Metab.* 2013;98(2):571-580.
255. McClung MR, Grauer A, Boonen S, et al. Romosozumab in postmenopausal women with low bone mineral density. *N Engl J Med.* 2014;370(5):412-420.
256. Cosman F, Lane NE, Bolognese MA, et al. Effect of transdermal teriparatide administration on bone mineral density in postmenopausal women. *J Clin Endocrinol Metab.* 2010;95(1):151-158.
257. Henriksen K, Andersen JR, Riis BJ, et al. Evaluation of the efficacy, safety and pharmacokinetic profile of oral recombinant human parathyroid hormone [rhPTH(1-31)NH(2)] in postmenopausal women with osteoporosis. *Bone.* 2013;53(1):160-166.
258. Horwitz MJ, Augustine M, Kahn L, et al. A comparison of parathyroid hormone-related protein (1-36) and parathyroid hormone (1-34) on markers of bone turnover and bone density in postmenopausal women: the PrOP study. *J Bone Miner Res.* 2013;28(11):2266-2276.
259. Esbrit P, Alcaraz MJ. Current perspectives on parathyroid hormone (PTH) and PTH-related protein (PTHrP) as bone anabolic therapies. *Biochem Pharmacol.* 2013;85(10):1417-1423.
260. Shaffer EA. Epidemiology and risk factors for gallstone disease: has the paradigm changed in the 21st century? *Curr Gastroenterol Rep.* 2005;7(2):132-140.
261. Marjoribanks J, Farquhar C, Roberts H, Lethaby A. Long term hormone therapy for perimenopausal and postmenopausal women. *Cochrane Database System Rev.* 2012;7:CD004143.
262. Cirillo DJ, Wallace RB, Rodabough RJ, et al. Effect of estrogen therapy on gallbladder disease. *JAMA.* 2005;293(3):330-339.
263. Santen RJ, Allred DC, Ardoin SP, et al; Endocrine Society. Postmenopausal hormone therapy: an Endocrine Society scientific statement. *J Clin Endocrinol Metab.* 2010;95(7 suppl 1):S1-S66.
264. Liu B, Beral V, Balkwill A, Green J, Sweetland S, Reeves G; Million Women Study Collaborators. Gallbladder disease and use of transdermal versus oral hormone replacement therapy in postmenopausal women: prospective cohort study. *BMJ.* 2008;337:a386.
265. Uhler ML, Marks JW, Voigt BJ, Judd HL. Comparison of the impact of transdermal versus oral estrogen on biliary markers of gallstone formation in postmenopausal women. *J Clin Endocrinol Metab.* 1998;83(2):410-414.
266. Wang HH, Liu M, Clegg DJ, Portincasa P, Wang DQ. New insights into the molecular mechanisms underlying effects of estrogen on cholesterol gallstone formation. *Biochim Biophys Acta.* 2009;1791(11):1037-1047.
267. Morimoto LM, Newcomb PA, Hampton JM, Trentham-Dietz A. Cholecystectomy and endometrial cancer: a marker of long-term elevated estrogen exposure? *Int J Gynecol Cancer.* 2006;16(3):1348-1353.
268. Racine A, Bijon A, Fournier A, et al. Menopausal hormone therapy and risk of cholecystectomy: a prospective study based on the French E3N cohort. *CMAJ.* 2013;185(7):555-561.
269. Friel NA, Chu CR. The role of ACL injury in the development of posttraumatic knee osteoarthritis. *Clin Sports Med.* 2013;32(1):1-12.
270. Hochberg MC, Altman RD, April KT, et al; American College of Rheumatology. American College of Rheumatology 2012 recommendations for the use of nonpharmacologic and pharmacologic therapies in osteoarthritis of the hand, hip, and knee. *Arthritis Care Res (Hoboken).* 2012;64(4):465-474.
271. Block JA, Shakoor N. Lower limb osteoarthritis: biomechanical alterations and implications for therapy. *Curr Opin Rheumatol.* 2010;22(5):544-550.
272. Block JA, Oegema TR, Sandy JD, Plaas A. The effects of oral glucosamine on joint health: is a change in research approach needed? *Osteoarthritis Cartilage.* 2010;18(1):5-11.
273. Vlad SC, LaValley MP, McAlindon TE, Felson DT. Glucosamine for pain in osteoarthritis: why do trial results differ? *Arthritis Rheum.* 2007;56(7):2267-2277.
274. Scott DL, Wolfe F, Huizinga TW. Rheumatoid arthritis. *Lancet.* 2010;376(9746):1094-1108.
275. Edwards NL. Crystal deposition diseases. In: Goldman L, Schafer A, eds. *Goldman's Cecil Medicine.* 24th ed. Maryland Heights, MO: Saunders; 2012:1737-1743.

Chapter 4

276. Sowers M, Luborsky J, Perdue C, Araujo KL, Goldman MB; SWAN. Thyroid stimulating hormone (TSH) concentrations and menopausal status in women at the mid-life: SWAN. *Clin Endocrinol (Oxf)*. 2003;58(3):340-347.
277. Hollowell JG, Staehling NW, Flanders WD, et al. Serum TSH, and thyroid antibodies in the United States population (1988 to 1994): National Health and Nutrition Examination Survey (NHANES III). *J Clin Endocrinol Metab*. 2002;87(2):489-499.
278. Ladenson PW, Singer PA, Ain KB, et al. American Thyroid Association guidelines for detection of thyroid dysfunction. *Arch Intern Med*. 2000;160(11):1573-1575. Erratum in: *Arch Intern Med*. 2001;161(2):284.
279. US Preventive Services Task Force. Screening for thyroid disease: recommendation statement. *Ann Intern Med*. 2004;140(2):125-127.
280. Beaulieu M-D. Screening for thyroid disorders and thyroid cancer in asymptomatic adults. In: Canadian Task Force on the Periodic Health Examination. *Canadian Guide to Clinical Preventive Health Care*. Ottawa, ON, Canada: Canada Communication Group; 1994:611-618.
281. Garber JR, Cobin RH, Gharib H, et al; American Association of Clinical Endocrinologists and American Thyroid Association Taskforce on Hypothyroidism in Adults. Clinical practice guidelines for hypothyroidism in adults: cosponsored by the American Association of Clinical Endocrinologists and the American Thyroid Association. *Endocr Pract*. 2012;18(6):988-1028. Erratum in: *Endocr Pract*. 2013;19(1):175.
282. Cooper DS, Biondi B. Subclinical thyroid disease. *Lancet*. 2012;379(9821):1142-1154.
283. Biondi B, Wartofsky L. Treatment with thyroid hormone. *Endocr Rev*. 2014;35(3):433-512.
284. Persani L. Clinical review: central hypothyroidism: pathogenic, diagnostic, and therapeutic challenges. *J Clin Endocrinol Metab*. 2012;97(9):3068-3078.
285. Aggarwal N, Razvi S. Thyroid and aging or the aging thyroid? An evidence-based analysis of the literature. *J Thyroid Res*. 2013;2013:481287.
286. Shifren J, Desindes S, McIlwain M, Doros G, Mazer NA. A randomized, open-label, crossover study comparing the effects of oral versus transdermal estrogen therapy on serum androgens, thyroid hormones, and adrenal hormones in naturally menopausal women. *Menopause*. 2007;14(6):985-994.
287. Tahboub R, Arafah BM. Sex steroids and the thyroid. *Best Pract Res Clin Endocrinol Metab*. 2009;23(6):769-780.
288. Taylor PN, Razvi S, Pearce SH, Dayan CM. Clinical review: a review of the clinical consequences of variation in thyroid function within the reference range. *J Clin Endocrinol Metab*. 2013;98(9):3562-3571.
289. Hyland KA, Arnold AM, Lee JS, Cappola AR. Persistent subclinical hypothyroidism and cardiovascular risk in the elderly: the Cardiovascular Health Study. *J Clin Endocrinol Metab*. 2013;98(2):533-540.
290. Pasqualetti G, Tognini S, Polini A, Caraccio N, Monazni F. Is subclinical hypothyroidism a cardiovascular risk factor in the elderly? *J Clin Endocrinol Metab*. 2013;98(6):2256-2266.
291. LeGrys VA, Funk MJ, Lorenz CE, et al. Subclinical hypothyroidism and risk for incident myocardial infarction among postmenopausal women. *J Clin Endocrinol Metab*. 2013;98(6):2308-2317.
292. Rodondi N, den Elzen WP, Bauer DC, et al; Thyroid Studies Collaboration. Subclinical hypothyroidism and the risk of coronary heart disease and mortality. *JAMA*. 2010;304(12):1365-1374.
293. Razvi S, Weaver JU, Butler TJ, Pearce SHS. Levothyroxine treatment of subclinical hypothyroidism, fatal and nonfatal cardiovascular events, and mortality. *Arch Intern Med*. 2012;172(10):811-817.
294. Bahn RS, Burch HB, Cooper DS, et al; American Thyroid Association and American Association of Clinical Endocrinologists. Hyperthyroidism and other causes of thyrotoxicosis: management guidelines of the American Thyroid Association and American Association of Clinical Endocrinologists. *Endocr Pract*. 2011;17(3):456-520. Erratum in: *Endocr Pract*. 2013;19(2):384.
295. Burch HB, Burman KD, Cooper DS. A 2011 survey of clinical practice patterns in the management of Graves' disease. *J Clin Endocrinol Metab*. 2012;97(12):4549-4558.
296. Collet TH, Gussekloo J, Bauer DC, et al; Thyroid Studies Collaboration. Subclinical hyperthyroidism and the risk of coronary heart disease and mortality. *Arch Intern Med*. 2012;172(10):799-809.
297. Bauer DC, Ettinger B, Nevitt MC, Stone KL; Study of Osteoporotic Fractures Research Group. Risk for fracture in women with low serum levels of thyroid-stimulating hormone. *Ann Intern Med*. 2001;134(7):561-568.
298. Surks MI, Ortiz E, Daniels GH, et al. Subclinical thyroid disease: scientific review and guidelines for diagnosis and management. *JAMA*. 2004;291(2):228-238.
299. Greenspan SL, Greenspan FS. The effect of thyroid hormone on skeletal integrity. *Ann Intern Med*. 1999;130(9):750-758.
300. American Thyroid Association (ATA) Guidelines Taskforce on Thyroid Nodules and Differentiated Thyroid Cancer; Cooper DS, Doherty GM, Haugen RB, et al. Revised American Thyroid Association management guidelines for patients with thyroid nodules and differentiated thyroid cancer. *Thyroid*. 2009;19(11):1167-1214.
301. Gharib H, Papini E, Paschke R, et al; AACE/AME/ETA Task Force on Thyroid Nodules. American Association of Clinical Endocrinologists, Associazione Medici Endocrinologi, and European Thyroid Association Medical guidelines for clinical practice for the diagnosis and management of thyroid nodules: executive summary of recommendations. *Endocr Pract*. 2010;16(3):468-475.
302. Mirfakhraee S, Mathews D, Peng L, Woodruff S, Zigman JM. A solitary hyperfunctioning thyroid nodule harboring thyroid carcinoma: review of the literature. *Thyroid Res*. 2013;6(1):7.
303. Sethi NK, Harden CL. Epilepsy in older women. *Menopause Int*. 2008;14(2):85-87.
304. Herzog AG. Catamenial epilepsy: definition, prevalence, pathophysiology and treatment. *Seizure*. 2008;17(2):151-159.
305. Erel CT, Brincat M, Gambacciani M. et al. EMAS position statement: managing the menopause in women with epilepsy. *Maturitas*. 2010;66(3):327-328. Erratum in: *Maturitas*. 2011;69(2):e3.
306. Herzog AG, Coleman AE, Jacobs AR, et al. Interictal EEG discharges, reproductive hormones, and menstrual disorders in epilepsy. *Ann Neurol*. 2003;54(5):625-637.
307. Herzog AG. Disorders of reproduction in patients with epilepsy: primary neurological mechanisms. *Seizure*. 2008;17(2):101-110.
308. Klein P, Serje A, Pezzullo JC. Premature ovarian failure in women with epilepsy. *Epilepsia*. 2001;42(12):1584-1589.
309. Harden CL, Koppel BS, Herzog AG, Nikolov BG, Hauser WA. Seizure frequency is associated with age of menopause in women with epilepsy. *Neurology*. 2003;61(4):451-455.
310. Harden CL, Pulver MC, Ravdin L, Jacobs AR. The effect of menopause and perimenopause on the course of epilepsy. *Epilepsia*. 1999;40(10):1402-1407.
311. Herzog AG, Fowler KM, Smithson SD, et al; Progesterone Trial Study Group. Progesterone vs placebo therapy for women with epilepsy: a randomized clinical trial. *Neurology*. 2012;78(24):1959-1966.
312. Harden CL, Herzog AG, Nikolov BG, et al. Hormone replacement therapy in women with epilepsy: a randomized, double-blind, placebo-controlled study. *Epilepsia*. 2006;47(9):1447-1451.
313. Herzog AG, Blum AS, Farina EL, et al. Valproate and lamotrigine level variation with menstrual cycle phase and oral contraceptive use. *Neurology*. 2009;72(10):911-914.
314. Shorvon SD, Tallis RC, Wallace HK. Antiepileptic drugs: coprescription of proconvulsant drugs and oral contraceptives: a national study of antiepileptic drug prescribing practice. *J Neurol Neurosurg Psychiatry*. 2002;72(1):114-115.
315. Sabers A, Ohman I, Christensen J, Tomson T. Oral contraceptives reduce lamotrigine plasma levels. *Neurology*. 2003;61(4):570-571.
316. Harden CL. Issues for mature women with epilepsy. *Int Rev Neurobiol*. 2008;83:385-395.
317. Tomson T, Lukic S, Ohman I. Are lamotrigine kinetics altered in menopause? Observations from a drug monitoring database. *Epilepsy Behav*. 2010;19(1):86-88.
318. Feldkamp J, Becker A, Witte OW, Scharff D, Scherbaum WA. Long-term anticonvulsant therapy leads to low bone mineral density—evidence for direct drug effects of phenytoin and carbamazepine on human osteoblast-like cells. *Exp Clin Endocrinol Diabetes*. 2000;108(1):37-43.
319. Harden CL. Menopause and bone density issues for women with epilepsy. *Neurolology*. 2003;61(6 suppl 2):S16-S22.
320. Pedrera JD, Canal ML, Carvajal J, et al. Influence of vitamin D administration on bone ultrasound measurements in patients on anticonvulsant therapy. *Eur J Clin Invest*. 2000;30(10):895-899.
321. Townsend EA, Miller VM, Prakash YS. Sex differences and sex steroids in lung health and disease. *Endocr Rev*. 2012;33(1):1-47.
322. Dimitropoulou C, Drakopanagiotakis F, Catravas JD. Estrogen as a new therapeutic target for asthma and chronic obstructive pulmonary disease. *Drug News Perspect*. 2007;20(4):241-252.
323. Subbarao P, Mandhane PJ, Sears MR. Asthma: epidemiology, etiology and risk factors. *CMAJ*. 2009;181(9):E181-E190.
324. Melero Moreno C, López-Viña A, García-Salmones Martín M, Cisneros Serrano C, Jareño Esteban J, Ramirez Prieto MT; Grupo de Asma de Neumomadrid. Factors related with the higher percentage of hospitalizations due to asthma amongst women: the FRIAM study. *Arch Bronconeumol*. 2012;48(7):234-239.

325. Real FG, Svanes C, Omenaas ER, et al. Lung function, respiratory symptoms, and the menopausal transition. *J Allergy Clin Immunol.* 2008;121(1):72-80.
326. Jarvis D, Leynaert B. The association of asthma, atopy and lung function with hormone replacement therapy and surgical cessation of menstruation in a population-based sample of English women. *Allergy.* 2008;63(1):95-102.
327. Zemp E, Schikowski T, Dratva J, Schindler C, Probst-Hensch N. Asthma and the menopause: a systematic review and meta-analysis. *Maturitas.* 2012;73(3):212-217.
328. Foschino Barbaro MP, Costa VR, Resta O, et al. Menopausal asthma: a new biological phenotype? *Allergy.* 2010;65(10):1306-1312.
329. Romieu I, Fabre A, Fournier A, et al. Postmenopausal hormone therapy and asthma onset in the E3N cohort. *Thorax.* 2010;65(4):292-297.
330. Barr RG, Wentowski CC, Grodstein F, et al. Prospective study of postmenopausal hormone use and newly diagnosed asthma and chronic obstructive pulmonary disease. *Arch Intern Med.* 2004;164(4):379-386.
331. Hepburn MJ, Dooley DP, Morris MJ. The effects of estrogen replacement therapy on airway function in postmenopausal, asthmatic women. *Arch Intern Med.* 2001;161(22):2717-2721.
332. Kos-Kudła B, Ostrowska Z, Marek B, Ciesielska-Kopacz N, Kajdaniuk D, Kudła M. Effects of hormone replacement therapy on endocrine and spirometric parameters in asthmatic postmenopausal women. *Gynecol Endocrinol.* 2001;15(4):304-311.
333. Centers for Disease Control and Prevention. *Leading Causes of Death by Race/Ethnicity, All Females—United States, 2009.* Centers for Disease Control and Prevention Web site. Published 2009. www.cdc.gov/Women/lcod/2009/09_race_women.pdf. Accessed May 23, 2014.
334. Canadian Cancer Society. *Cancer Statistics at a Glance.* Canadian Cancer Society Web site. Published 2013. www.cancer.ca/en/cancer-information/cancer-101/cancer-statistics-at-a-glance/?region=on. Accessed May 23, 2014.
335. American Cancer Society, Surveillance Research. *Estimated New Cancer Cases by Sex and Age (Years), 2013.* American Cancer Society Web site. Published 2013. www.cancer.org/acs/groups/content/@epidemiologysurveilance/documents/document/acspc-037114.pdf. Accessed May 23, 2014.
336. Canadian Cancer Society's Advisory Committee on Cancer Statistics. *Canadian Cancer Statistics 2013.* Toronto, ON: Canadian Cancer Society; 2013. Published May 2013. www.cancer.ca/~/media/cancer.ca/CW/publications/Canadian%20Cancer%20Statistics/canadian-cancer-statistics-2013-EN.pdf. Accessed May 23, 2014.
337. Centers for Disease Control and Prevention. *Cancer Prevention and Control: Cancer and Women.* Centers for Disease Control and Prevention Web site. www.cdc.gov/cancer/dcpc/resources/features/WomenAndCancer. Updated May 8, 2014. Accessed May 23, 2014.
338. American Cancer Society. *Cancer Facts and Figures 2013.* Atlanta, GA: American Cancer Society; 2013.
339. Calle EE, Kaaks R. Overweight, obesity and cancer: epidemiological evidence and proposed mechanisms. *Nat Rev Cancer.* 2004;4(8):579-591.
340. Hursting SD, Hursting MJ. Growth signals, inflammation, and vascular perturbations: mechanistic links between obesity, metabolic syndrome, and cancer. *Arterioscler Thromb Vasc Biol.* 2012;32(8):1766-1770.
341. Maddison AR, Asada Y, Urquhart R. Inequity in access to cancer care: a review of the Canadian literature. *Cancer Causes Control.* 2011;22(3):359-366.
342. Morris AM, Rhoads KF, Stain SC, Birkmeyer JD. Understanding racial disparities in cancer treatment and outcomes. *J Am Coll Surg.* 2010;211(1):105-113.
343. Nelson DE, Jarman DW, Rehm J, et al. Alcohol-attributable cancer deaths and years of potential life lost in the United States. *Am J Public Health.* 2013;103(4):641-648.
344. Lemanne D, Cassileth B, Gubili J. The role of physical activity in cancer prevention, treatment, recovery, and survivorship. *Oncology (Williston Park).* 2013;27(6):580-585.
345. Pharoah PD, Day NE, Duffy S, Easton DF, Ponder BA. Family history and the risk of breast cancer: a systematic review and meta-analysis. *Int J Cancer.* 1997;71(5):800-809.
346. Foulkes WD. Inherited susceptibility to common cancers. *N Engl J Med.* 2008;359(20):2143-2153.
347. Schorge JO, Modesitt SC, Coleman RL, et al. SGO White Paper on ovarian cancer: etiology, screening and surveillance. *Gynecol Oncol.* 2010;119(1):7-17.
348. Koornstra JJ, Mourits MJ, Sijmons RH, Leliveld AM, Hollema H, Kleibeuker JH. Management of extracolonic tumours in patients with Lynch syndrome. *Lancet Oncol.* 2009;10(4):400-408.
349. Jemal A, Center MM, DeSantis C, Ward EM. Global patterns of cancer incidence and mortality rates and trends. *Cancer Epidemiol Biomarkers Prev.* 2010;19(8):1893-1907.
350. Siegel R, Naishadham D, Jemal A. Cancer statistics, 2013. *CA Cancer J Clin.* 2013;63(1):11-30.
351. Public Health Agency of Canada. *Canadian Cancer Statistics 2012: Breast Cancer.* Public Health Agency of Canada Web site. www.phac-aspc.gc.ca/cd-mc/cancer/breast_cancer-cancer_du_sein-eng.php. Modified October 7, 2013. Accessed May 23, 2014.
352. Glass AG, Lacey JV Jr, Carreon D, Hoover RN. Breast cancer incidence, 1980-2006: combined roles of menopausal hormone therapy, screening mammography, and estrogen receptor status. *J Natl Cancer Inst.* 2007;99(15):1152-1161.
353. Howe HL, Wu K, Ries LA, et al. Annual report to the nation on the status of cancer, 1975-2003, featuring cancer among US Hispanic/Latino populations. *Cancer.* 2006;107(8):1711-1742.
354. Haas JS, Kaplan CP, Gerstenberger EP, Kerlikowske K. Changes in the use of postmenopausal hormone therapy after the publication of clinical trial results. *Ann Intern Med.* 2004;140(3):184-188.
355. Ravdin PM, Cronin KA, Howlader N, et al. The decrease in breast-cancer incidence in 2003 in the United States. *N Engl J Med.* 2007;356(16):1670-1674.
356. Colditz GA, Rosner B. Cumulative risk of breast cancer to age 70 years according to risk factor status: data from the Nurses' Health Study. *Am J Epidemiol.* 2000;152(10):950-964.
357. Chlebowski RT, Chen Z, Anderson GL, et al. Ethnicity and breast cancer: factors influencing differences in incidence and outcome. *J Natl Cancer Inst.* 2005;97(6):439-448.
358. American Cancer Society. *Breast Cancer Facts and Figures* 2013-2014. Atlanta, GA: American Cancer Society; 2013.
359. Campeau PM, Foulkes WD, Tischkowitz MD. Hereditary breast cancer: new genetic developments, new therapeutic avenues. *Hum Genet.* 2008;124(1):31-42.
360. National Cancer Institute. *Breast Cancer Risk Assessment Tool.* National Institutes of Health Web site. www.cancer.gov/bcrisktool/Default.aspx. Modified May 16, 2011. Accessed May 23, 2014.
361. Chlebowski RT, Anderson GL, Lane DS, et al; Women's Health Initiative Investigators. Predicting risk of breast cancer in postmenopausal women by hormone receptor status. *J Natl Cancer Inst.* 2007;99(22):1695-1705.
362. Endogenous Hormones and Breast Cancer Collaborative Group; Key TJ, Appleby PN, Reeves GK, et al. Sex hormones and risk of breast cancer in premenopausal women: a collaborative reanalysis of individual participant data from seven prospective studies. *Lancet Oncol.* 2013;14(10):1009-1019.
363. Chlebowski RT, Hendrix SL, Langer RD, et al; WHI investigators. Influence of estrogen plus progestin on breast cancer and mammography in healthy postmenopausal women: the Women's Health Initiative Randomized Trial. *JAMA.* 2003;289(24):3243-3253.
364. Boyd NF, Guo H, Martin LJ, et al. Mammographic density and the risk and detection of breast cancer. *N Engl J Med.* 2007;356(3):227-236.
365. Tamimi RM, Hankinson SE, Chen WY, Rosner B, Colditz GA. Combined estrogen and testosterone use and risk of breast cancer in postmenopausal women. *Arch Intern Med.* 2006;166(14):1483-1489.
366. Cummings SR, Tice JA, Bauer S, et al. Prevention of breast cancer in postmenopausal women: approaches to estimating and reducing risk. *J Natl Cancer Inst.* 2009;101(6):384-398.
367. Rohan TE, Negassa A, Chlebowski RT, et al. Conjugated equine estrogen and risk of benign proliferative breast disease: a randomized controlled trial. *J Natl Cancer Inst.* 2008;100(8):563-571. Erratum in: *J Natl Cancer Inst.* 2008;100(10):754.
368. Kerlikowske K, Ichikawa L, Miglioretti DL, et al; National Institutes of Health Breast Cancer Surveillance Consortium. Longitudinal measurement of clinical mammographic breast density to improve estimation of breast cancer risk. *J Natl Cancer Inst.* 2007;99(5):386-395.
369. Fournier A, Boutron-Ruault MC, Claver-Chapelon F. Breast cancer and hormonal therapy in postmenopausal women. *N Engl J Med.* 2009;360(22):2366-2367.
370. Beral V; Million Women Study Collaborators. Breast cancer and hormone-replacement therapy in the Million Women Study. *Lancet.* 2003;362(9382):419-427. Erratum in: *Lancet.* 2003;362(9390):1160.
371. Schairer C, Lubin J, Troisi R, Sturgeon S, Brinton L, Hoover R. Menopausal estrogen and estrogen-progestin replacement therapy and breast cancer risk. *JAMA.* 2000;283(4):485-491. Erratum in: *JAMA.* 2000;284(20):2597.

372. Calle EE, Feigelson HS, Hildebrand JS, Teras LR, Thun MJ, Rodriguez C. Postmenopausal hormone use and breast cancer associations differ by hormone regimen and histologic subtype. *Cancer*. 2009;115(5):936-945. Erratum in: *Cancer*. 2009;115(7):1587.
373. Chlebowski RT, Anderson GL, Gass M, et al; WHI Investigators. Estrogen plus progestin and breast cancer incidence and mortality in postmenopausal women. *N Engl J Med*. 2010;304(15):1684-1692.
374. Li CI, Malone KE, Porter PL, et al. Relationship between menopausal hormone therapy and risk of ductal, lobular, and ductal-lobular breast carcinomas. *Cancer Epidemiol Biomarkers Prev*. 2008;17(1):43-50. Erratum in: *Cancer Epidemiol Biomarkers Prev*. 2009;18(1):2803.
375. Reeves GK, Beral V, Green J, Gathani T, Bull D; Million Women Study Collaborators. Hormonal therapy for menopause and breast-cancer risk by histological type: a cohort study and meta-analysis. *Lancet Oncol*. 2006;7(11):910-918.
376. Bélisle S, Blake J, Basson RL, et al; Menopause Guidelines Committee. Canadian Consensus Conference on menopause, 2006 update. *J Obstet Gynaecol Can*. 2006;28(2 suppl 1):S7-S94.
377. Fournier A, Berrino F, Clavel-Chapelon F. Unequal risks for breast cancer associated with different hormone replacement therapies: results from the E3N cohort study. *Breast Cancer Res Treat*. 2008;107(1):103-111. Erratum in: *Breast Cancer Res Treat*. 2008;107(2):307-308.
378. Beral V, Reeves G, Bull D, Green J; Million Women Study Collaborators. Breast cancer risk in relation to the interval between menopause and starting hormone therapy. *J Natl Cancer Inst*. 2011;103(4):296-305.
379. LaCroix AZ, Chlebowski RT, Manson JE, et al; WHI Investigators. Health outcomes after stopping conjugated equine estrogens among postmenopausal women with prior hysterectomy: a randomized controlled trial. *JAMA*. 2011;305(13):1305-1314.
380. Wingo PA, Austin H, Marchbanks PA, et al. Oral contraceptives and the risk of death from breast cancer. *Obstet Gynecol*. 2007;110(4):793-800. Erratum in: *Obstet Gynecol*. 2008;111(2 pt 1):454.
381. Cibula D, Gompel A, Mueck AO, et al. Hormonal contraception and risk of cancer. *Hum Reprod Update*. 2010;16(6):631-650.
382. DiSaia PJ, Brewster WR, Ziogas A, Anton-Culver H. Breast cancer survival and hormone replacement therapy: a cohort analysis. *Am J Clin Oncol*. 2000;23(6):541-545.
383. Fletcher AS, Erbas B, Kavanagh AM, Hart S, Rodger A, Gertig DM. Use of hormone replacement therapy (HRT) and survival following breast cancer diagnosis. *Breast*. 2005;14(3):192-200.
384. Holmberg L, Iversen OE, Rudenstam CM, et al; HABITS Study Group. Increased risk of recurrence after hormone replacement therapy in breast cancer survivors. *J Natl Cancer Inst*. 2008;100(7):75-482. Erratum in: *J Natl Cancer Inst*. 2008;100(9):685.
385. Brezden CB, Phillips KA, Abdolell M, Bunston T, Tannock IF. Cognitive function in breast cancer patients receiving adjuvant chemotherapy. *J Clin Oncol*. 2000;18(14):2695-2701.
386. Li CI, Daling JR, Porter PL, Tang MT, Malone KE. Relationship between potentially modifiable lifestyle factors and risk of second primary contralateral breast cancer among women diagnosed with estrogen receptor-positive invasive breast cancer. *J Clin Oncol*. 2009;27(32):5312-5318.
387. Hartmann LC, Sellers TA, Frost MH, et al. Benign breast disease and the risk of breast cancer. *N Engl J Med*. 2005;353(3):229-237.
388. Hwang ES, Miglioretti DL, Ballard-Barbash R, Weaver DL, Kerlikowski K; National Cancer Institute Breast Cancer Surveillance Consortium. Association between breast density and subsequent breast cancer following treatment for ductal carcinoma in situ. *Cancer Epidemiol Biomarkers Prev*. 2007;16(12):2587-2593.
389. Walsh T, Casadei S, Coats KH, et al. Spectrum of mutations in BRCA1, BRCA2, CHEK2, and TP53 in families at high risk of breast cancer. *JAMA*. 2006;295(12):1379-1388.
390. Rebbeck TR, Lynch HT, Neuhausen SL, et al; Prevention and Observation of Surgical End Points Study Group. Prophylactic oophorectomy in carriers of BRCA1 or BRCA2 mutations. *N Engl J Med*. 2002;346(21):1616-1622.
391. Rebbeck TR, Friebel T, Wagner T, et al; the Prose Study Group. Effect of short-term hormone replacement therapy on breast cancer risk reduction after bilateral prophylactic oophorectomy in BRCA1 and BRCA2 mutation carriers: the PROSE Study Group. *J Clin Oncol*. 2005;23(31):7804-7810.
392. Metcalfe KA, Birenbaum-Carmeli D, Lucinski J, et al; Hereditary Breast Cancer Clinical Study Group. International variation in rates of uptake of preventive options in BRCA1 and BRCA2 mutation carriers. *Int J Cancer*. 2008;122(9):2017-2022.
393. Chang-Claude J, Andrieu N, Rookus M, et al; Epidemiological Study of Familial Breast Cancer (EMBRACE); Gene Etude Prospective Sein Ovaire (GENEPSO); Genen Omgeving studie van de werkgroep Hereditair Borstkanker Onderzoek Nederland (GEO-HEBON); International BRCA1/2 Carrier Cohort Study (IBCCS) collaborators group. Age at menarche and menopause and breast cancer risk in the International BRCA1/2 Carrier Cohort Study. *Cancer Epidemiol Biomarkers Prev*. 2007;16(4):740-746.
394. Carney PA, Miglioretti DL, Yankaskas BC, et al. Individual and combined effects of age, breast density, and hormone replacement therapy use on the accuracy of screening mammography. *Ann Intern Med*. 2003;138(3):168-175. Erratum in: *Ann Intern Med*. 2003;138(9):771.
395. American Cancer Society. *Breast Cancer: Early Detection*. www.cancer.org/acs/groups/cid/documents/webcontent/003165-pdf.pdf. Revised January 28, 2014. Accessed May 27, 2014.
396. National Cancer Institute. *Mammograms*. National Institutes of Health Web site. www.cancer.gov/cancertopics/factsheet/detection/mammograms. Reviewed March 25, 2014. Accessed May 27, 2014.
397. Bevers TB, Anderson BO, Bonaccio E, et al; National Comprehensive Cancer Network. NCCN clinical practice guidelines in oncology: breast cancer screening and diagnosis. *J Natl Compr Cancer Netw*. 2009;7(10):1060-1096. Erratum in: *J Natl Compr Cancer Netw*. 2010;8(2):xxxvii.
398. US Preventive Services Task Force. Screening for breast cancer: US Preventive Services Task Force recommendation statement. *Ann Intern Med*. 2009;151(10):716-726. Erratum in: *Ann Intern Med*. 2010;152(10)688; *Ann Intern Med*. 2010;152(3):199-200.
399. Pisano ED, Gatonis C, Hendrick E, et al; Digital Mammographic Imaging Screening Trial (DMIST) Investigators Group. Diagnostic performance of digital versus film mammography for breast-cancer screening. *N Engl J Med*. 2005;353(17):1773-1783. Erratum in: *N Engl J Med*. 2006;355(17):1840.
400. Odle TG. Breast ultrasound. *Radiol Technol*. 2007;78:222M-242M.
401. Fabian CJ, Kimler BF, Zalles CM, et al. Short-term breast cancer prediction by random periareolar fine-needle aspiration cytology and the Gail risk model. *J Natl Cancer Inst*. 2000;92(15):1217-1227.
402. Saslow D, Boetes C, Burke W, et al; American Cancer Society Breast Cancer Advisory Group. American Cancer Society guidelines for breast screening with MRI as an adjunct to mammography. *CA Cancer J Clin*. 2007;57(2):75-89.
403. Lehman CD. Screening MRI for women at high risk for breast cancer. *Semin Ultrasound CT MR*. 2006;27(4):333-338.
404. Kriege M, Brekelmans CTM, Boetes C, et al; Magnetic Resonance Imaging Screening Study Group. Efficacy of MRI and mammography for breast-cancer screening in women with a familial or genetic predisposition. *N Engl J Med*. 2004;351(5):427-437.
405. Tilanus-Linthorst MM, Obdeijn IM, Bartels KC, de Koning HJ, Oudkirk M. First experiences in screening women at high risk for breast cancer with MR imaging. *Breast Cancer Res Treat*. 2000;63(1):53-60.
406. Sprague BL, Trentham-Dietz A, Egan KM, Titus-Ernstoff L, Hampton JM, Newcomb PA. Proportion of invasive breast cancer attributable to risk factors modifiable after menopause. *Am J Epidemiol*. 2008;168(4):404-411.
407. West-Wright CN, Henderson KD, Sullivan-Halley J, et al. Long-term and recent recreational physical activity and survival after breast cancer: the California Teachers Study. *Cancer Epidemiol Biomarkers Prev*. 2009;18(11):2851-2859.
408. Prentice RL, Caan B, Chlebowski RT, et al. Low-fat dietary pattern and risk of invasive breast cancer: the Women's Health Initiative Randomized Controlled Dietary Modification Trial. *JAMA*. 2006;295(6):629-642.
409. Larsson SC, Giovannucci E, Wolk A. Folate and risk of breast cancer: a meta-analysis. *J Natl Cancer Inst*. 2007;99(1):64-76.
410. Key J, Hodgson S, Omar RZ, et al. Meta-analysis of studies of alcohol and breast cancer with consideration of the methodological issues. *Cancer Causes Control*. 2006;17(6):759-770.
411. Allen NE, Beral V, Casabonne D, et al; Million Women Study Collaborators. Moderate alcohol intake and cancer incidence in women. *J Natl Cancer Inst*. 2009;101(5):296-305.
412. Chen WY, Colditz GA, Rosner B, et al. Use of postmenopausal hormones, alcohol, and risk for invasive breast cancer. *Ann Intern Med*. 2002;137(10):798-804.
413. Garland CF, Garland FC, Gorham ED, et al. The role of vitamin D in cancer prevention. *Am J Public Health*. 2006;96(2):252-261.
414. Cauley JA, Chlebowski RT, Wactawski-Wende J, et al. Calcium plus vitamin D supplementation and health outcomes five years after active intervention ended: The Women's Health Initiative. *J Womens Health (Larchmt)*. 2013;22(11):915-929.

415. Bardia A, Hartmann LC, Vachon CM, et al. Recreational physical activity and risk of postmenopausal breast cancer based on hormone receptor status. *Arch Intern Med.* 2006;166(22):2478-2483.

416. Gotay CC. Behavior and cancer prevention. *J Clin Oncol.* 2005;23(2):301-310.

417. Muti P, Rogan E, Cavalieri E. Androgens and estrogens in the etiology and prevention of breast cancer. *Nutr Cancer.* 2006;56(2):247-252.

418. Fisher B, Cosantino JP, Wickerham DL, et al. Tamoxifen for prevention of breast cancer: report of the National Surgical Adjuvant Breast and Bowel Project P-1 Study. *J Natl Cancer Inst.* 1998;90(18):1371-1388.

419. Cuzick J, Forbes JF, Sestak I, et al; International Breast Cancer Intervention Study I Investigators. Long-term results of tamoxifen prophylaxis for breast cancer—96-month follow-up of the randomized IBIS-I trial. *J Natl Cancer Inst.* 2007;99(4):272-282.

420. Powles TJ, Ashley S, Tidy A, Smith IE, Dowsett M. Twenty-year follow-up of the Royal Marsden randomized, double-blinded tamoxifen breast cancer prevention trial. *J Natl Cancer Inst.* 2007;99(4):283-290.

421. Gail MH, Costantino JP, Bryant J, et al. Weighing the risks and benefits of tamoxifen treatment for preventing breast cancer. *J Natl Cancer Inst.* 1999;91(21):1829-1846. Erratum in: *J Natl Cancer Inst.* 2000;92(3):275.

422. Goetz MP, Schaid DJ, Wickerham DL, et al. Evaluation of CYP2D6 and efficacy of tamoxifen and raloxifene in women treated for breast cancer chemoprevention: results from the NSABP P1 and P2 clinical trials. *Clin Cancer Res.* 2011;17(21):6944-6951.

423. Cauley JA, Norton L, Lippman ME, et al. Continued breast cancer risk reduction in postmenopausal women treated with raloxifene: 4-year results from the MORE trial. Multiple outcomes of raloxifene evaluation. *Breast Cancer Res Treat.* 2001;65(2):125-134.

424. Lippman ME, Krueger KA, Eckert S, et al. Indicators of lifetime estrogen exposure: effect on breast cancer incidence and interaction with raloxifene therapy in the multiple outcomes of raloxifene evaluation study participants. *J Clin Oncol.* 2001;19(12):3111-3116.

425. Martino S, Cauley JA, Barrett-Connor E, et al; CORE Investigators. Continuing outcomes relevant to Evista: breast cancer incidence in postmenopausal osteoporotic women in a randomized trial of raloxifene. *J Natl Cancer Inst.* 2004;96(23):1751-1761.

426. Barrett-Connor E, Grady D, Sashegyi A, et al; MORE Investigators (Multiple Outcomes of Raloxifene Evaluation). Raloxifene and cardiovascular events in osteoporotic postmenopausal women: four-year results from the MORE (Multiple Outcomes of Raloxifene Evaluation) randomized trial. *JAMA.* 2002;287(7):847-857.

427. Vogel VG, Costantino JP, Wickerham DL, et al; National Surgical Adjuvant Breast and Bowel Project (NSABP). Effects of tamoxifen vs raloxifene on the risk of developing invasive breast cancer and other disease outcomes: the NSABP Study of Tamoxifen and Raloxifene (STAR) P-2 trial. *JAMA.* 2006;295(23):2727-2741. Erratum in: *JAMA.* 2006;296(24):2926; *JAMA.* 2007;298(9):973.

428. Land SR, Wickerham DL, Costantino JP, et al. Patient-reported symptoms and quality of life during treatment with tamoxifen or raloxifene for breast cancer prevention: the NSABP Study of Tamoxifen and Raloxifene (STAR) P-2 trial. *JAMA.* 2006;295(23):2742-2751.

429. Vogel VG, Costantino JP Wickerham DL, et al; National Surgical Adjuvant Breast and Bowel Project. Update of the National Surgical Adjuvant Breast and Bowel Project Study of Tamoxifen and Raloxifene (STAR) P-2 Trial: preventing breast cancer. *Cancer Prev Res (Phila).* 2010;3(6):696-706.

430. Vogel VG, Costantino JP, Wickerham DL, et al. Carcinoma in situ outcomes in National Surgical Adjuvant Breast and Bowel Project Breast Cancer Chemoprevention Trials. *J Natl Cancer Inst Monogr.* 2010;2010(41):181-186.

431. Runowicz CD, Costantino JP, Wickerham DL, et al. Gynecologic conditions in participants in the NSABP breast cancer prevention study of tamoxifen and raloxifene (STAR). *Am J Obstet Gynecol.* 2011;205(6):535.e1-e5.

432. Barrett-Connor E, Mosca L, Collins P, et al; Raloxifene Use for The Heart (RUTH) Trial Investigators. Effects of raloxifene on cardiovascular events and breast cancer in postmenopausal women. *N Engl J Med.* 2006;355(2):125-137.

433. Jordan VC. Optimising endocrine approaches for the chemoprevention of breast cancer beyond the Study of Tamoxifen and Raloxifene (STAR) trial. *Eur J Cancer.* 2006;42(17):2909-2913.

434. Evista [package insert]. Indianapolis, IN: Eli Lilly; 2011.

435. Cuzick J, DeCensi A, Arun B, et al. Preventive therapy for breast cancer: a consensus statement. *Lancet Oncol.* 2011;12(5):496-503.

436. Visvanathan K, Hurley P, Bantug E, et al. Use of pharmacologic interventions for breast cancer risk reduction: American Society of Clinical Oncology clinical practice guideline. *J Clin Oncol.* 2013;31(23):2942-2962.

437. National Comprehensive Cancer Network. *NCCN Clinical Practice Guidelines in Oncology (NCCN Guidelines): Breast Cancer.* Version 2.2013. March 11, 2013. http://infooncos.es/wp-content/uploads/2011/10/breast_cancer_2.2013.pdf. Accessed May 27, 2014.

438. Freedman AN, Yu B, Gail MH, et al. Benefit/risk assessment for breast cancer chemoprevention with raloxifene or tamoxifen for women age 50 years or older. *J Clin Oncol.* 2011;29(17):2327-2333.

439. Cuzick J, Sestak I, Bonanni B, et al; SERM Chemoprevention of Breast Cancer Overview Group. Selective oestrogen receptor modulators in prevention of breast cancer: an updated meta-analysis of individual participant data. *Lancet.* 2013;381(9880):1827-1834.

440. Breast International Group (BIG) 1-98 Collaborative Group; Thürlimann B, Keshaviah A, Coates AS, et al. A comparison of letrozole and tamoxifen in postmenopausal women with early breast cancer. *N Engl J Med.* 2005;353(26):2747-2757. Erratum in: *N Engl J Med.* 2006;354(20):2200.

441. Coates AS, Keshaviah A, Thürlimann B, et al. Five years of letrozole compared with tamoxifen as initial adjuvant therapy for postmenopausal women with endocrine-responsive early breast cancer: update of study BIG 1-98. *J Clin Oncol.* 2007;25(5):486-492.

442. Coombes RC, Hall E, Gibson JL, et al; Intergroup Exemestane Study. A randomized trial of exemestane after two to three years of tamoxifen therapy in postmenopausal women with primary breast cancer. *N Engl J Med.* 2004;350(11):1081-1092. Erratum in: *N Engl J Med.* 2004;351(213):2461; *N Engl J Med.* 2006;355(16):1746.

443. Dowsett M, Cuzick J, Ingle J, et al. Meta-analysis of breast cancer outcomes in adjuvant trials of aromatase inhibitors versus tamoxifen. *J Clin Oncol.* 2010;28(3):509-518.

444. Goss PE, Ingle JN, Alés-Martínez JE, et al; NCIC CTG MAP.3 Study Investigators. Exemestane for breast-cancer prevention in postmenopausal women. *N Engl J Med.* 2011;364(25):2381-2391. Erratum in: *N Engl J Med.* 2011;365(14):1361.

445. Brufsky A, Harker WG, Beck JT, et al. Zoledronic acid inhibits adjuvant letrozole-induced bone loss in postmenopausal women with early breast cancer. *J Clin Oncol.* 2007;25(7):829-836.

446. Gnant MF, Mlineritsch B, Luschin-Ebengreuth G, et al; Austrian Breast and Colorectal Cancer Study Group. Zoledronic acid prevents cancer treatment-induced bone loss in premenopausal women receiving adjuvant endocrine therapy for hormone-responsive breast cancer: a report from the Austrian Breast and Colorectal Cancer Study Group. *J Clin Oncol.* 2007;25(7):820-828.

447. Kauff ND, Satagopan JM, Robson ME, et al. Risk-reducing salpingo-oophorectomy in women with a BRCA1 or BRCA2 mutation. *N Engl J Med.* 2002;346(21):1609-1615.

448. Domchek SM, Friebel TM, Singer CF, et al. Association of risk-reducing surgery in BRCA1 or BRCA2 mutation carriers with cancer risk and mortality. *JAMA.* 2010;304(9):967-975.

449. Eisen A, Lubinski J, Gronwald J, et al; Hereditary Breast Cancer Clinical Study Group. Hormone therapy and the risk of breast cancer in BRCA1 mutation carriers. *J Natl Cancer Inst.* 2008;100(19):1361-1367.

450. Yap OW, Matthews RP. Racial and ethnic disparities in cancers of the uterine corpus. *J Natl Med Assoc.* 2006;98(12):1930-1933.

451. American Cancer Society. *Uterine Sarcoma.* American Cancer Society Web site. www.cancer.org/acs/groups/cid/documents/webcontent/003145-pdf.pdf. Revised May 20, 2014. Accessed May 28, 2014.

452. Bokhman JV. Two pathogenetic types of endometrial carcinoma. *Gynecol Oncol.* 1983;15(1):10-17.

453. Creasman WT, Morrow CP, Bundy BN, Homesley HD, Graham JE, Heller PB. Surgical pathologic spread patterns of endometrial cancer. A Gynecologic Oncology Group Study. *Cancer.* 1987;60(8 suppl):2035-2041.

454. Levine RL, Cargile CB, Blazes MS, van Rees B, Kurman RJ, Ellenson LH. PTEN mutations and microsatellite instability in complex atypical hyperplasia, a precursor lesion to uterine endometrioid carcinoma. *Cancer Res.* 1998;58(15):3254-3258.

455. Emons G, Fleckenstein G, Hinney B, Huschmand A, Heyl W. Hormonal interactions in endometrial cancer. *Endocr Relat Cancer.* 2000;7(4):227-242.

456. Clement PB, Young RH. Non-endometrioid carcinomas of the uterine corpus: a review of their pathology with emphasis on recent advances and problematic aspects. *Adv Anat Pathol.* 2004;11(3):117-142.

457. Amant F, Moerman P, Neven P, Timmerman D, Van Limbergen E, Vergote I. Endometrial cancer. *Lancet.* 2005;366(9484):491-505.

458. Hamilton CA, Cheung MK, Osann K, et al. Uterine papillary serous and clear cell carcinomas predict for poorer survival compared to grade 3 endometrioid corpus cancers. *Br J Cancer.* 2006;94(5):642-646.

Chapter 4

459. Leslie KK, Thiel KW, Goodheart MJ, De Geest K, Jia Y, Yang S. Endometrial cancer. *Obstet Gynecol Clin North Am*. 2012;39(2):255-268.
460. Merisio C, Berretta R, De Ioris A, et al. Endometrial cancer in patients with preoperative diagnosis of atypical endometrial hyperplasia. *Eur J Obstet Gynecol Reprod Biol*. 2005;122(1):107-111.
461. Trimble CL, Kauderer J, Zaino R, et al. Concurrent endometrial carcinoma in women with a biopsy diagnosis of atypical endometrial hyperplasia: a Gynecologic Oncology Group study. *Cancer*. 2006;106(4):812-819.
462. Lacey JV Jr, Ioffe OB, Ronnett BM, et al. Endometrial carcinoma risk among women diagnosed with endometrial hyperplasia: the 34-year experience in a large health plan. *Br J Cancer*. 2008;98(1):45-53.
463. Lacey JV Jr, Sherman ME, Rush BB, et al. Absolute risk of endometrial carcinoma during 20-year follow-up among women with endometrial hyperplasia. *J Clin Oncol*. 2010;28(5):788-792.
464. Mariani A, Dowdy SC, Keeney GL, Long HJ, Lesnick TG, Podratz KC. High-risk endometrial cancer subgroups: candidates for target-based adjuvant therapy. *Gynecol Oncol*. 2004;95(1):120-126.
465. Felix AS, Weissfeld JL, Stone RA, et al. Factors associated with type I and type II endometrial cancer. *Cancer Causes Control*. 2010;21(11):1851-1856.
466. Matsuzaki S, Fukaya T, Suzuki T, Murakami T, Sasano H, Yajima A. Oestrogen receptor alpha and beta mRNA expression in human endometrium throughout the menstrual cycle. *Mol Hum Reprod*. 1999;5(6):559-564.
467. Deroo BJ, Korach KS. Estrogen receptors and human disease. *J Clin Invest*. 2006;116(3):561-570.
468. Wang Q, Li X, Wang L, Feng YH, Zeng R, Gorodeski G. Antiapoptotic effects of estrogen in normal and cancer human cervical epithelial cells. *Endocrinology*. 2004;145(12):5568-5579.
469. Mishra GD, Cooper R, Tom SE, Kuh D. Early life circumstances and their impact on menarche and menopause. *Womens Health (Lond Engl)*. 2009;5(2):175-190.
470. Setiawan VW, Pike MC, Karageorgi S, et al; Australian National Endometrial Cancer Study Group. Age at last birth in relation to risk of endometrial cancer: pooled analysis in the Epidemiology of Endometrial Cancer Consortium. *Am J Epidemiol*. 2012;176(4):269-278.
471. Pocobelli G, Doherty JA, Voigt LF, et al. Pregnancy history and risk of endometrial cancer. *Epidemiology*. 2011;22(5):638-645.
472. Phipps AI, Doherty JA, Voigt LF, et al. Long-term use of continuous-combined estrogen-progestin hormone therapy and risks of endometrial cancer. *Cancer Causes Control*. 2011;22(12):1639-1646.
473. Hill DA, Weiss NS, Beresford SA, et al. Continuous combined hormone replacement therapy and risk of endometrial cancer. *Am J Obstet Gynecol*. 2000;183(6):1456-1461.
474. Chubak J, Tworoger SS, Yasui Y, Ulrich CM, Stanczyk FZ, McTiernan A. Associations between reproductive and menstrual factors and postmenopausal sex hormone concentrations. *Cancer Epidemiol Biomarkers Prev*. 2004;13(8):1296-1301.
475. Shang Y, Brown M. Molecular determinants for the tissue specificity of SERMs. *Science*. 2002;295(5564):2465-2468.
476. Jones ME, van Leeuwen FE, Hoogendoorn WE, et al. Endometrial cancer survival after breast cancer in relation to tamoxifen treatment: pooled results from three countries. *Breast Cancer Res*. 2012;14(3):R91.
477. Barsalou A, Dayan G, Anghel SI, Alaoui-Jamali M, Van de Velde P, Mader S. Growth-stimulatory and transcriptional activation properties of raloxifene in human endometrial Ishikawa cells. *Mol Cell Endocrinol*. 2002;190(1-2):65-73.
478. Cummings SR, Eckert S, Krueger KA, et al. The effect of raloxifene on risk of breast cancer in postmenopausal women: results from the MORE randomized trial. Multiple Outcomes of Raloxifene Evaluation. *JAMA*. 1999;281(23):2189-2197.
479. DeMichele A, Troxel AB, Berlin JA, et al. Impact of raloxifene or tamoxifen use on endometrial cancer risk: a population-based case-control study. *J Clin Oncol*. 2008;26(25):4151-4159.
480. Bulun SE, Chen D, Lu M, et al. Aromatase excess in cancers of breast, endometrium and ovary. *J Steroid Biochem Mol Biol*. 2007;106(1-5):81-96.
481. Sasaki M, Tanaka Y, Kaneuchi M, Sakuragi N, Dahiya R. Polymorphisms of estrogen receptor alpha gene in endometrial cancer. *Biochem Biophys Res Commun*. 2002;297(3):558-564.
482. Iwamoto I, Fujino Y, Douchi T, Nagata Y. Association of estrogen receptor alpha and beta3-adrenergic receptor polymorphisms with endometrial cancer. *Obstet Gynecol*. 2003;102(3):506-511.
483. Wedrén S, Lovmar L, Humphreys K, et al. Estrogen receptor alpha gene polymorphism and endometrial cancer risk—a case-control study. *BMC Cancer*. 2008;8:322.
484. Anderson KE, Anderson E, Mink PJ, et al. Diabetes and endometrial cancer in the Iowa women's health study. *Cancer Epidemiol Biomarkers Prev*. 2001;10(6):611-616.
485. Furberg AS, Thune I. Metabolic abnormalities (hypertension, hyperglycemia and overweight), lifestyle (high energy intake and physical inactivity) and endometrial cancer risk in a Norwegian cohort. *Int J Cancer*. 2003;104(6):669-676. Erratum in: *Int J Cancer*. 2003;104(6):799.
486. Schouten LJ, Goldbohm RA, van den Brandt PA. Anthropometry, physical activity, and endometrial cancer risk: results from the Netherlands Cohort Study. *J Natl Cancer Inst*. 2004;96(21):1635-1638.
487. Lucenteforte E, Bosetti C, Talamini R, et al. Diabetes and endometrial cancer: effect modification by body weight, physical activity and hypertension. *Br J Cancer*. 2007;97(7):995-998.
488. Augustin LS, Dal Maso L, Franceschi S, et al. Association between components of the insulin-like growth factor system and endometrial cancer risk. *Oncology*. 2004;67(1):54-59.
489. Zheng W, Cao P, Zheng M, Kramer EE, Godwin TA. p53 overexpression and bcl-2 persistence in endometrial carcinoma: comparison of papillary serous and endometrioid subtypes. *Gynecol Oncol*. 1996;61(2):167-174.
490. Lax SF, Kendall B, Tashiro H, Slebos RJ, Hedrick L. The frequency of p53, K-ras mutations, and microsatellite instability differs in uterine endometrioid and serous carcinoma: evidence of distinct molecular genetic pathways. *Cancer*. 2000;88(4):814-824.
491. Hecht JL, Mutter GL. Molecular and pathologic aspects of endometrial carcinogenesis. *J Clin Oncol*. 2006;24(29):4783-4791.
492. Doll A, Abal M, Rigau M, et al. Novel molecular profiles of endometrial cancer—new light through old windows. *J Steroid Biochem Mol Biol*. 2008;108(3-5):221-229.
493. Lagarda H, Catasus L, Arguelles R, Matias-Guiu X, Prat J. K-ras mutations in endometrial carcinomas with microsatellite instability. *J Pathol*. 2001;193(2):193-199.
494. Enomoto T, Inoue M, Perantoni AO, et al. K-ras activation in premalignant and malignant epithelial lesions of the human uterus. *Cancer Res*. 1991;51(19):5308-5314.
495. Mutter GL, Lin MC, Fitzgerald JT, et al. Altered PTEN expression as a diagnostic marker for the earliest endometrial precancers. *J Natl Cancer Inst*. 2000;92(11):924-930.
496. Moreno-Bueno G, Hardisson D, Sánchez C, et al. Abnormalities of the APC/beta-catenin pathway in endometrial cancer. *Oncogene*. 2002;21(52):7981-7990.
497. Scholten AN, Creutzberg CL, van den Broek LJ, Noordijk EM, Smit VT. Nuclear beta-catenin is a molecular feature of type I endometrial carcinoma. *J Pathol*. 2003;201(3):460-465.
498. Hinkula M, Pukkala E, Kyyrönen P, Kauppila A. Grand multiparity and incidence of endometrial cancer: a population-based study in Finland. *Int J Cancer*. 2002;98(6):912-915.
499. Li X, Qi X, Zhou L, et al. P2X(7) receptor expression is decreased in epithelial cancer cells of ectodermal, uro-genital sinus, and distal paramesonephric-duct origin. *Purinergic Signal*. 2009;5(3):351-368.
500. Czarnecka AM, Klemba A, Semczuk A, et al. Common mitochondrial polymorphisms as risk factor for endometrial cancer. *Int Arch Med*. 2009;2(1):33.
501. Calle EE, Rodriguez C, Walker-Thurmond K, Thun MJ. Overweight, obesity, and mortality from cancer in a prospectively studied cohort of US adults. *N Engl J Med*. 2003;348(17):1625-1638.
502. Epplein M, Reed SD, Voigt LF, Newton KM, Holt VL, Weiss NS. Risk of complex and atypical endometrial hyperplasia in relation to anthropometric measures and reproductive history. *Am J Epidemiol*. 2008;168(6):563-570.
503. Park SL, Goodman MT, Zhang ZF, Kolonel LN, Henderson BE, Setiawan VW. Body size, adult BMI gain and endometrial cancer risk: the multiethnic cohort. *Int J Cancer*. 2010;126(2):490-499.
504. Reeves KW, Carter GC, Rodabough RJ, et al. Obesity in relation to endometrial cancer risk and disease characteristics in the Women's Health Initiative. *Gynecol Oncol*. 2011;121(2):376-382.
505. Lu L, Risch H, Irwin ML, et al. Long-term overweight and weight gain in early adulthood in association with risk of endometrial cancer. *Int J Cancer*. 2011;129(5):1237-1243.
506. Siegel R, Ward E, Brawley O, Jemal A. Cancer statistics, 2011: the impact of eliminating socioeconomic and racial disparities on premature cancer deaths. *CA Cancer J Clin*. 2011;61(4):212-236.

DISEASE RISK

507. Evans T, Sany O, Pearmain P, Ganesan R, Blann A, Sundar S. Differential trends in the rising incidence of endometrial cancer by type: data from a UK population-based registry from 1994 to 2006. *Br J Cancer*. 2011;104(9): 1505-1510.

508. Bakkum-Gamez JN, Gonzalez-Bosquet J, Laack NN, Mariani A, Dowdy SC. Current issues in the management of endometrial cancer. *Mayo Clin Proc*. 2008;83(1):97-112.

509. Kaaks R, Lukanova A, Kurzer MS. Obesity, endogenous hormones, and endometrial cancer risk: a synthetic review. *Cancer Epidemiol Biomarkers Prev*. 2002;11(12):1531-1543.

510. Allen NE, Key TJ, Dossus L, et al. Endogenous sex hormones and endometrial cancer risk in women in the European Prospective Investigation into Cancer and Nutrition (EPIC). *Endocr Relat Cancer*. 2008;15(2):485-497.

511. Nestler JE, Powers LP, Matt DW, et al. A direct effect of hyperinsulinemia on serum sex hormone-binding globulin levels in obese women with the polycystic ovary syndrome. *J Clin Endocrinol Metab*. 1991;72(1):83-89.

512. Friberg E, Mantzoros CS, Wolk A. Diabetes and risk of endometrial cancer: a population-based prospective cohort study. *Cancer Epidemiol Biomarkers Prev*. 2007;16(2):276-280.

513. Weiderpass E, Brismar K, Bellocco R, Vainio H, Kaaks R. Serum levels of insulin-like growth factor-I, IGF-binding protein 1 and 3, and insulin and endometrial cancer risk. *Br J Cancer*. 2003;89(9):1697-1704.

514. Moore SC, Gierach GL, Schatzkin A, Matthews CE. Physical activity, sedentary behaviours, and the prevention of endometrial cancer. *Br J Cancer*. 2010;103(7):933-938.

515. Conroy MB, Sattelmair JR, Cook NR, Manson JE, Buring JE, Lee IM. Physical activity, adiposity, and risk of endometrial cancer. *Cancer Causes Control*. 2009;20(7):1107-1115.

516. John EM, Koo J, Horn-Ross PL. Lifetime physical activity and risk of endometrial cancer. *Cancer Epidemiol Biomarkers Prev*. 2010;19(5): 1276-1283.

517. Arem H, Irwin ML, Zhou Y, Lu L, Risch H, Yu H. Physical activity and endometrial cancer in a population-based case-control study. *Cancer Causes Control*. 2011;22(2):219-226.

518. Ollikainen M, Abdel-Rahman WM, Moisio AL, et al. Molecular analysis of familial endometrial carcinoma: a manifestation of hereditary nonpolyposis colorectal cancer or a separate syndrome? *J Clin Oncol*. 2005;23(21):4609-4616.

519. Boltenberg A, Furgyik S, Kullander S. Familial cancer aggregation in cases of adenocarcinoma corporis uteri. *Acta Obstet Gynecol Scand*. 1990;69(3): 249-258.

520. Gruber SB, Thompson WD. A population-based study of endometrial cancer and familial risk in younger women. Cancer and Steroid Hormone Study Group. *Cancer Epidemiol Biomarkers Prev*. 1996;5(6):411-417.

521. Kazerouni N, Schairer C, Friedman HB, Lacey JV Jr, Greene MH. Family history of breast cancer as a determinant of the risk of developing endometrial cancer: a nationwide cohort study. *J Med Genet*. 2002;39(11):826-832.

522. Setiawan VW, Monroe KR, Goodman MT, Kolonel LN, Pike MC, Henderson BE. Alcohol consumption and endometrial cancer risk: the multiethnic cohort. *Int J Cancer*. 2008;122(3):634-638.

523. Lesko SM, Rosenberg L, Kaufman DW, et al. Cigarette smoking and the risk of endometrial cancer. *N Engl J Med*. 1985;313(10):593-596.

524. Viswanathan AN, Feskanich D, De Vivo I, et al. Smoking and the risk of endometrial cancer: results from the Nurses' Health Study. *Int J Cancer*. 2005;114(6):996-1001.

525. Cui X, Rosner B, Willett WC, Hankinson SE. Antioxidant intake and risk of endometrial cancer: results from the Nurses' Health Study. *Int J Cancer*. 2011;128(5):1169-1178.

526. Goldstein SR. Modern evaluation of the endometrium. *Obstet Gynecol*. 2010;116(1):168-176.

527. Guido RS, Kanbour-Shakir A, Rulin MC, Christopherson WA. Pipelle endometrial sampling. Sensitivity in the detection of endometrial cancer. *J Reprod Med*. 1995;40(8):553-555.

528. Creasman W. Revised FIGO staging for carcinoma of the endometrium. *Int J Gynaecol Obstet*. 2009;105(2):109.

529. Horn LC, Schnurrbusch U, Bilek K, Hentschel B, Einenkel J. Risk of progression in complex and atypical endometrial hyperplasia: clinicopathologic analysis in cases with and without progestogen treatment. *Int J Gynecol Cancer*. 2004;14(2):348-353.

530. Lai CH, Huang HJ. The role of hormones for the treatment of endometrial hyperplasia and endometrial cancer. *Curr Opin Obstet Gynecol*. 2006; 18(1):29-34.

531. Gallos ID, Ganesan R, Gupta JK. Prediction of regression and relapse of endometrial hyperplasia with conservative therapy. *Obstet Gynecol*. 2013; 121(6):1165-1171.

532. Randall TC, Kurman RJ. Progestin treatment of atypical hyperplasia and well-differentiated carcinoma of the endometrium in women under age 40. *Obstet Gynecol*. 1997;90(3):434-440.

533. Suh-Burgmann E, Hung YY, Armstrong MA. Complex atypical endometrial hyperplasia: the risk of unrecognized adenocarcinoma and value of preoperative dilation and curettage. *Obstet Gynecol*. 2009;114(3): 523-529.

534. Chiva L, Lapuente F, González-Cortijo L, et al. Sparing fertility in young patients with endometrial cancer. *Gynecol Oncol*. 2008;111(2 suppl): S101-S104.

535. Reed SD, Newton KM, Garcia RL, et al. Complex hyperplasia with and without atypia: clinical outcomes and implications of progestin therapy. *Obstet Gynecol*. 2010;116(2 pt 1):365-373.

536. Rotman M, Azziz H, Halpern J, Schwartz D, Sohn C, Choi K. Endometrial carcinoma. Influence of prognostic factors on radiation management. *Cancer*. 1993;71(4 suppl):1471-1479.

537. Aalders JG, Thomas G. Endometrial cancer—revisiting the importance of pelvic and para aortic lymph nodes. *Gynecol Oncol*. 2007;104(1):222-231.

538. Chan JK, Wu H, Cheung MK, Shin JY, Osann K, Kapp DS. The outcomes of 27,063 women with unstaged endometrioid uterine cancer. *Gynecol Oncol*. 2007;106(2):282-288.

539. Smith DC, Macdonald OK, Lee CM, Gaffney DK. Survival impact of lymph node dissection in endometrial adenocarcinoma: a surveillance, epidemiology, and end results analysis. *Int J Gynecol Cancer*. 2007;18(2):255-261.

540. Mariani A, Dowdy SC, Cliby WA, et al. Prospective assessment of lymphatic dissemination in endometrial cancer: a paradigm shift in surgical staging. *Gynecol Oncol*. 2008;109(1):11-18.

541. Benedetti Panici P, Basile S, Maneschi F, et al. Systematic pelvic lymphadenectomy vs. no lymphadenectomy in early-stage endometrial carcinoma: randomized clinical trial. *J Natl Cancer Inst*. 2008;100(23): 1707-1716.

542. Orr JW Jr, Taylor PT Jr. Surgical management of endometrial cancer: how much is enough? *Gynecol Oncol*. 2008;109(1):1-3.

543. ASTEC study group, Kitchener H, Swart AM, Qian Q, Amos C, Parmar MK. Efficacy of systematic pelvic lymphadenectomy in endometrial cancer (MRC ASTEC trial): a randomised study. *Lancet*. 2009;373(9658):125-136. Erratum in: *Lancet*. 2009;373(9677):1764.

544. Barton DP, Naik R, Herod J. Efficacy of systemic pelvic lymphadenectomy in endometrial cancer (MRC ASTEC Trial): a randomized study. *Int J Gynecol Cancer*. 2009;19(8):1465.

545. Todo Y, Kato H, Kaneuchi M, Watari H, Takeda M, Sakuragi N. Survival effect of para-aortic lymphadenectomy in endometrial cancer (SEPAL study): a retrospective cohort analysis. *Lancet*. 2010;375(9721):1165-1172. Erratum in: *Lancet*. 2010;376(9741):594.

546. Kilgore LC, Partridge EE, Alvarez RD, et al. Adenocarcinoma of the endometrium: survival comparisons of patients with and without pelvic node sampling. *Gynecol Oncol*. 1995;56(1):29-33.

547. Frumovitz M, Slomovitz BM, Singh DK, et al. Frozen section analyses as predictors of lymphatic spread in patients with early-stage uterine cancer. *J Am Coll Surg*. 2004;199(3):388-393.

548. Cragun JM, Havrilesky LJ, Calingaert B, et al. Retrospective analysis of selective lymphadenectomy in apparent early-stage endometrial cancer. *J Clin Oncol*. 2005;23(16):3668-3675.

549. Case AS, Rocconi RP, Straughn JM Jr, et al. A prospective blinded evaluation of the accuracy of frozen section for the surgical management of endometrial cancer. *Obstet Gynecol*. 2006;108(6):1375-1379.

550. Keys HM, Roberts JA, Brunetto V, et al; Gynecologic Oncology Group. A phase III trial of surgery with or without adjunctive external pelvic radiation therapy in intermediate risk endometrial adenocarcinoma: a Gynecologic Oncology Group study. *Gynecol Oncol*. 2004;92(3):744-751. Erratum in: *Gynecol Oncol*. 2004;94(1):241-242.

551. Creutzberg CL, van Putten WL, Koper PC, et al. Surgery and postoperative radiotherapy versus surgery alone for patients with stage-1 endometrial carcinoma: multicentre randomised trial. PORTEC Study Group. Post Operative Radiation Therapy in Endometrial Carcinoma. *Lancet*. 2000; 355(9213):1404-1411.

552. Kong A, Johnson N, Cornes P, et al. Adjuvant radiotherapy for stage I endometrial cancer. *Cochrane Database Syst Rev*. 2007;(2):CD003916. Update in: *Cochrane Database Syst Rev*. 2012;3:CD003916.

Chapter 4

553. ASTEC/EN.5 Study Group, Blake P, Swart AM, et al. Adjuvant external beam radiotherapy in the treatment of endometrial cancer (MRC ASTEC and NCIC CTG EN.5 randomized trials): pooled trial results, systematic review, and meta-analysis. *Lancet.* 2009;373(9658):137-146.

554. Nout RA, Smit VT, Putter H, et al; PORTEC Study Group. Vaginal brachytherapy versus pelvic external beam radiotherapy for patients with endometrial cancer of high-intermediate risk (PORTEC-2): an open-label, non-inferiority, randomised trial. *Lancet.* 2010;375(9717):816-823.

555. Nout RA, Putter H, Jürgenliemk-Schulz IM, et al. Quality of life after pelvic radiotherapy or vaginal brachytherapy for endometrial cancer: first results of the randomized PORTEC-2 trial. *J Clin Oncol.* 2009;27(21):3547-3556.

556. Aapro MS, van Wijk FH, Bolis G, et al; European Organisation for Research and Treatment of Cancer Gynecological Cancer Group. Doxorubicin versus doxorubicin and cisplatin in endometrial carcinoma: definitive results of a randomized study (55872) by the EORTC Gynaecological Cancer Group. *Ann Oncol.* 2003;14(3):441-448.

557. Fleming GF, Brunetto VL, Cella D, et al. Phase III trial of doxorubicin plus cisplatin with or without paclitaxel plus filgrastim in advanced endometrial carcinoma: a Gynecologic Oncology Group Study. *J Clin Oncol.* 2004;22(11):2159-2166.

558. Thigpen JT, Brady MF, Homesley HD, et al. Phase III trial of doxorubicin with or without cisplatin in advanced endometrial carcinoma: a Gynecologic Oncology Group study. *J Clin Oncol.* 2004;22(19):3902-3908.

559. Randall ME, Filiaci VL, Muss H, et al; Gynecologic Oncology Group Study. Randomized phase III trial of whole-abdominal irradiation versus doxorubicin and cisplatin chemotherapy in advanced endometrial carcinoma: a Gynecologic Oncology Group Study. *J Clin Oncol.* 2006;24(1):36-44.

560. Chao CK, Grigsby PW, Perez CA, Mutch DG, Herzog T, Camel HM. Medically inoperable stage I endometrial carcinoma: a few dilemmas in radiotherapeutic management. *Int J Radiat Oncol Biol Phys.* 1996;34(1):27-31.

561. Nguyen TV, Petereit DG. High-dose-rate brachytherapy for medically inoperable stage I endometrial cancer. *Gynecol Oncol.* 1998;71(2):196-203.

562. Lachance JA, Darus CJ, Rice LW. Surgical management and postoperative treatment of endometrial carcinoma. *Rev Obstet Gynecol.* 2008;1(3):97-105.

563. Madalinska JB, van Beurden M, Bleiker EM, et al. The impact of hormone replacement therapy on menopausal symptoms in younger high-risk women after prophylactic salpingo-oophorectomy. *J Clin Oncol.* 2006;24(22):3576-3582.

564. Suriano KA, McHale M, McLaren CE, Li KT, Re A, DiSaia PJ. Estrogen replacement therapy in endometrial cancer patients: a matched control study. *Obstet Gynecol.* 2001;97(4):555-560.

565. Barakat RR, Bundy BN, Spirtos NM, Bell J, Mannel RS; Gynecologic Oncology Group Study. Randomized double-blind trial of estrogen replacement therapy versus placebo in stage I or II endometrial cancer: a Gynecologic Oncology Group Study. *J Clin Oncol.* 2006;24(4):587-592.

566. Reid RL. Progestins in hormone replacement therapy: impact on endometrial and breast cancer. *J SOGC.* 2000;22(9):677-681.

567. Beral V, Bull D, Reeves G; Million Women Study Collaborators. Endometrial cancer and hormone-replacement therapy in the Million Women Study. *Lancet.* 2005;365(9470):1543-1551.

568. Bernstein L. The risk of breast, endometrial and ovarian cancer in users of hormonal preparations. *Basic Clin Pharmacol Toxicol.* 2006;98(3):288-296.

569. Anderson GL, Judd HL, Kaunitz AM, et al; Women's Health Initiative Investigators. Effects of estrogen plus progestin on gynecologic cancers and associated diagnostic procedures: the Women's Health Initiative randomized trial. *JAMA.* 2003;290(13):1739-1748.

570. American Cancer Society. *What Are the Key Statistics About Cervical Cancer?* American Cancer Society Web site. www.cancer.org/cancer/cervicalcancer/detailedguide/cervical-cancer-key-statistics. Revised January 31, 2014. Accessed May 27, 2014.

571. Canadian Cancer Society. *Cervical Cancer Statistics.* Canadian Cancer Society Web site. Published 2014. www.cancer.ca/en/cancer-information/cancer-type/cervical/statistics/?region=qc. Accessed May 27, 2014.

572. American Cancer Society. *Cervical Cancer: Prevention and Early Detection.* American Cancer Society Web site. www.cancer.org/acs/groups/cid/documents/webcontent/003167-pdf.pdf. Revised February 4, 2014. Accessed May 27, 2014.

573. National Cancer Institute. *Cancer Health Disparities.* National Cancer Institute Web site. www.cancer.gov/cancertopics/factsheet/disparities/cancer-health-disparities. Reviewed March 11, 2008. Accessed May 27, 2014.

574. Freeman HP, Wingrove BK. *Excess Cervical Cancer Mortality: A Marker for Low Access to Health Care in Poor Communities.* Rockville, MD: National Cancer Institute, Center to Reduce Cancer Health Disparities; 2005. NIH Pub. No. 05-5282.

575. Dunne EF, Unger ER, Sternberg M, et al. Prevalence of HPV infection among females in the United States. *JAMA.* 2007;297(8):813-819.

576. Smith JS, Green J, Berrington de Gonzalez A, et al. Cervical cancer and use of hormonal contraceptives: a systematic review. *Lancet.* 2003;361(9364):1159-1167.

577. Yasmeen S, Romano PS, Pettinger M, et al. Incidence of cervical cytological abnormalities with aging in the Women's Health Initiative: a randomized controlled trial. *Obstet Gynecol.* 2006;108(2):410-419.

578. Lacey JV Jr, Brinton LA, Barnes WA, et al. Use of hormone replacement therapy and adenocarcinomas and squamous cell carcinomas of the uterine cervix. *Gynecol Oncol.* 2000;77(1):149-154.

579. Arbyn M, Bergeron C, Klinkhamer P, Martin-Hirsch P, Siebers AG, Bulten J. Liquid compared with conventional cervical cytology: a systematic review and meta-analysis. *Obstet Gynecol.* 2008;111(1):167-177.

580. Committee on Practice Bulletins—Gynecology. ACOG Practice Bulletin Number 131: screening for cervical cancer. *Obstet Gynecol.* 2012;120(5):1409-1420.

581. Saslow D, Solomon D, Lawson HW, et al; ACS-ASCCP-ASCP Cervical Cancer Guideline Committee. American Cancer Society, American Society for Colposcopy and Cervical Pathology, and American Society for Clinical Pathology screening guidelines for the prevention and early detection of cervical cancer. *CA Cancer J Clin.* 2012;62(3):147-172.

582. Moyers VA; US Preventive Services Task Force. Screening for cervical cancer: US Preventive Task Force recommendation statement. *Ann Intern Med.* 2012;156(12):880-891. Erratum in: *Ann Intern Med.* 2013;158(11):852.

583. Saslow D, Castle PE, Cox JT, et al; Gynecologic Cancer Advisory Group, Garcia F. American Cancer Society guideline for human papillomavirus (HPV) vaccine use to prevent cervical cancer and its precursors. *Ca Cancer J Clin.* 2007;57(1):7-28.

584. Villa LL, Costa RL, Petta CA, et al. Prophylactic quadrivalent human papillomavirus (types 6, 11, 16, and 18) L1 virus-like particle vaccine in young women: a randomised double-blind placebo-controlled multicentre phase II efficacy trial. *Lancet Oncol.* 2005;6(5):271-278.

585. Villa LL, Costa RL, Petta CA, et al. High sustained efficacy of a prophylactic quadrivalent human papillomavirus type 6/11/16/18 L1 virus-like particle vaccine through 5 years of follow-up. *Br J Cancer.* 2006;95(11):1459-1466.

586. Markowitz LE, Hariri S, Lin C, et al. Reduction in human papillomavirus (HPV) prevalence among young women following HPV vaccine introduction in the United States, National Health and Nutrition Examination Surveys, 2003-2010. *J Infect Dis.* 2013;208(3):385-393.

587. Rodríguez AC, Schiffman M, Herrero R, et al. Longitudinal study of human papillomavirus persistence and cervical intraepithelial neoplasia grade 2/3: critical role of duration of infection. *J Natl Cancer Inst.* 2010;102(5):315-324.

588. Committee opinion no. 588: human papillomavirus vaccination. *Obstet Gynecol.* 2014;123(3):712-718.

589. Howlader N, Noone AM, Krapcho M, et al, eds. *SEER Cancer Statistics Review, 1975-2010.* Bethesda, MD: National Cancer Institute; 2013.

590. Landen CN Jr, Birrer MJ, Sood AK. Early events in the pathogenesis of epithelial ovarian cancer. *J Clin Oncol.* 2008;26(6):995-1005.

591. Crum CP, McKeon FD, Xian W. The oviduct and ovarian cancer: causality, clinical implications, and "targeted prevention." *Clin Obstet Gynecol.* 2012;55(1):24-35.

592. Jazaeri AA, Bryant JL, Park H, et al. Molecular requirements for transformation of fallopian tube epithelial cells into serous carcinoma. *Neoplasia.* 2011;13(10):899-911.

593. Quirk JT, Natarajan N. Age-specific ovarian cancer incidence rate patterns in the United States. *Gynecol Oncol.* 2005;99(1):248-250.

594. Ramus SJ, Harrington PA, Pye C, et al. Contribution of BRCA1 and BRCA2 mutations to inherited ovarian cancer. *Hum Mutat.* 2007;28(12):1207-1215.

595. Chen S, Parmigiani G. Meta-analysis of BRCA 1 and BRCA 2 penetrance. *J Clin Oncol.* 2007;25(11):1329-1333.

596. South SA, Vance H, Farrell C, et al. Consideration of hereditary nonpolyposis colorectal cancer in BRCA mutation-negative familial ovarian cancers. *Cancer.* 2009;115(2):324-333.

597. Langseth H, Hankinson SE, Siemiatycki J, Weiderpass E. Perineal use of talc and risk of ovarian cancer. *J Epidemiol Community Health.* 2008;62(4):358-360.

598. Muscat JE, Huncharek MS. Perineal talc use and ovarian cancer: a critical review. *Eur J Cancer Prev.* 2008;17(2):139-146.

599. Gertig DM, Hunter DJ, Cramer DW, et al. Prospective study of talc use and ovarian cancer. *J Natl Cancer Inst.* 2000;92(3):249-252.

600. Whysner J, Mohan M. Perineal application of talc and cornstarch powders: evaluation of ovarian cancer risk. *Am J Obstet Gynecol.* 2000;182(3):720-724.

601. Huncharek M, Muscat J, Onitilo A, Kupelnick B. Use of cosmetic talc on contraceptive diaphragms and risk of ovarian cancer: a meta-analysis of nine observational studies. *Eur J Cancer Prev.* 2007;16(5):422-429.
602. Pearce CL, Templeman C, Rossing MA, et al; Ovarian Cancer Association Consortium. Association between endometriosis and risk of histological subtypes of ovarian cancer: a pooled analysis of case-control studies. *Lancet Oncol.* 2012;13(4):385-394.
603. Collaborative Group on Epidemiological Studies of Ovarian Cancer; Beral V, Doll R, Hermon C, Peto R, Reeves G. Ovarian cancer and oral contraceptives: collaborative reanalysis of data from 45 epidemiological studies including 23,257 women with ovarian cancer and 87,303 controls. *Lancet.* 2008;371(9609):303-314.
604. Jordan SJ, Siskind V, C Green A, Whiteman DC, Webb PM. Breastfeeding and risk of epithelial ovarian cancer. *Cancer Causes Control.* 2010;21(1):109-116.
605. Kjaer SK, Mellemkjaer L, Brinton LA, Johansen C, Gridley G, Olsen JH. Tubal sterilization and risk of ovarian, endometrial and cervical cancer. A Danish population-based follow-up study of more than 65,000 sterilized women. *Int J Epidemiol.* 2004;33(3):596-602.
606. Purdie DM, Siskind V, Bain CJ, Webb PM, Green AC. Reproduction-related risk factors for mucinous and nonmucinous epithelial ovarian cancer. *Am J Epidemiol.* 2001;153(9):860-864.
607. Lacey JV Jr, Mink PJ, Lubin JH, et al. Menopausal hormone replacement therapy and risk of ovarian cancer. *JAMA.* 2002;288(3):334-341. Erratum in: *JAMA.* 2002;288(20):2544.
608. Beral V; Million Women Study Collaborators, Bull D, Green J, Reeves G. Ovarian cancer and hormone replacement therapy in the Million Women Study. *Lancet.* 2007;369(9574):1703-1710.
609. Mørch LS, Løkkegaard E, Andreasen AH, Krüger-Kjaer S, Lidegaard O. Hormone therapy and ovarian cancer. *JAMA.* 2009;302(3):298-305.
610. Rossing MA, Cushing-Haugen KL, Wicklund KG, Doherty JA, Weiss NS. Menopausal hormone therapy and risk of epithelial ovarian cancer. *Cancer Epidemiol Biomarkers Prev.* 2007;16(12):2548-2556.
611. Swerdlow AJ, Jones ME. Ovarian cancer risk in premenopausal and perimenopausal women treated with tamoxifen: a case-control study. *Br J Cancer.* 2007;96(5):850-855.
612. Goff BA, Mandel L, Muntz HG, Melancon CH. Ovarian cancer diagnosis. *Cancer.* 2000;89(10):2068-2075.
613. Twombly R. Cancer killer may be "silent" no more. *J Natl Cancer Inst.* 2007;99(18):1359-1361.
614. Rossing MA, Wicklund KG, Cushing-Haugen KL, Weiss NS. Predictive value of symptoms for early detection of ovarian cancer. *J Natl Cancer Inst.* 2010;102(4):222-229.
615. Partridge E, Kreimer AR, Greenlee RT, et al; PLCO Project Team. Results from four rounds of ovarian cancer screening in a randomized trial. *Obstet Gynecol.* 2009;113(4):775-782.
616. Buys SS, Partridge E, Black A, et al; PLCO Project Team. Effect of screening on ovarian cancer mortality: the Prostate, Lung, Colorectal and Ovarian (PLCO) Cancer Screening Randomized Controlled Trial. *JAMA.* 2011;305(22):2295-2303.
617. Rossing MA, Cushing-Haugen KL, Wicklund KG, Doherty JA, Weiss NS. Recreational physical activity and risk of epithelial ovarian cancer. *Cancer Causes Control.* 2010;21(4):485-491.
618. McGuire V, Felberg A, Mills M, et al. Relation of contraceptive and reproductive history to ovarian cancer risk in carriers and noncarriers of BRCA1 gene mutations. *Am J Epidemiol.* 2004;160(7):613-618.
619. Kwon JS, Tinker A, Pansegrau G, et al. Prophylactic salpingectomy and delayed oophorectomy as an alternative for BRCA mutation carriers. *Obstet Gynecol.* 2013;121(1):14-24.
620. Henley JS, Richards TB, Underwood MJ, Sunderam CR, Plescia M, McAfee TS; Centers for Disease Control and Prevention (CDC). Lung cancer incidence trends among men and women—United States, 2005-2009. *MMWR Morb Mortal Wkly Rep.* 2014;63(1):1-5.
621. American Cancer Society. *Lung Cancer (Non-Small Cell).* American Cancer Society Web site. www.cancer.org/acs/groups/cid/documents/webcontent/003115-pdf.pdf. Revised April 30, 2014. Accessed May 28, 2014.
622. Canadian Cancer Society. *Lung Cancer Statistics.* Canadian Cancer Society Web site. Published 2014. www.cancer.ca/en/cancer-information/cancer-type/lung/statistics/?region=bc#ixzz2upLOQHBV. Accessed May 28, 2014.
623. Chlebowski RT. Menopausal hormone therapy, hormone receptor status, and lung cancer in women. *Semin Oncol.* 2009;36(6):566-571.
624. Siegfried JM, Hershberger PA, Stabile LP. Estrogen receptor signaling in lung cancer. *Semin Oncol.* 2009;36(6):524-531.
625. Chlebowski RT, Schwartz AG, Wakelee H, et al; Women's Health Initiative Investigators. Oestrogen plus progestin and lung cancer in postmenopausal women: a post-hoc analysis of a randomised controlled trial. *Lancet.* 2009;374(9697):1243-1251.
626. Olsson H, Bladström A, Ingvar C. Are smoking-associated cancers prevented or postponed in women using hormone replacement therapy? *Obstet Gynecol.* 2003;102(3):565-570.
627. Schwartz AG, Wenzlaff AS, Prysak GM, et al. Reproductive factors, hormone use, estrogen receptor expression and risk of non small-cell lung cancer in women. *J Clin Oncol.* 2007;25(36):5785-5792.
628. Rodriguez C, Spencer Feigelson H, Deka A, et al. Postmenopausal hormone therapy and lung cancer risk in the Cancer Prevention Study II nutrition cohort. *Cancer Epidemiol Biomarkers Prev.* 2008;17(3):655-660.
629. Katcoff H, Wenzlaff AS, Schwartz AG. Survival in women with NSCLC: the role of reproductive history and hormone use. *J Thorac Oncol.* 2014;9(3):355-361.
630. Ramchandran K, Patel JD. Sex differences in susceptibility to carcinogens. *Semin Oncol.* 2009;36(6):516-523.
631. Patel JD. Lung cancer: a biologically different disease in women? *Womens Health (Lond Engl).* 2009;5(6):685-691.
632. Cote ML, Yoo W, Wenzlaff AS, et al. Tobacco and estrogen metabolic polymorphisms and risk of non-small cell lung cancer in women. *Carcinogenesis.* 2009;30(4):626-635.
633. Bouchardy C, Benhamou S, Schaffar R et al. Lung cancer mortality risk among breast cancer patients treated with anti-estrogens. *Cancer.* 2011;117(6):1288-1295.
634. Brenner H, Chang-Claude J, Seiler CM, Stürmer T, Hoffmeister M. Case-control study supports extension of surveillance interval after colonoscopic polypectomy to at least 5 yr. *Am J Gastroenterol.* 2007;102(8):1739-1744.
635. American Cancer Society. *Colorectal Cancer.* American Cancer Society Web site. www.cancer.org/acs/groups/cid/documents/webcontent/003096-pdf.pdf. Revised January 31, 2014. Accessed May 28, 2014.
636. Mills KT, Bellows CFC, Hoffman AE, Kelly TN, Gagliardi G. Diabetes mellitus and colorectal cancer prognosis: a meta-analysis. *Dis Colon Rectum.* 2013;56(11):1304-1319.
637. Nimptsch K, Bernstein AM, Giovannucci E, Fuchs CS. Willett WC, Wu K. Dietary intake of red meat, poultry, and fish during high school and risk of colorectal adenomas in women. *Am J Epidemiol.* 2013;178(2):172-183.
638. Doubeni CA., Major JM, Laiyemo AO, et al. Contribution of behavioral risk factors and obesity to socioeconomic differences in colorectal cancer Incidence. *J Natl Cancer Inst.* 2012;104(18):1353-1362.
639. Bardou M, Barkun AN, Martel M. Republished: obesity and colorectal cancer. *Postgrad Med J.* 2013;89(1055):519-533.
640. Cho E, Lee JE, Rimm EB, Fuchs CS, Giovannucci EL. Alcohol consumption and the risk of colon cancer by family history of colorectal cancer. *Am J Clin Nutr.* 2012;95(2):413-419.
641. Zgaga L, Agakov F, Theodoratou E, et al. Model selection approach suggests causal association between 25-hydroxyvitamin D and colorectal cancer. *PLoS One.* 2013;8(5):e63475.
642. Lagerstedt Robinson K, Liu T, Vandrovcova J, et al. Lynch syndrome (hereditary nonpolyposis colorectal cancer) diagnostics. *J Natl Cancer Inst.* 2007;99(4):291-299.
643. Kohlmann W, Gruber SB. Lynch syndrome. In: Pagon RA, Adam MP, Bird TD, et al, eds. *GeneReviews [Internet].* Seattle, WA: University of Washington, Seattle; 1993-2014. www.ncbi.nlm.nih.gov/books/NBK1211/. Updated May 22, 2014. Accessed May 28, 2014.
644. Lynch PM. When and how to perform genetic testing for inherited colorectal cancer syndromes. *J Natl Compr Canc Netw.* 2013;11(12):1577-1583.
645. Half E, Bercovich D, Rozen P. Familial adenomatous polyposis. *Orphanet J Rare Dis.* 2009;4:22.
646. Wei MY, Garland CF, Gorham ED, Mohr SB, Giovannucci E. Vitamin D and prevention of colorectal adenoma: a meta-analysis. *Cancer Epidemiol Biomarkers Prev.* 2008;17(11):2958-2969.
647. Holick MF. Vitamin D deficiency. *N Engl J Med.* 2007;357(3):266-281.
648. Rex DK, Johnson DA, Anderson JC, Shoenfeld PS, Burke CA, Inadomi JM; American College of Gastroenterology. American College of Gastroenterology guidelines for colorectal cancer screening 2009 [corrected]. *Am J Gastroenterol.* 2009;104(3):739-750. Erratum in: *Am J Gastroenterol.* 2009;104(6):1613.
649. Khan AF. The role of fecal occult blood testing in colorectal cancer screening. In: *Benchmarks.* National Cancer Institute Web site. Published March 26, 2010. http://benchmarks.cancer.gov/2010/03/the-role-of-fecal-occult-blood-testing-in-colorectal-cancer-screening. Accessed May 28, 2014.

Chapter 4

650. US Preventive Services Task Force. Screening for colorectal cancer: US Preventive Services Task Force recommendation statement. *Ann Intern Med.* 2008;149(9):627-637.
651. Whitlock EP, Lin JS, Liles E, Beil TL, Fu R. Screening for colorectal cancer: a targeted systematic review for the US Preventive Services Task Force. *Ann Intern Med.* 2008;149(9):638-658.
652. Panteris V, Haringsma J, Kuipers EJ. Colonoscopy perforation rate, mechanisms and outcome: from diagnostic to therapeutic colonoscopy. *Endoscopy.* 2009; 41(11): 941-951.
653. Gatto NM, Frucht H, Sundararajan V, Jacobsen JS, Grann VR, Neugat AI. Risk of perforation after colonoscopy and sigmoidoscopy: a population-based study. *J Natl Cancer Inst.* 2003;95(3):230-236.
654. Arora G, Mannalithara A, Singh G, Gerson LB, Triadafilopoulos G. Risk of perforation from a colonoscopy in adults: a large population-based study. *Gastrointest Endosc.* 2009;69(3 pt 2):654-664.
655. Sagawa T, Kakizaki S, Iizuka H, et al. Analysis of colonoscopic perforations at a local clinic and a tertiary hospital. *World J Gastroenterol.* 2012;18(35): 4898-4904.
656. Bielwaska B, Day AG, Lieberman DA, Hookey LC. Risk factors for early colonoscopic perforation include non-gastroenterologist endoscopists: a multivariable analysis. *Clin Gastroenterol Hepatol.* 2014;12(1):85-92.
657. Winawer SJ, Stewart ET, Zauber AG, et al. A comparison of colonoscopy and double-contrast barium enema for surveillance after polypectomy. National Polyp Study Work Group. *N Engl J Med.* 2000;342(24):1766-1772.
658. Ferrucci JT. Double-contrast barium enema: use in practice and implications for CT colonography. *AJR Am J Roentgenol.* 2006;187(1):170-173.
659. Pickhardt PJ, Choi JR, Hwang I, et al. Computed tomographic virtual colonoscopy to screen for colorectal neoplasia in asymptomatic adults. *N Engl J Med.* 2003;349(23):2191-2200.
660. Iafrate F, Iussich G, Correale L, et al. Adverse events of computed tomography colonography: an Italian National Survey. *Dig Liver Dis.* 2013; 45(8):645-650.
661. Umar A, Boland CR, Terdiman JP, et al. Revised Bethesda guidelines for hereditary nonpolyposis colorectal cancer (Lynch syndrome) and microsatellite instability. *J Natl Cancer Inst.* 2004;96(4):261-268.
662. Beresford SA, Johnson KC, Ritenbaugh NL, et al. Low-fat dietary pattern and risk of colorectal cancer: the Women's Health Initiative Randomized Controlled Dietary Modification Trial. *JAMA.* 2006;295(6):643-654.
663. Lanza E, Schatzkin A, Daston C, et al, PPT Study Group. Implementation of a 4-y, high-fiber, high-fruit-and-vegetable, low-fat dietary intervention: results of dietary changes in the Polyp Prevention Trial. *Am J Clin Nutr.* 2001;74(3):387-401.
664. Park Y, Hunter DJ, Spiegelman D, et al. Dietary fiber intake and risk of colorectal cancer: a pooled analysis of prospective cohort studies. *JAMA.* 2005;294(22):2849-2857.
665. Longacre TA, Fenoglio-Preiser CM. Mixed hyperplastic adenomatous polyps/serrated adenomas. A distinct form of colorectal neoplasia. *Am J Surg Pathol.* 1990;14(6):524-537.
666. Lieberman DA, Rex DK, Winawer SJ, Giardello FM, Johnson DA, Levin TR; United States Multi-Society Task Force on Colorectal Cancer. Guidelines for colonoscopy surveillance after screening and polypectomy: a consensus update by the US Multi-Society Task force on Colorectal Cancer. *Gastroenterology.* 2012;143(3):844-857.
667. Nishihara R, Lochhead P, Kuchiba A, et al. Aspirin use and risk of colorectal cancer according to BRAF mutation status. *JAMA.* 2013;309(24):2563-2571.
668. Ishikawa H, Wakabayashi K, Suzuki S, et al. Preventive effects of low-dose aspirin on colorectal adenoma growth in patients with familial adenomatous polyposis: double-blind, randomized clinical trial. *Cancer Med.* 2013; 21(1):50-56.
669. Razzak AA, Oxentenko AS, Vierkant RA, et al. Associations between intake of folate and related micronutrients with molecularly defined colorectal cancer risks in the Iowa Women's Health Study. *Nutr Cancer.* 2012;64(7):899-910.
670. Williams JL, Ji P, Ouyang N, Kopelovich L, Rigas B. Protein nitration and nitrosylation by NO-donating aspirin in colon cancer cells: relevance to its mechanism of action. *Exp Cell Res.* 2011;317(10):1359-1367.
671. Chlebowski RT, Wactawski-Wende J, Ritenbaugh C, et al; Women's Health Initiative Investigators. Estrogen plus progestin and colorectal cancer in postmenopausal women. *N Engl J Med.* 2004;350(10):991-1004.
672. Simon MS, Chlebowski RT, Wactawski-Wende J, et al. Estrogen plus progestin and the colorectal cancer incidence and mortality. *J Clin Oncol.* 2012;30(32):3983-3990. Erratum in: *J Clin Oncol.* 2013;31(16):2063.
673. Tamburrino A, Piro G, Carbone C, Tortora G, Melisi D. Mechanisms of resistance to chemotherapeutic and anti-angiogenic drugs as novel targets for pancreatic cancer therapy. *Front Pharmacol.* 2013;4:56.
674. Jemal A, Bray F, Center MM, Ferlay J, Ward E, Forman D. Global cancer statistics. *CA Cancer J Clin.* 2011;61(2):69-90. Erratum in: *CA Cancer J Clin.* 2011;61(2):134.
675. Yadav D, Lowenfels AB. The epidemiology of pancreatitis and pancreatic cancer. *Gastroenterology.* 2013;144(6):1252-1261.
676. Navarro Silvera SA, Miller AB, Rohan TE. Hormonal and reproductive factors and pancreatic cancer risk: a prospective cohort study. *Pancreas.* 2005;30(4):369-374.
677. Heuch I, Jacobsen BK, Albrektsen G. Kvåle G. Reproductive factors and pancreatic cancer risk: a Norwegian cohort study. *Br J Cancer.* 2008; 98(1):189-193.
678. Prizment AE, Anderson KE, Hong CP, Folsom AR. Pancreatic cancer incidence in relation to female reproductive factors: Iowa Women's Health Study. *JOP.* 2007;8(1):16-27.
679. Teras LR, Patel AV, Rodriguez C, Thun MJ, Calle EE. Parity, other reproductive factors, and risk of pancreatic cancer mortality in a large cohort of US women (United States). *Cancer Causes Control.* 2005;156(9): 1035-1040.
680. Stevens RJ, Roddam AW, Green J, et al; Million Women Study Collaborators. *Cancer Epidemiol Biomarkers Prev.* 2009;18(5):1457-1460.
681. Lin Y, Tamakoshi A, Kawamura T, et al; JACC Study Group, Japan Collaborative Cohort. A prospective cohort study of cigarette smoking and pancreatic cancer in Japan. *Cancer Causes Control.* 2002;13(3):249-254.
682. Batabyal P, Vander Hoorn S, Christophi C, Nikfarjam M. Association of diabetes mellitus and pancreatic adenocarcinoma: a meta-analysis of 88 studies. *Ann Surg Oncol.* 2014;21(7):2453-2462.
683. Chan JM, Wang F, Holly EA. Vegetable and fruit intake and pancreatic cancer in a population-based case-control study in the San Francisco bay area. *Cancer Epidemiol Biomarkers Prev.* 2005;14(9):2093-2097.
684. Coughlin SS, Calle EE, Patel AV, Thun MJ. Predictors of pancreatic cancer mortality among a large cohort of United States adults. *Cancer Causes Control.* 2000;11(10):915-923.
685. Larsson SC, Permert J, Håkansson N, Näslund I, Bergkvist L, Wolk A. Overall obesity, abdominal adiposity, diabetes and cigarette smoking in relation to the risk of pancreatic cancer in two Swedish population-based cohorts. *Br J Cancer.* 2005;93(11):1310-1315.
686. Lin Y, Yagya K, Ueda J, Kurosawa M, Tamakoshi Am Kikuchi S; JACC Study Group. Active and passive smoking and risk of death from pancreatic cancer: findings from the Japan Collaborative Cohort Study. *Pancreatology.* 2013;13(3):279-284.
687. Bao Y, Giovannucci EL, Kraft P, et al. Inflammatory plasma markers and pancreatic cancer risk: a prospective study of five US cohorts. *Cancer Epidemiol Biomarkers Prev.* 2013;22(5):855-861.
688. Garber JE, Offit K. Hereditary cancer predisposition syndromes. *J Clin Oncol.* 2005;23(2):276-292.
689. Elashoff M, Matveyenko AV, Gier B, Elashoff R, Butler PC. Pancreatitis, pancreatic, and thyroid cancer with glucagon-like peptide-1-based therapies. *Gastroenterology.* 2011;141(1):150-156.
690. Khorana AA, Fine RL. Pancreatic cancer and thromboembolic disease. *Lancet Oncol.* 2004;5(11):655-663.
691. Lee E, Horn-Ross PL, Rull RP, et al. Reproductive factors, exogenous hormones, and pancreatic cancer risk in the CTS. *Am J Epidemiol.* 2013; 178(9):1403-1413.
692. Arem H, Reedy J, Sampson J, et al. The Healthy Eating Index 2005 and risk for pancreatic cancer in the NIH-AARP study. *J Natl Cancer Inst.* 2013; 105(17):1298-1305.
693. Bao Y, Hu FB, Giovannucci EL, et al. Nut consumption and risk of pancreatic cancer in women. *Br J Cancer.* 2013;109(11):2911-2916.
694. Han X, Li J, Brasky TM, et al. Antioxidant intake and pancreatic cancer risk; the Vitamins and Lifestyle (VITAL) Study. *Cancer.* 2013;119(7):1314-1320.
695. Skinner HG, Michaud DS, Giovannucci E, Willett WC, Colditz GA, Fuchs CS. Vitamin D intake and the risk of pancreatic cancer in two cohort studies. *Cancer Epidemiol Biomarkers Prev.* 2006;15(9):1688-1695.
696. Stolzenberg-Solomon RZ, Vieth R, Azad A, et al. A prospective nested case-control study of vitamin D status and pancreatic cancer risk in male smokers. *Cancer Res.* 2006;66(20):10213-10219.
697. Eide MJ, Weinstock MA. Public health challenges in sun protection. *Dermatol Clin.* 2006;24(1):119-124.

698. Poochareon VN, Cockerell CJ. The war against skin cancer: the time for action is now. *Arch Dermatol.* 2005;141(4):499-501.
699. Little EG, Eide MJ. Update on the current state of melanoma incidence. *Dermatol Clin.* 2012;30(3):355-361.
700. Balch CM, Buzaid AC, Soong SJ, et al. Final version of the American Joint Committee on Cancer staging system for cutaneous melanoma. *J Clin Oncol.* 2001;19(16):3635-3648.
701. American Cancer Society. *Melanoma Skin Cancer.* www.cancer.org/acs/groups/cid/documents/webcontent/003120-pdf.pdf. Revised January 9, 2014. Revised May 30, 2013. Accessed May 29, 2014.
702. Werner RN, Sammain A, Erdmann R, Hartmann V, Stockfleth E, Nast A. The natural history of actinic keratosis: a systematic review. *Br J Dermatol.* 2013;169(3):502-518.
703. Lowe NJ. An overview of ultraviolet radiation, sunscreens, and photo-induced dermatoses. *Dermatol Clin.* 2006;24(1):9-17.

CHAPTER 5

Clinical Evaluation and Counseling

As women move through the menopause transition, regular health examinations provide them with opportunities to collaborate with healthcare professionals to evaluate their health and improve their health practices at midlife, leading toward healthy aging. Some experts are questioning the value of the periodic health examination in reducing all-cause, cardiovascular, or cancer mortality. For example, a systematic meta-analysis and qualitative synthesis concluded that general health checks are unlikely to be beneficial in reducing morbidity or mortality.[1] Nonetheless, the annual evaluation and counseling visit often remains the standard of care. Some studies have found that the periodic health exam has allayed patient fears and anxieties and actually avoided excessive use of the healthcare system. The exam was found to be consistent with their values and the second principle of evidence-based medicine—that evidence alone is not enough to make a clinical decision.[2,3] Above all, the perimenopausal health visit provides the opportunity to screen for diseases at risk, diagnose preclinical disease that may already be present, and educate on all aspects for enhancement of future quality of life (QOL).

The exam should be tailored to the individual woman and also to the known physical and psychological changes of midlife and menopause. Each woman experiences menopause in a unique way. Some women will have troublesome symptoms; others will have few or no symptoms. Most women's experiences and views of menopause are not consistent with the negative associations linked with menopause in the past.

A useful way for women and their healthcare professionals to view menopause is as a sentinel event that presents a unique opportunity to identify menopause-related issues, receive appropriate anticipatory guidance, plan preventive care, diagnose early disease, and determine the need for intervention, if any.

During the transition from the reproductive years through menopause and beyond, women may experience many physical changes, most of which are expected outcomes of menopause and aging. Therefore, it is essential that women receive accurate information about these physiologic changes as well as about the management of menopause symptoms and how to reduce the risk of diseases that become more common with aging.

In general, the clinical evaluation includes (Table 1)[4]

- A detailed medical history, including psychological, social, obstetric, surgical, sexual, and family history. Obtaining an immunization history is important for midlife women.

- Physical examination, including vital signs, height, weight, body mass index (BMI), waist circumference, and thyroid, breast, and pelvic examinations.

- Laboratory testing (when indicated and per accepted guidelines)—such as fasting lipids (total; high-density lipoprotein cholesterol; low-density lipoprotein cholesterol; and triglycerides); fasting glucose; Papanicolaou (Pap) test; high-risk human papillomavirus (HPV) screen; thyroid; urine screens; screens for sexually transmitted infections (STIs), including hepatitis C and HIV in high-risk populations; vaginal pH; and fecal immunochemical and occult blood tests.

- Problem-oriented testing (eg, wet mount, yeast culture, urine culture)

- Other age- and risk-appropriate tests, such as screening for cancer of the skin, breast, cervix, and colon; eye screening (including vision and glaucoma); hearing; and bone density

Clinicians will want to consider the appropriate approach for each individual patient. Because the focus here is on specific menopause-related issues, it does not include all the possible elements of a comprehensive physical examination and preventive care.

History gathering

A comprehensive, 9-page menopause health questionnaire has been developed by the North American Menopause Society (NAMS) that can assist clinicians in gathering a

Chapter 5

Table 1. Elements of a Comprehensive Evaluation

Presenting history (reason for visit)

Family history
- Heart disease
- Cancer of the breast, uterus, ovary, cervix, lung, skin (melanoma), or colon
- Osteoporosis and fractures
- Diabetes mellitus
- Thyroid problems

Personal history
- Menopausal age/Menstrual pattern
- Menopausal: vasomotor symptoms and palpitations
- Particulars of pregnancies
- Gynecologic operations including removal of ovaries
- Vaginal bleeding
- Diet/Nutrition assessment
- Physical activity/Exercise
- Tobacco, alcohol, and other drug use
- Use of complementary and alternative medicine
- Breasts
- Heart disease
- Thromboembolic episodes
- Liver disease
- Diabetes
- Osteoporosis and fractures
- Allergies and contraindications to drugs
- Family relationships and personal problems
- Domestic violence and abuse
- Psycho-socio-cultural: Nervousness, irritability, insomnia, and depression
- Sexual relations: Frequency, change in desire, pain, satisfaction, partner problem

Physical examination
- Blood pressure
- Height, weight, body mass index
- Oral cavity
- Glands of neck and thyroid
- Breasts and axilla
- Skin, hair
- Abdominal examination
- Pelvic examination

Adapted from Utian WH.[4]

menopause-focused history. It is available on the NAMS website (www.menopause.org).

Medical history

A complete medical history of a perimenopausal or postmenopausal woman will include information from these areas:

Symptom history. Questions about symptoms in general, including those that could be related to menopause, should be asked. Symptoms should be rated according to frequency, severity, duration, and associated distress. The National Institutes of Health once attributed only vasomotor symptoms (VMS), painful intercourse, and possibly sleep disturbance to menopause; however, women often report many additional physical and psychological complaints at the time of the menopause transition. Whether these perceived changes are related to menopause or aging, potential areas for discussion in addition to VMS (usual and atypical), difficulty sleeping, and dyspareunia include moodiness, anxiety, depression, urinary symptoms, sexual issues (desire, arousal, orgasm), hair and skin changes, weight gain, joint pain, cognitive function, and memory, all of which are frequently mentioned at midlife examinations. Numerous symptom inventories can be used to evaluate menopausal women. The most widely used is the 21-question Greene Climacteric Scale, which is easily administered and scored.[5]

Gynecologic history. Review a woman's menstrual history, age at menarche, description of menses throughout her reproductive life, current menstrual history, and date of final menses, if applicable. Note all gynecologic problems, including ovarian cysts, polycystic ovarian syndrome, fibroids, infertility, endometriosis, STIs, abnormal Pap tests, diethylstilbestrol exposure in utero, and gynecologic surgery.

It is important to establish the date and results of the patient's last clinical breast and pelvic examinations as well as health screens such as Pap tests, mammograms, and tests for cholesterol, glucose, and bone density because guidelines about frequency of these screens continue to change.

Obstetric history. Establish the number of pregnancies, full-term births, premature births, abortions, and living children; the woman's age at time of first birth; and significant complications during pregnancy or delivery. Women with a history of gestational diabetes have a 7-fold risk of developing type 2 diabetes mellitus (DM) later in life.[6] Women who had a pregnancy complicated by preeclampsia may be at increased risk of cardiovascular disease.[7]

History of serious illness. Exploring a woman's self-perceived and objective health status provides a framework within which to approach menopause and aging. Put special emphasis on cardiovascular disease (CVD), DM, cancer (especially breast), obesity, and osteoporosis, although any serious medical condition is relevant. Review hospitalizations.

Surgical history. Obtain a full history of all patient surgeries.

Medication history. An accurate medication list from patients is critical and often difficult to obtain.[8] Studies show that errors are common. Asking patients to bring their medications and supplements or at least a list to their

CLINICAL EVALUATION AND COUNSELING

appointment can be helpful. Document medication allergies and current and past hormone use (hormonal contraceptives, menopausal hormone therapy [HT]). It is useful to ask specifically about previous strategies to deal with symptoms attributed to menopause. For all medications—especially those used for menopause-related symptoms—ask about duration of use, effectiveness, adverse events (AEs), and reasons for stopping.

Sexual history. Sexuality is important to midlife women and may be adversely affected by the menopause transition.[9] A complete sexual history requires a nonjudgmental attitude. Many women will not discuss sexual concerns unless asked. Often clinicians avoid discussions on sexuality because they lack the skills to deal with these issues, are uncomfortable with the topic, have no knowledge of available interventions, or feel that they do not have time to address such concerns.[10] Practical guidance does exist for this sometimes-challenging undertaking.[11] Be sensitive to the woman's specific situation. Do not make assumptions about sexual orientation, context, or values.

Psychological history. It is important to elicit a woman's history of depression, anxiety, psychotherapy, and other mental health issues. Studies indicate that the likelihood of depressed mood in the menopause transition is approximately 30% to 300% greater compared with that during premenopause.[12] Women who have had hormone-related mood issues such as premenstrual syndrome, premenstrual dysphoric disorder, and postpartum depression are at risk for exacerbation of mood disorders during perimenopause. Women with a history of depression are nearly 5 times more likely to have a diagnosis of major depression in the menopause transition, whereas women with no history of depression are 2 to 4 times more likely to report depressed mood compared with premenopausal women. The increased risk decreases after perimenopause. The menopause transition may be an increased period of vulnerability for some women, with added risk factors including poor sleep, hot flashes, and stressful or negative life events. Because women often present to their primary care or other professionals before consulting a mental health professional, conducting an initial assessment of psychological health should be a routine component of the periodic exam.

Social history

Marital status; occupation; tobacco (current and previous), alcohol, and illicit drug use; family status; life stresses; and living situation all affect a woman's health. Her financial status and access to care may be relevant issues to explore. Ask her whether she feels safe at home. The open-ended question, "What are the stresses in your life?" can be revealing.

Family history

In taking the family history, be especially attentive to breast, ovarian, and colon cancer; CVD; thromboembolic disease; DM; and osteoporosis (including fracture), as well as the age when each disease was diagnosed. These have health implications for midlife women. The age at which a woman's first-degree female relatives reached menopause may help predict her age at menopause but is not definitive.

Physical examination

The physical examination should include measurement of height, weight, and blood pressure (BP) as well as pelvic and breast examinations.

Height

Current height and her maximal adult height are important components of the clinical evaluation. Height loss greater than 1.5 in (3.8 cm) may be associated with vertebral compression fractures and thus osteoporosis. The preferred method for height measurement is a stadiometer. Height should be measured (without shoes) during each visit and, ideally, at approximately the same time of day. Women lose up to 0.24 in (6 mm) of height over the course of a day.

Weight and body mass index

Recording a woman's weight is another essential component of clinical evaluation. Clinicians should always be aware that weight is a sensitive subject for many women. The BMI provides a measure of adiposity that is relatively independent of height. The formula for calculating BMI is

$$\text{BMI (in kg/m}^2\text{)} = \frac{\text{weight in kg}}{(\text{height in meters})^2}$$

Many electronic health records calculate BMI automatically.

Sometimes BMI is expressed simply as the number (without kg/m^2). Web-based calculators are also available.[13] The US National Library of Medicine has established definitions to classify BMI (Table 2),[14] and once it has been calculated, the woman's weight classification can be determined (ie, normal, underweight, obese). The BMI is helpful to frame discussions with women about weight and quantify any obesity-associated risks.

In addition to BMI, the presence of central obesity out of proportion to total body fat is an independent predictor of type 2 DM, CVD, and total mortality.[15] The waist circumference (measured parallel to the ground, just above the iliac crest, while a woman is standing and after exhaling) can be measured for the initial assessment of obesity and then to monitor the success of any weight loss treatment. A waist circumference of 35 in or more (88 cm) in women is associated with increased risk for type 2 DM, dyslipidemia, hypertension, and CVD. Waist circumference measurement is most useful in women who fall in the normal or overweight BMI category.[16]

The waist-to-hip ratio (WHR) is an alternative measure to classify body fat distribution as *android* obesity (fat in the waist and stomach, or "apple-shaped") or *gynecoid* obesity (fat in the hips, or "pear-shaped"). The ratio estimates the amount of intra-abdominal fat, which is greater with android obesity. A WHR greater than 0.85 is indicative of android obesity, whereas a WHR of less than 0.75 is indicative of gynecoid obesity. The Nurses' Health Study found that women with a WHR of 0.74 or higher had a 2-fold increase in heart disease risk.[17] In addition, waist circumference was found to be an independent factor associated with risk of coronary heart disease in women. Because measuring the waist alone is just as accurate, however, the WHR is no longer recommended by the American Heart Association.[18]

Obesity is a fundamental health parameter.[19] Data from the third National Health and Nutrition Examination Survey indicate that risk for type 2 DM increases dramatically when BMI exceeds 27 and as overweight (particularly android obesity) increases.[20] The increase in obesity observed over the past decade in the United States has been accompanied by a 25% increase in the prevalence of type 2 DM.[21] In the third National Health and Nutrition Examination Survey, higher body weight was also associated with a greater risk of gallstones and cholecystectomy.[20]

Increasing body weight also elevates the risk for osteoarthritis. Persons with a BMI of 30 or more have a markedly increased risk for knee osteoarthritis. Conversely, increased body weight seems to offer protection against the development of osteoporosis.

Obesity, in general, is associated with increased incidence and mortality from certain cancers.[22] Accumulating evidence recognizes obesity as a chronic inflammatory disease, and chronic inflammation is increasingly being acknowledged as an etiology in several cancers including esophageal, liver, colon, postmenopausal breast, and endometrial. Additional association has been found between obesity, inflammation, and other cancers such as prostate, renal, gastric, pancreatic, and gallbladder, further suggesting that inflammation might be important in the obesity-cancer link.[23]

An estimated 34% to 56% of cases of endometrial cancer are associated with increased body weight (BMI >29). Almost one-half of breast cancer cases among postmenopausal women occur in those with a BMI greater than 29. In the Nurses' Health Study, women gaining more than 20 lb (9 kg) from age 18 to midlife doubled their risk for breast cancer compared with women who maintained stable weight.[24] Compared with women of normal weight, obese women have a higher mortality rate from cancers of the endometrium, cervix, gallbladder, colon, ovary, and breast (in postmenopausal women). These findings with respect to mortality were for the most part corroborated in a large prospective study of 900,000 participants in North America in which the optimal BMI was 22.5 to 25; BMI below optimal was often associated with smoking-related disease.[25]

Please see Chapter 2 for more about midlife body weight changes.

Blood pressure testing

Hypertension is an important parameter in determining cardiovascular and stroke risk for women. Women are nearly as likely as men to develop hypertension during their lifetimes; however, in people aged 65 years and older, women are more likely than men to have high BP.[26] The incidence of hypertension in women aged 55 to 64 years is 53.3% (in men, 54%), increasing to 69.3% (in men, 64%) in women aged 65 to 74 years and 78.5% (in men, 66.7%) in women aged 75 years and older. Blood pressure should be measured during every visit. The designation *prehypertension*—BP in the range of 120-139 mm Hg/80-89 mm Hg—identifies women who probably need lifestyle interventions to reduce their BP and who must be followed closely.

Please see Chapter 4 for more on BP and cardiovascular health.

Clinical breast examination

The clinical breast examination is a time-honored ritual in women's health that has been challenged in the wake of scant data in support of a reduction in breast cancer mortality.[27] The American Cancer Society (ACS) and the American Congress of Obstetricians and Gynecologists (ACOG) recommend yearly examinations for women aged older than 40 years. However, the Cochrane Collaboration and the US Preventive Services Task Force (USPSTF) state that there is a lack of evidence to support this practice. The latter group reaffirmed this position in 2009 and recommends biennial mammograms for women aged 50 to 74 years, recommends against teaching self-breast examinations, and states that there is insufficient evidence to assess benefits and harms of clinical breast examination.[28] In a center with a low rate of false positives, well-trained nurses spent 8 to 10 minutes on the clinical breast examination.[29] Until more evidence clarifies the risks of clinical breast examination, a cautious approach is to continue providing a clinical breast examination for perimenopausal and postmenopausal women.

Please see Chapter 4 for information on breast cancer.

Pelvic examination

ACOG recommends that all women have a periodic pelvic examination once they turn 21 years old.[30] There is not enough evidence to support a routine internal examination in an asymptomatic, healthy patient who is younger than 21 years; however, an external-only genital exam is acceptable. The evidence does not support or refute an annual pelvic examination or speculum and bimanual examination in women aged 21 years and older. The decision to perform a complete pelvic examination should be a decision shared between a patient and her healthcare professional.

The ACS previously had recommended a yearly pelvic exam but has no recommendations for it in their 2012 guidelines.[31] New Pap guidelines have led to reconsideration of this practice because it does not seem valuable in an asymptomatic woman.[32] Nevertheless, a thorough and sensitive pelvic examination of the perimenopausal and postmenopausal woman provides an opportunity to screen for disease and to assess the vulvovaginal area, in which some of the most troublesome effects of low estrogen are manifest.

Start the pelvic examination with a disciplined look at the external genitalia. The distribution of pubic hair reflects androgen levels. Pale, thin epithelium at the introitus extending into the vagina suggests lack of estrogen. A damp cotton-tipped swab can be used to evaluate the sensitivity of the introitus just distal to the hymen. This step is especially important for the woman who is experiencing dyspareunia. If a woman experiences any pain from a gentle touch in the absence of visible lesions, vestibulodynia (also called vulvar vestibulitis) should be suspected. This condition is characterized by a positive swab test, tenderness localized within the vulvar vestibule, and dyspareunia. A visible clitoris and labia minora that are not attenuated help rule out the vulvar dystrophies

Please see Chapter 2 for more on midlife vaginal changes and Chapter 3 for more on the genitourinary syndrome of menopause and other vulvar and vaginal clinical issues.

Decreased pelvic support, as evidenced by the presence of bladder, uterine, or rectal descensus, should be recorded and correlated with symptoms. Using a warm and narrow speculum minimizes the discomfort of this part of the examination. Visualization of the cervix allows identification of polyps and the opportunity to obtain a Pap test with or without concurrent HPV testing (depending on the current guidelines for the individual patient).

Please see Chapter 4 for more on cervical cancer.

A vaginal pH obtained with a cotton-tipped applicator from the vaginal sidewall can provide information on estrogen status, if necessary. A high vaginal pH suggests a low estrogen level or some form of vaginitis. Please see Chapter 2 for more on midlife vaginal changes and Chapter 3 for more on other vulvar and vaginal clinical issues.

The bimanual pelvic examination can provide information on the internal reproductive organs and the capacity of the vagina. Masses and/or sources of pain may be identified. Women with symptomatic vaginal atrophy can be counseled about the availability of low-dose vaginal estrogen products, an oral selective estrogen-receptor modulator (ospemifene), and vaginal physical therapy.

Please see Chapter 3 for more on vulvar and vaginal clinical issues.

Rectal examination

The rectal examination may or may not be indicated. With the more widespread use of colonoscopy, the value of this uncomfortable examination has come into question. Any lesions around the anus should be noted and evaluated. If a fecal occult blood test (FOBT) or fecal immunochemical testing is desired, it may be preferable to obtain stool samples from home in case any tearing during the digital examination would invalidate an office sample. Please see Chapter 4 for information on colorectal cancer.

Table 2. Body Mass Index Classification for Women

Classification	BMI, kg/m²
Underweight	<18.5
Normal weight	18.5-24.9
Overweight	25.0-29.9
Obese	30.0-39.9
Morbidly obese	≥40.0

US National Library of Medicine, National Institutes of Health.[14]

Other examinations

Other examinations may be appropriate, and discussion in the medical literature about which ones add value will no doubt continue. These examinations are part of comprehensive healthcare that, time permitting, the menopause clinician may address. As with any clinician, menopause specialists must know when they can diagnose and treat and when they should refer.

Skin examination. A skin examination requires time and expertise, and a clinician performing a physical examination of any sort has the opportunity to observe the skin. Although the USPSTF states that there is insufficient evidence to recommend for or against routine screening for skin cancer by primary care professionals, the median age at diagnosis of malignant melanoma is 53 years.[33] Menopausal women may also have concerns about changes in their hair, too little or too much, and the possible relationship to menopause.

Please see Chapter 2 for information on midlife skin changes and Chapter 4 for information on skin cancer.

Eye examination. A fundosopic eye examination is not in the repertoire of most menopause clinicians. However, they should encourage their patients to have regular eye examinations and, in particular, to be screened for glaucoma at least every 3 years. Please see Chapter 2 for more on midlife ocular changes.

Dental/Oral examination. The oral cavity is a source of health issues for the aging woman, and the menopause clinician can easily do a superficial assessment of dental hygiene and encourage appropriate dental care. Please see Chapter 2 for more on midlife dental and oral cavity changes.

Auditory examination. The prevalence of hearing impairment increases beyond age 50 years. Audiometric testing should be performed on all persons who report hearing

Chapter 5

impairment or who demonstrate it in the office. Simply whispering a question out of the sight of the patient can easily be incorporated into the visit. Referral to a specialist for more specific testing and use of hearing aids may need to be considered. Please see Chapter 2 for more on midlife hearing changes.

Identification of modifiable health-risk factors

Menopause is an identifiable milestone for all women and provides an excellent opportunity for a woman and her healthcare professionals to review her overall health and her personal risk for disease. An important element of a menopause-related therapeutic plan is lifestyle modification. Asking about physical activity; weight changes; diet; stress management; use of caffeine, alcohol, tobacco, and "recreational" (illegal) drugs; seat belt use; and safe sex practices is critical in helping every woman to manage her present and future well-being.

Overweight and obesity

Weight management is an important strategy for perimenopausal and postmenopausal women. Higher weight and level of body fat are associated with adverse health consequences, including type 2 DM, CVD, stroke, hypertension, some cancers, osteoarthritis, and premature mortality.

Longitudinal studies show that midlife women gain weight, although the factors contributing to this are not fully understood. Sedentary women, women who quit smoking, and those who are already overweight have been shown to be particularly at risk. Of note, overweight women who lose just 10% of their body weight can reap many health benefits, including a significant lowering of BP.

Plotting a woman's weight over time gives a woman and her clinician the opportunity to identify and discuss trends. Inasmuch as women typically gain weight quite slowly at midlife, it is often beneficial to demonstrate to them that gaining "only a couple of pounds" every year can add up over a decade.

Decreasing caloric intake and increasing physical activity to avoid further weight gain are appropriate for almost all women at or above a healthy weight. Weight loss is indicated for those who are overweight or obese. Weight gain and weight loss involve the complex interaction of numerous physical, social, and emotional factors, and it is difficult for people to change their eating habits and lifestyle.[19]

Being underweight is also of concern. There is little information about eating disorders in midlife women or their psychological and physical associations. According to the multiethnic Study of Women's Health Across the Nation (SWAN) of menopause and aging, rates of dissatisfaction with eating patterns, regular binge eating, and marked fear of weight gain were 29.3%, 11%, and 9.2%, respectively.[34] Black women were more likely than white women to report fasting. High BMI (or waist circumference), depressive symptoms, past depression, and history of childhood/adolescence abuse were significantly associated with binge eating and preoccupation with eating, shape, and weight subscale scores in SWAN. Women who weigh less than 127 pounds (57.7 kg) have an increased risk of osteoporosis.

Please see Chapter 2 for more on midlife body weight changes.

Unhealthy diet

A complete nutrition history requires a food diary; however, this exercise may not always be feasible. Asking women if they eat 5 to 7 servings of fruits and vegetables a day is a good way to assess those aspects of diet and provides an opportunity for education. Or one can ask what fruit and vegetables are in the house. Remind women that juices are very high in sugar and calories and that it is better to eat the entire fruit. Determine what vitamins, minerals, and other nutritional supplements are used. Be sure to ask about dietary restrictions.

Physical inactivity

Regular physical activity can help prevent CVD, obesity, type 2 DM, and cancer and maintain musculoskeletal strength and mental well-being. Women who exercise sleep better, are less depressed, and are more able to maintain a healthy weight.[35] Practitioners should encourage midlife women to assess or reassess the benefits of exercise (not just weight loss) and explain that regular physical activity has an immediate effect on stress level and mood.

Questions to elicit the level of activity are an important component of the evaluation. Sedentary women should also be screened for CVD before starting any exercise regimen.

Stress

Although menopause has not been shown to raise stress levels, women at midlife may face many stressors.[36] Stress negatively affects QOL, produces various unpleasant symptoms such as sleep disturbances and decreased libido, and may aggravate some medical conditions, including CVD.[37] Sometimes just asking a woman whether there are any particular stresses in her life can provide an opening to hear about her specific concerns and allow discussion of stress-reducing strategies.

Mind-body medicine, one form of complementary and alternative medicine, focuses on the interactions among the brain, mind, body, and behavior as well as the ways in which emotional, mental, social, spiritual, and behavioral factors can directly affect health. Various stress-reduction techniques are widely used by US adults.[38] The data supporting their effectiveness are mixed.

Encourage women to identify their own life stressors, to seek and find stress-relieving strategies that work for them, and to take time to relax every day.

Substance abuse

All categories of substance abuse, including tobacco, caffeine, alcohol, prescription drugs (including benzodiazepines, opiates, and psychostimulants), and recreational drugs (such as marijuana and cocaine) are important habits to identify when taking a woman's history.

Tobacco. Smoking cessation is the most important change a woman can make for her lifelong health.[39,40] Smoking is a significant independent risk factor for early natural menopause,[41] which places smokers at increased risk for associated diseases. Although smoking has not been associated with altered levels of estrogen either premenopause or postmenopause, postmenopausal smokers who use oral HT have lower serum estrone and estradiol levels than nonsmokers.

The 3 leading smoking-related causes of death in women are lung cancer, heart disease, and chronic lung disease. There are many other AEs of smoking as well.

- *Other cancers.* Women who smoke have an increased risk for cancers other than lung cancer, including cancers of theoral cavity, pharynx, larynx, esophagus, pancreas, kidney, bladder, and uterine cervix. Use of snuff and tobacco also causes cancers of the oral cavity, esophagus, and larynx.

- *Bone loss.* Smoking during adolescence and early adulthood may impede the achievement of optimal peak bone mass. Smoking is also associated with more rapid bone loss in women and higher fracture rates. In the Nurses' Health Study, hip fracture risk increased linearly with greater cigarette consumption.[42] The mechanisms by which smoking might affect bone mass are not known, although some evidence suggests that some components of cigarette smoke interfere with estrogen metabolism.

- *Oral health.* Smoking cigarettes, as well as use of snuff and chewing tobacco, jeopardizes oral and dental health for several reasons. It has a direct influence on gingival tissues caused by the heat and chemical constituents of tobacco smoke. Smoking may also increase the likelihood of infection and periodontitis by inhibiting tissue oxygen levels, limiting gingival blood supply, and impairing antibacterial immune response.

- *Vasomotor symptoms.* Women who smoke cigarettes generally experience more hot flashes than nonsmokers, and the risk increases with the amount smoked.[43,44] Anecdotal observations suggest that stopping smoking may lower the hot flash risk, but no study has specifically tested the effects of smoking cessation on the severity and rate of hot flashes. A study on gene variants reported that certain variants are associated with more frequent and severe hot flashes in smokers compared with nonsmokers.[45]

Alcohol. Drinking alcohol has been associated with risks and benefits, depending on the amount consumed.[46] In perimenopausal and postmenopausal women, the effect of alcohol on endogenous estrogen levels remains unclear. Although some studies have suggested that alcohol consumption may lower estrogen levels, one study in postmenopausal women using HT found that acute alcohol consumption was associated with significantly sustained elevations in circulating estradiol up to levels 300% higher than those seen typically with HT use.[47]

Moderate alcohol consumption appears to lower the risk of hip fractures in women aged 65 years and older, possibly because it increases calcitonin excretion, which may inhibit bone resorption. In addition, there is some evidence that light to moderate alcohol use is associated with reduced CVD risk, better cognitive function, and perhaps reduced risk of dementia. In the Nurses' Health Study, women who consumed 75 g of alcohol per week or more had significantly higher bone mineral density at the lumbar spine than nondrinkers, although alcohol intake of less than 75 g per week was also of benefit.[48] This positive association was observed among current users and never users of HT. However, alcohol consumption was not associated with a higher femoral bone mineral density.

Women are more affected by alcohol than men because of many factors, such as having less water in their bodies to dilute the alcohol, fewer enzymes to digest the alcohol, typically smaller body size, and hormonal differences that may affect absorption. Death rates from alcohol abuse are 50% to 100% higher for women than for men.[49] Women and men who drink have a higher risk of many forms of cancer. Women who consume 1 or 2 drinks daily may be at increased risk for breast cancer.[50] There are several mechanisms postulated for this observation, including effects on estradiol and the estrogen receptor.[51]

Risks often associated with excessive alcohol use include cirrhosis, cardiac failure secondary to cardiomyopathy, accidents, and victimization by physical, sexual, and emotional abuse.

Physical markers for recognizing alcohol abuse include frequent gastrointestinal disturbances, difficulty controlling health problems such as hypertension or type 2 DM, and unexplained seizures. Abnormal laboratory results consistent with alcoholism are an elevated γ-glutamyltransferase level or elevated mean corpuscular volume.

Drinking moderate amounts of alcohol can cause hair and skin to appear dull and can worsen acne and dandruff. Alcohol might lead to weight gain through its low nutritional caloric content. Those who abuse alcohol may suffer from malnutrition. Moderate alcohol consumption is also associated with insomnia, even when consumed a long time before bed.

Traditional markers for alcoholism include tolerance, withdrawal symptoms, loss of control over drinking, social decline, and impaired working skills. Some of these symptoms may be confused with menopause-related symptoms. Clinicians should always be on guard for addictive disorders.[52]

There are a variety of screening tools that are useful in clinical settings, such as the well-known 4-question CAGE questionnaire, the Michigan Alcohol Screening Test (geriatric version), the Alcohol-Related Problems Survey, and the Alcohol Use Disorders Identification Test.[53]

Caffeine. Caffeine-containing drinks (coffee, tea, colas, soft drinks) may have a negative effect on health. Caffeine ingestion may trigger hot flashes and can contribute to insomnia, even when consumed hours before bedtime. Caffeine is a natural diuretic, which increases dehydration and also may act as a bladder irritant. Caffeine has been proposed as a risk factor for bone loss in postmenopausal women; however, many of the studies linking caffeine to bone loss were confounded by covariates. A few studies have found a benefit from caffeine consumption, including a positive effect on Parkinson disease, some cancers, and a possible neuroprotective role in cognition and Alzheimer disease.[54,55]

Women are often unaware of the effects of caffeine or its sources. Clinicians are advised to include a discussion about caffeine with patients who consume large amounts.

Prescription drugs. Perimenopausal and postmenopausal women are more likely to abuse prescription medications if they have another identified chemical dependency such as alcohol or nicotine. Some women obtain prescriptions for medications from several clinicians, none of whom is aware of prescriptions from the others. Often there is a history of repeated refill requests for reasons such as a lost prescription or the alleged use of the prescription by family members or friends.

Women who are abusing mood-altering drugs may have many physical concerns consistent with menopause symptoms. These include mood changes, vasomotor instability, and insomnia. A primary psychiatric problem such as a depressive or anxiety disorder may also be part of the clinical picture.

To detect problematic drug use, it is helpful to look for preoccupation with a particular drug in conjunction with an entire lifestyle that seems to be centered on drug procurement and use. Address concerns about use of alcohol or other drugs (including prescription medications) in an immediate and direct fashion. Beginning with a statement such as "I'm concerned about you" can be very effective. If a physician is uncomfortable dealing with these types of issues, referral to a skilled professional is recommended. This could include a physician or counselor who is experienced in dealing with addictive disorders.

Recreational drugs. Identification of women with alcohol or illegal drug dependence requires a careful history. It is important to be knowledgeable about and willing to make inquiries about illegal drug use and to evaluate women for common comorbid issues such as anxiety and depression. However, responses may vary from candid honesty to complete misrepresentation. Specific questions such as "how much" and "how often" might yield more honest responses than yes-or-no questions.

Diagnostic and screening tests

Screening tests come in many forms. Although one typically thinks of laboratory testing first, simple questions or questionnaires clearly fall into this category as well. A screening test should be simple to perform, readily available, and used to identify a disease or condition with a preclinical state amenable to treatment.[56] Screening tests should have the appropriate balance of sensitivity (identifies most of those who have the condition) and specificity (excludes those who do not have the condition). Diagnostic testing should be highly specific and generally follows use of a screening tool or suspected abnormality.

Clinicians may find themselves in the role of the primary care physician or the consultant. The applicability of some of the screening strategies discussed may be dictated by the role the practitioner is playing in the continuum of the woman's care.

Blood chemistries

Historically, many tests, including blood chemistries, have been performed to screen for asymptomatic disease. There are few tests that should be performed in the asymptomatic patient without elevated risk factors for a particular disease process. For instance, screening for anemia, chronic kidney disease, or thyroid dysfunction without symptoms or risk factors is discouraged.

Bone health

Bone health is multifaceted, and evaluation should go beyond assessing bone density. Either by questionnaire or oral history, at-risk (eg, postmenopausal, small stature, positive family history) patients should be screened for the ability to perform load-bearing exercise, appropriate diet and calcium intake, risk for vitamin-D deficiency, fall risk and stability, sarcopenia (significantly diminished muscle mass), smoking status, use of medications that contribute to bone loss, and metabolic diseases. Evaluation for osteoporosis has become simpler. All women aged older than 65 years should undergo dual-energy x-ray absorptiometry (DXA). Women aged younger than 65 years would undergo testing if their risk of fracture equals or is greater than that of a 65-year-old. One approach is to use the FRAX calculator (www.shef.ac.uk/FRAX/) without bone density data and proceed with DXA if the patient's risk of a major osteoporotic fracture is calculated at or above 9.3%.[57]

Please see Chapter 4 for more on osteoporosis and bone health.

Breast health

The best time for a breast examination or mammogram is immediately after menses or HT-induced bleeding; however, most clinicians do not order mammography on a timed basis.

Mammography is a screening tool, but breast cancer may still be present despite a normal study. The false-negative rate for screening mammography is approximately 10% to 15%. All women should have a clinical breast examination and mammogram before beginning HT and at regular intervals thereafter. The USPSTF in 2009 recommended biannual mammograms for women aged between 50 and 74 years.[28] The American Congress of Obstetricians and Gynecologists (ACOG) recommends that women should have mammograms every 1 to 2 years beginning at age 40 and that women aged 50 years and older have annual mammograms.[58] The American Cancer Society (ACS) recommends a yearly mammogram and a clinical breast examination beginning at age 40.[31] In Canada, breast screening recommendations include a mammogram and clinical breast examination every 2 years in asymptomatic women aged 50 to 69 years.[59]

Ultrasound is often used to evaluate developing focal asymmetric densities on mammograms and any palpable masses of the breast. There is no role for screening ultrasonography when mammography is readily available.

The ACS guidelines recommend magnetic resonance imaging (MRI) as an adjunct to mammography for women at high risk for breast cancer[60]; however, this recommendation is controversial because MRI leads to an excessive number of recalls and biopsies for benign disease. It should not be considered for screening women of average risk.

Please see Chapter 4 for more on breast cancer.

Cardiovascular evaluation

Coronary heart disease (CHD) is the leading cause of death in women. All patients should be screened for modifiable risk factors such as smoking, obesity, atherogenic diet, sedentary lifestyle, and stress. It may be helpful to use a standardized risk assessment such as a Framingham-based global CHD risk calculator as a screening tool in lower-risk women (no evidence of cardiovascular disease and without DM) to help quantify risk for the patient and identify those who will have the greatest benefit from intervention.[61] In addition to a complete history and physical exam, recommendations for screening include serial BP measurements, fasting glucose, and a fasting lipid profile. There is insufficient evidence to recommend routine electrocardiograms, C-reactive protein, advanced lipid testing, or imaging (eg, coronary calcium scoring assessment) as screening tools.[62,63]

Please see Chapter 4 for more on cardiovascular health.

Cervical evaluation

Pelvic examinations, Pap tests with HPV DNA testing, endometrial biopsy, ultrasound, hysteroscopy and/or saline hysterography, colposcopy, and cervical biopsy are effective methods for the evaluation of gynecologic disease, when indicated.[64]

In 2012, 2 different groups—the USPSTF and a partnership among the ACS, the American Society for Colposcopy and Cervical Pathology (ASCCP), and the American Society for Clinical Pathology (ASCP)—issued new recommendations for cervical cancer screening. There is some variation between the USPSTF and the partnered societies[65]:

- Cervical cancer screening should begin at the age of 21.
- Women aged between 21 and 29 years should be screened with cytology every 3 years.
- The ACS/ASCCP/ASCP guidelines say that women aged 30 years and older should be screened with cytology and HPV testing (co-testing) every 5 years (preferred) or cytology alone every 3 years (acceptable). In contrast, the USPSTF recommends that women aged 30 to 65 years should be screened by either cytology every 3 years or cotesting every 5 years.
- Women with certain risk factors may need to be screened more frequently. These risk factors include HIV, immunosuppression, diethylstilbestrol exposure in utero, or history of treatment for cervical intraepithelial neoplasia 2 or higher (CIN 2+) severity.

Screening may cease for

- Women who have had a hysterectomy with removal of the cervix who do not have a history of a high-grade precancerous lesion (CIN 2+) or cervical cancer.
- Women aged 65 years or older with evidence of adequate negative prior screening and no history of CIN 2+ within the last 20 years. Adequate negative prior screening is defined as 3 consecutive negative cytology results or 2 consecutive negative co-tests within the 10 years before cessation of screening, with the most recent test occurring within the past 5 years.

Screening should not be resumed for any reason, even if a woman reports having a new sexual partner. Please see Chapter 4 for more on cervical cancer.

Colorectal evaluation

For women aged 50 years and over with an average risk for colorectal cancer, the ACS recommends selecting 1 of these 5 screening options: annual FOBT, flexible sigmoidoscopy every 5 years, annual FOBT plus flexible sigmoidoscopy every 5 years, double-contrast barium enema every 5 years, or colonoscopy every 10 years.[66] The American College of Gastroenterology recommends that black persons begin screening at age 45 because of their higher risk for colon cancer.[67]

Please see Chapter 4 for more on colorectal cancer.

Depression

Depression should be considered when women present with moodiness or depressive symptoms at the time of menopause. Studies have indicated that menopause may be a vulnerable time for some women, especially those with a history of depression. The risk of depression appears to decrease after menopause.[68] Symptoms of depression may be more difficult to recognize in older populations because women may attribute them to the aging process or to chronic disease. Using a formal screening tool such as the Geriatric Depression Scale significantly improves the likelihood of detection.[69]

Diabetes mellitus

The USPSTF recommends screening (eg, fasting glucose) asymptomatic adult patients for DM who have BPs (treated or untreated) higher than 135/80 mm Hg.[70] With the burden that DM places on the health of the individual person and the entire population, appropriate screening should be performed.

Hormonal evaluation

At present, there is no single test of ovarian function that will predict or confirm menopause. Usually, a woman's medical and menstrual history and symptoms are sufficient to confirm menopause. However, tests of nonovarian hormone levels (eg, thyroid-stimulating hormone [TSH]) may be necessary to rule out other causes of symptoms (eg, thyroid disease).

Tests of ovarian function—follicle-stimulating hormone (FSH), estradiol, luteinizing hormone (LH), total and free testosterone (or bioavailable testosterone), inhibin, antimüllerian hormone (AMH), and prolactin—can be important tests for differentiating various causes of amenorrhea, such as primary ovarian insufficiency, hypothalamic hypogonadotropic amenorrhea, and polycystic ovary syndrome. No tests are routinely recommended for confirming menopause. They are also not recommended in premenopausal women for predicting the time of menopause.

Women often ask for baseline and/or intermittent hormone testing based on their own research or on the insistence of some compounding pharmacists or clinicians that no meaningful treatment decisions can be made without this information. This view implies that a careful patient history is inadequate. There is no scientific basis for this practice, either to have medication dosages titrated so that a woman's estrogen or progesterone levels reach a specified "target" value or to have a specific ratio (often called "hormonal balancing") correlated with improved symptom relief or better safety as claimed. Recommended practice is to titrate medication doses on the basis of a woman's report of symptom relief and AEs. Baseline testing of hormone levels is seldom necessary (Table 3).

Estrogen levels. There are few circumstances in which estrogen levels need to be measured. Estradiol and estrone levels are erratic during perimenopause. Postmenopausal women not using HT can be assumed to have low estrogen levels. Women who do not respond to HT may be tested to determine whether there is suboptimal drug absorption. If so, using a different route of administration may be advisable.

Commercial salivary testing for estrogen has not been proven accurate or reliable, and desired levels of hormones in postmenopausal women have not been established. Urinary estrogen levels, although useful in research, are not commonly used clinically. There is no indication for salivary or urinary hormone testing in clinical practice.

Progesterone levels. Progesterone production depends on the integrity of the menstrual cycle. Early in the menopause transition, progesterone levels are usually normal. In anovulatory cycles, progesterone levels are very low. During the menopause transition, progesterone is often lower than in normal-cycling women, even during ovulatory cycles.[71] Measuring progesterone has very limited value in confirming perimenopause or menopause when used as an isolated test. Generally, an endometrial biopsy to look for secretory endometrium can be useful in women with irregular menses. There are no valid reasons to test for baseline progesterone levels before initiating HT. It may be useful for documenting ovulation in perimenopausal women with irregular menses.

Testosterone levels contribute little to the diagnosis of menopause because testosterone levels do not change significantly during the menopause transition (from 4 y before to 2 y afterward). A woman who has undergone bilateral oophorectomy can be presumed to have lower levels of testosterone. Laboratory testing of testosterone levels should be used to rule out a testosterone-excess state (either endogenous or secondary to testosterone treatment) rather than to diagnose testosterone insufficiency.

Measuring women's testosterone levels in clinical practice is problematic. Serum testosterone levels reflect only a fraction of the total intracellular amount formed in situ by adrenal precursors such as dehydroepiandrosterone and androstenedione. Measuring total and free or bioavailable testosterone may provide only a limited view of a woman's androgen status. Measurement of dehydroepiandrosterone sulfate may contribute to a more complete picture of androgen activity, but this has not been proven. Measurement of the testosterone metabolites androsterone and androstenediol has also been proposed as a more complete measure of androgenic activity, but it also has not been established or correlated with androgen-related conditions or symptoms.[72]

A further challenge for the clinician is identifying a commercial assay that can accurately measure the low serum testosterone levels found in women. Free or bioavailable testosterone values are derived from the total serum testosterone level, and they are useless if the total serum measurement is inaccurate. Liquid chromatography-tandem mass spectrometry techniques for commercially measuring steroids have become the gold standard for measuring testosterone. Baseline or posttreatment free or bioavailable testosterone levels should always be correlated with clinical findings. Laboratory values do not always correlate with therapeutic effect, so dosing of testosterone treatment

Clinical Evaluation and Counseling

Table 3. Reasons to Order Hormone Testing in Clinical Practice

Estradiol	To assess absorption in women with persistent vasomotor symptoms on HT
Prolactin	To differentiate causes of oligomenorrhea or galactorrhea
TSH	To differentiate causes of oligomenorrhea, atypical hot flashes, sleep disorders, fatigue, and weight changes

Abbreviations: HT, hormone therapy; TSH, thyroid-stimulating hormone.

should be based on symptom improvement as long as testosterone values remain within normal range.

Assays to measure testosterone in saliva are available. However, these assays are unreliable and inaccurate, especially for assessing the very low ranges seen in women. Furthermore, salivary concentrations of testosterone represent only a small fraction of the amount in circulation, and accurate measurement is limited by the imprecision of available assays. Their use in clinical practice is not recommended.[73]

Pituitary hormones. Because natural menopause is a retrospective diagnosis (ie, 12 mo of consecutive amenorrhea for which there is no other physiologic or pathologic cause), serum FSH levels have been evaluated as a laboratory marker that would potentially allow earlier diagnosis of menopause as well as impending menopause. Government-approved self-tests measure 2 urine FSH levels. In laboratory tests, these tests compared favorably with serum FSH tests.

It is generally accepted that a woman has reached menopause if she has consistently elevated levels of FSH greater than 30 mIU/mL (IU/L). The difficulty in using FSH as a marker of menopause is that, in perimenopausal women, FSH levels in the postmenopausal range can return to premenopausal ranges a few days, weeks, or months later. A single measurement of FSH greater than 30 mIU/mL (IU/L) in a perimenopausal woman is not considered to be a definitive diagnosis of menopause; several FSH measurements consistently greater than 30 mIU/mL (IU/L) over a prolonged period of time may be necessary.[74] Furthermore, FSH levels in perimenopausal women are frequently normal or can be elevated even while serum estradiol levels are still in a premenopausal range. This seeming paradox underscores the shortcomings of using FSH determination alone as a marker of menopause.

Hormonal contraceptives and HT lower FSH levels, making it difficult to diagnose menopause in women who use them. A study of perimenopausal women taking oral contraceptives concluded that measuring FSH on the seventh pill-free day was not a sensitive test for confirming menopause.[75] A serum FSH-to-LH ratio greater than 1 or estradiol less than 20 pg/mL (73 pmol/L) on the seventh pill-free day was found to more accurately reflect menopause status.

Much of the research on ovarian function tests comes from efforts to assess fertility. Follicle-stimulating hormone has been used as an indicator of "ovarian reserve," a term coined to reflect the remaining reproductive capacity of the ovary. Measuring FSH in the early follicular phase has been used to predict the likelihood of a successful response to infertility treatment and correlates better with treatment outcome than age does.

Antimüllerian hormone (AMH) is a protein hormone expressed by granulosa cells of small ovarian follicles during the reproductive years. Levels of AMH reflect the size of the follicular pool in the ovary, so AMH is a reliable marker of ovarian reserve.[76] Antimüllerian hormone levels have been used primarily to assess ovarian reserve in women seeking fertility assessment. It does not vary with phases of the menstrual cycle, so it can be drawn at any time in the cycle. Levels of AMH are especially useful in predicting ovarian response in patients undergoing in vitro fertilization. Antimüllerian hormone gradually declines with age as the number of primordial follicles declines, becoming undetectable at menopause.[77] Measurements of AMH have been proposed as a means of predicting age at menopause.

Changes in FSH levels seem to be preceded by a decline in ovarian production of inhibin B. A lower fertility rate was observed in women who had a normal FSH level on day 3 but a low inhibin B level compared with women in whom both FSH and inhibin B levels were normal. As inhibin B levels decline, FSH levels rise. Inhibin B levels are normal in hypothalamic amenorrhea but very low in menopause. The average level of inhibin B in primary ovarian insufficiency is only slightly higher than after menopause at the normal age. Production of inhibin A does not decrease until close to menopause.

Although tests of ovarian reserve were designed to predict the success of infertility treatment in older women at risk for infertility, this testing is likely associated with the onset of the menopause transition. The Stages of Reproductive Aging Workshop (SWAN) proposed a staging system for menopause and discussed the relation between FSH levels and perimenopausal stages.[78] An elevated early follicular FSH in 1 cycle is sufficient to place a woman in the late reproductive stage. However, FSH levels can be highly variable in the perimenopausal transition. Elevations of estradiol suppress FSH, limiting the predictive value of a low FSH level. Thus, measuring FSH and estradiol together in the early follicular phase is more informative. However, neither of these tests will definitively predict menopause. Please see Chapter 1 for more about menopause stages.

The elevation of LH associated with menopause is a late occurrence, much later than the increase in FSH. Luteinizing hormone has limited value in confirming perimenopause or menopause.

Genetic testing

ACOG and the USPSTF recommend that primary care providers screen women who have family members with breast, ovarian, tubal, or peritoneal cancer with one of several screening tools designed to identify a family history that may be associated with an increased risk for potentially harmful mutations in breast cancer susceptibility genes (*BRCA1* or *BRCA2*).[28,79] Women with positive screening results should receive genetic counseling and, if indicated after counseling, BRCA testing. Given the implications of a positive finding for the patient, testing should not be performed without the appropriate resources to support the patient.

Lifestyle

Evaluating the patient's lifestyle will likely provide important insight not typically uncovered with laboratory studies. Areas to consider evaluating include level of daily activity and exercise, dietary choices and eating disorders, sleep habits, personal safety, level of desired sexual activity, support network, alcohol use, tobacco use, nonprescription medications, supplements, and fall risk.

Ovarian evaluation

The bimanual pelvic examination has not been proven to be an effective screening test for ovarian cancer. Serum CA-125 levels and transvaginal ultrasound examinations have been used to identify ovarian cancer in women at high risk for the disease. Unfortunately, because of high false-positive and false-negative results and lack of effect on mortality, use of transvaginal ultrasound and CA-125 as screening tools is not recommended.[80,81] Please see Chapter 4 for more on ovarian cancer.

Pelvic evaluation

Pelvic ultrasound may be used to evaluate the ovaries, bladder, uterus, cervix, and the area of the fallopian tubes. Sonohysterography—transvaginal ultrasound with saline infused transcervically to distend the uterine cavity—can better visualize the endometrial cavity and identify focal lesions such as endometrial polyps and submucous fibroids. Ultrasound evaluation should be considered a diagnostic test rather than a routine screening tool.

Sexually transmitted infections

Perimenopausal and postmenopausal women may remain at risk for STIs and may not be as knowledgeable about infection risks or as willing to take steps to minimize these risks as are younger women. Additionally, vaginal atrophy increases the risk of contracting an STI.

Screening may include testing for chlamydia, gonorrhea, hepatitis B virus, hepatitis C virus, HPV, herpes simplex virus, and syphilis, based on risk factors.[82,83] The USPSTF recommends screening adults up to age 65 for HIV regardless of risk factors. Older adults at risk should also be tested.

Please see Chapter 3 for more on sexually transmitted infections.

Thyroid function

The primary function of the thyroid gland is to produce hormones that regulate metabolism, primarily by increasing the basal metabolism rate. Thyroid hormones also affect protein synthesis, carbohydrate and lipid metabolism, and absorption of vitamins. These hormones are regulated through a complex interaction of the hypothalamus, pituitary, and thyroid glands. Much of this regulatory function is controlled by TSH, which is secreted by the anterior pituitary gland.[84,85]

The thyroid gland takes iodine from the circulating blood, combines it with the amino acid tyrosine, and converts it to the thyroid hormones triiodothyronine (T_3) and thyroxine (T_4). The thyroid gland stores T_3 and T_4 until they are released into the bloodstream under the influence of TSH from the pituitary gland. Most thyroid hormones are bound to proteins. Hence, dialysis assessment of the free portion of thyroid hormone (eg, free T_3, free T_4) is desirable for accurate portrayal of thyroid function.

The USPSTF has stated that it could not determine the balance of benefits and risks of screening asymptomatic adults for thyroid disease.[86] However, all women first presenting with irregular menses or vasomotor symptoms should have a thyroid evaluation because these symptoms may have their origin in a thyroid abnormality. A TSH level using a sensitive TSH assay is the most appropriate initial test. If the TSH level is abnormal, then thyroid function should be evaluated further.

Women taking thyroxine supplements should have their serum TSH levels monitored annually and when there is any change in HT use. Measurement of free thyroxine levels is generally not indicated for assessing the adequacy of thyroxine supplements. Free T_4 levels are typically not checked, but there is a small percentage of women who may need to take extra T_3, especially women who are depressed and on thyroid medication.

Please see Chapter 4 for more on thyroid disease.

Urinalysis

A urinalysis can help identify potential medical causes for incontinence. For example, the presence of hematuria may suggest bladder pathology (eg, stones or bladder cancer) and should be investigated. A urinalysis may also be used to screen for early signs of disease, blood in the urine, or urinary tract infection. This test may be suggested as well if the woman has signs of DM or kidney disease. Measuring a postvoid residual within 15 minutes of voiding is recommended to evaluate for urinary retention and overflow incontinence.[87]

Uterine evaluation

Procedures used to evaluate the endometrium in perimenopausal women with abnormal uterine bleeding and in postmenopausal women in whom endometrial evaluation is indicated are determined by patient preference, the clinician's training and skill, cost, and access.

- *Endometrial biopsy.* An endometrial biopsy provides an inexpensive, office-based endometrial evaluation with sensitivity ranging from 60% to 97% in diagnosing endometrial cancer.[88]

- *Transvaginal ultrasound.* A probe inserted into the vagina produces images to measure the thickness of the endometrium and evaluate the uterine and adnexal anatomy. For a postmenopausal woman experiencing abnormal uterine bleeding, transvaginal ultrasonography can be used to exclude malignancy, provided that the entire endometrium can be visualized, the endometrial-myometrial interface is distinct, and the echo is less than 5 mm.[89] ACOG recommends that when an endometrial thickness of 4 mm or less is found, endometrial sampling is not required, unless abnormal bleeding persists.[90]

  Using transvaginal ultrasound with saline infused transcervically to distend the uterus, a sonohysterography can better visualize the endometrial cavity and identify focal lesions such as endometrial polyps and submucous fibroids.

- *Hysteroscopy.* A small flexible or rigid endoscope is inserted into the vagina and through the cervix to allow a direct view of the uterine lining. The uterus is distended with carbon dioxide or fluid for better visualization. Hysteroscopy may be useful in identifying and taking biopsies of (or removing) endometrial polyps and submucous fibroids.

- *Dilation and curettage.* In this surgical procedure, the cervix is dilated and the uterine lining is blindly sampled by scraping or by suction and scraping. This procedure is performed much less frequently than endometrial biopsy because it usually requires anesthesia. Dilation and curettage is often performed with operative hysteroscopy.

Please see Chapter 3 for more on abnormal uterine bleeding and Chapter 4 for more on endometrial cancer.

Vulvovaginal evaluation

The pelvic examination should include an assessment for vulvovaginal atrophy whether vaginal problems have been disclosed. Friability and pallor of the vaginal epithelium should be noted, along with any bleeding from low levels of trauma (eg, speculum insertion). Biopsy may be indicated for visible lesions or persistent symptoms to rule out vulvar dystrophy or vulvar neoplasia.[91]

Vaginal fluid should also be examined, noting the amount and character. If the diagnosis of vulvovaginal atrophy is uncertain, vaginal pH can be assessed. An increase in vaginal pH of 5 or above is a sign of estrogen loss and atrophic changes, provided presence of pathogens (eg, Trichomonas) has been ruled out. If concern is raised about an abnormal discharge, a wet smear or cultures may be considered.

Please see Chapter 3 for more on vulvar and vaginal clinical issues.

Other evaluations

A dental examination and cleaning is recommended at least yearly, preferably twice yearly. Removing the biofilm is important in reducing tooth and gum disease. Problems with teeth and gums indicate increased risk for postmenopausal osteoporosis.[92] Eye examinations are recommended periodically between ages 40 and 65, with annual examinations after age 65 to screen for vision problems, glaucoma, and macular degeneration.

Counseling issues

There are many issues to consider when counseling women about healthy aging and the menopause transition, especially related to health risks and options to reduce those risks. Some decisions warrant a greater focus on the woman's perspective, preferences, and values. Managing patients during the menopause transition should involve addressing their concerns on the basis of scientific evidence while also being respectful of their individual priorities.

Social and cultural aspects of care

Menopause marks a new, vital developmental milestone in the life of a woman. Health status is determined by many factors beyond bodily health, including education, income, social status, housing, employment, health services, community support, spirituality, the environment, and personal health practices.

Differences among social and cultural backgrounds also have implications for the way women experience the menopause transition and for their future health and well-being. Risk factors, morbidity and mortality patterns, and access to healthcare differ among various populations.

United States. There are approximately 40 million postmenopausal women in the United States.[93] The percentage of non-Hispanic white women older than 65 years is almost twice that of any other racial or ethnic group. Nearly one-third of adult women are included in racial and ethnic minorities. This includes more than 3.5 million black, 1 to 2 million Hispanic, and 1 million Asian women. Almost 10% of the US population are foreign born. Nearly 15% are estimated to speak a foreign language at home. Millions of US-born residents follow the traditions and beliefs of other cultures. About 1 in 3 US residents is multiethnic, multiracial, or multicultural; by midcentury, about 47% of the population will be nonwhite.[94] These findings underscore the importance of being aware of social and cultural differences and their potential effect on health.

Canada. Canadian healthcare professionals face similar social and cultural challenges in meeting the needs of an increasingly diverse population. Sources of immigration to Canada have also shifted, with an increasing number of immigrants from Eastern Asia, Central and South America, the Middle East, and Africa. Although there is a lack of an ethnospecific national database, analyses suggest that women who were recent immigrants to Canada reported better health and were less likely to engage in risky health behaviors such as smoking and regular alcohol consumption than are Canadian-born women. However, over time, non-European immigrants were twice as likely as people born in Canada to report deterioration in their health.[95]

Ethnicity and menopause. Variations exist across racial and ethnic groups in the frequency and severity of menopause-related symptoms, attitudes toward menopause, use of menopausal HT, and the healthcare system.

SWAN, a multisite, longitudinal, epidemiologic study of several ethnic groups of US women, including black, Chinese, Japanese, Hispanic, and white women, was designed to examine group differences with respect to the menopause transition.[96] In general, women's attitudes toward menopause were neutral to positive. Although previous results showed ethnic differences on all 5 domains of the Medical Outcomes Short Form Health Survey, further analysis, after adjusting for variables, suggested that most of the differences were not because of culture. Socioeconomic, health, and psychosocial stress factors had a substantial effect on attitudes toward menopause. The study found, for example, that less-acculturated Hispanic women reported more bodily pain and more significant effects from their physical health and emotional problems on social functioning than did white women. Additionally, Japanese women were less likely to report low vitality or that role functioning was affected by emotional problems.

SWAN also found differences in menopause symptoms across ethnic groups, although hot flashes and night sweats were reported by most women. Sixty percent more black women than white women reported such symptoms, and Chinese and Japanese women are about 40% less likely than white women to report hot flashes.[97]

Women who experience surgical menopause may have higher symptom frequency than those who experience natural menopause. Women who are obese and women who smoke may have more hot flashes. Social factors may also play a role in explaining the variability of particular symptoms and the meaning attached to menopause as a phase of life. Such factors include socioeconomic status, definitions of women's social position across the life cycle, prevalent ideas about body and sexual functioning, and norms related to femininity and aging.

Whether menopause is accepted as a natural phase of life or considered to be a medical condition requiring treatment varies from woman to woman and from clinician to clinician. Variations in how information is shared will influence how symptoms are tolerated and interventions are perceived.[98] It is helpful to ask a woman directly how she views menopause and how she feels about it.

Cross-cultural counseling. Effective counseling requires that the clinician be aware of any cultural beliefs that can affect a woman's view of menopause and various treatment options. As always, delivery of healthcare must respect each woman as a unique individual. One study in black women reported that only 14% identified their healthcare professional as the primary source of information on menopause; 60% identified their family and friends as the primary source, with literature second at 20%.[99] In contrast, 67% of white women relied on literature as their primary source, with their healthcare professional second at 17%. Barriers such as education, income level, health insurance status, cultural values, and transportation may hamper access to care.

Lesbian health

Estimates of same-sex relationships among women in the United States vary, although data suggest that up to 5% of women have their primary emotional and sexual relationships with other women, and an estimated 2.3 million women identify themselves as lesbian.[100] According to the National Gay and Lesbian Task Force, 500,000 to 1 million women aged 65 years and older are lesbian or bisexual.[101] Many clinicians assume that all women they are caring for are heterosexual. Only about a third of older lesbian women have shared their sexual orientation with their healthcare professional.

Lesbian women may be celibate or sexually active with women, men, or both. Lesbians reflect the same demographic attributes as other women in the general population as they relate to age at menopause, education, religious preference, and other socioeconomic characteristics.[102]

Lesbians and heterosexual women do not always face the same health issues.[103] Approximately 12% of lesbians express a lack of confidence that they will receive appropriate and unbiased treatment from medical personnel. Before 1990, evidenced-based recommendations for the healthcare of lesbians were uncommon. However, between 1990 and 2000, increased attention was focused on this area of study, and research is available to guide decisions for healthcare in this population.[104] Although 70% of lesbians are in partnered relationships, studies show that they access healthcare services less frequently than heterosexual women because insurance benefits through the partner are not available to them without a legally recognized marriage.[103]

Clinical Evaluation and Counseling

For a lesbian woman to receive appropriate healthcare, her sexual orientation and lifestyle must be known and understood by her healthcare professional (Table 4). Often, clinicians do not ask the appropriate questions. In a Canadian survey of nearly 500 lesbians asked about their healthcare experiences, only 24% had been asked by a healthcare professional about their sexual orientation; this low proportion has remained the same over the last 25 years.[105] However, 97% of lesbians and gay men revealed their sexual orientation when questioned about it by their healthcare professionals.

Studies have shown that lesbians who disclose their sexual orientation to their healthcare professionals are more likely to seek healthcare services and express a better sense of personal comfort and improved communication.[105] This implies that it is possible for the healthcare professional to discuss this topic without offense and that women will appreciate the inclusive approach. Women respond well to language free of heterosexual assumptions. In addition, it is important not to assume that the sexual relations of a lesbian are exclusively with other women. Asking all patients the open-ended question "Do you have sex with men, women, or both?" provides an open, nonjudgmental environment for women to discuss their sexuality.

Substance abuse. The National Household Survey on Drug Abuse found women who reported same-sex partners were more likely to have substance abuse health issues.[103] Other studies have reported similar findings, and some studies have found that lesbians and bisexual women were more likely to experience negative consequences from drinking and were more likely to use marijuana than heterosexual women.

Cancer. Gynecologic cancers may be a greater risk for lesbians than for heterosexual women because of the prevalence of risk factors such as smoking, high BMI, and nulliparity in this population.[103] Many lesbians have not taken oral contraceptives, which are known to reduce the risk of ovarian and uterine cancers. Lesbians often underestimate their risk of developing cancer, particularly cervical cancer, perhaps because they rarely have heterosexual intercourse; thus, many lesbians do not think they need a gynecologic examination. Although rates of physical examinations in this population have increased over the past 20 years, as many as 10% of lesbians still do not undergo routine Pap tests.[104] Studies have found that lesbians are at risk for HPV and abnormal Pap tests. Routine screening Pap tests are an important part of a lesbian woman's health evaluation.

Breast cancer statistics based on sexual orientation have not been reported; however, estimates suggest a higher risk of the disease among lesbians.[103] Many factors influence this finding, including that lesbians are less likely to be screened with mammograms and breast examinations.[106]

Table 4. Counseling Lesbian Patients

- Use a questionnaire that includes questions about sexual orientation, such as
  - Are you in a relationship?
  - Are you sexually active?
  - Do you have a partner or partners?
  - Is your partner a man or a woman?
- Instill trust that the information will be treated with respect and confidentiality
- Use language free of heterosexual assumptions until sexual orientation is known
- Don't assume that sexual relations are exclusively with other women
- Respect the role of the lesbian partner in her life regarding health-related decisions, treating her as a spouse
  - Instead of asking for the spouse's name, ask, "Who would you like to have involved in the discussion of your treatment and surgery?"
  - Give her partner complete access if the patient is hospitalized; if needed, suggest obtaining a durable power of attorney or healthcare power of attorney
  - Be aware of insurance issues, especially when the partner is the only one working and the employer does not recognize the patient as a family member

However, the Women's Health Initiative showed no difference in the rate of breast cancer among the lesbian and bisexual participants compared with heterosexual women.[107]

Please see Chapter 4 for more on gynecologic and breast cancers.

Sexually transmitted infections. Relatively few data are available to address the risk of STIs among lesbians. This is problematic because it makes it difficult for clinicians and healthcare organizations to give comprehensive and context-specific information to women and their partners regarding screening and protection.[103] Lesbians often underestimate their need for risk reduction of STIs.[108] Data on the prevalence of STIs within a woman-to-woman sexual encounter are limited. There is evidence that lesbians who engage in high-risk behaviors are less likely than heterosexual women to practice safe sex. Lesbians and their partners, however, are at risk of contracting STIs. Many types of STIs, including trichomoniasis, chlamydia, HPV, and herpes, can be passed between female partners through digital-vaginal or digital-anal contact and through sharing of penetrative sex devices.[103] Please see Chapter 3 for more on sexually transmitted infections.

Abuse. Clinicians are advised to be alert to the possibility of current or previous physical or sexual abuse in their lesbian patients. It is estimated that approximately 38% of lesbians have been sexually abused in childhood. An estimated 40% reported sexual assault, similar to women in the general population. Lesbian intimate partner violence (IPV) does occur and is less likely to be reported.[108] Psychological abuse occurs more frequently than physical abuse.[103] The prevalence of depression may be higher among lesbians, given the stresses they encounter in today's culture.[103,104]

Clinicians are encouraged to examine their biases regarding sexual orientation. If they or their staff are uncomfortable obtaining an in-depth sexual history and providing clinical care for lesbians, referral to clinicians who are comfortable providing this care is advised.

Intimate partner violence and sexual violence

Violence toward women is a serious public health concern. Studies find that women are often not asked about IPV and sexual violence by their healthcare professionals because clinicians are often uncomfortable opening discussions about violence with their patients.[109] The 2010 National Intimate Partner and Sexual Violence Survey measures 5 types of intimate partner and sexual violence, including sexual violence, physical violence, stalking, psychological aggression, and control of reproductive or sexual health.[110] Additionally, the survey measures 5 types of sexual violence, including acts of rape, and types of sexual violence other than rape (sexual coercion; being made to penetrate someone else; unwanted sexual contact; noncontact unwanted sexual experiences) and stalking. According to the report on survey results, approximately 1 in 4 women in the United States have experienced severe physical violence by an intimate partner at some point in their lifetime, and nearly 1 in 5 women (18%) have been raped in their lifetimes.[111] Where psychological aggression was used, the most commonly reported behaviors among women were expressive forms such as being called derogatory names such as ugly, fat, crazy, or stupid (64.3%); witnessing a partner act angry in a way that seemed dangerous (57.9%); or being insulted or humiliated (58.0%). Some women are ordered to report their location at all times (61.7%).

Additionally, according to the report, women who are victims of IPV, sexual violence, and stalking are more likely to experience short-term and long-term chronic disease and other significant effects on their health such as posttraumatic stress disorder, asthma, DM, irritable bowel syndrome, headaches, chronic pain, difficulty with sleeping, activity limitations, poor physical health, and poor mental health than women who did not experience these forms of violence.[111]

The USPSTF released a recommendation in 2013 regarding screening for IPV. It stated that although abuse of middle-aged women and abuse and neglect of elderly and vulnerable adults can have equally devastating consequences as they do in younger women, there is currently not enough evidence to provide guidance about how primary care clinicians can effectively screen older women.[112] Organizations, including NAMS, the American Medical Association, ACOG, the Society of Obstetricians and Gynaecologists of Canada, and the Registered Nurses' Association of Ontario, recommend that routine universal screening for abuse be part of all evaluations. Additionally, screening as a part of standard patient care is required by hospitals obtaining accreditation from the Joint Commission.

Detecting abuse can be difficult because women are often reluctant to disclose their experience. An environment of openness, safety, and trust may help to facilitate disclosure. Displaying posters and print materials about IPV and sexual violence in public and private areas (such as in the washroom) around the office gives women the opportunity to read the information, educating them about options for responding to violence. Many women are not aware of community outreach groups, safe shelters, or the full range of services available and how to contact them.[113] Posting contact and help information in the restroom allows women to write down the information discretely.

Resources have been designed by the Centers for Disease Control and Prevention and by ACOG to help clinicians feel more at ease when broaching the subject of abuse with a patient.[114,115] The Women's Experience With Battering scale may be an appropriate screening tool for patients because it covers physical and psychological violence, it can be self-administered, and it requires only 2 minutes to complete.[116] Other reliable scales that are easy to administer are the Partner Violence Screen and the brief Women Abuse Screening Tool.[117]

Woman Abuse: Screening, Identification and Initial Response is a guide created by the Registered Nurses' Association of Ontario that provides comprehensive information for healthcare professionals to develop the knowledge and skills necessary to screen and respond appropriately and effectively to abuse.[118]

These validated tools may be used, or clinicians may develop their own approaches (Table 5) as part of a health history that includes

- Conducting interviews in private, with no friends, relatives, or caregivers present

- Mentioning any reporting requirements or other limits to professional-patient confidentiality before screening

- Explaining that all women are being asked about abuse because it is so prevalent in society and has significant health consequences

- Informing women that they can expect to be screened each time a health history is taken

- Using a flexible approach tailored to each person, using direct and nonjudgmental language that is culturally and linguistically appropriate

- Giving a clear message that violence is unacceptable

Before initiating screening, the practitioner needs to inform the woman of the scope and limitations of confidentiality. In most US states and Canadian provinces, confidentiality cannot be guaranteed if child abuse or neglect is suspected, if there is a possibility of the woman harming herself or others, or if documents are subpoenaed by the courts.

Documentation must be comprehensive and legible and must accurately reflect the screening process. In the medical record, include a safety check, direct quotations of what the woman describes, direct observations made by the practitioner, and referrals that were made and information given. Again, women need to be aware before screening that the interaction will be documented and will become part of their permanent health record.

If abuse is suspected, document the incident and physical examination findings, including photographs, as well as any treatments. In many US states, clinicians are required to report elder abuse and IPV to government authorities. Disclosure of any health information to any individual or organization outside the healthcare team requires the woman's consent except in cases for which disclosure is required by law.

Health promotion and lifestyle modification

The menopause transition is an appropriate time for a comprehensive review of a woman's overall health, for assessment of risk factors for disease, and for counseling about options for health promotion and disease prevention. Clinicians can use the NAMS Menopause Health Questionnaire in whole or in part to gain information about basic health status and knowledge from patients.[119]

Although smoking may be the single greatest preventable cause of illness and premature death, clinicians also need to stress the importance of other factors to overall health (Table 6). The healthcare professional can be a powerful voice for reducing risk factors on an individual, community, and policy level.[120,121] The economic consequences of behavioral risk factors place a tremendous burden on society in terms of lost productivity and increased demands on health and social services.

Counseling to promote behavior change often requires more than brief advice. Effective interventions usually involve behavioral counseling techniques, multiple contacts, and use of other resources.

Motivational interviewing can make behavioral counseling more efficient and effective, but there is controversy about the optimal technique and how healthcare professionals should be trained.[122,123] Identifying a patient's key concerns or fears is often an effective place to start.

Adjuncts to counseling include interventions by multiple healthcare team members including nurses, health educators, physical therapists, and pharmacists and the use of other communication strategies (eg, telephone-, video-, or computer-assisted learning; self-help guides; handouts;

Table 5. Suggested Questions for Detecting Abuse and Suggested Responses

Questions

- Have you ever been emotionally or physically abused by your partner or someone important to you?
- Within the last year, have you been pushed or shoved, hit, slapped, kicked, or otherwise physically hurt by someone?
- Do you (or did you ever) feel controlled by or isolated by your partner?
- Within the past year, has anyone forced you to have sexual activities?
- Are you afraid of your partner or anyone else?
- Do you feel you are in danger? Is it safe to go home?
- Has any of this happened to you in a previous relationship?

Responses

If a woman discloses abuse

- Acknowledge the abuse
- Validate the woman's experience
- Assess her immediate health needs and treat accordingly
- Assess her immediate safety
- Explore her options
- Have available a contact list of services concerned with violence against women
- Refer her to the appropriate services with the woman's consent
- Document the interaction

If a woman denies abuse and the clinician suspects otherwise

- Discuss what has been observed and explain continued concern about her health and safety
- Offer educational information about the health effects and prevalence of abuse
- Explain that abusers can escalate their abuse over time
- Highlight referral services
- Document the woman's responses

mailings). Email communication has been shown to improve satisfaction and the relationships between the patient and professional; however, it is important to use a secure email system.[124]

Counseling on diet. Dietary guidelines developed in the United States and Canada recommend that nutrient needs be met primarily through a diet that is high in whole-

Chapter 5

Table 6. Lifestyle Counseling Issues for Midlife Women

Substance use

- Tobacco cessation
- Alcohol/Drug safety (eg, avoid use while driving, swimming, boating)
- Alcohol/Drug abuse

Diet and exercise

- Limit fat and cholesterol intake
- Maintain caloric balance
- Consume a diet based on whole grains, fruits, vegetables, water
- Ensure adequate vitamin and mineral intake, especially calcium
- Emphasize importance of regular physical activity

Injury prevention

- Wear lap/shoulder belts in the car
- Institute fall prevention methods
- Wear appropriate helmet and other safety equipment when riding a motorcycle, bicycle, or all-terrain vehicle
- Have an adequate number of smoke and carbon monoxide detectors at home
- Ensure safe storage or removal of firearms
- Set water heater thermostat between 120°F (49°C) and 130°F (54°C) or lower
- Train household members to deliver cardiopulmonary resuscitation

Sexual behavior

- Institute prevention of sexually transmitted infections
- Avoid high-risk sexual behavior
- Use condoms or female barrier or both
- Prevent unintended pregnancies with appropriate contraception

Dental health

- Stress importance of regular dental visits
- Floss and brush with fluoride toothpaste daily

grain products, vegetables, and fruits and low in saturated fats and cholesterol.[125,126] In some instances, fortified foods and dietary supplements such as vitamin D may be useful sources of nutrients for consuming recommended amounts. However, dietary supplements cannot replace a healthy diet.

Examples of eating patterns that exemplify dietary guidelines are the *Dietary Guidelines for Americans:* the Dietary Approaches to Stop Hypertension (DASH) diet; the Atkins, Zone, and Ornish diets; the Lifestyle, Exercise, Attitudes, Relationships, and Nutrition (LEARN) diet; and Canada's Food Guide.[126-129] All these eating plans are designed so that most people can meet dietary recommendations across a range of calorie levels. Although originally developed to study the effects of an eating pattern on the prevention and treatment of hypertension, the DASH plan is one example of a balanced eating plan consistent with the 2015 Dietary Guidelines for Americans and diet recommendations of the American Heart Association.[128,130]

The recommended calorie intake will differ for persons based on age, sex, and activity level. It may be helpful to point out that just 20 extra calories a day results in 2 pounds of weight gain a year and 10 pounds in 5 years.[131] This calculation reinforces the fact that discipline is required just to maintain weight.

Please see Chapter 7 for more on vitamins and minerals.

Counseling on exercise. Guidelines suggest 30 minutes daily of moderate exercise equivalent to brisk walking (which can be intermittent).[132] For adults attempting to lose weight or maintain weight loss, at least 60 minutes of physical activity is recommended most days of the week. When performed regularly, activities such as brisk walking, running, aerobics, dancing, swimming, tennis, and strength training provide numerous health benefits.

Despite these recommendations, more than one-third of US women aged 45 years and older do not participate in leisure-time physical activity.[133] Less than 20% participate in regular, sustained physical activity of at least 30 minutes, 5 or more times per week. Reports in Canada are similar—only 15% of Canadian women aged 40 to 54 years are sufficiently active; 23% are inactive.[134] The percentage of those physically inactive increases as Canadian women age; 72% of women aged older than 70 years are inactive.

Women benefit from guidance regarding which types and level of physical activity are appropriate and can be encouraged to incorporate exercise into their daily routine for the rest of their lives. Brief interventions by healthcare professionals can be effective in increasing physical activity in the short term. For exercise to be sustained a year later, follow-up sessions at 3- to 6-month intervals are required after the initial discussion. It is also helpful to provide written information about the benefits of regular activity and local opportunities available.

The 3 basic exercise types are

- *Strength training* (eg, resistance exercises, weight-bearing exercises). This type of exercise, using free weights or weight machines, provides muscle resistance. Early in life, strength training promotes higher bone mass; later in life, it can have a modest effect on slowing bone loss.

CLINICAL EVALUATION AND COUNSELING

Older women in particular need these exercises to build strength, thereby improving balance to prevent falls.

- *Aerobic.* The cardiovascular and respiratory systems benefit from aerobic exercises, including brisk walking, jogging, swimming, rowing, and cycling. Low-impact aerobics are easier on the joints than high-impact aerobics and thus may be a better choice for women at midlife and beyond.

- *Flexibility.* Exercises such as yoga and stretching help maintain flexibility and reduce stiffness with aging. Improving flexibility and balance can also decrease the risk of falls and resultant fractures.

Current activity level, physical condition, preferences, and personal circumstances are key determinants of individual exercise prescriptions. For example, if a woman has been sedentary, advice can include starting slowly and progressing gradually. Regimens can begin with strength exercises that engage all muscle groups, to be performed 3 times per week on alternate days for a minimum of 10 to 12 weeks, then reduced to 2 times per week, with aerobic exercise added to the program. Resistance training for 20 minutes, 2 to 3 times a week on nonconsecutive days, also helps to reduce insulin resistance and facilitates weight loss.

A written prescription for exercise to outline physical activity goals can be helpful, and follow-up at appropriate intervals may be more important than the length of each session. Women should be encouraged to put some mental effort into planning an exercise program. Finding ways to make exercise a permanent part of daily life will help ensure a healthier future. One way is to suggest partnering with a friend for regular walks or other physical activities.

Smoking cessation. Smoking cessation is the most effective strategy for smokers to enhance the quality and duration of their lives. Nearly all smokers acknowledge that tobacco use is harmful to their health, but they underestimate the magnitude of their risk. The nicotine in tobacco is as addictive as heroin or cocaine. Tobacco use delivers nicotine to the brain quickly and effectively, causing a rapid onset and maintenance of addiction. This results in both a physiologic and psychological dependence on tobacco, which explains the continued use of tobacco products despite the known health risks.

On average, women gain about 5 pounds after quitting smoking, an amount that can be controlled through diet and exercise. Smoking cessation is not a single event but a process that involves a change in lifestyle, personal values, social groups, perceptions, and coping skills. Several attempts are usually required before a smoker truly quits.

A clinician's most important first step in identifying tobacco dependence is screening for tobacco use and offering minimal smoking cessation interventions (lasting 1-3 min) to all smokers at every opportunity. Prominently displaying "Quit smoking" posters and easily accessible cessation materials deliver a strong message to patients that cessation assistance is available. Labeling each patient's chart with smoking status reminds healthcare professionals to consistently integrate smoking cessation into their care. Progress can also be made by assessing each smoker's readiness to quit and helping her move closer to the stage of quitting.

Intensive intervention is appropriate for all smokers willing to participate and includes smoking history, motivation to quit, identification of high-risk situations, and help with problem-solving strategies for those situations. Proactive telephone, group, or individual counseling are all effective smoking cessation interventions.

Healthcare professionals can offer a variety of prescription and nonprescription smoking cessation aids. The use of pharmacologic therapy approximately doubles the long-term abstinence rates over those produced by placebo. Government-approved, first-line medications for smoking cessation include slow-release bupropion and nicotine replacement therapy (NRT). Nicotine replacement therapy is available in gum, lozenges, transdermal patch, and vapor inhaler with a prescription in the United States and without a prescription in Canada. Other NRT options (eg, nasal spray and sublingual tablets) have been demonstrated to be effective. Varenicline is a selective nicotinic-receptor agonist that is also government approved for smoking cessation.[135] In one study, varenicline and slow-release bupropion were found to be superior to placebo in promoting abstinence from smoking during 7 weeks of active treatment, and varenicline (1 mg, twice daily) was most effective for smoking abstinence for 1 year. Despite the efficacy demonstrated in the research studies, only 6.75% of those who cease smoking use NRT.[136] Most smokers stop abruptly when they are ready.

Nonpharmacologic interventions to assist with smoking cessation include self-help books and materials, individual counseling, hypnosis, group programs, and mutual aid and self-help group support. A combination of behavior-modification techniques and prescription drug therapy seems to be the most successful approach. Because of the high rate of relapse in the first 3 months after quitting, a greater emphasis on follow-up care and training in relapse prevention may improve long-term quit rates.

Importance of listening and building trust

Healthcare professionals can play an important role in motivating and facilitating behavior change. They often have repeated contacts with women over many years and provide continuity of care that contributes to a relationship of trust between the healthcare professional and patient. Studies have shown that patients expect clinicians to provide preventive health information and recommendations and that this advice is a strong motivator for health-promoting behavior.

Four categories of behavioral theories have contributed to the understanding of behavior change and compliance with counseling recommendations. These are communication, rational belief, a self-regulative system, and social learning

Chapter 5

models. Each has a slightly different perspective about risky health behaviors, but all refer to similar components: illness cognition, risk perception, motivation to change, acquisition of coping strategies, and appraisal of results. Most counseling strategies use a combination of components from complementary theories to form a theoretical framework.

Behavioral counseling strategies address complex behaviors that are part of daily living. They vary in intensity and scope according to the person, and they require repeated action by the healthcare professional and the recipient to achieve health improvement. Effective counseling interventions are goal oriented and patient centered and require active participation from the clinician and the patient.

Listening and building trust are primary avenues toward fulfilling clinicians' counseling responsibilities (Table 7). Actively listening to each woman's account of her menopause experience is significant to identify individual health beliefs, to motivate a change in behavior and level of commitment, to determine the best management approach, and to build trust in the therapeutic relationship. This approach places greater emphasis on the woman's role and promotes a partnership of exploration versus a prescriptive interaction with the clinician.

The USPSTF and the Canadian Task Force on Preventive Health Care have adopted a construct for behavioral counseling interventions called the *Five As*, chosen because it was found to have the highest degree of empirical support for each of its elements and because of its use in existing literature (Table 8).[123]

Counseling about medications

When counseling a woman regarding treatment for menopause-related symptoms, the goal is to fully inform her

---

Table 7. Clinician Counseling Responsibilities

- Develop satisfactory clinical relationships through communication and listening.
- Provide all the information necessary for an informed decision.
- Provide unbiased, factual, and comprehensive information on the risks and benefits of any therapeutic initiative.
- Elicit and include the woman's preferences in any recommendations.
- Periodically evaluate treatment continuance and adjust the regimen as needed.
- Regardless of treatment continuance, the clinician still has an ethical and legal responsibility. To fulfill this responsibility, the clinician must understand the woman's comprehension of the instructions and capacity to follow the instructions.

Table 8. The *Five As* of Behavioral Counseling

- Assess: Ask about or determine health risks or other factors affecting the woman's choice of goals, behavior changes, or interventions. Be aware of any cultural issues surrounding interactions and avoid judgmental statements and questions.
- Advise: Provide personalized, specific advice on behavioral changes, including information on her personal risks and benefits for choosing or not choosing to follow a recommendation. Avoid medical jargon that might not be understood.
- Agree: Partner with the woman to jointly select appropriate treatment goals and methods based on her interest and willingness. Through open-ended questions or reflective statements, encourage the woman to speak spontaneously, allowing time for response.
- Assist: Encourage the woman to achieve mutually agreed-on goals by providing various levels of support, including reading material and media training.
- Arrange: Schedule follow-up as appropriate to provide ongoing educational updates or to adjust the treatment plan as goals, desires, and changes are evident.

Adapted from Whitlock EP, et al.[123]

---

about options and encourage her to take an active part in the decision-making process. The healthcare community must be able to provide available resources to allow women to be functional consumers of the healthcare system.[137] A woman who has more confidence in her ability to participate and who experiences fewer barriers to participation is more likely to take an active role in the healthcare encounter and, in turn, be more satisfied with the decisions made. Her priorities for treatment options and her concerns are key.

The clinician should be able to present accurate and current information about treatment options in order to help the woman reach the outcomes she desires. The clinician can also reinforce the fact that menopause is a natural event, not a disease, and that perimenopause is a phase in a woman's life. Some women may experience menopause-associated symptoms that interfere with their daily lives. These women may be uncertain about what is happening to their bodies and need to understand the hormonal changes involved at menopause. Many changes may be related to aging, not menopause. Even asymptomatic women need to understand possible changes to their risk profiles at this time in their lives. Culture may influence communication style. Skills and sensitivity in communicating with women from different cultural backgrounds are essential. The important consideration is that the treatment regimen is mutually agreed on by patient and clinician. Such a process leads to the woman following the treatment plan to achieve her own goals.

Some women will navigate the menopause transition with absolutely no symptoms, and some may seek interventions from their healthcare professional. But regardless of the strategies, the discussion of menopause between the patient and clinician will allow a time for finding personal meaning during this multidimensional period in her life. There is no universal menopause experience other than the physiologic change marking the end of the reproductive period. However, the menopause transition and the time afterward are important periods for implementing behavioral changes to ensure healthy aging.

Please see Chapter 7 for information on nonprescription therapy options and Chapter 8 for prescription therapies.

Quality-of-life assessment tools

Quality of life has become increasingly valued as a therapeutic outcome, and yet there is no universal agreement on what QOL is and how it can be quantified. The World Health Organization defines QOL as a person's perception of his or her life status in the context of the culture and value systems in which he or she lives and in relation to his or her goals, expectations, standards, and concerns.[138] This definition can be applied to postmenopausal women.

A midlife woman's perception of her QOL is not limited to menopause-related symptoms. It involves a more global sense of well-being across the physical, cognitive, and emotional-functioning domains. Additionally, assessment of a woman's perceived QOL is becoming more valued as a therapeutic outcome and may be a determinant of her adherence to a recommended plan of care.

The importance of broadband assessments of the effective practice of menopausal medicine has been recognized in the growing literature on QOL.[139] Indeed, effects of a variety of therapies, including pharmaceuticals, devices, and behavioral interventions, on QOL is of growing interest. Assessment of QOL as related to each intervention is important to the patient, the clinician, and health insurers. Traditional objective measures of the efficacy of medical therapies and interventions, such as incidence of AEs and morbidity or death rates, do not measure a person's own sense of overall life satisfaction and are not, in themselves, adequate indicators of treatment success.

There are several aspects of QOL that have been studied in relation to the menopause transition and postmenopause. Health-related QOL (HRQOL) refers to the perceptions one has about QOL as it is affected by health and is often assessed by measures of physical functioning, emotional functioning, and role limitations.[140] Menopause-specific QOL (MSQOL) reflects the effects that symptoms experienced during the menopausal transition and early postmenopause have on QOL.[141] Measures of MSQOL include women's evaluations of the effect of symptoms by assessing bother, interference, or burden associated with their symptoms. General QOL (GQOL) refers to a woman's perception of her position in life in context of the culture and social systems in which she lives and in relation to her goals, standards, and concerns.[138] General QOL denotes individual perceptions and is not an objective measure of QOL. Efforts to assess GQOL in ways appropriate for midlife women have culminated in development of the Utian Quality of Life (UQOL) scale specific to this population.[142]

The comprehensive clinical evaluation may include use of validated QOL questionnaires that consider the symptom profile and well-being. No single questionnaire serves this purpose. For adequate measurement of QOL, an instrument needs to incorporate contemporary language, be applicable to the specific population being studied, and have normal values for different populations. It also must show change over time or with different interventions.

Failure to use adequately validated rating scales has been a major problem in menopause research. Standardized menopause-specific instruments that measure symptoms of the menopause transition and postmenopause need to satisfy factor-analysis criteria, include subscales measuring different aspects of symptoms, have sound psychometric properties, and be standardized across populations of women. The MSQOL uses measures to assess bother and interference with multiple dimensions of daily life that are linked to symptoms reported by women during the menopausal transition and are exemplified by the Menopause-Specific Quality of Life (MENQOL) Questionnaire and the Women's Health Questionnaire (WHQ).[143-146]

The earliest large, randomized, clinical trials of HT included several varieties of QOL measures. Among these are measures of HRQOL, such as the MS36, an instrument reflecting health-related effects on functional capacity.[147] Other trials have incorporated measures of MSQOL, such as the MENQOL Questionnaire and the WHQ.[143,145] To date, a limited number of scales, such as the UQOL scale, have incorporated measures reflecting GQOL.[142]

Thus, the MENQOL Questionnaire, the Greene Climacteric Scale, and the UQOL apply to perimenopausal and postmenopausal populations.[5,142,143] An ideal assessment can best be generated by a combination of a validated HRQOL menopause symptom profile (eg, Greene Climacteric Scale) and a GQOL instrument (eg, UQOL). This allows clarification of the relationship between each instrument and change over time.

To date, the effects of HT on GQOL are not supported by data adequate to determine therapeutic effects. There is clearly a need for further studies on menopause and menopause-related therapies using appropriate and validated QOL instruments.

Generic quality-of-life scales

Researchers tend to use menopause-specific instruments in menopause-related research. Nonetheless, a few generic instruments are still being widely used.

- The SF-36 is a pure symptom inventory and is used to evaluate QOL in older populations with chronic disease.[147] Frequently used as a symptom profile survey, it has been validated with 8 domains, 4 of each summarizing overall measures of physical health (physical functioning, role physical, bodily pain, general health) and mental health (vitality, social functioning, role emotional, mental health).

- The EuroQOL EQ-5D is a multidimensional instrument that measures 5 dimensions—mobility, self-care, usual activities, pain/discomfort, and anxiety/depression—each at 3 levels (no problem to extreme problem).[148] In addition, it includes a visual analog scale ranging from the worst imaginable state to the best imaginable state.

Menopause-specific quality-of-life scales

- The Greene Climacteric Scale uses factor analysis to categorize symptoms into 3 groups—vasomotor, somatic, and psychological—and consists of 21 symptoms, each rated on a 4-point scale of severity.[5] Its validity has been proven over time.

- The WHQ is based on a factor analysis of 36 symptoms reported by a general population sample from southeast England. There are 8 subscales; 4 are identical to the Greene Climacteric Scale with 32 symptoms. It is used as a comparative measure, with demonstrated construct validity.[145,146]

- The Menopausal Symptom List is based on a factor analysis of 56 symptoms from a general population sample of Australian women.[149] There are 3 subscales—vasosomatic, general somatic, and psychological. The psychological subscale includes the anxiety and depression subscales of the Greene Climacteric Scale and the WHQ. The final version has 25 symptoms, each rated on a 6-point scale of frequency and severity.

- The Menopause Rating Scale is based on a factor analysis of 3 dimensions of severity—somatic, psychological, and urogenital symptoms—from a sample of German women.[150] The final scale consists of 11 symptoms, each rated on a 5-point severity scale. The women were retested for 1.5 years with a high degree of stability in all 3 subscales.

- The MENQOL Questionnaire is an early hybrid, largely measuring HRQOL but incorporating some domains of GQOL.[143] It has been validated in a perimenopausal population. A modified MENQOL-Intervention Questionnaire has been subsequently developed and recommended by the developers for use when AEs of an intervention might negatively affect a woman's QOL.[144]

Global quality-of-life menopause-specific scale

- The UQOL is based on a 2-stage factorial process.[142] Principal components analysis is followed by factor analysis using 40 questions from a sample of Americans living in the East and Midwest of the United States. The final scale consists of 23 items, each rated on a 5-point Likert scale. It should be used in combination with a standardized measure of climacteric symptoms. The UQOL is validated in multiple languages.[151,152]

References

1. Krogsbøll LT, Jørgensen KJ, Grønhøj Larsen C, Gøtzsche PC. General health checks in adults for reducing morbidity and mortality from disease: Cochrane systemic review and meta-analysis. *BMJ.* 2012;345:e7191.
2. Kermott CA, Kuhle CS, Faubion SS, Johnson RE, Hensrud DD, Murad MH. The diagnostic yield of the first episode of a periodic health evaluation: a descriptive epidemiology study. *BMC Health Serv Res.* 2012;12:137.
3. Guyatt GH, Haynes RB, Jaeschke RZ, et al. Users' Guides to the Medical Literature: XXV. Evidence-based medicine: principles for applying the Users' Guides to patient care. Evidence-Based Medicine Working Group. *JAMA.* 2000;284(10):1290-1296.
4. Utian WH. *Change Your Menopause! Why One Size Does Not Fit All.* Cleveland, OH: Utian Press; 2011.
5. Greene JG. A factor analytic study of climacteric symptoms. *J Psychosom Res.* 1976;20(5):425-430.
6. Bellamy L, Casas JP, Hingorani AD, Williams D. Type 2 diabetes mellitus after gestational diabetes: a systematic review and meta-analysis. *Lancet.* 2009;373(9677):1773-1779.
7. Brown MC, Best KE, Pearce MS, Waugh J, Robson SC, Bell R. Cardiovascular disease in women with pre-eclampsia: systematic review and meta-analysis. *Eur J Epidemiol.* 2013;28(1):1-19.
8. Halapy H, Kertland H. Ascertaining problems with medication histories. *Can J Hosp Pharm.* 2012;65(5):360-367.
9. Woods NF, Mitchell ES, Smith-Di Julio K. Sexual desire during the menopausal transition and early postmenopause: observations from the Seattle Midlife Women's Health Study. *J Womens Health (Larchmt).* 2010;19(2):209-218.
10. Berman L, Berman J, Felder S, et al. Seeking help for sexual function complaints: what gynecologists need to know about the female patient's experience. *Fertil Steril.* 2003;79(3):572-576.
11. Althof SE, Rosen RC, Perelman MA, Rubio-Aurioles E. Standard operating procedures for taking a sexual history. *J Sex Med.* 2013;10(1):26-35.
12. Freeman EW. Associations of depression with the transition to menopause. *Menopause.* 2010;17(4):823-827.
13. National Heart, Lung, and Blood Institute. *Calculate Your Body Mass Index.* National Institutes of Health Web site. www.nhlbi.nih.gov/guidelines/obesity/BMI/bmicalc.htm. Accessed June 10, 2014.
14. US National Library of Medicine, National Institutes of Health. *Body Mass Index.* www.nlm.nih.gov/medlineplus/ency/article/007196.htm. Updated May 16, 2014. Accessed June 10, 2014.
15. Orzano AJ, Scott JG. Diagnosis and treatment of obesity in adults: an applied evidence-based review. *J Am Board Fam Pract.* 2004;17(5):359-369.
16. Weight-Control Information Network (WIN). *Understanding Adult Overweight and Obesity.* National Institute of Diabetes and Digestive and Kidney Diseases Web site. http://win.niddk.nih.gov/publications/understanding.htm. Modified January 31, 2014. Accessed June 10, 2014.
17. Rexrode KM, Carey VJ, Hennekens CH, et al. Abdominal adiposity and coronary heart disease in women. *JAMA.* 1998;280(21):1843-1848.
18. American Heart Association. *Frequently Asked Questions (FAQs) About BMI.* American Heart Association Web site. www.heart.org/HEARTORG/GettingHealthy/WeightManagement/BodyMassIndex/Frequently-Asked-Questions-FAQs-about-BMI_UCM_307892_Article.jsp. Updated March 17, 2014. Accessed June 10, 2014.
19. National Institutes of Health, National Heart, Lung, and Blood Institute, North American Association for the Study of Obesity. *The Practical Guide: Identification, Evaluation, and Treatment of Overweight and Obesity in Adults.* October 2000. www.nhlbi.nih.gov/guidelines/obesity/prctgd_c.pdf. Accessed June 10, 2014.
20. Centers for Disease Control and Prevention. *National Health and Nutrition Examination Survey.* Centers for Disease Control and Prevention Web site. www.cdc.gov/nchs/nhanes.htm. Updated May 29, 2014. Accessed June 10, 2014.

21. Cowie CC, Rust KF, Byrd-Holt DD, et al. Prevalence of diabetes and impaired fasting glucose in adults in the US population: National Health and Nutrition Examination Survey 1999-2002. *Diabetes Care.* 2006;29(6):1263-1268.
22. Calle EE, Rodriguez C, Walker-Thurmond K, Thun MJ. Overweight, obesity, and mortality from cancer in a prospectively studied cohort of US adults. *N Engl J Med.* 2003;348(17):1625-1638.
23. Ramos-Nino ME. The role of chronic inflammation in obesity-associated cancers. *ISRN Oncol.* 2013;2013:697521.
24. Eliassen AH, Colditz GA, Rosner B, Willett WC, Hankinson SE. Adult weight change and risk of postmenopausal breast cancer. *JAMA.* 2006;296(2):193-201.
25. Prospective Studies Collaboration; Whitlock G, Lewington S, Sherliker P, et al. Body-mass index and cause-specific mortality in 900,000 adults: collaborative analyses of 57 prospective studies. *Lancet.* 2009;373(9669):1083-1096.
26. Centers for Disease Control and Prevention. *High Blood Pressure Facts.* Centers for Disease Control and Prevention Web site. www.cdc.gov/bloodpressure/facts.htm. Updated March 17, 2014. Accessed June 10, 2014.
27. Barton MB, Elmore JG. Pointing the way to informed medical decision making: test characteristics of clinical breast examination. *J Natl Cancer Inst.* 2009;101(18):1223-1225.
28. US Preventive Services Task Force. Screening for breast cancer: US Preventive Services Task Force recommendation statement. *Ann Intern Med.* 2009;151(10):716-726, W-236. Erratum in: *Ann Intern Med.* 2010;152(3):199-200; *Ann Intern Med.* 2010;152(10):688.
29. Chiarelli AM, Majpruz V, Brown P, Thériault M, Shumak R, Mai V. The contribution of clinical breast examination to the accuracy of breast screening. *J Natl Cancer Inst.* 2009;101(18):1236-1243.
30. Committee on Gynecologic Practice. Committee opinion no. 534: well-woman visit. *Obstet Gynecol.* 2012;120(2 pt 1):421-424.
31. American Cancer Society. *American Cancer Society Guidelines for the Early Detection of Cancer.* American Cancer Society Web site. www.cancer.org/healthy/findcancerearly/cancerscreeningguidelines/american-cancer-society-guidelines-for-the-early-detection-of-cancer. Revised May 3, 2013. Accessed June 10, 2014.
32. Westhoff CL, Jones HE, Guiahi M. Do new guidelines and technology make the routine pelvic examination obsolete? *J Womens Health (Larchmt).* 2011;20(1):5-10.
33. Centers for Disease Control and Prevention. *Skin Cancer Screening (PDQ).* Centers for Disease Control and Prevention Web site. www.cancer.gov/cancertopics/pdq/screening/skin/patient. Updated March 5, 2014. Accessed June 10, 2014.
34. Marcus MD, Bromberger JT, Wei HL, Brown C, Kravitz HM. Prevalence and selected correlates of eating disorder symptoms among a multiethnic community sample of midlife women. *Ann Behav Med.* 2007;33(3):269-277.
35. Jakicic JM, Marcus BH, Gallagher KI, Napolitano M, Lang W. Effect of exercise duration and intensity on weight loss in overweight, sedentary women: a randomized trial. *JAMA.* 2003;290(10):1323-1330.
36. Simpson EE, Thompson W. Stressful life events, psychological appraisal and coping style in postmenopausal women. *Maturitas.* 2009;63(4):357-364.
37. Hunter M, Rendall M. Bio-psycho-socio-cultural perspectives on menopause. *Best Pract Res Clin Obstet Gynaecol.* 2007;21(2):261-274.
38. Barnes PM, Bloom B, Nahin R. *Complementary and Alternative Medicine Use Among Adults and Children: United States, 2007.* National Health Statistics Reports No. 12. Hyattsville, MD: National Center for Health Statistics; 2008. http://nccam.nih.gov/sites/nccam.nih.gov/files/news/nhsr12.pdf. Accessed June 10, 2014.
39. Women and smoking: a report of the Surgeon General. Executive summary. *MMWR Recomm Rep.* 2002;51(RR-12):i-iv; 1-13.
40. Health Canada. *Canadian Tobacco Use Monitoring Survey (CTUMS): Summary of Annual Results for 2012.* www.hc-sc.gc.ca/hc-ps/tobac-tabac/research-recherche/stat/_ctums-esutc_2012/ann_summary-sommaire-eng.php. Modified October 1, 2013. Accessed June 10, 2014.
41. Sun L, Tan L, Yang F, et al. Meta-analysis suggests that smoking is associated with an increased risk of early natural menopause. *Menopause.* 2012;19(2):126-132.
42. Cornuz J, Feskanich D, Willett WC, Colditz GA. Smoking, smoking cessation, and risk of hip fracture. *Am J Med.* 1999;106(3):311-314.
43. Sutter G, Schmelter T, Gude K, Schaefers M, Gerlinger C, Archer DF. Population pharmacokinetic/pharmacodynamic evaluation of low-dose drospirenone with 17β-estradiol in postmenopausal women with moderate to severe vasomotor symptoms. *Menopause.* 2014;21(3):236-242.
44. Gallicchio L, Miller SR, Visvanathan K, et al. Cigarette smoking, estrogen levels, and hot flashes in midlife women. *Maturitas.* 2006;53(2):133-143.
45. Butts SF, Freeman EW, Sammel MD, Queen K, Lin H, Rebbeck TR. Joint effects of smoking and gene variants involved in sex steroid metabolism in late reproductive-aged women. *J Clin Endocrinol Metab.* 2012;97(6):1032-1042.
46. Di Castelnuovo AD, Costanzo S, Bagnardi V, Donati MB, Iacoviello L, de Gaetano G. Alcohol dosing and total mortality in men and women: an updated meta-analysis of 34 prospective studies. *Arch Intern Med.* 2006;166(22):2437-2445.
47. Ginsburg ES, Mello NK, Mendelson JH, et al. Effects of alcohol ingestion on estrogens in postmenopausal women. *JAMA.* 1996;276(21):1747-1751.
48. Feskanich D, Korrick SA, Greenspan SL, Rosen HN, Colditz GA. Moderate alcohol consumption and bone density among postmenopausal women. *J Womens Health.* 1999;8(1):65-73.
49. US Dept of Health and Human Services. National Institutes of Health. National Institute on Alcohol Abuse and Alcoholism. *Alcohol: A Woman's Health Issue.* http://pubs.niaaa.nih.gov/publications/brochurewomen/Woman_English.pdf. Revised June 2008. Accessed June 10, 2014.
50. Zhang SM, Lee IM, Manson JE, Cook NR, Willett WC, Buring JE. Alcohol consumption and breast cancer risk in the Women's Health Study. *Am J Epidemiol.* 2007;165(6):667-676.
51. Dumitrescu RG, Shields PG. The etiology of alcohol-induced breast cancer. *Alcohol.* 2005;35(3):213-225.
52. Fiellin DA, Reid MC, O'Connor PG. Outpatient management of patients with alcohol problems. *Ann Intern Med.* 2000;133(10):815-827.
53. Sorocco KH, Ferrell SW. Alcohol use among older adults. *J Gen Psychol.* 2006;133(4):453-467.
54. Ross GW, Abbott RD, Petrovitch H, et al. Association of coffee and caffeine intake with the risk of Parkinson disease. *JAMA.* 2000;283(20):2674-2679.
55. Rosso A, Mossey J, Lippa CF. Caffeine: neuroprotective functions in cognition and Alzheimer's disease. *Am J Alzheimers Dis Other Demen.* 2008;23(5):417-422.
56. Hennekens CH, Buring JE. *Epidemiology in Medicine.* Mayrent SL, ed. Boston, MA: Little, Brown; 1987.
57. Helmrich G. Screening for osteoporosis. *Clin OB Gyn.* 2013;56(4):659-666.
58. American Congress of Obstetricians and Gynecologists. Annual mammograms now recommended for women beginning at age 40. July 20, 2011. ACOG Web site. www.acog.org/About ACOG/News Room/News Releases/2011/Annual Mammograms Now Recommended for Women Beginning at Age 40.aspx. Accessed June 10, 2014.
59. Public Health Agency of Canada. *Guidelines for Monitoring Breast Screening Program Performance.* 2nd ed. Report from the Evaluation Indicators Working Group. March 2007. www.phac-aspc.gc.ca/publicat/2007/gmbspp-ldsppdcs/pdf/gmbspp-ldsppdcs_e.pdf. Accessed June 10, 2014.
60. Saslow D, Boetes C, Burke W, et al; American Cancer Society Breast Cancer Advisory Group. American Cancer Society guidelines for breast screening with MRI as an adjunct to mammography. *CA Cancer J Clin.* 2007;57(2):75-89. Erratum in: *CA Cancer J Clin.* 2007;57(3):185.
61. Viera AJ, Sheridan SL. Global risk of coronary heart disease: assessment and application. *Am Fam Phys.* 2010;82(3):265-274.
62. Moyer VA; US Preventive Services Task Force. Screening for coronary heart disease with electrocardiography: US Preventive Task Force recommendation statement. *Ann Intern Med.* 2012;157(7):512-518.
63. Mosca L, Benjamin EJ, Berra K, et al. Effectiveness-based guidelines for the prevention of cardiovascular disease in women—2011 update: a guideline from the American Heart Association. *Circulation.* 2011;123(11):1243-1262.
64. Wright TC Jr, Massad LS, Dunton CJ, Spitzer M, Wilkinson EJ, Solomon D; 2006 American Society for Colposcopy and Cervical Pathology-sponsored Consensus Conference. 2006 consensus guidelines for the management of women with abnormal cervical cancer screening tests. *Am J Obstet Gynecol.* 2007;197(4):346-355.
65. American Congress of Obstetricians and Gynecologists. New cervical cancer screening recommendations from the US Preventive Services Task Force and the American Cancer Society/American Society for Colposcopy and Cervical Pathology/American Society for Clinical Pathology. March 14, 2012. ACOG Web site. www.vcom.edu/obgyn/files/New%20Cervical%20Cancer%20Screening%20Recommendations%20March%202012.pdf. Accessed June 10, 2014.
66. American Cancer Society. *American Cancer Society Recommendations for Colorectal Cancer Early Detection.* American Cancer Society Web site. www.cancer.org/cancer/colonandrectumcancer/moreinformation/colonandrectumcancerearlydetection/colorectal-cancer-early-detection-acs-recommendations. Revised June 6, 2014. Accessed June 10, 2014.

Chapter 5

67. Rex DK, Johnson DA, Anderson JC, Schoenfeld PS, Burke CA, Inadomi JM; American College of Gastroenterology. American College of Gastroenterology guidelines for colorectal cancer screening 2009 [corrected]. *Am J Gastroenterol*. 2009;104(3):739-750. Erratum in: *Am J Gastroenterol*. 2009;104(6):1613.
68. Freeman EW, Sammel MD, Boorman DW, Zhang R. Longitudinal pattern of depressive symptoms around natural menopause. *JAMA Psychiatry*. 2014;71(1):36-43.
69. Rodda J, Walker Z, Carter J. Depression in older adults. *BMJ*. 2011;343:d5219.
70. Norris SL, Kansagara D, Bougatsos C, Fu R; US Preventive Services Task Force. Screening adults for type 2 diabetes: a review of the evidence for the US Preventive Services Task Force. *Ann Intern Med*. 2008;148(11):855-868.
71. Hale GE, Hughes CL, Burger HG, Robertson DM, Fraser IS. Atypical estradiol secretion and ovulation patterns caused by luteal out-of-phase (LOOP) events underlying irregular ovulatory menstrual cycles in the menopausal transition. *Menopause*. 2009;16(1):50-59.
72. Labrie F, Luu-The V, Labrie C, Simard J. DHEA and its transformation into androgens and estrogens in peripheral target tissues: intracrinology. *Front Neuroendocrinol*. 2001;22(3):185-212.
73. Bachmann G, Bancroft J, Braunstein G, et al; Princeton. Female androgen insufficiency: the Princeton consensus statement on definition, classification, and assessment. *Fertil Steril*. 2002;77(4):660-665.
74. Stellato RK, Crawford SL, McKinlay SM, Longcope C. Can follicle-stimulating hormone be used to define menopausal status? *Endocr Pract*. 1998;4(3):137-141.
75. Creinin MD. Laboratory criteria for menopause in women using oral contraceptives. *Fertil Steril*. 1996;66(1):101-104.
76. Dewailly D, Andersen CY, Balen A, et al. The physiology and clinical utility of anti-Mullerian hormone in women. *Hum Reprod Update*. 2014;20(3):370-385.
77. Sowers MR, Eyvazzadeh AD, McConnell D, et al. Anti-mullerian hormone and inhibin B in the definition of ovarian aging and the menopause transition. *J Clin Endocrinol Metab*. 2008;93(9):3478-3483.
78. Soules MR, Sherman S, Parrott E, et al. Executive summary: Stages of Reproductive Aging Workshop (STRAW) Park City, Utah, July, 2001. *Menopause*. 2001;8(6):402-407.
79. American College of Obstetricians and Gynecologists; ACOG Committee on Practice Bulletins—gynecology; ACOG Committee on Genetics; Society of Gynecologic Oncologists. ACOG Practice Bulletin No.103: hereditary breast and ovarian cancer syndrome. *Obstet Gynecol*. 2009;113(4):957-966.
80. American College of Obstetricians and Gynecologists. ACOG Committee Opinion No. 477: the role of the obstetrician-gynecologist in the early detection of epithelial ovarian cancer. *Obstet Gynecol*. 2011;177(3):742-746.
81. Moyer VA; US Preventive Services Task Force. Screening for ovarian cancer: US Preventive Services Task Force reaffirmation recommendation statement. *Ann Intern Med*. 2012;157(12):900-904.
82. American College of Obstetricians and Gynecologists. ACOG Committee Opinion. Routine human immunodeficiency virus screening. *Obstet Gynecol*. 2008;112(2 pt 1):401-403.
83. Moyer VA; US Preventive Services Task Force. Screening for HIV: US Preventive Services Task Force recommendation statement. *Ann Intern Med*. 2013;159(1):51-60.
84. Ladenson PW, Singer PA, Ain KB, et al. American Thyroid Association guidelines for detection of thyroid dysfunction. *Arch Intern Med*. 2000;160(11):1573-1575. Erratum in: *Arch Intern Med*. 2001;161(2):284.
85. Surks MI, Ortiz E, Daniels GH, et al. Subclinical thyroid disease: scientific review and guidelines for diagnosis and management. *JAMA*. 2004;291(2):228-238.
86. US Preventive Services Task Force. Screening for thyroid disease: recommendation statement. *Ann Intern Med*. 2001;140(2):125-127.
87. Ho MH, Bhatia NN. Lower urinary tract disorders in postmenopausal women. In: Lobo RA, ed. *Treatment of the Postmenopausal Woman: Basic and Clinical Aspects*. 3rd ed. San Diego, CA: Academic Press; 2007:693-737.
88. Dijkhuizen FP, Mol BW, Brölmann HA, Heinz AP. The accuracy of endometrial sampling in the diagnosis of patients with endometrial carcinoma and hyperplasia: a meta-analysis. *Cancer*. 2000;89(8):1765-1772.
89. Goldstein SR. The role of transvaginal ultrasound or endometrial biopsy in the evaluation of the menopausal endometrium. *Am J Obstet Gynecol*. 2009;201(1):5-11.
90. American College of Obstetricians and Gynecologists. ACOG Committee Opinion No. 426: the role of transvaginal ultrasonography in the evaluation of postmenopausal bleeding. *Obstet Gynecol*. 2009;113(2 pt 1):462-464.
91. Bachmann G, Cheng RF, Rovner E. Vulvovaginal complaints. In: Lobo RA, ed. *Treatment of the Postmenopausal Woman: Basic and Clinical Aspects*. 3rd ed. San Diego, CA: Academic Press; 2007:263-269.
92. Buencamino MC, Palomo L, Thacker HL. How menopause affects oral health, and what we can do about it. *Cleve Clin J Med*. 2009;76(8):467-475.
93. US Census Bureau. Age and sex composition in the United States: 2011. US Census Bureau Web site. www.census.gov/population/age/data/2011comp.html. Revised November 28, 2012. Accessed June 10, 2014.
94. Shrestha LB, Heisler EJ. *The Changing Demographic Profile of the United States*. Congressional Research Service Report for Congress. www.fas.org/sgp/crs/misc/RL32701.pdf. March 31, 2011. Accessed June 10, 2014.
95. Statistics Canada. *Healthy Today, Healthy Tomorrow? Findings From the National Population Health Survey (82-618-M)*. Statistics Canada Web site. http://www5.statcan.gc.ca/olc-cel/olc.action?objId=82-618-M&objType=2&lang=en&limit=1. Modified June 10, 2014. Accessed June 10, 2014.
96. Avis NE, Colvin A, Bromberger JT, et al. Change in health-related quality of life over the menopausal transition in a multiethnic cohort of middle-aged women: Study of Women's Health Across the Nation. *Menopause*. 2009;16(5):860-869.
97. *Highlights of Women's Health Research for ORWH 20th Anniversary: Focus on the Menopause Transition*. July 22, 2010. www.swanstudy.org/docs/SWAN_Highlights_ORWH.pdf. Accessed June 10, 2014.
98. Obermeyer CM. Menopause across cultures: A review of the evidence. *Menopause*. 2000;7(3):184-192.
99. Sharps PW, Phillips J, Oguntimalide L, Saling J, Yun S. Knowledge, attitudes, perceptions and practices of African-American women toward menopausal health. *J Natl Black Nurses Assoc*. 2003;14(2):9-15.
100. Marrazzo JM, Stine K. Reproductive health history of lesbians: implications for care. *Am J Obstet Gynecol*. 2004;190(5):1298-1304.
101. Grant JM, Koskovich G, Somjen Frazer M, Bjerk S; Services and Advocacy for GLBT Elders (SAGE). *Outing Age 2010: Public Policy Issues Affecting Lesbian, Gay, Bisexual and Transgender Elders*. Washington, DC: The National Gay and Lesbian Task Force; 2010. www.thetaskforce.org/downloads/reports/reports/outingage_final.pdf. Accessed June 10, 2014.
102. Utian W. Lesbian women traversing menopause [editorial]. *Menopause Management*. 2009;18:11-12.
103. Dibble SL, Robertson PA. *Lesbian Health 101: A Clinician's Guide*. San Francisco, CA: UCSF Nursing Press; 2010.
104. Roberts SJ. Health care recommendations for lesbian women. *J Obstet Gynecol Neonatal Nurs*. 2006;35(5):583-591.
105. Steele LS, Tinmouth JM, Lu A. Regular health care use by lesbians: a path analysis of predictive factors. *Fam Pract*. 2006;23(6):631-636.
106. Dibble SL, Roberts SA, Nussey B. Comparing breast cancer risk between lesbians and their heterosexual sisters. *Womens Health Issues*. 2004;14(2):60-68.
107. Valanis BG, Bowen DJ, Bassford T, Whitlock E, Charney P, Carter RA. Sexual orientation and health: comparisons in the Women's Health Initiative sample. *Arch Fam Med*. 2000;9(9):843-853.
108. Marrazzo JM, Coffey P, Bingham A. Sexual practices, risk perception and knowledge of sexually transmitted disease risk among lesbian and bisexual women. *Perspect Sex Reprod Health*. 2005;37(1):6-12.
109. Klap R, Tang L, Wells K, Starks SL, Rodriguez M. Screening for domestic violence among adult women in the United States. *J Gen Intern Med*. 2007;22(5):579-584.
110. Centers for Disease Control and Prevention. *The National Intimate Partner and Sexual Violence Survey*. Centers for Disease Control and Prevention Web site. www.cdc.gov/violenceprevention/nisvs. Updated February 26, 2014. Accessed June 10, 2014.
111. Centers for Disease Control and Prevention. National Center for Injury Prevention and Control. Division of Violence Prevention. *NISVS: 2010 Summary Report Findings*. www.cdc.gov/violenceprevention/nisvs/2010_report.html. Updated February 26, 2014. Accessed June 10, 2014.
112. US Preventive Services Task Force. Screening for intimate partner violence and abuse of elderly and vulnerable adults: US Preventive Services Task Force Recommendation Statement. AHRQ Publication No. 12-05167-EF-2. January 2013. www.uspreventiveservicestaskforce.org/uspstf12/ipvelder/ipvelderfinalrs.htm. Accessed June 10, 2014.
113. Family Violence Prevention Fund. *National Consensus Guidelines on Identifying and Responding to Domestic Violence Victimization in Health Care Settings*. San Francisco, CA: Family Violence Prevention Fund; 2004. www.futureswithoutviolence.org/userfiles/file/Consensus.pdf. Updated February 2004. Accessed June 10, 2014.

114. Basile KC, Hertz MF, Back SE. *Intimate Partner Violence and Sexual Violence Victimization Assessment Instruments for Use in Healthcare Settings: Version 1.0*. Atlanta, GA: Centers for Disease Control and Prevention, National Center for Injury Prevention and Control; 2007. www.cdc.gov/ncipc/pub-res/images/ipvandsvscreening.pdf. Accessed June 10, 2014.

115. ACOG Committee Opinion No. 518: Intimate partner violence. *Obstet Gynecol*. 2012;119(2 pt 1):412-417.

116. Coker AL, Pope BO, Smith PH, Sanderson M, Hussey JR. Assessment of clinical partner violence screening tools. *J Am Med Womens Assoc*. 2001;56(1):19-23.

117. Halpern LR, Perciaccante VJ, Hayes C, Susarla S, Dodson TB. A protocol to diagnose intimate partner violence in the emergency department. *J Trauma*. 2006;60(5):1101-1105.

118. Registered Nurses' Association of Ontario. *Woman Abuse: Screening, Identification and Initial Response*. Toronto, Canada: Registered Nurses' Association of Ontario, 2005. http://rnao.ca/sites/rnao-ca/files/BPG_Woman_Abuse_Screening_Identification_and_Initial_Response.pdf. Revised 2012. Accessed June 10, 2014.

119. North American Menopause Society. Menopause Health Questionnaire. North American Menopause Society Web site. Published July 2005. www.menopause.org/docs/default-document-library/questionnaire.pdf?sfvrsn=0. Accessed May 14, 2014.

120. Wild RA, Taylor EL, Knehans A. The gynecologist and the prevention of cardiovascular disease. *Am J Obstet Gynecol*. 1995;172(1 pt 1):1-13.

121. Smedley BD, Syme SL; Committee on Capitalizing on Social Science and Behavioral Research to Improve the Public's Health. Promoting health: intervention strategies from social and behavioral research. *Am J Health Promot*. 2001;15(3):149-166.

122. Miller WR, Yahne CE, Moyers TB, Martinez J, Pirritano M. A randomized trial of methods to help clinicians learn motivational interviewing. *J Consult Clin Psychol*. 2004;72(6):1050-1062.

123. Whitlock EP, Orleans CT, Pender N, Allan J. Evaluating primary care behavioral counseling interventions: an evidence-based approach. *Am J Prev Med*. 2002;22(4):267-284.

124. Mehta NB, Jain AK. Internet-based clinician-patient communications. *Menopause Management*. 2009;18:13-16.

125. US Dept of Health and Human Services. *Dietary Guidelines for Americans, 2015*. DietaryGuidelines.gov Web site. www.health.gov/dietaryguidelines/2015.asp. Updated June 10, 2014. Accessed June 10, 2014.

126. Health Canada. *Eating Well With Canada's Food Guide*. Health Canada Web site. www.hc-sc.gc.ca/fn-an/food-guide-aliment/index-eng.php. Modified September 1, 2011. Accessed June 10, 2014.

127. Appel LJ, Brands MW, Daniels SR, Karanja N, Elmer PJ, Sacks FM; American Heart Association. Dietary approaches to prevent and treat hypertension: a scientific statement from the American Heart Association. *Hypertension*. 2006;47(2):296-308.

128. US Dept of Health and Human Services. *Nutrition and Weight Status*. HealthyPeople.gov Web site. www.healthypeople.gov/2020/topicsobjectives2020/overview.aspx?topicid=29. Updated June 10, 2014. Accessed June 10, 2014.

129. Gardner CD, Kiazand A, Alhassan S, et al. Comparison of the Atkins, Zone, Ornish, and LEARN diets for change in weight and related risk factors among overweight premenopausal women. The A to Z Weight Loss Study: a randomized trial. *JAMA*. 2007;297(9):969-977.

130. American Heart Association Nutrition Committee; Lichtenstein AH, Appel LJ, Brands M, et al. Diet and lifestyle recommendations revision 2006: a scientific statement from the American Heart Association Nutrition Committee. *Circulation*. 2006;114(1):82-96. Erratum in: *Circulation*. 2006;114(1):e27; *Circulation*. 2006;114(23):e629.

131. Brown WJ, Williams L, Ford JH, Ball K, Dobson AJ. Identifying the energy gap: magnitude and determinants of 5-year weight gain in midage women. *Obes Res*. 2005;13(8):1431-1441. Erratum in: *Obes Res*. 2006;14(2):342.

132. National Heart, Lung, and Blood Institute. *Guide to Physical Activity*. National Institutes of Health Web site. www.nhlbi.nih.gov/health/public/heart/obesity/lose_wt/phy_act.htm. Accessed June 10, 2014.

133. US Dept of Health and Human Services. *Nutrition, Physical Activity, and Obesity*. HealthyPeople.gov Web site. www.healthypeople.gov/2020/LHI/nutrition.aspx?tab=data#PA_2_4. Updated June 10, 2014. Accessed June 10, 2014.

134. Bryan S, Walsh P. Physical activity and obesity in Canadian women. *BMC Womens Health*. 2004;4(suppl 1):S6.

135. Nides M, Oncken C, Gonzales D, et al. Smoking cessation with varenicline, a selective alpha4beta2 nicotinic receptor partial agonist: results from a 7-week, randomized, placebo- and bupropion-controlled trial with 1-year follow-up. *Arch Intern Med*. 2006;166(15):1561-1568.

136. Moore D, Aveyard P, Connock M, Wang D, Fry-Smith A, Barton P. Effectiveness and safety of nicotine replacement therapy assisted reduction to stop smoking: systematic review and meta-analysis. *BMJ*. 2009;338:b1024.

137. Rigby AJ, Ma J, Stafford RS. Women's awareness and knowledge of hormone therapy post-Women's Health Initiative. *Menopause*. 2007;14(5):853-858.

138. World Health Organization Division of Mental Health and Prevention of Substance Abuse. *WHOQOL: Measuring Quality of Life*. Geneva, Switzerland: World Health Organization; 1997.

139. Utian WH, Woods NF. Impact of hormone therapy on quality of life after menopause. *Menopause*. 2013;20(10):1098-1105.

140. Avis NE, Assmann SF, Kravitz HM, Ganz PA, Ory M. Quality of life in diverse groups of midlife women: assessing the influence of menopause, health status and psychosocial and demographic factors. *Qual Life Res*. 2004;13(5):933-946.

141. Schneider HP, MacLennan AH, Feeny D. Assessment of health-related quality of life in menopause and aging. *Climacteric*. 2008;11(2):93-107.

142. Utian WH, Janata JW, Kingsberg SA, Schluchter M, Hamilton JC. The Utian Quality of Life (UQOL) Scale: development and validation of an instrument to quantify quality of life through and beyond menopause. *Menopause*. 2002;9(6):402-410.

143. Hilditch JR, Lewis J, Peter A, et al. A menopause-specific quality of life questionnaire: development and psychometric qualities. *Maturitas*. 1996;24(3):161-175. Erratum in: *Maturitas*. 1996;25(3):231.

144. Lewis JE, Hilditch JR, Wong CJ. Further psychometric property development of the Menopause-Specific Quality of Life questionnaire and development of a modified version, MENQOL-Intervention questionnaire. *Maturitas*. 2005;50(3):209-221.

145. Hunter M. The Women's Health Questionnaire (WHQ): a measure of mid-aged women's perceptions of their emotional and physical health. *Psychol Health*. 1992;7(1):45-54.

146. Hunter M. The Women's Health Questionnaire (WHQ): the development, standardization and application of a measure of mid-aged women's emotional and physical health. *Qual Life Res*. 2000;9(1 suppl):733-738.

147. Ware JE Jr, Sherbourne CD. The MOS 36-item short-form health survey (SF-36). I. Conceptual framework and item selection. *Med Care*. 1992;30(6):473-483.

148. Kind P. The EuroQoL instrument: an index of health-related quality of life. In: Spilker B, ed. *QOL and Pharmacoeconomics in Clinical Trials*. 2nd ed. Philadelphia, PA: Lippincott-Raven; 1996:191-201.

149. Perz JM. Development of the menopause symptom list: a factor analytic study of menopause associated symptoms. *Women Health*. 1997;25(1):53-69.

150. Schneider HP, Heinemann LA, Rosemeier HP, Potthoff P, Behre HM. The Menopause Rating Scale (MRS): reliability of scores of menopausal complaints. *Climacteric*. 2000;3(1):59-64.

151. Chen PL, Chao HT, Chou KR, et al. The Chinese Utian Quality of Life Scale for women around menopause: translation and psychometric testing. *Menopause*. 2012;19(4):438-447.

152. Pimenta F, Leal I, Maroco J, Rosa B, Utian WH. Adaptation of the Utian quality of life scale to Portuguese using a community sample of Portuguese women in premenopause, perimenopause, and postmenopause. *Menopause*. 2013;20(5):532-539.

Chapter 6

Complementary and Alternative Medicine

Complementary and alternative medicine (CAM) refers to a group of diverse medical and healthcare systems, practices, and products generally considered to be distinct from biomedicine. Although an increasing number of physicians are referring patients to CAM practitioners, many continue to view CAM as unconventional or even unscientific. What each CAM therapy may offer in the way of treating menopause symptoms varies; research evidence for some is nonexistent, for others equivocal at best.

Integrative medicine

There are 4 evidence-based CAM whole-medical systems for which there is research demonstrating efficacy in the treatment of menopause patients: naturopathy, homeopathy, Chinese medicine, and Ayurveda.

Whole-medical systems are built on complete structures of theory and practice. These systems have evolved apart from and, in some cases, earlier than biomedical approaches. Examples that developed in Western cultures include naturopathy and homeopathy. Examples that developed in non-Western cultures include Chinese medicine and Ayurveda.[1,2]

These systems are prime examples of *integrative medicine*, defined by the National Center for Complementary and Alternative Medicine as combining CAM and biomedical interventions.[3] They can provide primary care for some medical complaints. For others, they enhance the effects of biomedicine. Regardless, they are most effective when their practice is integrated into the provision of biomedicine. In some states, practitioners of these systems work side-by-side with allopathic physicians in hospitals, integrative medicine clinics, research centers, and outpatient medical clinics, as well as in private practice.

These systems have several characteristics in common with each other and with biomedicine, and some that distinguish them from each other:

- Internally consistent theories of health and disease, methods of assessment, and therapies that address primary, secondary, and tertiary prevention.

- Individualized treatments. For example, an integrative medicine practitioner with 10 different menopause patients might treat each patient differently, basing treatments on a patient's unique constellation of signs and symptoms (eg, hot flashes, insomnia, mood changes, musculoskeletal symptoms). Treatments focus on the principal complaint but also address other signs and symptoms that may exist independent of menopause.

- Treatments designed to address signs and symptoms but also the underlying imbalance that causes the signs and symptoms.

- Holistic philosophies that addresses the whole person physically, mentally, emotionally, and spiritually.

- Internally integrative. The systems offer a host of therapies to treat the patient, combining nutrition, exercise, bodywork, herbs, nutritional supplements, and other therapies for a more comprehensive intervention.

- Practitioners who are teachers and who guide patients to enhanced lifestyle choices by providing education, multidisciplinary referrals, and individual support as part of their total intervention. In many cases, the quality of the interaction with the practitioner becomes part of the therapeutic intervention.

- A philosophy of self-healing in which the intervention normalizes physiologic functions so that the body can heal itself and return to homeostasis.

These characteristics can result in comprehensive treatments for various conditions because integrative medicine practitioners may engage any number of interventions to treat a single sign or symptom. However, they also complicate research design because it is challenging to study these systems as they are actually practiced. Generally, researchers overlay a Western research design on a system and study the effect of one component of the system at a time, such as a single homeopathic remedy, a single acupuncture protocol, or a single herb. Because this is not how these systems are actually practiced, study results provide an incomplete picture of the possible full therapeutic benefit of these systems. Studying such systems as they are practiced would make statistical analysis difficult, and sample sizes would have to be quite large to demonstrate significance.

When evaluating the quality of research on integrative medicine, it is worth noting that some issues can complicate translating the available data on the therapeutic benefit of integrative medicine systems:

- As with pharmaceuticals, treatment effect may decline with time after cessation of therapy. This is to be expected and does not necessarily demonstrate a shortcoming of the intervention, although duration of effect is always a goal.

- The definitions for premenopausal, perimenopausal, and postmenopausal vary from study to study; studies have different inclusion and exclusion criteria.

- The period of treatment and the number of treatments vary from study to study; some studies may be of insufficient duration to demonstrate a therapeutic effect.

- Each study uses different objective and subjective assessments to determine therapeutic effect (eg, estradiol and follicle-stimulating hormone [FSH] levels, quality-of-life [QOL] measures, diaries, etc), making comparison among studies difficult.

- A common mistake in analyzing research on integrative medicine is to preclude review of each system's scientific journals. Although there is a wide range in the quality of research among these systems, well-designed studies published in less commonly read journals do exist.

Whole medical systems

Naturopathy and homeopathy

In naturopathic medicine, disease is viewed as a manifestation of alterations in the processes by which the body naturally heals itself. Naturopathic physicians provide primary care diagnosis and therapy. Formal training for the Doctor of Naturopathy (ND) degree mirrors the course work of allopathic physicians (MDs) and osteopathic physicians (DOs), including in such areas as minor surgery, clinical pharmacology, and obstetrics, as well as classroom and clinical instruction in most of the CAM modalities. Training takes 4 years in the United States. Seventeen states, the District of Columbia, and the US territories of Puerto Rico and the US Virgin Islands license or regulate NDs.

The North American Board of Naturopathic Examiners administers the examination that is accepted by some states as one criterion for licensure. The Council of Naturopathic Medical Education (CNME) accredits naturopathic colleges, of which there are 5 schools in the United States and 2 in Canada. The Association of Accredited Naturopathic Medical Colleges is the member organization of those schools that have been accredited by CNME. The American Association of Naturopathic Physicians is the discipline's primary national professional association.

Naturopathic physicians employ an array of healing practices, including clinical nutrition; homeopathy; acupuncture; herbal medicine; hydrotherapy; spinal and soft-tissue manipulation; physical therapies involving electric currents, ultrasound, and light therapy; therapeutic counseling; and pharmacology. Most often, naturopathic physicians function as collaborators with internists, family care practitioners, and gynecologists, providing for a responsible medical care continuum. As with other CAM services, naturopathic services are not covered by all health insurance policies.

Homeopathy is an unconventional Western system that is based on the principle that "like cures like" (ie, large doses of a particular substance may produce symptoms of an illness; very small doses will cure it). Minute doses of specially prepared plant extracts and minerals are used to stimulate the body's defense mechanisms and healing processes to treat illness. The approach focuses on the links among a person's physical, emotional, and mental symptoms.

Clinical trials with homeopathic or naturopathic remedies have resulted in contradictory findings; however, 4 meta-analyses and systematic reviews that evaluated only high-quality trials showed that homeopathy has more than a placebo effect.[4-7]

Three randomized, double-blind, placebo-controlled trials have been conducted evaluating a homeopathic complex remedy; black cohosh/multibotanicals/soy/hormone therapy (HT); and isoflavone clover extract.[8-10] The homeopathic complex versus placebo trial evaluated 102 symptomatic perimenopausal and postmenopausal women using the Menopause Rating Scale II as the primary endpoint.[8] The women were randomized to receive different orders of remedy and placebo. Symptoms were evaluated after 12 weeks. The researchers concluded that there was no clinically significant improvement of menopause symptoms after 12 or 24 weeks' treatment with the complex remedy.

A 1-year trial with 351 symptomatic women aged 45 to 55 years using the Wiklund Vasomotor Symptom Subscale to measure rate and intensity of vasomotor symptoms (VMS) was conducted, but researchers found no difference in the score between herbal intervention and placebo at 3, 6, or 12 months.[9] In fact, at 12 months, the multibotanical plus soy intervention was significantly worse than placebo ($P=.016$). However, HT versus placebo was significant, with –4.06 VMS per day ($P<.001$). The researchers acknowledged that the lack of significant effect could be because of not incorporating the whole-person approach used by naturopathic physicians.

Tice and associates compared 2 dietary red clover supplements with placebo in 252 symptomatic women aged 45 to 60 years.[10] The women were evaluated for 12 weeks by measuring the frequency of hot flashes. They did not find any clinical effect on hot flashes.

A 2010 study used the homeopathic remedy BRN-01 in a multicenter, randomized, double-blind, placebo-controlled trial involving 108 women aged older than 50 years to assess hot flash score and QOL.[11] BRN-01 contains 5 products: *Actaea racemosa*, *Arnica montana*, *Glonoinum*, *Lachesis mutus*, and *Sanguinaria canadensis*. The study found a significant reduction in hot flash score and improvement in QOL. The supplement was well tolerated.

Several small studies using the whole-person approach showed promise in improving menopause symptoms. Homeopathic therapy including *Sepia*, *Lachesis*, *Calacrea carb*, *Lycopodium*, and sulphur was shown to be effective in decreasing menopause symptoms.[12] A "potential benefit" of combination botanicals for menopause symptoms was found in 8 women by using the Modified Kupperman Index.[13]

A retrospective cohort study using chart review compared improvement of menopause symptoms treated by an ND with an MD.[14] Patients treated with naturopathy were 7 times more likely to report improvement in insomnia than conventionally treated patients. There were no differences in anxiety, hot flashes, menstrual changes, and vaginal dryness between the 2 cohorts. Naturopathy was felt to be an effective alternative to conventional therapy for menopause symptoms.

More evidence is needed from large, well-designed trials and for longer durations before recommendations can be made, because botanicals take longer than estrogen therapy (ET) to work (Table 1).[15] Clinical trial results are contradictory, and systematic reviews and meta-analyses have not found homeopathy to be a definitively proven treatment for any medical condition, although homeopathic remedies generally seem to be safe.[15-17]

Chinese medicine

Chinese medicine comprises a host of ancient healing principles historically practiced in Asian cultures. More than 3,000 years old, Chinese medicine uses various therapeutic techniques to promote health and prevent disease, as well as treat acute and chronic health issues and address pain syndromes. Chinese medicine views all phenomena in the universe from the perspective of the interaction of *yin* and *yang*. Culturally, these are very complex concepts, but one simplistic way to look at them is the interaction of matter and energy or form and function. Therapies focus on promoting energetic homeostasis through the manipulation of *qi*, commonly conceptualized in the West as *energy*. When yin and yang are out of balance, illness occurs. To treat this imbalance, practitioners manipulate qi to restore the balance.

Chinese medicine practitioners employ an array of healing therapies, including Chinese dietary therapy; herbal medicine; acupuncture; tuina (a type of bodywork); exercise; and *qigong*, a type of energy therapy. Although an energy-based medical system, students of Chinese medicine receive training in biomedical diagnostics, anatomy and physiology, clinical nutrition, and basic pharmacology.

Table 1. Recommendations for Use of Complementary and Alternative Therapies in Menopause and in Future Research

- Evidence from randomized trials that CAM therapies improve menopause symptoms or have the same benefits as HT is poor
- The safety of CAM therapies needs to be evaluated
- There is concern about interactions of CAM therapies with other treatments, because these may have potentially fatal consequences
- Safety of CAM therapies in women with cancer is unknown
- CAM therapies should not be used in women with premature ovarian failure who generally will benefit from estrogen-based therapy until the average age of natural menopause
- Non-estrogen-based treatments are not as effective as estrogen for hot flashes

Research agenda

- Well-designed, adequately powered, RCTs are required
- There needs to be standardization of chemical preparations, eligibility criteria and clinical endpoints, so that comparisons can be made between studies
- The stability of the chemical preparations needs to be evaluated

Abbreviations: CAM, complementary and alternative; HT, hormone therapy; RCT, randomized, controlled trial.
Rees M.[15]

In the United States, most master's-level training takes 3 to 4 years. In the past 10 years, several schools have also begun to offer clinically based doctoral-level training. The doctoral degree designation is typically Doctor of Oriental Medicine. Licensure differs from state to state, and licenses include Licensed Acupuncturist, Registered Acupuncturist, and Acupuncture Physician. The National Certification Commission for Acupuncture and Oriental Medicine administers the board exam. Depending on what exams an applicant sits for, passage may result in the Diplomate of Acupuncture, Diplomate of Chinese Herbology, or Diplomate of Oriental Medicine. Most states require attendance at an accredited school and passage of the national board as criteria for licensure. Some states, such as California, administer their own licensing exam.

The Accreditation Commission for Acupuncture and Oriental Medicine, the national organization of all 58 accredited US colleges, accredits Chinese medicine schools in the United States. The Council of Colleges of Acupuncture and Oriental Medicine is the national organization of all

Chapter 6

58 accredited US colleges. The American Association of Acupuncture and Oriental Medicine is the primary national professional association.

Anecdotal evidence supports the effectiveness of Chinese medicine in relieving VMS, disturbed sleep, altered mood, and musculoskeletal pain and in enhancing libido and addressing cognitive changes.

Although significant research evidence exists to support the use of Chinese medicine to treat menopause symptoms, many studies are poorly designed: for example, testing different acupuncture protocols for a single condition with an inadequate sample size; no blinding (it is difficult to double blind, because an acupuncturist may be able to determine what is being treated based on the point selection protocol); no comparison to a control group; inadequate subjective or objective assessments of the intervention; or too few treatments to achieve a therapeutic dose.

Acupuncture. Acupuncture involves stimulating specific anatomic points in the body for therapeutic purposes, usually by puncturing the skin with a needle. Acupuncture is widely practiced in North America.

Comparing acupuncture studies is complicated by the fact that each study uses its own unique point selection protocol; many studies use sham acupuncture as a control. As represented in the literature, sham acupuncture may be shallow needle insertion, selection of points with no known empirical activity, or the use of retractable needles that do not penetrate the skin. Regardless, an increasing number of studies suggest that sham acupuncture is not inert; it does have some therapeutic effect and so cannot be considered useful as a placebo control. Thus, there is an inherent problem if a study shows no significant difference between true and sham acupuncture because they are essentially both therapeutic, although one expects sham acupuncture to be less effective than a true acupuncture treatment.

A prospective, randomized, sham-controlled trial (n=29) found that true acupuncture significantly reduced severity of nocturnal hot flashes compared to sham acupuncture. There was no significant difference in frequency between true and sham acupuncture. Both true and sham acupuncture improved sleep, but there was no significant difference between the two.[18]

One randomized, sham-controlled, pilot study (n=29) found that true acupuncture significantly decreased the severity but not the frequency of hot flashes compared with sham acupuncture.[19]

A prospective, randomized, single-blind, sham-controlled clinical trial (n=103) found that medical acupuncture was no better at reducing hot flashes than sham acupuncture.[20] However, both treatments did cause a reduction in hot flashes, suggesting a clear benefit to the treatments.

One multicenter, randomized, single-blind, controlled study with 2 parallel arms (n=267) found that acupuncture resulted in a decrease in hot flash frequency and intensity, improvement in sleep, and reduction in musculoskeletal pain at 12 weeks from baseline, but this improvement disappeared at follow-up at 6 and 12 months.[21]

Another multicenter, randomized, controlled trial (RCT) compared true acupuncture plus usual care to usual care (n=175).[22] This study found significant improvements in frequency and severity of hot flashes, as well as improvements in psychological, somatic, and urogenital dimensions of menopause.

A randomized, single-blind, controlled study (n=53) compared true acupuncture to sham acupuncture.[23] True acupuncture resulted in a significant decrease in hot flash severity, as well as a significant increase in estradiol and decrease in luteinizing hormone levels, with no change in FSH levels, compared with sham acupuncture.

One randomized, single-blind, sham-controlled pilot study (n=33) compared true acupuncture to sham acupuncture and to a waiting control with regard to VMS, QOL, and the hypothalamic-pituitary-adrenal axis (HPA).[24] This study demonstrated an improvement in VMS in both true acupuncture and sham acupuncture groups. Participants receiving true acupuncture showed lower urinary measures of total cortisol metabolites and dehydroepiandrosterone compared to the other 2 groups, showing a possible mechanism of action of acupuncture with regard to the HPA.

A 4-arm RCT looked at the combination of acupuncture and traditional Chinese herbal medicine in the treatment of menopause symptoms.[25] This study found that true acupuncture was superior to sham acupuncture, Chinese herbal medicine, and sham Chinese herbal medicine in reduction of hot flash frequency and severity.

Another study looked at the effect of acupuncture on sleep disturbance in postmenopausal women.[26] In a randomized, sham-controlled, double-blind study (n=18), sleep scores were assessed after participants received either true acupuncture or sham acupuncture. Treatment with true acupuncture resulted in significantly improved sleep compared with sham acupuncture.

Two studies researched the use of acupuncture in patients with estrogen-responsive breast cancer to treat the musculoskeletal symptoms associated with taking aromatase inhibitors, which often chemically induce menopausal symptoms. The first, a randomized, single-blind, sham-controlled trial (n=51), found that true acupuncture resulted in a significant improvement of joint pain compared with sham acupuncture.[27] The second, a dual-center, randomized, blind, controlled trial (n=51), found an improvement in musculoskeletal symptoms but no significant difference between true and sham acupuncture.[28]

Chinese herbal therapy. One double-blind, randomized, placebo-controlled study (n=310) found that the classical herbal formulation *Zhi Bai Di Huang Wan* was able to reduce hot flashes significantly compared with placebo.[29]

Hormone therapy was more effective than Chinese herbal medicine in reducing hot flashes in that study.

In another randomized, controlled group, participants (n=47) were given either *Geng Nian Le*, an herbal formula for perimenopausal depression, or tibolone.[30] Depression scores decreased for both groups. Follicle-stimulating hormone levels decreased in both groups, and estradiol increased in both groups, all at significant levels.

A randomized, double-blind, controlled study (n=108) of the Chinese herbal formula *Er Xian Tang* found that the formulation significantly reduced the mean frequency of hot flashes as well as their severity in the treatment group compared with the control group.[31]

Moxibustion. Moxibustion is a Chinese medical intervention that involves the burning of moxa (Eurasian *Artemisia*) above the body surface of acupuncture points. A randomized, waiting-list, controlled clinical trial on the use of moxibustion to treat hot flashes (n=51) found that 4 weeks of moxibustion therapy resulted in reductions in frequency and severity of hot flashes compared with the waiting-list control group.[32]

Chinese dietary therapy. In the United States, most Chinese medicine schools devote less time in the curriculum to Chinese dietary therapy than they do to herbs and acupuncture, although it is considered an important field of study in China. Possibly as a result, there is a dearth of literature on the use of Chinese dietary therapy to treat menopause symptoms. Much of the literature on food and menopause focuses on 1 food (eg, soy) or 1 distillation of a food (eg, soy isoflavones) rather than the effects of patterns of eating, which is more difficult to measure. Typically, Chinese dietary therapy focuses on the energetics of food rather than on what micronutrients they contain, so some foods are considered warming, others are cooling. Some are considered energetically drying, others are moistening. With this in mind, many Chinese medicine practitioners often recommend avoiding warming foods such as coffee, soda, alcohol, or very spicy foods and other substances such as marijuana that could exacerbate menopause symptoms.[33] They would recommend consuming more cooling foods, such as pears, watermelons, and cucumbers. These recommendations are part of the tradition of Chinese medicine, although there appears to be very little in the literature at this time to support these recommendations.

Qigong. A preliminary observational, controlled study with perimenopausal women found that participants (n=35) practicing qigong over a 12-week period for 30 minutes a day showed an improvement in sleep and somatic symptoms compared with a control group that received only visitation by a nurse in a community health examination counseling setting.[34] The longer the participants practiced the qigong, the greater was the improvement in sleep quality.

Although the results of many studies on Chinese medicine are equivocal, evidence suggests that this system can be helpful in reducing menopause symptoms in women. This, coupled with its relative safety, makes Chinese medicine a valuable component of integrative medicine in improving the QOL of menopause patients.

Ayurveda

Ayurveda is a system of healing that originated in India more than 3,000 years ago. In Sanskrit, *ayur* means *life* or *living*, and *veda* means *science* or *knowledge*, so Ayurveda is "the science of life." Ayurvedic practitioners receive training in nutrition, detoxification and purification techniques, herbal remedies, yoga, breathing exercises, meditation, and massage therapy.

Training in Ayurveda may range from 250 to 2,500 hours in the United States, depending on the school. There is no clearly defined scope of practice for practitioners. Curricula differ dramatically from school to school.

At present, no organization accredits Ayurvedic training programs in the United States, nor does any board certify Ayurvedic practitioners. No states in the United States license Ayurveda. Although no official body exists to accredit schools, the National Ayurvedic Medical Association, the primary national professional organization, has 11 member schools and requires them to offer a minimum of 500 hours of training in order to become members of the organization. However, there are approximately 50 schools of Ayurveda in the United States. The Council for Ayurveda Credentialing formed in 2011 but has yet to publish criteria for school accreditation.

Ayurvedic treatments have been developed in India for diseases such as diabetes mellitus, cardiovascular conditions, and neurologic disorders. However, there is an inherent challenge to the design of clinical trials for evaluating alternative individualized medicine using Western standardized treatment methodology. The question exists whether significant effect can be calculated for individualized treatment plans. Studies of the effect of Ayurveda on symptoms of menopause are scant.

Yoga

Publications on trials of yoga for menopause symptoms have included a trial of self-assessed as well as physiologic measures of hot flashes using *Hatha* yoga.[35] This pilot trial had 12 symptomatic perimenopausal and postmenopausal women exposed to a 10-week yoga program. Researchers found "improvement in symptoms perceptions and well being" that "warrant further study of yoga for menopausal symptoms."

In 2008, researchers published 2 reports on 120 patients randomly divided into an integrated approach of yoga therapy and a control group that featured physical activity. One report addressed menopause symptoms based on the Greene Climacteric Scale. The researchers reported significant difference in VMS between the groups (*P*<.05) as well as a significant decrease in Perceived Stress Scales scores (*P*<.001).[36] In the second report, they evaluated cognitive functions between the 2 groups. They used the 6-letter cancellation test checklist to measure attention and concentration and the Punit Govil Intelligence Memory Scale to evaluate cognitive function. They found superiority of the integrated approach of yoga therapy over physical activity (*P*<.001).[37] Suggestions for future investigation included larger studies, as well as studies of neurohormonal functions during the yoga therapy.

Biologically based practices

Isoflavones

The most studied of the botanicals for menopause-related conditions are isoflavones, sometimes called *phytoestrogens*. They are plant-derived compounds with estrogen-like biologic activity and a chemical structure similar to that of estradiol. Isoflavones are a class of *phytochemicals*, a broad group of nonsteroidal compounds of diverse structure that bind to estrogen receptors (ERs) in animals and human beings (Figure).

Isoflavones have greater affinity for ER-β than for ER-α and possess estrogen-agonist and estrogen-antagonist properties.[38] The isoflavones include the biochemicals genistein, daidzein, glycitein, biochanin A, and formononetin. Genistein and daidzein are found in high amounts in soybeans and soy products as well as in red clover, kudzu, and the American groundnut.

Perimenopausal and postmenopausal women are confronted with numerous foods and supplements referred to by a variety of terms including *plant estrogens*, *soy*, *soy protein*, and *isoflavones*. Unfortunately, the terms are often incorrectly used interchangeably.

Soy. Soy is the most widely used isoflavone-containing food. The term *soy* usually refers to a product derived from the whole soy (or soya) bean. Soy protein refers to a product derived by extracting the protein from the whole bean.

Soy protein is a rich source of isoflavones. The primary isoflavones of soybeans are genistein, daidzein, and glycitein. The whole soybean contains about equal amounts of genistein and daidzein, with only traces of glycitein.

Some soy supplements are made from the germ of the soybean (soy germ). The germ of the soybean differs from the whole soybean in that it has a higher concentration of isoflavones, with daidzein being about 4 times greater than that of genistein and relatively high concentrations of glycitein.

The relative amounts of daidzein and genistein are thought to be determinants of the therapeutic efficacy of soy supplementation. Individual isoflavones such as genistein may have different therapeutic outcomes when administered alone compared with the same amounts administered with all 3 isoflavones in a supplement.

Because scientific publications over the last few decades have suggested potential health benefits of dietary soy and isoflavones, US sales of soy food have increased—from $1 billion in 1996 to $5.2 billion in 2011.[39] The most dramatic increase occurred between 2008 and 2011, with the biggest gains occurring in sales of soy milk and energy bars. Newer categories of soy foods include soy-based drinks, drinkable cultured soy, soy dairy-free frozen desserts, and energy bars, all of which have shown strong and steady growth in sales.

Soy food intake has been assessed specifically among midlife US women. A 2002 telephone survey of 886 women aged 45 to 65 years who were members of the Group Health Cooperative in Washington State found that 22.9% used dietary soy.[40] Breast cancer survivors were 6 times as likely as the overall survey respondents to report use of dietary soy, and women using HT were half as likely to report its use.

The isoflavone content of each soy food can vary considerably, depending on growing conditions and processing (Table 2).[41] Many soy foods are manufactured from fermentation of soy beans (eg, miso and tempeh). This process tends to concentrate the isoflavones. In contrast, heating and cooking processes that remove fats, taste, and color also tend to remove isoflavones.

Soy and other isoflavone supplements are regulated in the United States as dietary supplements. Their effectiveness has not been well established, and they are not monitored for purity, amount of active ingredient, or health claims.

Figure. Primary Isoflavones (Phytoestrogens) in Soy and the Origin of Equol

Isoflavones can exert estrogenic and antiestrogenic effects, depending on their concentration, the concentration of endogenous sex hormones, and the specific end organ involved. Some effects of these molecules may result from interactions with pathways of cellular activity that do not involve the estrogen receptors. In addition, it is not clear whether the putative health effects in human beings are attributable to isoflavones alone or to isoflavones plus other components in whole foods or to the generally more healthy diet and lifestyle that women consuming soy may follow.

Equol. Equol is a nonsteroidal estrogen that binds to both ERs but with a high affinity for ER-β; thus, it is often designated as an ER-β agonist. Equol is a metabolite of the isoflavones daidzein and daidzin. It is produced by the intestinal bacterial flora in only some adult patients. Approximately 30% of North American women can metabolize daidzein to equol in contrast with Asia, where rates are as high as 60%.[42]

Equol has 2 isomers, *S-equol* and *R-equol*. Only S-equol is detected in the plasma of equol-producing women and thought to have any biologic activity. Research opportunities in the menopause health area concern the potential benefits of equol and the as-yet-unanswered issue of whether equol is merely a marker for some beneficial effect of gut flora on steroid metabolism.[43]

Health effects. The health effects of soy and soy isoflavones on midlife women are mixed. Soy-based isoflavones are modestly effective in relieving menopause symptoms; supplements providing higher proportions of genistein or increased in S-equol may provide more benefits.[44] Whether soy has cardiovascular benefits is still uncertain, and data suggest that timing of the treatment may be influential.

Vasomotor symptoms. There has been a major effort to determine whether and to what extent soy or soy isoflavones provide benefits in the control of menopause-related VMS. The original basis for that effort was the observation that only 10% to 20% of Asian women have hot flashes, whereas 70% to 80% of North American women experience them. It seemed reasonable to speculate that the isoflavones present in the high soy diets of Asian women were providing some protection from VMS by reducing the effect of the more potent estradiol in the premenopausal years and then providing some weak estrogenic support in the postmenopausal years, such that, effectively, there may not be such a severe drop in estrogen effect in Asian women at the time of menopause.

There have been a large number of studies intended to evaluate the effect of soy or soy isoflavones on VMS. Small benefits were found in about half the trials, and no benefits in the other half. There is no clear explanation for the conflicting outcomes; however, most of the trials had notable limitations. One report on 14 trials of the effect of isoflavones on hot flashes compared with placebo showed that 11 of the trials showed efficacy at doses of 50 mg to 60 mg at 12 weeks if baseline number of hot flashes were at least 4 per day.[38] Women experiencing more than 4 hot flashes per day did not show improvement over placebo.

Table 2. Isoflavone Content of Foods

Food	Mean isoflavones per 100 g of food, mg
Miso soup (mix, dry)	69.84
Soy flour	172.55
Soy hot dog	1.00
Soy milk (original, vanilla)	10.73
Soy protein isolate	91.05
Soy sauce (soy + wheat; shoyu)	1.18
Soybeans (green, raw, edamame)	48.95
Soybeans (mature, sprouted, raw)	34.39
Tempeh	60.61
Tofu (silken)	18.04
Tofu yogurt	16.30

Bhagwat S, et al.[41]

Among the more comprehensive trials, a 12-week double-blind, prospective study randomized 60 healthy postmenopausal women (aged 40-69 y) to either a placebo group or a group that was given a soy drink containing 60 mg of soy isoflavones daily.[45] Hot flashes and night sweats were significantly decreased in the soy isoflavone-treated group compared with placebo.

A 12-month trial of 351 women aged 45 to 55 years, 52% of whom were perimenopausal and 48% postmenopausal, received a multibotanical intervention and were then put on a soy diet of 12 g to 20 g of soy protein daily. Both interventions were compared with traditional menopausal HT.[9] The results of the interventions on hot flashes and night sweats showed that the addition of the soy diet had no effect, whereas HT was highly effective. However, the doses of soy protein in this study seemed to be lower than what is used in many other trials.

A 2012 meta-analysis and systematic review of randomized trials to determine the effect of extracted or synthesized soy isoflavones provides a reasonable estimate of the beneficial effects on menopausal hot flashes.[44] Soy isoflavones were found to be significantly more effective than placebo in reducing the frequency and severity of hot flashes. Isoflavone supplements providing more than 18.8 mg of genistein were more than twice as potent as lower doses.

A study conducted at Johns Hopkins University focused specifically on the effects of soy isoflavones on QOL in postmenopausal women.[46] Participants were given either 20 g of soy protein containing 160 mg of total isoflavones or a taste-matched placebo made from whole-milk protein. There was significant improvement in 4 QOL subscales in women using soy protein: vasomotor, psychosexual, physical, and sexual. No changes were seen in the placebo group.

Red clover is another source of isoflavones that has been studied mainly for hot flashes. Six trials of 2 types of red clover isoflavones, Promensil (40 mg/d, 80-82 mg/d, and 160 mg/d) and Rimostil (57 mg/d), provided data for a meta-analysis.[47] The combined weighted mean difference in the number of daily hot flashes for red clover isoflavones compared with placebo was not statistically significant. Quality of trials and type of red clover isoflavone did not influence results.

Research in isoflavone treatment of menopause symptoms is focusing on the individual isoflavone components genistein and equol. It has been reported that genistein given alone has beneficial effects on hot flashes.[48] One group studied 236 women with hot flashes. The women in the treatment group (n=119) were given tablets that contained 27 mg of total isoflavone, 98% of which was reported to be genistein. In addition, the tablets contained 400 IU of vitamin D and 500 mg of calcium carbonate. At 12 months, the number of hot flashes experienced by the women in the placebo group was about 4.2 per day, about what they had been at baseline. The number of hot flashes in the treated group steadily declined from about 4.4 to about 1.9 per day, a 56.4% reduction ($P<.001$).

Vaginal dryness. Two studies have explored the potential benefits of isoflavones for the treatment of postmenopausal vaginal dryness, suggesting no clinical benefit. A group of investigators at Helsinki University conducted a double-blind, crossover trial of isoflavone treatment that consisted of 114 mg of isoflavones daily for 3 months.[49] The investigators concluded that the isoflavones had no effect on subjective perception of vaginal dryness or on objective findings in the vagina.

A randomized, crossover study of perimenopausal and postmenopausal women in Bangkok given either placebo or 25 g of soy daily found that a soy-rich diet did not relieve urogenital symptoms, restore vaginal epithelium, or improve the vaginal health of these women.[50]

Bone metabolism. Evidence shows no benefits of soy or soy isoflavones on postmenopausal bone loss. One study reported that for postmenopausal women (mean age, 55 y), consumption of soy containing either 52 mg or 96 mg of isoflavones daily for 15 months had no benefits for bone mineral density (BMD) compared with soy protein having only traces of isoflavones.[51] Another major study found no effect on BMD in postmenopausal women given a soy protein supplement that provided 99 mg of isoflavones per day.[52]

One group of researchers used a novel approach, capable of detecting small effects on bone metabolism: they labeled the bones of postmenopausal women with calcium 41, a long-lived radiotracer, and then measured the urinary excretion of the labeled calcium compared with the unlabeled calcium.[53] In a crossover design, they compared daily intakes of 0 mg, 97.5 mg, and 135.5 mg of isoflavones. Additionally, they compared those effects with those of 1 woman who took HT. None of the doses of soy isoflavones had any effect, whereas the woman given HT had a major change in the urinary ratio of labeled-to-unlabeled calcium.

An Italian study showed that genistein significantly decreased urinary excretion of pyridinoline and deoxypyridinoline, increased levels of bone-specific alkaline phosphatase and insulin-like growth factor 1, and did not change endometrial thickness compared with placebo.[54] A later Italian study found that 54 mg of genistein per day given to postmenopausal women not only increased BMD in the lumbar spine and femoral neck but also improved the "stiffness index," a measure of bone strength.[55] These observations, however, have not been confirmed by other investigators.

It is possible that the failure of isoflavones to prevent bone loss in the human studies is because of the low number of equol producers in the study groups.[42] A 1-year Japanese study of 75 mg of isoflavones per day (38 mg daidzin; 0.6 mg daidzein; 8.6 mg genistin; 0.2 mg genistein; 24 mg glycitin with glycitein) compared with placebo analyzed results according to equol status.[56] There was no effect on spinal BMD comparing equol producers and nonproducers, but there was a significant benefit on total hip and femoral neck BMD in the equol producers.

A 1-year trial of 10 mg of natural equol supplements per day for 93 non-equol-producing, postmenopausal Japanese women resulted in some inhibition of urine bone resorption markers and significantly less bone loss at the hip, although there was no effect on the spine.[57] However, the effects are clearly less than those reported with low-dose estrogen, and no fracture data are available for isoflavones.

Cognitive function. Initially, there were several reports indicating that soy and soy isoflavones might have favorable effects on cognitive function in postmenopausal women. Researchers reported the results of a trial in which postmenopausal women aged 55 to 74 years were treated for 6 months with 110 mg of soy isoflavones per day.[58] The study found a significant improvement in category fluency and a trend toward improvement in verbal memory among the soy isoflavone-treated women compared with those given placebo.

The results of a double-blind, placebo-matched trial in which postmenopausal women aged 51 to 66 years were treated with 60 mg of soy isoflavones per day showed significant improvement in mental flexibility and planning ability.[59] Later, another study found similar improvements in cognitive function of postmenopausal women treated with 60 mg of soy isoflavones per day.[60]

Despite some early positive findings, most later reports do not support a cognitive benefit from soy isoflavones.

Postmenopausal women were treated in 1 large trial with soy protein containing 99 mg of isoflavones per day or milk protein (as the placebo).[52] The women were subjected to a variety of cognitive function measures, and no differences were found between the treatment and placebo groups.

In a study of Chinese postmenopausal women, researchers administered 80 mg day of soy isoflavones per day or a placebo for 6 months.[61] No differences were found between the treatment and placebo groups in tests of memory, executive function, attention, motor control, language, and visual perception, nor in a global cognitive function assessment.

A study at Washington State University compared the effects on postmenopausal women of soy milk with those of cow's milk and a placebo control.[62] Soy isoflavones did not improve a variety of cognitive function measures and indeed were associated with a decline in verbal working memory.

The most comprehensive trial was the determination of the cognitive effects of long-term soy isoflavones treatment on postmenopausal women in the Women's Isoflavone Soy Health (WISH) study.[63] Women in the treatment arm were given 91 mg of soy isoflavones daily, and primary cognitive endpoints were compared with a control group at 2.5 years. There was no significant effect of treatment on global cognition. There was, however, significant improvement in visual memory.

Some earlier studies had suggested that there might be a "window of opportunity" for cognitive benefits with better results if initiated soon after menopause, but not too soon. The issue remains uncertain; the WISH study results found a nonsignificant trend based on time since menopause. The post hoc analysis suggested that women between 5 and 10 years postmenopause were more likely to show cognitive benefits from soy treatment compared with those women less than 5 years from menopause and those more than 10 years from menopause. There was also a nonsignificant trend for women with surgical menopause to perform worse on soy supplements than on placebo.

Similarly, the question of whether equol-producing status influences the potential cognitive benefits of soy remains somewhat uncertain. In the WISH study, analyses comparing consistent equol producers with women receiving placebo found a favorable trend for consistent equol producers that was not statistically significant.

Coronary heart disease. There has been intense research on the potential benefit of soy protein and soy isoflavones on plasma lipids and lipoproteins as a means of reducing coronary heart disease (CHD).

On the basis of animal research and human epidemiologic evidence, many experts believed that consumption of soy protein and soy isoflavones could potentially reduce plasma cholesterol concentrations and thereby reduce the risk of CHD. In 1999, the US Food and Drug Administration (FDA) approved the health claim that 25 g of soy protein per day, as part of a diet low in saturated fat and cholesterol, may reduce the risk of heart disease. Shortly thereafter, the American Heart Association (AHA) recommended dietary soy protein and isoflavones for decreasing the risk of CHD.[64] As more data accumulated, however, the AHA reversed its recommendation and concluded that soy and soy isoflavones had such small effects on plasma lipid profiles that they probably did not reduce CHD risk.[65]

There have been 2 well-controlled studies that seem to have placed the subject in proper perspective. One study concluded that the regular intake of high levels of soy protein (>50 g/d) had just a modest effect on blood cholesterol levels and only in patients with elevated low-density lipoprotein cholesterol (LDL-C) levels (>4.14 mmol/L), although soy protein was potentially helpful when used to replace animal products in the diet.[66]

The second study administered 25.6 g of soy protein containing 99 mg of isoflavones to postmenopausal women daily for 12 months.[52] The study found no significant effect of the soy supplementation on plasma concentrations of total cholesterol, LDL-C, high-density lipoprotein cholesterol (HDL-C), triglycerides, or lipoprotein(a).

These conclusions were consistent with a clinical review that concluded that soy protein and soy isoflavone extracts caused only very small reductions in total plasma cholesterol concentrations—primarily in the LDL-C fraction—and no changes in the HDL-C fraction and that these decreases were likely too small to be clinically beneficial.[67] This finding was consistent with the AHA advisory on soy and cardiovascular health, which reviewed 22 RCTs to compare isolated soy-protein isoflavones with milk and other proteins.[65] They reported that soy reduced plasma concentrations of LDL-C about 3% on average, with no significant effects on HDL-C, triglycerides, lipoprotein(a), or blood pressure. The panel also considered 19 studies involving purified soy isoflavone extract and found no consistent effects on LDL-C or other plasma lipid risk factors. The overall conclusion was that any cardiovascular benefit from soy protein or isoflavone supplements would be "minimal at best."

Investigators from Johns Hopkins reported a significant decrease in LDL-C particle number, a stronger indicator of CHD progression than LDL-C plasma concentration.[68] Additionally, although isoflavone treatment of postmenopausal women tends not to improve plasma lipid concentrations, isoflavones do result in significant improvement in arterial compliance and arterial stiffness, measurements closely associated with degree of atherosclerosis.[69]

There are good data from the double-blind, placebo-controlled WISH study that was designed to determine whether isoflavone-containing soy protein treatment reduces the progression of atherosclerosis in postmenopausal women to an extent greater than its minimal effect on plasma lipids.[70] The trial involved 350 postmenopausal women aged 45 to 92 years without diabetes mellitus or prevalent cardiovascular disease. The women were randomized to 2 evenly divided doses of 25 g soy protein containing 91 mg of aglycone isoflavones equivalents or placebo for 2.7 years. The endpoint was the progression over the 2.7 years in carotid artery intima-media thickness. Although isoflavone-containing soy supplementation failed to reduce the progression of atherosclerosis in the carotid artery, among a subgroup of women at low cardiovascular risk who were randomized within 5 years of menopause, soy isoflavones supplementation resulted in a 68% lower rate of progression of carotid artery intima-media thickness. This finding suggests that a "timing hypothesis," now generally accepted as relating to the postmenopausal atheroprotective effects of estrogen, may also apply to soy isoflavones.

Whether equol-producing capacity is a determinant of soy's cardiovascular benefits is uncertain. One study found that pasta enriched with soy germ isoflavones improved markers of cardiovascular risk for equol producers, whereas 2 other studies found no effect of equol-producing capacity on cardiovascular benefits.[71-73] Equol-producing capacity has been shown to be associated with favorable vascular function among women being treated with tibolone even when not being given soy supplements.[74] No support for the role of equol-producing capacity was found in the WISH study.[70]

Breast effects. The literature on the effects of soy and soy isoflavones on breast cancer risk is extensive and often conflicting. Meta-analyses are useful to understand the current status of the question.

A 2006 meta-analysis of soy intake and breast cancer risk evaluated 18 epidemiologic studies (12 case-control and 6 cohort) performed between 1978 and 2004.[75] High soy intake was associated with modestly reduced breast cancer risk. Among the 10 studies that stratified by menopause status, the inverse association between soy exposure and breast cancer risk was stronger in premenopausal women. In these studies, risk estimate levels, measures of soy exposure, and controls for confounding factors varied considerably. The researchers concluded that soy intake may be associated with a small reduction in breast cancer but that the results should be interpreted with caution and that recommendation for isoflavone supplementation to prevent breast cancer are premature. Competitive binding of the weaker isoflavones to the ER may reduce the effect of estradiol in the premenopausal woman.

Another meta-analysis of 8 trials conducted among Asian women and 11 trials in Western populations showed a significant trend of decreasing breast risk with increasing soy food consumption in Asian women.[76] Compared with the lowest soy food intake (≤5 mg/d), risk was intermediate with moderate intake (approximately 10 mg/d) and lowest with high intake (≥20 mg/d). Soy intake was unrelated to breast cancer in the trials conducted in low-consuming Western populations, whose average highest and lowest isoflavone intake levels were approximately 0.8 mg to 15 mg daily, respectively.

Equol is produced by most nonhuman species but not by most humans. Data suggest that equol is not a strong antioxidant nor a chemopreventive agent in animal and cellular models.[77-79] In observational studies of Western populations, little association of breast cancer risk in relation to equol has been suggested.[80] In contrast, in Asian populations that have higher prevalence of soy consumption and equol producers, equol may be associated with lower breast cancer risk.[80-81]

Because an increase in hot flashes is common among breast cancer survivors, there has been high interest in whether soy might be useful or harmful for such patients. Generally, there has been concern about the use of soy because genistein was found to stimulate breast cancer cells in rodents.[82] In a study to determine the effect of soy intake on survival and recurrence of breast cancer among a group of 5,042 breast cancer survivors in China, soy protein or soy isoflavone intake was found to be inversely associated with mortality and recurrence.[83]

Uterine effects. Soy and soy isoflavones are likely safe for the uterus, and some observational studies show reduced endometrial cancer risk in women with higher dietary intake of these products.

A case-control study that included 424 cases of endometrial cancer and 398 controls suggested a decreased cancer risk in lean women taking isoflavones.[84] In another study involving 500 cases and 470 controls in non-Asian women, the highest quartile of total isoflavone intake was associated with lower endometrial cancer risk.[85] In a third case-control study in China with 832 cases and 842 controls, soy food consumption was inversely associated with endometrial cancer risk, particularly among women with higher body mass index and waist-to-hip ratio.[86]

Soy and soy isoflavones may have small benefits in the treatment of VMS in the short term (12 wk) but not for longer periods (6-12 mo), and there appears to be no benefit for symptoms of vaginal dryness. Evidence suggests that equol is more effective than the usual mixture of soy isoflavones in the treatment of menopause symptoms. There is good evidence that using soy for the treatment of VMS does not have a harmful effect on either the breast or the endometrium and that intake of soy isoflavone may be safe for breast cancer survivors. With the possible exception of genistein given alone, neither soy nor soy isoflavones appears to prevent postmenopausal bone loss.

Herbal therapies

Some people prefer taking herbs and nutritional supplements over pharmaceuticals because they hold the mistaken belief that they are natural and therefore safer. However, herbs and supplements are drugs. Their active ingredients may be less concentrated than drugs, but they can still cause adverse events (AEs) and interactions with other substances. Some herbs and nutritional supplements are contraindicated in pregnancy.

Another concern with herbs and supplements is their overall quality. Are they tested for pesticide residue, aluminum, heavy metals, and other toxic substances? Do they contain adulterants? The quality or strength of herbs may differ from season to season and from growing region to growing region. Is an herb listed on an ingredient label the identified herb or some alternative purported to have similar effects? Does the formulation have unlabeled pharmaceuticals? There have been cases of counterfeit herbal formulations produced in China that have spurious labeling.

A number of herbs, including black cohosh and dong quai, plus a wide variety of multiherbal products, have been used to treat acute menopause-related symptoms.

Many dietary supplements containing mixtures of various herbs are advertised for relief of menopause-related symptoms. Although anecdotal evidence may support efficacy, there are scant clinical trial data to document safety or efficacy for most.

Many women and some healthcare professionals believe that herbal therapies are safer than prescription drugs because they are "natural," but herbs can have beneficial pharmacologic effects as well as AEs. Clinical trials are needed to document the safety and efficacy of these products; however, in the meantime, millions of women will continue to use these products, and a primary goal should be to help them do so safely.

Marketed herb products are regulated in the United States as dietary supplements. Many manufacturers employ rigorous quality-control measures and produce high-quality products; however, for less rigorous manufacturers, there remain problems in the marketplace with regard to purity, levels of active and marker compounds, and health claims.

Please see Chapter 7 for more information on government regulation of dietary supplements.

Black cohosh. Preparations made from the rhizomes (underground stems) of black cohosh (botanical name, *Cimicifuga racemosa* or *Actaea racemosa*) have been used by North American Indians for medicinal purposes for hundreds of years.[87] Europeans have been using this native North American plant to treat menopause-related symptoms for more than 50 years. In 1989, the German Federal Institute for Drugs and Medical Devices approved black cohosh for menopause-related complaints as well as for premenstrual syndrome (PMS) and dysmenorrhea. Although several of the plant's constituents have been identified, its precise mechanism of action is unknown. Serotinergic mechanisms have been proposed to explain some of its actions.[88]

Black cohosh comes in many formulations including capsules (with extract or powdered rhizomes), tablets, liquid tincture, and extracts that can be mixed in water or dry root for tea.[89] Recommended doses for extracts (most of the products in the US market) range from 40 mg to 80 mg and should have a standardized 1 mg of 27-deoxyactein. Tincture use is 2 mL to 4 mL, 3 times a day.

Results are inconclusive in clinical trials comparing black cohosh with estrogen and/or placebo for treating hot flashes. A 12-month, phase 2 trial failed to find any benefit for a daily dose of 128 mg ethanolic extract of black cohosh.[90] Another 12-month study failed to find any benefit for daily 160 mg ethanolic extract of black cohosh over placebo in relieving hot flashes.[9] One trial found that a fixed combination of black cohosh and St. John's wort was better than placebo in treating menopause symptoms, including those with a strong psychological component and hot flashes specifically.[91]

Several trials have compared black cohosh extract with conjugated estrogens or placebo with varying results. One trial found that black cohosh and estrogen had similar effects with regard to the Menopause Rating Scale and reduction in hot flashes and night sweats.[92] A phase 3, 4-week trial evaluating the efficacy of 40 mg black cohosh extract daily and placebo failed to find any difference between them.[93]

Several meta-analysis studies have been performed to look for more evidence of efficacy of preparations containing black cohosh. One such study employed 3 databases and found a 26% (range, 11%-40%) improvement of VMS in preparations using black cohosh versus placebo; however, there was significant heterogeneity in these formulations and doses.[94] Dose-dependent effects on hot flashes have been reported in a 180-patient, 12-week trial.[95]

A trial comparing topical estradiol and black cohosh found them equally effective in the 136 women in each treatment arm that completed the trial.[96] There was no placebo arm, which limits the study results.

An 8-week randomized trial of black cohosh versus placebo for the treatment of hot flashes in women diagnosed with breast cancer who had completed their primary treatment (N=85) found a decrease in sweating but not in hot flash frequency or severity among the women taking black cohosh.[97] These findings should be viewed carefully, however, because they may be confounded by the large number (n=59) of women taking tamoxifen, a drug known to induce hot flashes. This study provides useful information about black cohosh in women with a history of breast cancer taking tamoxifen but should not be considered relevant for women going through a natural menopause. Changes in FSH and luteinizing hormone blood levels did not differ between the treatment and placebo groups.

A 24-week clinical trial that evaluated the effects of black cohosh (39 mg/d or 127.3 mg/d) on vaginal cytology and reproductive hormone levels found that its benefit in relieving hot flashes was not associated with systemic estrogen-agonistic effects for either dose.[98]

A 3-month trial examining the effect of black cohosh (160 mg/d) on lipids, fibrinogen, glucose, and insulin in

CHAPTER 6

women aged 45 to 55 years concluded that there were no statistical differences between herbal groups and placebo.[99]

No vaginal bleeding has been reported with black cohosh in study periods of up to 6 months. One study found no increases in endometrial thickness as measured by ultrasound after 52 weeks of treatment.[100] Some experts believe that longer trials are required to ensure endometrial safety.

The incidence of AEs with black cohosh is relatively low, particularly with single-agent supplements. Adverse events include occasional gastrointestinal (GI) discomfort, nausea, vomiting, dizziness, frontal headache, and bradycardia. The GI disturbances are primarily with first use.[101]

There have been more than 50 case reports that suggest a possible link between liver failure and black cohosh use. This prompted the Australian Therapeutic Goods Authority and Health Canada to require cautionary statements on all retail black cohosh product labels. The *US Pharmacopeia* Supplements Panel has recommended a cautionary warning on black cohosh products regarding liver effects.[102]

Toxicity may be caused by adulteration with other species of cohosh related to black cohosh. A specific product labeled as black cohosh that initially was assessed as having a probable causal association with 4 serious AEs reported in Canada subsequently was shown to contain the wrong species of cohosh. Using high-performance liquid chromatography analysis and mass spectrometry, it was found that the suspect product did not contain authentic black cohosh (*Actaea racemosa*) but probably the Asian species *Actaea cimicifuga* L. Because of many such suspect accounts, a cause-and-effect relationship between black cohosh and liver failure cannot be stated with certainty. However, practitioners should be alert to the possibility and counsel patients to report any untoward symptoms promptly. Used with caution, high-quality black cohosh products are relatively safe and can be tried in doses of 40 mg or 80 mg per day. It works for some women but not for all.

In 2010, a review of 69 cases of suspected black cohosh-induced liver disease found that the assessed data raised serious doubts about the causality of black cohosh in these cases.[103] Inconsistencies in the reported data included uncertainty of product, undisclosed indication, and inadequate evaluation of alcohol abuse.

Cranberry. The juice of cranberries (*Vaccinium macrocarpon*) has long been used as a home remedy for urinary tract infections.[104] Although it was formerly thought to work by acidification of the urine, research demonstrates that it works primarily by preventing bacterial adherence to the urinary epithelia. In a 1994 study of older women (mean age, 78.5 y), cranberry juice recipients had significantly lower odds of having bacteriuria with pyuria than they did when they received a placebo (27% vs 42%).[105] One 6-month study found that 500 mg of cranberry extract daily was similar in effectiveness to 100 mg trimethoprim for the prevention of recurrent urinary tract infections in women aged 45 years or older and was better tolerated.[106] Further studies have not favored those recommendations for all. A 2014 study found no benefit over placebo in women with multiple sclerosis who had urinary disorders.[107]

Dong quai. This aromatic herb, also known as *Angelica sinensis*, Chinese angelica, tang kuei, or dang gui, has been used as a medicinal herb in China for at least 1,200 years. Among Chinese therapies, it is the most extensively used herb for treating gynecologic conditions. It is also used to stimulate the circulation. Some practitioners caution against using dong quai in women who have heavy menstrual flow because it tends to increase bleeding.

The only double-blind efficacy trial to date (N=71) found that 4.5 g of dong quai used daily for 6 months was no more helpful than placebo in relieving hot flashes.[108] Practitioners trained in traditional Chinese medicine counter that dong quai is not meant to be used alone but rather in an individually tailored mixture of herbs. A 6-month trial of the combination of dong quai and astragalus (*Astragalus membranaceus*) found a significant reduction in mild hot flashes, but the combination was no better than placebo for relief of moderate to severe hot flashes or night sweats.[109]

Dong quai can trigger heavy uterine bleeding and should not be used in women who have fibroids, hemophilia, or other blood-clotting problems. It is contraindicated for use with anticoagulants.

Evening primrose oil. This plant, also called *Oenothera biennis*, produces seeds that are rich in oils containing γ-linolenic acid. Preparations made from the oils are reported to improve atopic eczema, reduce hypercholesterolemia, and relieve mastalgia. Evening primrose oil is also promoted for the relief of hot flashes; however, the only RCT found no benefit over placebo for treating menopause-related hot flashes in 56 women.[110]

Reported AEs include inflammation, thrombosis, immunosuppression, nausea, and diarrhea. It may increase the risk of seizures in patients diagnosed with schizophrenia who are taking antipsychotics. It should not be used with phenothiazines.

Ginkgo. This herb, also known as *Ginkgo biloba*, has been used as a medicinal agent for at least 3 millennia. Standardized extracts of the leaf have been used to treat many conditions, including vertigo, tinnitus, intermittent claudication, short-term memory loss, macular degeneration, and asthma. Ginkgo is thought to act by dilating blood vessels, reducing blood viscosity, modifying neurotransmitters, and acting as a potent antioxidant.

The primary use of ginkgo is to treat cerebral function disorders, including age-related cognitive decline, and to slow the progress of neurodegenerative disorders such as Alzheimer disease. A federally funded, multicenter trial of 3,069 participants over 6 years failed to find that 240 mg of ginkgo extract daily resulted in less cognitive decline in older adults with normal cognition or with mild cognitive impairment.[111] Another study found that ginkgo at 120 mg twice daily was not effective in reducing the rate of dementia or Alzheimer disease.[112] A Cochrane review reported trials showing improvement in cognition, activities of daily living, and mood, although these effects were small, and unsatisfactory methodology and publication biases cannot be excluded.[113] The review concludes that the evidence that ginkgo has predictable and clinically significant benefit for people with dementia or cognitive impairment is inconsistent and unreliable.

The most serious AE purportedly associated with ginkgo use is bleeding. However, whether ginkgo actually increases the risk of bleeding is not known. The most common AEs reported with ginkgo use are GI distress and headache. Large doses may cause restlessness, anxiety, allergic skin reactions, sleep disturbances, and GI upset, including diarrhea, nausea, and vomiting.

Ginseng. The most common types of ginseng are Asian (Korean or Chinese) ginseng (*Panax ginseng*) and American ginseng (*Panax quinquefolius*). Eleuthero, sometimes referred to as Siberian ginseng (*Eleutherococcus senticosus*), is not a true ginseng because it is not in the *Panax* genus. The various types of ginseng exhibit different effects. It is the multibranched root of these perennial, shade-loving plants that is used in botanical medicine.

Preparations of Asian ginseng root have been held in high esteem in traditional Chinese medicine for thousands of years. Marketers of ginseng supplements have promoted the products for women and men to build stamina and resistance to disease, although there is no strong documentation for these claims.

Ginseng contains more than a dozen terpenoids, especially a group of compounds called ginsenosides. Ginseng may exert estrogenic effects, although the plant does not actually contain phytoestrogens.

Ginseng has been studied for menopause-related complaints.[114] An RCT of ginseng found that a ginseng extract had no overall effect on VMS or serum hormone levels, although there was improvement in subsets involving depression, general health, and well-being. A review of several further trials confirms this outcome.[115]

Although ginseng is generally well tolerated, reported AEs have included nervousness, insomnia, dizziness, and hypertension. Mastalgia with diffuse breast nodularity also has been reported. Case reports have associated ginseng with uterine bleeding.[116,117]

In one RCT, 2 weeks of American ginseng administration to 20 women receiving warfarin significantly reduced the INR compared with placebo.[118] Practitioners should counsel patients to exercise caution if taking anticoagulant therapy. Some experts contraindicate the use of ginseng with antihypertensives or stimulants, including dietary supplement remedies containing ma huang, ephedrine, or guarana.

Kava. Kava rhizome, also known as *Piper methysticum*, is used for treating anxiety, hot flashes, and sleep disruption. Active constituents in kava include the kavalactones (also called kavapyrones). Kava is ingested as a tea or as a dietary supplement. A Cochrane review concluded that kava extract seems to be an effective symptomatic treatment option for anxiety compared with placebo.[119] In a small, open study of kava in perimenopausal women, significant improvements were seen in anxiety symptoms on several scales of anxiety, depression, and climacteric symptoms.[120]

Kava has been linked with cases of severe hepatotoxicity, including active liver failure, cholestatic hepatitis, and cirrhosis of the liver. As a result, some countries (Canada, United Kingdom, Germany, Australia) have banned kava supplements. In March 2002, FDA issued a warning recommending that kava products not be used before consulting a physician. FDA has not concluded whether kava has a causal relationship to liver disease. Although kava is still sold in the United States, many manufacturers stopped selling it because of concerns of possible litigation and inability to obtain product liability insurance. Given the hepatotoxicity concerns, it may be advisable to avoid use altogether.

Licorice. The root of the licorice plant, also known as *Glycyrrhiza glabra*, contains coumarins, flavonoids, and terpenoids. The most well-known ingredients of licorice are glycyrrhizinic acid and its derivatives.

Licorice is mostly used for its anti-inflammatory, antibacterial, antiviral, and expectorant properties. Small amounts of licorice also are often included in Chinese medicine formulations for postmenopausal women. Any therapeutic benefit may be because of the mild estrogenic activity of compounds such as glabridin (similar to 17β-estradiol).[121]

Licorice root tinctures, extracts, capsules, and lozenges are available. Most licorice candies manufactured in the United States do not contain licorice but are flavored with anise, whereas imported candies usually contain real licorice. Licorice is also found in many teas and over-the-counter cough remedies sold in the United States.

In Chinese medicine, licorice is always used as part of a mixture. The synergistic effects of mixtures, and perhaps dose limitations, may prevent AEs. Most reported cases of licorice-induced AEs have been from licorice-containing candies, gums, laxatives, or chewing tobacco, not from the use of licorice as herbal medicine.

Large, chronic doses of licorice may result in pseudoprimary aldosteronism, with symptoms that may include edema, hypertension, and hypokalemia. Cardiac arrhythmias and cardiac arrest, including 2 known deaths, have occurred in chronic consumers of licorice candy products. Cardiomyopathy, hypokalemic myopathy, and pulmonary edema have also been reported. Hypokalemia caused by licorice may be potentiated by the use of diuretics, so the combination should be avoided.

Sage. Some women use sage, or *Salvia officinalis*, to help with hot flashes and night sweats. An open, multicenter clinical trial recruited 71 women who had been menopausal for at least 12 months and were having at least 5 hot flashes daily.[122] Women receiving the sage tablets reported a significant 50% decrease in the mean number of intensity-rated hot flashes within 4 weeks and 64% within 8 weeks, although study results are limited by absence of a placebo arm for comparison ($P<.0001$).

Although the teas and capsules are likely safe, the ethanolic extracts and essential oil are not generally recommended because of the toxicity of at least 1 of their components, a volatile oil called thujone. Prolonged or excessive doses of herbs that contain thujone can cause vomiting, vertigo, kidney damage, and convulsions.

St John's wort. In Germany, St. John's wort, also known as *Hypericum perforatum*, is the most popular treatment for mild to moderate depression, and a growing number of women are taking it alone in supplement form or in combination with black cohosh to ease hot flashes.

A randomized, placebo-controlled study included 100 premenopausal, perimenopausal, and postmenopausal women having active hot flashes.[123] Women received either St. John's wort or placebo for 8 weeks. The difference in hot flash severity and duration between groups was not significant on the fourth week of intervention; however, there was a statistically significant difference between the 2 groups on both outcomes by the eighth week of treatment in favor of St. John's wort ($P<.001$).

A 12-week trial found that 900 mg (300 mg 3 times/d) of St. John's wort extract significantly improved QOL and sleep parameters compared with placebo.[124] There was a nonsignificant trend in hot flash reduction. Another trial found the combination of black cohosh and St. John's wort to be more effective than placebo for relieving hot flashes.[91]

In a Cochrane review, 29 trials involving 5,498 patients using St. John's wort to treat mild to moderately severe depressive disorders were identified.[125] Most trials were 4 to 6 weeks long, with some lasting 6 months. The researchers concluded that the hypericum extracts tested in the included trials are superior to placebo in patients with major depression, are similarly effective as standard antidepressants, and have fewer AEs than standard antidepressants. Adverse events were reported by 26.3% of those receiving St. John's wort compared with 44.7% for antidepressants.

A review of common botanicals used for treatment of mood and anxiety disorders in perimenopausal and postmenopausal women found that 5 of 7 trials of St. John's wort for mild to moderate depression showed significant improvement.[126]

The results of several trials comparing St. John's wort with selective serotonin-reuptake inhibitors (SSRIs) were mixed. One randomized trial found that neither St. John's wort nor sertraline performed significantly better than placebo in treating patients with major depressive disorder.[127] Two studies comparing St. John's wort with SSRIs found it at least as effective as paroxetine and significantly more effective than fluoxetine for moderate to severe and major depression.[128,129] Other studies found it to be as efficacious as citalopram for moderate depression and paroxetine for preventing relapse after recovery from moderate to severe depression.[130,131] In several of the studies, St. John's wort was reported to be better tolerated than SSRIs in patients.

St. John's wort should not be used concomitantly with psychotropic medications. Taking it with SSRIs may result in the production of too much serotonin (called "serotonin syndrome") and subsequent dizziness, restlessness, and muscle twitching.

The usual dose of St. John's wort in supplement form is 300 mg to 600 mg (standardized to contain 3%-5% hyperforin, 0.3% hypericin, or both) 3 times daily. Onset of action occurs in 2 to 4 weeks.

Adverse GI events have been reported with St. John's wort, although dosing with food minimizes upset. Fatigue is also associated with its use, and in rare cases, it can increase sensitivity to sunlight. Combined with sunlight, it may also contribute to cataract formation.

St. John's wort may decrease serum levels of warfarin, digoxin, theophylline, indinavir, cyclosporine, and phenprocoumon.

Valerian. Preparations are made from the roots and underground plant parts of valerian, or *Valeriana officinalis*. This herb is used primarily to treat nervousness and insomnia and is recognized by the German health authorities and the World Health Organization for these purposes. A systematic review of valerian trials for improving sleep quality suggested that valerian might improve sleep quality without producing AEs.[132]

No substantial AEs of valerian have been noted with recommended doses, although long-term administration may be associated with headache, restlessness, sleeplessness, and cardiac disorders. Unlike other sedatives, it does not seem to interact with alcohol to intensify drowsiness.

Vitex. This herb, also known as chasteberry or *Vitex agnus-castus*, is commonly used for PMS, irregular menstruation, and cyclical mastalgia. It is approved by the German health authorities for all 3 conditions. Vitex is generally standardized to its iridoid glycoside content, calculated as agnuside. The combination of vitex and St. John's wort was found to be superior to placebo for reducing total PMS scores in perimenopausal women.[133] A 2-part study survey found that participants taking vitex experienced strong symptomatic relief of some common menopausal symptoms.[134,135] Trials have shown that it improves symptoms of PMS, normalizes luteal-phase length, and increases luteal-phase progesterone levels.[136] Some herbalists recommend the herb to reduce the heavy, irregular uterine bleeding experienced by some perimenopausal women.

Vitex is reputed to have a libido-reducing effect, and this effect is responsible for its other names: chaste-tree berry (or chasteberry) and monk's pepper. Although clinicians who recommend vitex indicate that this effect is rare, they advise that women with low libido should not be given this herb. Adverse events are mild and include nausea, headache, GI disturbances, menstrual disorders, acne, pruritus, and erythematous rash.[137]

Safety

These integrative medicine systems are relatively safe, but AEs may occur with their use. Acupuncture has been demonstrated to be a safe procedure, especially when used by competent practitioners.[138] Common AEs, such as local pain and bruising, minor bleeding, and lightheadedness, are transient and minor. Serious AEs are rare. A systematic analysis of 12 prospective studies that surveyed more than a million acupuncture treatments reported 6 serious AEs: 4 pneumothorax incidents and 2 broken needles.[139] Proper needling over the lung field prevents the occurrence of a pneumothorax. There is no research that suggests acupuncture is dangerous for treating menopause symptoms in women with cancer. Women should be advised to confirm that acupuncture treatments are being performed with sterile, disposable needles to prevent the risk of blood-borne infections, including hepatitis and HIV.

A number of AEs have been associated with herbal therapies and nutritional supplements. They can interact with prescription drugs, resulting in enhanced or diminished effects of the herb or supplement, the drug, or both. It is possible that a new effect may be observed that is not seen with either substance taken alone. However, the validity of many reported adverse herb-drug interactions is questionable because some of the products used were not tested for purity.

Pharmacokinetic interactions may also occur. Mucilage-rich herbs may interfere with drug absorption. For example, St. John's wort, commonly prescribed for mild depression, is an inducer of the hepatic enzyme CYP3A4. It has been shown to decrease the rate of metabolism of a number of drugs. Diuretic herbs that alter sodium resorption in the renal tubule can increase plasma levels of many drugs, including lithium. Pharmacodynamic interactions between agonists and antagonists at receptor sites are also possible, resulting in an inhibitory or additive effect.

Dramatic quantitative and qualitative differences in drug effects may result from genetic variability in metabolizing drugs or herbs or both.

Although many drug-herb or drug-nutritional supplement interactions are not likely to be clinically significant, caution should be exercised, particularly when prescribing drugs that have a narrow therapeutic index and serious toxicity (eg, warfarin) or when the medication is necessary for life (eg, cyclosporine). Women with a disease that can be fatal if undertreated (eg, epilepsy) also require close observation.

The American College of Obstetricians and Gynecologists has issued a warning that a number of herbs, in addition to nonsteroidal anti-inflammatory drugs, can cause excessive bleeding if they are taken by patients who are also taking anticoagulants.[140] Other herbs and supplements can reduce the effectiveness of anticoagulants.

Some herbs and supplements have hypoglycemic activity. Women who are taking insulin or oral hypoglycemics should closely monitor their blood glucose levels when adding such therapies to their daily regimen.

A number of herbs and nutritional supplements, including dong quai root (*radix Angelica sinensis*), evening primrose oil, ginkgo leaf (*folium Ginkgo bilobae*), ginger (*rhizome Zingiberis officinalis*), garlic (*Allium sativum*), ginseng (*radix Ginseng*), and feverfew (*Tanacetum parthenium*), have been found to inhibit platelet aggregation. Combining any of these with an anticoagulant such as warfarin, aspirin (including low-dose aspirin for cardiovascular benefits), or vitamin E is not recommended, unless a patient is closely monitored. These botanicals should be closely monitored in women experiencing abnormal uterine bleeding. Healthcare professionals should advise all women to discontinue any supplement with a blood-thinning effect 7 to 10 days before surgery; supplements can usually be resumed after discharge (Table 3).

Although integrative therapies are not as effective as HT, they may be an option because not all women can safely take HT. Pharmaceuticals can interact and result in serious AEs, as can integrative therapies.

There are several ways to improve patient safety. Patients should speak with practitioners specifically trained in herbs and nutrition and should not rely solely on information found on the Internet in order to self-prescribe. Physicians can support state licensure for providers who have graduated from accredited schools, passed national boards, and meet a minimum level of competency. Recommend that patients only purchase formulations labeled with the designation *good manufacturing practices* (GMP) to ensure adequate testing of ingredients. When taking a drug history, ask patients to include all herbs and nutritional supplements. All labeling should be in English.

Research local practitioners to whom you can refer. Consider receiving a treatment yourself in order to assess its effects and evaluate the quality of the practitioner. Review the criteria you would use to refer to another physician: How many years' experience does the practitioner have? Does the practitioner have expertise with the biomedical diagnosis? Is the practitioner licensed, if licensure exists in your area? Is the practitioner board certified, if the discipline offers board certification? What is the practitioner's reputation among physicians? What is his or her reputation in the community? Do not hesitate to call a practitioner and investigate these on your own. The ideal CAM practitioner will have respect for biomedicine, know his or her own limitations, and know when in turn to refer to others, including MDs, physical therapists, chiropractors, massage therapists, and other integrative medicine practitioners.

Not all CAM therapies are equal. There exist numerous other therapies and interventions for which there may be little or no scientific evidence of efficacy. Therapies such as crystal healing and sound healing, for example, although perhaps not inherently dangerous, may cause patients to develop unrealistic expectations that result in their not accessing therapies that are safe and proven effective. Patients may experience subjective amelioration of symptoms through a placebo effect. This raises the ethical question of whether the use of CAM therapies should be supported if scientifically proven interventions do not work and an intervention with no scientific evidence to support its use results in some subjective improvement, even if only a placebo effect.

Patient access of integrative medicine in the United States is common and growing. There is evidence that many patients do not inform physicians of their use of integrative medicine; they fear lack of approval, or worse, being told to stop using it. To enhance patient safety, clinicians should actively enquire regarding their patients' use of integrative medicine in a value-neutral way and determine whether a patient reports subjective improvement of symptoms.

Table 3. Precautions and Interactions When Using Herbs or Other Agents That May Interact With Anticoagulant Therapies

- Use is contraindicated in patients with active bleeding (eg, AUB, peptic ulcer, intracranial bleeding) or a history of bleeding (hemostatic disorders); with drug-related hemostatic problems; and in those taking prescription anticoagulant medications (eg, warfarin or antiplatelet agents such as ticlopidine, clopidogrel, dipyridamole).

- Caution is advised when using more than 1 OTC anticoagulant therapy, including aspirin (including low-dose aspirin for cardiovascular benefit), aspirin-containing products, NSAIDs, vitamin E, fish oil, dong quai, St. John's wort, evening primrose oil, feverfew, and the 4 Gs: garlic, ginger, Ginkgo biloba, and ginseng.

- Use should be discontinued 7 to 10 days before dental or surgical procedures; use can usually be resumed after discharge.

Abbreviations: AUB, abnormal uterine bleeding; NSAIDS, nonsteroidal anti-inflammatory drugs; OTC, over-the-counter.

References

1. Fugh-Berman A. Herbs, phytoestrogens, and other CAM therapies. In: Lobo RA, ed. *Treatment of the Postmenopausal Woman: Basic and Clinical Aspects*. 3rd ed. San Diego, CA: Academic Press; 2007:683-690.
2. Berman BM, Swyers JP, Hartnoll SM, Singh BB, Bausell B. The public debate over alternative medicine: the importance of finding a middle ground. *Altern Ther Health Med*. 2000;6(1):98-101.
3. National Center for Complementary and Alternative Medicine. *CAM Basics: Complementary, Alternative, or Integrative Health: What's in a Name?* National Institutes of Health Web site. http://nccam.nih.gov/sites/nccam.nih.gov/files/CAM_Basics_What_Are_CAIHA.pdf. October 2008. Updated May 2013. Accessed March 27, 2014.
4. Kleijnen J, Knipschild P, ter Riet G. Clinical trials of homeopathy. *BMJ*. 1991;302(6772):316-323. Erratum in: *BMJ*. 1991;302(6780):818.
5. Linde K, Scholz M, Ramirez G, Clausius N, Melchart D, Jonas WB. Impact of study quality on outcome in placebo-controlled trials of homeopathy. *J Clin Epidemiol*. 1999;52(7):631-636.
6. Shang A, Huwiler-Müntener K, Nartey L, et al. Are the clinical effects of homeopathy placebo effects? Comparative study of the effectiveness of placebo-controlled trials of homeopathy and allopathy. *Lancet*. 2005;366(9487):726-732.
7. Lüdtke R, Rutten AL. The conclusions on the effectiveness of homeopathy highly depend on the set of analyzed trials. *J Clin Epidemiol*. 2008;61(12):1197-1204.
8. von Hagens C, Schiller P, Godbillon B, et al. Treating menopausal symptoms with a complex remedy or placebo: a randomized controlled trial. *Climacteric*. 2012;15(4):358-367.
9. Newton KM, Reed SD, LaCroix AZ, Grothaus LC, Ehrlich K, Guiltinan J. Treatment of vasomotor symptoms of menopause with black cohosh, multibotanicals, soy, hormone therapy, or placebo: a randomized trial. *Ann Intern Med*. 2006;145(12):869-879.
10. Tice JA, Ettinger B, Ensrud K, Wallace R, Blackwell T, Cummings SR. Phytoestrogen supplements for the treatment of hot flashes: the Isoflavone Clover Extract (ICE) Study: a randomized controlled trial. *JAMA*. 2003;290(2):207-214.
11. Colau JC, Vincent S, Marijnen P, Allaert FA. Efficacy of a non-hormonal treatment, BRN-01, on menopausal hot flashes: a multicenter, randomized, double-blind, placebo-controlled trial. *Drugs R D*. 2012;12(3):429-440.
12. Nayak C, Singh V, Singh K, et al. Management of distress during climacteric years by homeopathic therapy. *J Altern Complement Med*. 2011;17(11):1037-1042.
13. Smolinski D, Wollner D, Orlowski J, Curcio J, Nevels J, Kim LS. A pilot study to examine a combination botanical for the treatment of menopausal symptoms. *J Altern Complement Med*. 2005;11(3):483-489.
14. Cramer EH, Jones P, Keenan NL, Thompson BL. Is naturopathy as effective as conventional therapy for the treatment of menopausal symptoms? *J Altern Complement Med*. 2003;9(4):529-538.
15. Rees M. Alternative treatments for the menopause. *Best Pract Res Clin Obstet Gynaecol*. 2009;23(1):151-161.
16. Linde K, Jonas WB, Melchart D, Willich S. The methodological quality of randomized controlled trials of homeopathy, herbal medicines and acupuncture. *Int J Epidemiol*. 2001;30(3):526-531.
17. Kronenberg F, Fugh-Berman A. Complementary and alternative medicine for menopausal symptoms: a review of randomized, controlled trials. *Ann Intern Med*. 2002;137(10):805-813.
18. Huang MI, Nir Y, Chen B, Schnyer R, Manber R. A randomized controlled pilot study of acupuncture for postmenopausal hot flashes: effect on nocturnal hot flashes and sleep quality. *Fertil Steril*. 2006;86(3):700-710.
19. Nir Y, Huang MI, Schnyer R, Chen B, Manber R. Acupuncture for postmenopausal hot flashes. *Maturitas*. 2007;56(4):383-395.
20. Vincent A, Barton DL, Mandrekar JN, et al. Acupuncture for hot flashes: a randomized, sham-controlled clinical study. *Menopause*. 2007;14(1):45-52.
21. Borud EK, Alraek T, White A, Grimsgaard S. The Acupuncture on Hot Flashes Among Menopausal Women study: observational follow-up results at 6 and 12 months. *Menopause*. 2010;17(2):262-268.
22. Kim KH, Kang KW, Kim DI, et al. Effects of acupuncture on hot flashes in perimenopausal and postmenopausal women—a multicenter randomized clinical trial. *Menopause*. 2010;17(2):269-280.
23. Sunay D, Ozdiken M, Arslan H, Seven A, Aral Y. The effect of acupuncture on postmenopausal symptoms and reproductive hormones: a sham controlled clinical trial. *Acupunct Med*. 2011;29(1):27-31.

24. Painovich JM, Shufelt CL, Azziz R, et al. A pilot randomized, single-blind, placebo-controlled trial of traditional acupuncture for vasomotor symptoms and mechanistic pathways of menopause. *Menopause*. 2012;19(1):54-61.
25. Nedeljkovic M, Tian L, Ji P, et al. Effects of acupuncture and Chinese herbal medicine (Zhi Mu 14) on hot flushes and quality of life in postmenopausal women: results of a four-arm randomized controlled pilot trial. *Menopause*. 2014;21(1):15-24.
26. Hachul H, Garcia TK, Maciel AL, Yagihara F, Tufik S, Bittencourt L. Acupuncture improves sleep in postmenopause in a randomized, double-blind, placebo-controlled study. *Climacteric*. 2013;16(1):36-40.
27. Crew KD, Capodice JL, Greenlee H, et al. Randomized, blinded, sham-controlled trial of acupuncture for the management of aromatase inhibitor-associated joint symptoms in women with early-stage breast cancer. *J Clin Oncol*. 2010;28(7):1154-1160.
28. Bao T, Cai L, Giles JT, et al. A dual-center randomized controlled double blind trial assessing the effect of acupuncture in reducing musculoskeletal symptoms in breast cancer patients taking aromatase inhibitors. *Breast Cancer Res Treat*. 2013;138(1):167-174.
29. Kwee SH, Tan HH, Marsman A, Wauters AM. The effect of Chinese herbal medicines (CHM) on menopausal symptoms compared to hormone replacement therapy (HRT) and placebo. *Maturitas*. 2007;58(1):83-90.
30. Qu F, Cai X, Gu Y, et al. Chinese medicinal herbs in relieving perimenopausal depression: a randomized, controlled trial. *J Altern Complement Med*. 2009;15(1):93-100.
31. Zhong LL, Tong Y, Tang GW, et al. A randomized, double-blind, controlled trial of a Chinese herbal formula (Er Xian decoction) for menopausal symptoms in Hong Kong perimenopausal women. *Menopause*. 2013;20(7):767-776.
32. Park JE, Lee MS, Jung S, et al. Moxibustion for treating menopausal hot flashes: a randomized clinical trial. *Menopause*. 2009;16(4):660-665.
33. Karaçam Z, Seker SE. Factors associated with menopausal symptoms and their relationship with the quality of life among Turkish women. *Maturitas*. 2007;58(1):75-82.
34. Yeh SC, Chang MY. The effect of Qigong on menopausal symptoms and quality of sleep for perimenopausal women: a preliminary observational study. *J Altern Complement Med*. 2012;18(6):567-575.
35. Booth-LaForce C, Thurston RC, Taylor MR. A pilot study of a Hatha yoga treatment for menopausal symptoms. *Maturitas*. 2007;57(3):286-295.
36. Chattha R, Raghuram N, Venkatram P, Hongasandra NR. Treating the climacteric symptoms in Indian women with an integrated approach to yoga therapy: a randomized controlled study. *Menopause*. 2008;15(5):862-870.
37. Chattha R, Nagarathna R, Padmalatha V, Nagendra HR. Effect of yoga on cognitive functions in climacteric syndrome: a randomized control study. *BJOG*. 2008;115(8):991-1000.
38. North American Menopause Society. The role of soy isoflavones in menopausal health: report of The North American Menopause Society/Wulf H. Utian Translational Science Symposium in Chicago, IL (October 2010). *Menopause*. 2011;18(7):732-753.
39. Soyfoods Association of North America. *Soy Products: Sales and Trends*. Soyfoods Association of North America Web site. www.soyfoods.org/products/sales-and-trends. Accessed March 27, 2014.
40. Newton KM, Buist DS, Keenan NL, Anderson LA, LaCroix AZ. Use of alternative therapies for menopause symptoms: results of a population-based survey. *Obstet Gynecol*. 2002;100(1):18-25. Erratum in: *Obstet Gynecol*. 2003;101(1):205.
41. Bhagwat S, Haytowitz DB, Holden J. *USDA Database for the Isoflavone Content of Selected Foods: Release 2.0*. US Department of Agriculture Web site. September 2008. www.ars.usda.gov/SP2UserFiles/Place/12354500/Data/isoflav/Isoflav_R2.pdf. Accessed March 27, 2014.
42. Setchell KD, Cole SJ. Method of defining equol-producer status and its frequency among vegetarians. *J Nutr*. 2006;136(8):2188-2193.
43. Vergne S, Sauvant P, Lamothe V, et al. Influence of ethnic origin (Asian v. Caucasian) and background diet on the bioavailability of dietary isoflavones. *Br J Nutr*. 2009;102(11):1642-1653.
44. Taku K, Melby MK, Kronenberg F, Kurzer MS, Messina M. Extracted or synthesized soybean isoflavones reduce menopausal hot flash frequency and severity: systematic review and meta-analysis of randomized controlled trials. *Menopause*. 2012;19(7):776-790.
45. Cheng G, Wilczek B, Warner M, Gustafsson JA, Landgren BM. Isoflavone treatment for acute menopausal symptoms. *Menopause*. 2007;14(3 pt 1):468-473.
46. Basaria S, Wisniewski A, Dupree K, et al. Effect of high-dose isoflavones on cognition, quality of life, androgens, and lipoprotein in post-menopausal women. *J Endocrinol Invest*. 2009;32(2):150-155.
47. Nelson HD, Vesco KK, Haney E, et al. Nonhormonal therapies for menopausal hot flashes: systematic review and meta-analysis. *JAMA*. 2006;295(17):2057-2071.
48. D'Anna R, Cannata ML, Atteritano M, et al. Effects of the phytoestrogen genistein on hot flushes, endometrium, and vaginal epithelium in postmenopausal women: a 1-year randomized, double-blind, placebo-controlled study. *Menopause*. 2007;14(3):648-655.
49. Nikander E, Rutanen EN, Nieminen P, Wahlström T, Ylikorkala O, Tiitinen A. Lack of effect of isoflavonoids on the vagina and endometrium in postmenopausal women. *Fertil Steril*. 2005;83(1):137-142.
50. Manonai J, Songchitsomboon S, Chanda K, Hong JH, Komindr S. The effect of a soy-rich diet on urogenital atrophy: a randomized, cross-over trial. *Maturitas*. 2006;54(2):135-140.
51. Gallagher JC, Satpathy R, Rafferty K, Haynatzka V. The effect of soy protein isolate on bone metabolism. *Menopause*. 2004;11(3):290-298.
52. Kreijkamp-Kaspers S, Kok L, Grobbee DE, et al. Effect of soy protein containing isoflavones on cognitive function, bone mineral density, and plasma lipids in postmenopausal women: a randomized controlled trial. *JAMA*. 2004;292(1):65-74.
53. Cheong JM, Martin BR, Jackson GS, et al. Soy isoflavones do not affect bone resorption in postmenopausal women: a dose-response study using a novel approach with 41Ca. *J Clin Endocrinol Metab*. 2007;92(2):577-582.
54. Marini H, Minutoli L, Polito F, et al. Effects of phytoestrogen genistein on bone metabolism in osteopenic postmenopausal women: a randomized trial. *Ann Intern Med*. 2007;146(12):839-847.
55. Atteritano M, Mazzaferro S, Frisina A, et al. Genistein effects on quantitative ultrasound parameters and bone mineral density in osteopenic postmenopausal women. *Osteoporos Int*. 2009;20(11):1947-1954.
56. Wu J, Oka J, Ezaki J, et al. Possible role of equol status in the effects of isoflavone on bone and fat mass in postmenopausal Japanese women: a double-blind, randomized, controlled trial. *Menopause*. 2007;14(5):866-874.
57. Tousen Y, Ezaki J, Fujii Y, Ueno T, Nishimuta M, Ishimi Y. Natural S-equol decreased bone resorption in postmenopausal, non-equol-producing Japanese women: a pilot randomized, placebo-controlled trial. *Menopause*. 2011;18(5):563-574.
58. Kritz-Silverstein D, Von Mühlen D, Barrett-Connor E, Bressel MA. Isoflavones and cognitive function in older women: the SOy and Postmenopausal Health In Aging (SOPHIA) Study. *Menopause*. 2003;10(3):196-202.
59. File SE, Hartley DE, Elsabagh S, Duffy R, Wiseman H. Cognitive improvement after 6 weeks of soy supplements in postmenopausal women is limited to frontal lobe function. *Menopause*. 2005;12(2):193-201.
60. Casini ML, Marelli G, Papaleo E, Ferrari A, D'Ambrosio F, Unfer V. Psychological assessment of the effects of treatment with phytoestrogens on postmenopausal women: a randomized, double-blind, crossover, placebo-controlled study. *Fertil Steril*. 2006;85(4):972-978.
61. Ho SC, Chan AS, Ho YP, et al. Effects of soy isoflavone supplementation on cognitive function in Chinese postmenopausal women: a double-blind, randomized, controlled trial. *Menopause*. 2007;14(3 pt 1):489-499.
62. Fournier LR, Ryan Borchers TA, Robison LM, et al. The effects of soy milk and isoflavone supplements on cognitive performance in healthy, postmenopausal women. *J Nutr Health Aging*. 2007;11(2):155-164.
63. Henderson VW, St John JA, Hodis HN, et al; WISH Research Group. Long-term soy isoflavone supplementation and cognition in women: a randomized, controlled trial. *Neurology*. 2012;78(23):1841-1848.
64. Erdman JW Jr. AHA science advisory: soy protein and cardiovascular disease: a statement for healthcare professionals from the Nutrition Committee of the AHA. *Circulation*. 2000;102(20):2555-2559.
65. Sacks FM, Lichtenstein A, Van Horn L, Harris W, Kris-Etherton P, Winston M; American Heart Association Nutrition Committee. Soy protein, isoflavones, and cardiovascular health: an American Heart Association Science Advisory for professionals from the Nutrition Committee. *Circulation*. 2006;113(7):1034-1044.
66. Lichtenstein AH, Jalbert SM, Adlercreutz H, et al. Lipoprotein response to diets high in soy or animal protein with and without isoflavones in moderately hypercholesterolemic subjects. *Arterioscler Thromb Vasc Biol*. 2002;22(11):1852-1858.
67. Dewell A, Hollenbeck PL, Hollenbeck CB. Clinical review: a critical evaluation of the role of soy protein and isoflavone supplementation in the control of plasma cholesterol concentrations. *J Clin Endocrinol Metab*. 2006;91(3):772-780.
68. Allen JK, Becker DM, Kwiterovich PO, Lindenstruth KA, Curtis C. Effect of soy protein-containing isoflavones on lipoproteins in postmenopausal women. *Menopause*. 2007;14(1):106-114.

69. Nestel PJ, Yamashita T, Sasahara T, et al. Soy isoflavones improve systemic arterial compliance but not plasma lipids in menopausal and perimenopausal women. *Arterioscler Thromb Vasc Biol.* 1997;17(12):3392-3398.
70. Hodis HN, Mack WJ, Kono N, et al; Women's Isoflavone Soy Health Research Group. Isoflavone soy protein supplementation and atherosclerosis progression in healthy postmenopausal women: a randomized controlled trial. *Stroke.* 2011;42(11):3168-3175.
71. Clerici C, Setchell KD, Battezzati PM, et al. Pasta naturally enriched with isoflavone aglycons from soy germ reduces serum lipids and improves markers of cardiovascular risk. *J Nutr.* 2007;137(10):2270-2278.
72. Vafeiadou K, Hall WL, Williams CM. Does genotype and equol-production status affect response to isoflavones? Data from a pan-European study on the effects of isoflavones on cardiovascular risk markers in post-menopausal women. *Proc Nutr Soc.* 2006;65(1):106-115.
73. Thorp AA, Howe PR, Mori TA, et al. Soy food consumption does not lower LDL cholesterol in either equol or nonequol producers. *Am J Clin Nutr.* 2008;88(2):298-304.
74. Törmälä R, Appt S, Clarkson TB, et al. Equol production capability is associated with favorable vascular function in postmenopausal women using tibolone; no effect with soy supplementation. *Atherosclerosis.* 2008;198(1):174-178.
75. Trock BJ, Hilakivi-Clarke L, Clarke R. Meta-analysis of soy intake and breast cancer risk. *J Natl Cancer Inst.* 2006;98(7):459-471.
76. Wu AH, Yu MC, Tseng CC, Pike MC Epidemiology of soy exposures and breast cancer risk. *Br J Cancer.* 2008;98(1):9-14.
77. Brown NM, Belles CA, Lindley SL, et al. The chemopreventive action of equol enantiomers in a chemically induced animal model of breast cancer. *Carcinogenesis.* 2010;31(5):886-893.
78. Brown NM, Belles CA, Lindley SL, et al. Mammary gland differentiation by early life exposure to enantiomers of the soy isoflavone metabolite equol. *Food Chem Toxicol.* 2010;48(11):3042-3050.
79. Magee PJ, Raschke M, Steiner C, et al. Equol: a comparison of the effects of the racemic compound with that of the purified S-enantiomer on the growth, invasion, and DNA integrity in breast and prostate cells in vitro. *Nutr Cancer.* 2006;54(2):232-242.
80. Lampe JW. Emerging research on equol and cancer. *J Nutr.* 2010;140(7):1369S-1372S.
81. Atkinson C, Frankenfeld CL, Lampe JW. Gut bacterial metabolism of the soy isoflavone daidzein: exploring the relevance to human health. *Exp Biol Med (Maywood).* 2005;230(3):155-170.
82. Helferich WG, Andrade JE, Hoagland MS. Phytoestrogens and breast cancer: a complex story. *Inflammopharmacology.* 2008;16(5):219-226.
83. Shu XO, Zheng Y, Cai H, et al. Soy food intake and breast cancer survival. *JAMA.* 2009;302(22):2437-2443.
84. Bandera EV, Williams MG, Sima C, et al. Phytoestrogen consumption and endometrial cancer risk: a population based case-control study in New Jersey. *Cancer Causes Control.* 2009;20(7):1117-1127.
85. Horn-Ross PL, John EM, Canchola AJ, Stewart SL, Lee MM. Phytoestrogen intake and endometrial cancer risk. *J Natl Cancer Inst.* 2003;95(15):1158-1164. Erratum in: *J Natl Cancer Inst.* 2006;98(20):1501.
86. Xu WH, Zheng W, Xiang YB, et al. Soya food intake and risk of endometrial cancer among Chinese women in Shanghai: population based case-control study. *BMJ.* 2004;328(7451):1285.
87. World Health Organization. *Rhizoma cimicifugae racemosae. WHO Monographs on Selected Medicinal Plants.* Vol. 2. Essential Medicines and Health Products Information Portal Web site. Published 2004. http://apps.who.int/medicinedocs/en/d/Js4927e/8.html#Js4927e.8. Accessed March 27, 2014.
88. Hajirahimkhan A, Dietz BM, Bolton JL. Botanical modulation of menopausal symptoms: mechanisms of action? *Planta Med.* 2013;79(7):538-553.
89. Rakel D, ed. *Integrative Medicine.* 3rd ed. Philadelphia, PA: Saunders; 2012.
90. Geller SE, Shulman LP, van Breemen RB, et al. Safety and efficacy of black cohosh and red clover for the management of vasomotor symptoms: a randomized controlled trial. *Menopause.* 2009;16(6):1156-1166.
91. Uebelhack R, Blohmer JU, Graubaum HJ, Busch R, Gruenwald J, Wernecke KD. Black cohosh and St. John's wort for climacteric complaints. *Obstet Gynecol.* 2006;107(2 pt 1):247-255.
92. Wuttke W, Gorkow C, Seidlová-Wuttke D. Effects of black cohosh (Cimicifuga racemosa) on bone turnover, vaginal mucosa, and various blood parameters in postmenopausal women: a double-blind, placebo-controlled, and conjugated estrogens-controlled study. *Menopause.* 2006;13(2):185-196.
93. Pockaj BA, Gallagher JG, Loprinzi CL, et al. Phase III double-blind, randomized, placebo-controlled crossover trial of black cohosh in the management of hot flashes: NCCTG Trial N01CC1. *J Clin Oncol.* 2006;24(18):2836-2841.
94. Shams T, Setia MS, Hemmings R, McCusker J, Sewitch M, Ciampi A. Efficacy of black cohosh-containing preparations on menopausal symptoms: a meta analysis. *Altern Ther Health Med.* 2010;16(1):36-44.
95. Schellenberg R, Saller R, Hess L, et al. Dose-dependent effects of the Cimicifuga racemosa extract Ze 450 in the treatment of climacteric complaints: a randomized, placebo-controlled study. *Evid Based Complement Alternat Med.* 2012;2012:260301.
96. Nappi RE, Malavasi B, Brundu B, Facchinetti F. Efficacy of Cimicifuga racemosa on climacteric complaints: a randomized study versus low-dose transdermal estradiol. *Gynecol Endocrinol.* 2005;20(1):30-35.
97. Jacobson JS, Troxel AB, Evans J, et al. Randomized trial of black cohosh for the treatment of hot flashes among women with a history of breast cancer. *J Clin Oncol.* 2001;19(10):2739-2745.
98. Liske E, Hänggi W, Henneicke-von Zepelin HH, Boblitz N, Wüstenberg P, Rahlfs VW. Physiologic investigation of a unique extract of black cohosh (Cimicifuga racemosae rhizoma): a 6-month clinical study demonstrates no systemic estrogenic effect. *J Womens Health Gend Based Med.* 2002;11(2):163-174.
99. Sprangler L, Newton KM, Grothaus LC, Reed SD, Ehrlich K, LaCroix AZ. The effects of black cohosh on lipids, fibrinogen, glucose and insulin. *Maturitas.* 2007;57(2):195-204.
100. Raus K, Brucker C, Gorkow C, Wuttke W. First-time proof of endometrial safety of the special black cohosh extract (Actaea or Cimicifuga racemosa extract) CR BNO 1055. *Menopause.* 2006;13(4):678-691.
101. Low Dog T, Powell KL, Weisman SM. Critical evaluation of the safety of Cimicifuga racemosa in menopause symptom relief. *Menopause.* 2003;10(4):299-313.
102. Mahady GB, Low Dog T, Barrett ML, et al. United States Pharmacopeia review of the black cohosh case reports of hepatotoxicity. *Menopause.* 2008;15(4 pt 1):628-638.
103. Teschke R. Black cohosh and suspected hepatotoxicity: inconsistencies, confounding variables, and prospective use of a diagnostic causality algorithm. A critical review. *Menopause.* 2010;17(2):426-440.
104. Kontiokari T, Sundqvist K, Nuutinen M, Pokka T, Koskela M, Uhari M. Randomised trial of cranberry-lingonberry juice and Lactobacillus GG drink for the prevention of urinary tract infections in women. *BMJ.* 2001;322(7302):1571.
105. Avorn J, Monane M, Gurwitz JH, Glynn RJ, Choodnovskiy I, Lipsitz LA. Reduction of bacteriuria and pyuria after ingestion of cranberry juice. *JAMA.* 1994;271(10):751-754.
106. McMurdo ME, Argo I, Phillips G, Daly F, Davey P. Cranberry or trimethoprim for the prevention of recurrent urinary tract infections? A randomized controlled trial in older women. *J Antimicrob Chemother.* 2009;63(2):389-395.
107. Gallien P, Amarenco G, Benoit N, et al. Cranberry versus placebo in the prevention of urinary infections in multiple sclerosis: a multicenter, randomized, placebo-controlled, double-blind trial. *Mult Scler.* 2014;20(9):1252-1259.
108. Hirata JD, Swiersz LM, Zell B, Small R, Ettinger B. Does dong quai have estrogenic effects in postmenopausal women? A double-blind, placebo-controlled trial. *Fertil Steril.* 1997;68(6):981-986.
109. Haines CJ, Lam PM, Chung TK, Cheng KF, Leung PC. A randomized, double-blind, placebo-controlled study of the effect of a Chinese herbal medicine preparation (Dang Gui Buxue Tang) on menopausal symptoms in Hong Kong Chinese women. *Climacteric.* 2008;11(3):244-251.
110. Chenoy R, Hussain S, Tayob Y, O'Brien PM, Moss MY, Morse PF. Effect of oral gamolenic acid from evening primrose oil on menopausal flushing. *BMJ.* 1994;308(6927):501-503.
111. Snitz BE, O'Meara ES, Carlson MC, et al; Ginkgo Evaluation of Memory (GEM) Study Investigators. Ginkgo biloba for preventing cognitive decline in older adults: a randomized trial. *JAMA.* 2009;302(24):2663-2670.
112. DeKosky ST, Williamson JD, Fitzpatrick AL, et al; Ginkgo Evaluation of Memory (GEM) Study Investigators. Ginkgo biloba for prevention of dementia: a randomized controlled trial. *JAMA.* 2008;300(19):2253-2262. Erratum in: *JAMA.* 2008;300(23):2730.
113. Birks J, Grimley Evans J. Ginkgo biloba for cognitive impairment and dementia. *Cochrane Database Syst Rev.* 2009;(1):CD003120.

114. Wiklund IK, Mattsson LA, Lindgren R, Limoni C. Effects of a standardized ginseng extract on quality of life and physiological parameters in symptomatic postmenopausal women: a double-blind, placebo-controlled trial. Swedish Alternative Medicine Group. *Int J Clin Pharmacol Res*. 1999;19(3):89-99.
115. Kim MS, Lim HJ, Yang HJ, Lee MS, Shin BC, Ernst E. Ginseng for managing menopause symptoms: a systematic review of randomized clinical trials. *J Ginseng Res*. 2013;37(1):30-36.
116. Kabalak AA, Soyal OB, Urfalioglu A, Saracoglu F, Gogus N. Menometrorrhagia and tachyarrhythmia after using oral and topical ginseng. *J Womens Health (Larchmt)*. 2004;13(7):830-833.
117. Greenspan EM. Ginseng and vaginal bleeding. *JAMA*. 249(15):2018.
118. Yuan CS, Wei G, Dey L, et al. Brief communication: American ginseng reduces warfarin's effect in healthy patients: a randomized, controlled trial. *Ann Intern Med*. 2004;141(1):23-27.
119. Pittler MH, Ernst E. Kava extract for treating anxiety. *Cochrane Database Syst Rev*. 2003;(1):CD003383.
120. Cagnacci A, Arangino S, Renzi A, Zanni AL, Malmusi S, Volpe A. Kava-Kava administration reduces anxiety in perimenopausal women. *Maturitas*. 2003;44(2):103-109.
121. Somjen D, Katzburg S, Vaya J, et al. Estrogenic activity of glabridin and glabrene from licorice roots on human osteoblasts and prepubertal rat skeletal tissues. *J Steroid Biochem Mol Biol*. 2004;91(4-5):241-246.
122. Bommer S, Klein P, Suter A. First time proof of sage's tolerability and efficacy in menopausal women with hot flushes. *Adv Ther*. 2011;28(6):490-500.
123. Abdali K, Khajehei M, Tabatabaee HR. Effect of St John's wort on severity, frequency, and duration of hot flashes in premenopausal, perimenopausal and postmenopausal women: a randomized, double-blind, placebo-controlled study. *Menopause*. 2010;17(2):326-331.
124. Al-Akoum M, Maunsell E, Verreault R, Provencher L, Otis H, Dodin S. Effects of Hypericum perforatum (St. John's wort) on hot flashes and quality of life in perimenopausal women: a randomized pilot trial. *Menopause*. 2009;16(2):307-314.
125. Linde K, Berner MM, Kriston L. St John's wort for major depression. *Cochrane Database Syst Rev*. 2008;(4):CD000448.
126. Geller SE, Studee L. Botanical and dietary supplements for mood and anxiety in menopausal women. *Menopause*. 2007;14(3 pt 1):541-549.
127. Hypericum Depression Trial Study Group. Effect of Hypericum perforatum (St John's wort) in major depressive disorder: a randomized controlled trial. *JAMA*. 2002;287(14):1807-1814.
128. Szegedi A, Kohnen R, Dienel A, Kieser M. Acute treatment of moderate to severe depression with hypericum extract WS 5570 (St John's wort): randomised controlled double blind non-inferiority trial versus paroxetine. *BMJ*. 2005;330(7490):503. Erratum in: *BMJ*. 2005;330(7494):759.
129. Fava M, Alpert J, Nierenberg AA, et al. A double-blind, randomized trial of St John's wort, fluoxetine, and placebo in major depressive disorder. *J Clin Psychopharmacol*. 2005;25(5):441-447.
130. Gastpar M, Singer A, Zeller K. Comparative efficacy and safety of a once-daily dosage of hypericum extract STW3-VI and citalopram in patients with moderate depression: a double-blind, randomised, multicentre, placebo-controlled study. *Pharmacopsychiatry*. 2006;39(2):66-75.
131. Anghelescu IG, Kohnen R, Szegedi A, Klement S, Kieser M. Comparison of Hypericum extract WS 5570 and paroxetine in ongoing treatment after recovery from an episode of moderate to severe depression: results from a randomized multicenter study. *Pharmacopsychiatry*. 2006;39(6):213-219.
132. Bent S, Padula A, Moore D, Patterson M, Mehling W. Valerian for sleep: a systematic review and meta-analysis. *Am J Med*. 2006;119(12):1005-1012.
133. van Die MD, Bone KM, Burger HG, Reece JE, Teede HJ. Effects of a combination of Hypericum perforatum and Vitex agnus-castus on PMS-like symptoms in late-perimenopausal women: findings from a subpopulation analysis. *J Altern Complement Med*. 2009;15(9):1045-1048.
134. Lucks BC, Sørensen J, Veal L. Vitex agnus-castus essential oil and menopausal balance: a self-care survey. *Complement Ther Nurs Midwifery*. 2002;8(3):148-154.
135. Chopin Lucks B. Vitex agnus castus essential oil and menopausal balance: a research update [Complement Therapies in Nursing and Midwifery 8 (2003) 148-154]. *Complement Ther Nurs Midwifery*. 2003;9(3):157-160.
136. Schellenberg R. Treatment for the premenstrual syndrome with agnus castus fruit extract: prospective, randomised, placebo controlled study. *BMJ*. 2001;322(7279):134-137.
137. Daniele C, Thompson Coon J, Pittler MH, Ernst E. Vitex agnus castus: a systematic review of adverse events. *Drug Saf*. 2005;28(4):319-332.
138. Vincent C. The safety of acupuncture. *BMJ*. 2001;323(7311):467-468.
139. White A. A cumulative review of the range and incidence of significant adverse events associated with acupuncture. *Acupunct Med*. 2004;22(3):122-133.
140. Committee on Practice Bulletins—Gynecology, American College of Obstetricians and Gynecologists. ACOG Practice Bulletin No. 84: Prevention of deep vein thrombosis and pulmonary embolism. *Obstet Gynecol*. 2007;110(2 pt 1):429-440.

CHAPTER 7

Nonprescription Options

There are many major nonprescription therapies considered for use by women at menopause and beyond, including vitamins, minerals, and other nonbotanical dietary supplements available over the counter (OTC). Some of these nonprescription therapies are recommended, when indicated, with appropriate oversight from a healthcare professional. However, the public frequently self-medicates with little guidance or knowledge of the efficacy or safety of the products they use. Few OTC therapies have the patient package inserts required by the US Food and Drug Administration (FDA) for all marketed prescription medications to provide vital information on how to take a drug safely, identify its adverse events (AEs), and avoid potentially dangerous interactions with other drugs.

Safety may not be mentioned at all in a nonprescription product's advertising or label, although the word *natural* is often seen and misinterpreted by the public to mean that they are safe and without risk. In addition, dietary supplements—a common type of OTC therapy—are regulated differently in the United States and Canada than prescription drugs with regard to allowed health claims. This can cause confusion among the public and sometimes healthcare professionals as well.

Government regulation of dietary supplements

Current FDA regulations for dietary supplements in the United States and Canada are essential information for healthcare professionals and patients.

There is a powerful tradition in the United States for empowerment of consumers to make their own choices about the benefits of their own healthcare programs and medications, as well as a tendency for FDA to view many of the purported benefits for dietary supplements, homeopathic remedies, and alternative medical therapies with a great deal of skepticism. The medical merits aside, most consumers believe that dietary supplements have real medical benefits, are for the most part safe, and are important to their diets to promote better health.

Hippocratic Oath
The North American Menopause Society recognizes that nonprescription therapies have not been proven to be as effective as prescription therapies for treating some health conditions. However, since the basic tenet of the Hippocratic Oath is to do no harm, and nonpharmacologic treatments typically do little harm, nonpharmacologic treatments are often suggested as first-line options because they appear to confer minimal risk.

The passage of the Dietary Supplement Health and Education Act (DSHEA) in 1994 may be viewed as a victory for the free market, consumer-choice advocates, and for those who viewed FDA action as paternalistic and too restrictive in its information and choices for patients, even if the purported benefits have little or no substantive efficacy data and even if some of the claims about the products are unsubstantiated. To a large degree, the act stripped FDA of almost all of its ability to regulate dietary supplements as well as the dietary supplement industry.

There is persistent confusion about supplements because the DSHEA defines the products that are subject to its provisions so broadly, even though the definition of what constitutes a dietary supplement is critical to potential regulation. There are, in fact, multiple definitions. For example, under section 201(ff)(1) of the act, a dietary supplement is defined as a *food* (not a drug) that contains one of a vitamin, a mineral, an herb, an amino acid, or any dietary substance used to supplement the human diet by increasing total dietary intake of the substance or any metabolite of any of the substances. Also, section 201(ff)(1)(E) of the act contains language so expansive that it theoretically could apply to any substance, so long as its intended use was as a supplement to food.

United States

In the United States, government regulations regarding whether a dietary supplement is effective and safe are so much less strict than those for prescription drugs that there is literally almost no way the 2 sets of regulations can be compared. Although food-and-drug law attorneys, as well as manufacturers of medical products, are under no illusions about the more lenient regulatory framework for dietary supplements, some physicians and many consumers fail to appreciate how severely the DSHEA restricted the power of FDA to regulate the quality of dietary supplements or to intervene when a potential safety issue arises regarding a particular product.

Under the DSHEA, the manufacturer (not FDA) is responsible for determining whether any representations or claims made about its products are substantiated by adequate evidence to show that they are not false or misleading. Dietary supplement marketers can make health claims for so-called natural conditions (eg, hot flashes, age-related memory loss) without providing documentation for efficacy and safety to the government. However, they cannot claim that a product prevents, treats, or cures a disease (eg, prevents heart attacks or osteoporosis, cures depression) unless FDA approves the claim. Because of this prohibition, manufacturers find other ways to convey what their supplements might do. For example, a dietary supplement pill for men will claim to "enhance male potency," whereas sildenafil citrate claims it treats erectile dysfunction.

> A drug that is FDA regulated can claim to "prevent, treat, mitigate, or cure a disease or a medical condition," but a supplement may not. Thus the difference between a claim of "enhancing male potency" with a nonregulated supplement versus "treating erectile dysfunction" with an FDA-approved product.

The DSHEA further states that the manufacturer (not FDA) is responsible for ensuring that labels on packages of dietary supplements are truthful and not misleading, that they contain enough information for consumers to make informed choices, that the serving size ("dose") is appropriate, and that all the dietary ingredients in the product are accurately listed.

Because the normal regulations for new prescription drugs or OTC drugs do not apply to dietary supplements, the normal FDA rules require drug manufacturers to prove that their products work (are effective) and are safe for their intended use. Demonstrating safety is not required before a dietary supplement is approved for sale. Under the DSHEA, dietary supplement manufacturers are responsible for substantiating the safety of the ingredients used in a product. FDA is responsible for taking action against any unsafe dietary supplement product after it reaches the market but can only intervene, if at all, if the degree of risk to public safety is significant or presents an unreasonable risk of illness or injury. FDA accomplishes its responsibilities through monitoring safety literature, dietary supplement AE reports, and product information.

Although a number of manufacturers employ rigorous quality-control measures, many products are not monitored for purity or level of active ingredient, nor in fact do they have to be. As a result, strength and quality can be unpredictable. If a product is suspected of causing harm, FDA can halt sales and have it analyzed.

Botanicals (eg, soy, isoflavones, black cohosh) are classified by FDA as a food, drug, or dietary supplement, depending on the intended use of the product. There are numerous quality-control concerns with some botanicals, including misidentification, "underlabeling" (ie, including prescription drugs in OTC products without listing them), adulteration, substitution, and contamination. In addition, analytic-method standards are lacking for many products, leading to difficulty when attempting to assess product quality. Marketers use different methods to determine the levels of active ingredient in their products.

To address these concerns, FDA established a rule, effective in 2007, for good manufacturing practices for dietary supplements.[1] This rule will help ensure that these products are produced in a quality manner, do not contain contaminants or impurities, and are accurately labeled. Manufacturers are required to evaluate the identity, purity, strength, and composition of their dietary supplements. Manufacturers are required to report all serious AEs to FDA.

In the United States, the designations "USP" (*United States Pharmacopeia*) and "NSF" (National Sanitation Foundation) are generally reliable indicators of good quality control. It is also preferable to choose specific brands that have been used in clinical trials.

Canada

In Canada, the term *natural health product* is used in place of *dietary supplement* as defined by the Natural Health Products Regulations, which came into effect in 2004. Natural health products include vitamins and minerals, probiotics, and other products such as amino acids and essential fatty acids. Also classified as natural health products are herbal products, homeopathic medicines, and complementary and alternative medicines such as traditional Chinese medicine. The Canadian definition of what constitutes a dietary supplement appears to be more expansive than that of FDA's; for example, FDA has not completely addressed the regulation of Chinese medicines.

It is the role of the Natural Health Products Directorate to ensure access to safe, effective, high-quality natural health products. The experience has been similar to that in the United States, with most of the responsibility placed on the government to prove that products are unsafe or ineffective. Canadian regulations require that all natural health products have a product license before they can be sold.

All licensed natural health products in Canada display a product identification number preceded by the prefix "NPN" (or "DIN-HM" for Drug Identification Number for homeopathic medicine), assigned once the product is authorized for sale. All manufacturers, packagers, labelers, and importers are required to obtain site licensing and practice product safety and quality. Standard labeling requirements ensure that customers can make informed choices. The Canadian adverse-reaction reporting system assists in issuing safety advisories to the public.

Canadian consumers are advised to purchase products displaying an NPN or DIN on their labels, which indicate that the products have undergone and passed a review of their formulation, labeling, and instructions for use.

Please see Chapter 6 for more information about complementary and alternative medicine.

Vitamins and minerals

The human body requires more than 45 vitamins and minerals to maintain health. Healthcare professionals prefer that women have a balanced diet rich in fruits and vegetables. However, the daily diet may not contain all the nutrients required for optimal health. Therefore, some women may benefit from a daily multivitamin and mineral supplement. However, the US Preventive Services Task Force (USPSTF) has stated that there is a lack of evidence that multivitamins or single-nutrient supplements prevent cancer or cardiovascular disease (CVD).[2] Furthermore, β-carotene and vitamin E each may carry more risk than benefit with regards to cancer and CVD.

Many studies have evaluated the diet as a whole using analytic methods such as dietary patterns. A 2009 study found that increased Mediterranean diet patterns (hazard ratio [HR], 0.63; 95% confidence interval [CI], 0.53-0.72) and high-quality diet patterns (HR, 0.63; 95% CI, 0.45-0.81) were each associated with a significantly lower risk of coronary heart disease (CHD).[3] Conversely, an increased consumption of trans fatty acids (relative risk [RR], 1.32; 95% CI, 1.16-1.48) and foods with a high glycemic index (RR, 1.32; 95% CI, 1.10-1.54) were associated with a significantly higher risk of diabetes mellitus (DM) and CHD.

Foods versus supplements

As stated in the *Dietary Guidelines for Americans, 2010*, nutrient needs should be met primarily through consuming foods or nutrient-fortified foods. Dietary supplements, although recommended in some cases, cannot replace a healthful diet. A balanced diet low in saturated fat and high in whole grains, fruits, and vegetables, with adequate water, vitamins, and minerals, contributes to good health.

Two eating patterns that embody the 2010 *Dietary Guidelines for Americans* are the US Department of Agriculture's Healthy Eating Index-2010 and the DASH (Dietary Approaches to Stop Hypertension) Eating Plan.[4,5] The DASH diet promotes intake of vegetables and fruits as well as low-fat dairy products, whole grains, chicken, fish, and nuts. Intake of fat, meat, sweets, and sodas should be minimized. The DASH diet provides more calcium, potassium, magnesium, and dietary fiber and less total fat, saturated fats, cholesterol, and sodium than the typical Western diet.[6] Adherence to the DASH diet is associated with reduced rates of DM, CHD, colorectal adenoma, and colorectal cancer.[7-11] A 2013 meta-analysis concluded that consumption of a DASH-like diet had a significant reverse linear association between the diet and CVD, CHD, stroke, and heart failure risk.[12]

Although diet patterns as a whole have been evaluated, there have been several studies that have identified food groups in relation to risk of disease. In the Nurses' Health Study, absolute quantity in fruit and vegetable intake was associated with a significantly lower risk of CHD, although the variety of fruit and vegetables did not appear to matter.[13] A 2013 Cochrane review also concluded that increasing fruit and vegetable intake can improve CVD risk factors, although more trials are needed to confirm this.[14] Greater fruit and vegetable intake lowered the risk of pancreatic cancer,[15] and greater consumption of fruits and vegetables lowered the risk of invasive bladder cancer among women.[16]

Daily recommended dietary intakes

Since 1994, the National Academy of Sciences in the United States and Health Canada have collaborated in the revision of the dietary reference standards known as Dietary Reference Intakes (DRIs). This provides a set of 4 nutrient-based reference values designed to replace the Recommended Dietary Allowances in the United States and the Recommended Nutrient Intakes in Canada. The DRIs include recommended intakes for individual persons, estimated average requirements, adequate intakes, and tolerable upper intake levels (Table 1).[17,18]

Several studies have examined the effect of antioxidant intake on disease. A 2013 review of randomized, controlled trials (RCTs) found that antioxidant vitamin supplementation had no effect on the incidence of major cardiovascular events, myocardial infarction (MI), stroke, total death, and cardiac death.[19] The relationship between dietary intake of supplemental antioxidant nutrients (including vitamins C and E and selenium, as well as carotenoids and vitamin A) and ovarian cancer was evaluated in 133,614 postmenopausal women enrolled in the Women's Health Initiative study.[20] Intake of dietary antioxidants, carotenoids, and vitamin A were not associated with a reduction in ovarian cancer risk.

A 2013 meta-analysis found that dietary intake of vitamin C and β-carotene, but not vitamins A and E, could

CHAPTER 7

Table 1. Recommended Daily Dietary Intakes for Women Aged 51-70 Years

Vitamins	
Vitamin A	700 µg
Vitamin B₁ (thiamin)	1.1 mg
Vitamin B₂ (riboflavin)	1.1 mg
Vitamin B₃ (niacin)	14 mg
Vitamin B₆ (pyridoxine)	1.5 mg
Vitamin B₉ (folate)	400 µg
Vitamin B₁₂ (cyanocobalamine)	2.4 µg
Vitamin C	
Nonsmokers	75 mg
Smokers	110 mg
Vitamin D	15 µg
Vitamin E (α-tocopherol)	15 mg
Minerals	
Calcium	1,200 mg
Magnesium	320 mg
Phosphorus	700 mg

National Academy of Sciences,[17] NAMS.[18]

reduce the risk of colorectal adenoma.[21] Again, the focus was on dietary and not supplemental intakes. A 2012 review of literature found that there was no evidence from clinical trials that supplementation with antioxidant vitamins (β-carotene, vitamin C, or vitamin E) prevents or slows the progression of age-related cataract.[22] The conclusion from a 2013 review of 26 studies showed no clear-cut evidence between vitamin supplementation and breast cancer prevention.[23]

The association between antioxidant vitamin intakes and cervical cancer risk was calculated for 144 cervical cancer cases and 288 age-matched, hospital-based controls.[24] Total intakes of vitamins A, C, and E were strongly and inversely associated with cervical cancer risk. This supports a role for increased dietary intake of antioxidant vitamins in decreasing the risk of cervical cancer. However, these associations need to be assessed in large prospective studies with long-term follow-up.

The relationships between intakes of selected dietary nutrients and food groups and risk of cervical cancer were evaluated in a hospital-based, case-control study including 239 cases diagnosed with squamous cell carcinoma of the cervix and 979 hospital patients with nonneoplastic diagnoses. Significant risk reductions of approximately 40% to 60% were observed in women in the highest versus lowest tertiles of dietary fiber and several antioxidants. A greater total fruit and vegetable intake significantly reduced the risk of cervical cancer (odds ratio [OR], 0.52; 95% CI, 0.34-0.77). This suggests that a diet rich in plant-based nutrients may be important in reducing the risk of cervical cancer.[25]

In a cross-sectional study using the National Health and Nutrition Examination Survey, nutrient intake was studied in relation to prevalent peripheral artery disease (PAD) in the US population.[26] Higher consumption of specific nutrients, including antioxidants (vitamins A, C, and E), vitamin B₆, fiber, folate, and omega-3 fatty acids may have a significant protective effect, irrespective of traditional CVD risk factors. These findings suggest but are not definitive that specific dietary supplementation may afford additional protection, above traditional risk factor modification, for the prevention of PAD.

In a review of 50 RCTs with 294,478 participants, supplementation with vitamins and antioxidants was not associated with reductions in the risk of major cardiovascular events.[27] There is little evidence to support the use of vitamin and antioxidant supplements for prevention of CVD, breast cancer, cataracts, or mortality, and there is a potential for harm at high intakes of these nutrients. There are several studies that indicate that isolated nutrients are not associated with reduced risk of cancer. Perhaps fruits and vegetables are protective against cancer because of interrelationships among nutrients only evident in an evaluation of complete dietary intake or because of other unknown constituents of these foods or because people who follow these dietary patterns have a healthier lifestyle in general. Therefore, the best advice to patients would be to make efforts to get these nutrients from dietary sources as part of an overall healthy diet pattern following the guidelines of the DASH diet and *Dietary Guidelines for Americans*.

Vitamins

Vitamins are any of various organic substances essential in small quantities to the nutrition of most animals and some plants. They act especially as coenzymes and precursors of coenzymes in the regulation of metabolic processes but do not provide energy or serve as building units. They are present in natural foodstuffs or, sometimes, are produced within the body.

Vitamin A. Vitamin A is necessary for the health of skin, vision, bone growth, and immune function. Vitamin A deficiency is associated with significant eye problems, including night blindness and conjunctival dryness. Two common types of vitamin A are retinol and β-carotene, which is a precursor to vitamin A.

The daily DRI of vitamin A for women aged 51 to 70 years is 700 µg (2,330 IU). The recommended intake may be increased in malabsorption syndromes associated with pancreatic insufficiency or in any condition in which fat malabsorption occurs, including diets that drastically restrict fat-containing foods. Absorption requires the presence of bile salts, pancreatic lipase, protein, and dietary fat. Requirements for vitamin A may also be increased in those receiving cholestyramine, colestipol, mineral oil, and neomycin.

Food sources include liver, eggs, sweet potato, pumpkin, carrots, spinach, collards, kale, turnip greens, egg yolk, milk, cheese, and butter.

As a fat-soluble vitamin, oversupplementation can cause buildup, with potential for toxic effects. Prolonged high doses may cause bleeding from the gums, dry or sore mouth, or drying, cracking, or peeling of the lips. Excessive intake (>10,000 IU/d) may stimulate bone loss, counteract the effects of calcium supplements, and can cause hypercalcemia, hair loss, and hepatotoxicity. The tolerable upper limit for vitamin A is 3,000 μg per day, and intakes above this should not be advised.

Studies in postmenopausal women have shown that too much vitamin A intake from retinol seems to increase the risk of hip fracture. Scientists believe that excessive amounts of vitamin A trigger an increase in osteoclasts, which break down bone. It may also interfere with absorption of vitamin D, which helps preserve bone. In general, vegetable sources of vitamin A (carotenoids) may be preferred for skeletal health and perhaps cancer prevention. There are limited data to support vitamin A supplementation for disease prevention. A 2014 report by the USPSTF concluded that vitamin A and β-carotene do not decrease the risk of CVD or cancer and that β-carotene actually has been shown to increase the risk of lung cancer in persons who smoke or have other high risks for lung cancer.[2]

Retinol is a form of vitamin A that is commonly used to treat acne, psoriasis, and other skin conditions. These synthetic products have the same negative effect on bone health. Their use has been linked to delayed bone growth in teens. Beta-carotene has not been linked to AEs on bone.

B vitamins. Vitamins B_1 (thiamin), B_2 (riboflavin), B_3 (niacin), B_5 (pantothenic acid), B_6 (pyridoxine), B_9 (folic acid), and B_{12} (cyanocobalamine) are water-soluble vitamins. Supplements are available either in combination or individually.

Simple nutritional deficiency of any one of the B vitamins is rare, inasmuch as inadequate nutritional intake usually results in multiple deficiencies. Supplementation may be necessary in the case of malnutrition because of inadequate dietary intake or in patients undergoing rapid weight loss. B vitamins may be supplemented after bariatric surgery. Older persons may also be at greater risk for deficiency of B vitamins.

Vitamin B_1 (thiamin). Vitamin B_1 is a coenzyme in the metabolism of carbohydrates and branched-chain amino acids. Food sources include whole-grain products, fortified cereals, legumes, pork, beef, yeast, and fresh vegetables. The DRI of thiamin for women aged 51 to 70 years is 1.1 mg. Increased doses may be needed with hemodialysis and in persons with malabsorption syndromes. There is no known toxicity.

Vitamin B_2 (riboflavin). Vitamin B_2 is a coenzyme in numerous reactions that are necessary for normal tissue respiration. It is also needed for activation of pyridoxine and for conversion of tryptophan to niacin. Absorption may be decreased when probenecid is used. Food sources are organ meats, milk, whole-grain breads, and fortified cereals. The DRI of riboflavin for women aged 51 to 70 years is 1.1 mg. Excess riboflavin can cause the urine to turn bright yellow. There is no known toxicity.

Vitamin B_3 (niacin, niacinamide). Niacin, after conversion to niacinamide, is a component of coenzymes necessary for tissue respiration, glycogenolysis, and lipid, amino acid, protein, and purine metabolism. Niacin (but not niacinamide) is used in the treatment of hyperlipidemia. It improves all major lipid parameters, reducing low-density lipoprotein cholesterol (LDL-C) and triglycerides and increasing high-density lipoprotein cholesterol (HDL-C). In a meta-analysis of 5 trials involving 432 patients, the difference in LDL-C and triglyceride reduction in women was greater than in men at all doses.[28] Food sources of vitamin B_3 (niacin) include meat, fish, poultry, enriched and whole-grain breads, and fortified cereals. The DRI of niacin for women aged 51 to 70 years is 14 mg.

Adverse events of excessive niacin intake include flushing, itching, and gastrointestinal (GI) discomfort. These are more commonly experienced when therapeutic rather than nutritional doses are taken, especially when beginning therapy. Niacin should be taken with the evening meal. Flushing may be minimized by taking aspirin 1 hour earlier, by increasing the niacin dose gradually, or by using the extended-release form.

Vitamin B_6 (pyridoxine). Vitamin B_6 acts as a coenzyme for various metabolic functions affecting protein, carbohydrate, and lipid use. It is involved in the conversion of tryptophan to niacin or serotonin and of glycogen to glucose, in the synthesis of γ-aminobutyric acid within the central nervous system, and in red blood cell (RBC) synthesis.

Food sources of pyridoxine are whole grains, fortified cereals, and organ meats. Pyridoxine supplements have been used to treat a variety of conditions (eg, premenstrual syndrome, depression, carpal tunnel syndrome, and diabetic neuropathy), with varied results. The DRI of pyridoxine for women aged 51 to 70 years is 1.5 mg. Recommended intakes may be increased if a woman is taking cycloserine, hydralazine, immunosuppressants, isoniazid, or estrogen-containing contraceptives. Increased intake is typically not required with standard doses of menopausal hormone therapy. Although it is generally nontoxic, high doses of pyridoxine (2-6 g/d) taken for several months have caused severe sensory neuropathy with residual weakness.

Vitamin B₉ (folate, folic acid). Vitamin B₉ is converted in the liver and plasma into its metabolically active form, tetrafolic acid, in the presence of ascorbic acid. This vitamin is necessary for normal erythropoiesis, synthesis, and metabolism of various amino acids and for other metabolic processes. Deficiency may produce megaloblastic and macrocytic anemias. Folate is a water-soluble B vitamin that plays a critical role in DNA synthesis, methylation, and repair. Imbalance in these functions may contribute to carcinogenesis, and data suggest that higher folate intake may be associated with decreased cancer risk.

Folate occurs naturally in food; dietary sources include dark green leafy vegetables, whole-grain breads, and fortified cereals. Folic acid is the synthetic form of folate that is found in supplements and added to fortified foods. Folic acid is almost completely absorbed, primarily in the upper duodenum, but absorption is impaired in malabsorption syndromes. Folic acid supplements are routinely recommended preconception and during pregnancy because this nutrient reduces the incidence of neural tube defects in the newborn.

The DRI of vitamin B₉ in women aged 51 to 70 years is 400 μg. Requirements may be increased in those receiving estrogen-containing contraceptives. No AEs other than allergic reactions have been reported with folic acid administration, even at doses up to 10 times the DRI for a month. Higher doses than the DRI are generally not recommended until the diagnosis of pernicious anemia has been ruled out, because higher doses correct the hematologic manifestations of pernicious anemia while allowing neurologic damage to progress irreversibly.

Vitamin B₁₂ (cyanocobalamin). Vitamin B₁₂ acts as a coenzyme for various metabolic functions. It is necessary for growth, hematopoiesis, and myelin synthesis. Dietary B₁₂ is released from the proteins to which it is bound by gastric acid and pancreatic proteases, then bound to intrinsic factor and absorbed from the lower half of the ileum. Food sources are fish, seafood, egg yolk, milk, and fermented cheeses. Bacteria found on vegetables may be a source of B₁₂ for vegans. Ordinary cooking temperatures will not cause loss of B₁₂ from foods, but severe heating should be avoided to maintain B₁₂ levels.

Deficiency may lead to macrocytic and megaloblastic anemias and possible irreversible neurologic damage (with pernicious anemia caused by either lack of or inhibition of intrinsic factor). Deficiency may be the result of inadequate nutrition or intestinal malabsorption. It can occur in vegans, because vitamin B₁₂ is found in animal protein and not in vegetables. Additional causes of deficiency are alcoholism, gastritis with achlorhydria, lack of intrinsic factor, and gastrectomy.

The oral route is useful for treating nutritional B₁₂ deficiency when absorption is normal, but it is not useful in small-bowel disease, in malabsorption syndromes, or after total gastrectomy or ileal resection. For treating deficiency resulting from lack of absorption, vitamin B₁₂ is given by injection (either intramuscularly or deep subcutaneously). It is also available in a sublingual dosage form. Vitamin B₁₂ plasma concentration determination is recommended before treatment of deficiency and between the fifth and seventh day of therapy.

The DRI of B₁₂ in women aged 51 to 70 years is 2.4 μg. Recommended intakes may need to be increased by those taking medications, most notably prolonged use of metformin and proton pump inhibitors. Patients aged older than 50 years and strict vegetarians should consume foods fortified with vitamin B₁₂ and vitamin B₁₂ supplements rather than attempting to get vitamin B₁₂ strictly from dietary sources.[29] Toxicity is not a problem, although hypokalemia is possible during the first 48 hours of treatment for megaloblastic anemia. B₁₂ administration may mask folic acid deficiency.

Selected studies relating B vitamins to women's health. There have been several studies that evaluated the role of B vitamins in women's health. The association between risk of colorectal cancer and vitamin B₆ intake, also assessed as blood levels of pyridoxal-5-phosphate (the active form of vitamin B₆), was evaluated in a meta-analysis of 13 studies.[30] Vitamin B₆ intake and blood pyridoxal-5-phosphate levels were inversely associated with the risk of colorectal cancer.

Dietary folate intake and pancreatic cancer were studied in the Prostate, Lung, Colorectal, and Ovarian Cancer Screening Trial cohort.[31] The highest quartile was associated with a significantly decreased pancreatic cancer risk among women (HR, 0.47; 95% CI, 0.23-0.94) compared with the lowest quartile of food folate.

The role of B vitamins in relation to cancer was evaluated in a large cohort study, with more than 16 years of follow-up, of 89,835 Canadian women aged 40 to 59 years. This large study provided little support for an association of dietary intake of thiamin, riboflavin, niacin, folate, or methionine with 5 major cancers (breast, endometrial, ovarian, colorectal, and lung) in women.[32]

In a 2-year clinical trial, higher doses of folic acid, pyridoxine, and cobalamine did not reduce the risk of cardiac events in 3,680 patients who had nondisabling cerebral infarction.[33]

Participants in the Women's Antioxidant and Folic Acid Cardiovascular Study, a randomized, double-blind, placebo-controlled trial of 5,442 women health professionals aged older than 40 years with a history of CVD or 3 or more risk factors for CVD, received a combination pill containing folic acid, vitamin B₆, and vitamin B₁₂ or a matching placebo.[34] After 7.3 years of treatment, the combination pill did not reduce a combined endpoint of total cardiovascular events among high-risk women, even though there was a significant reduction in homocysteine levels. Furthermore, an updated Cochrane review concluded that there was no evidence to suggest that homocysteine-lowering interventions in the form of supplements of vitamins B_6, B_9, or B_{12} given alone or in combination should be used for preventing cardiovascular events.[35]

Homocysteinemia may play an etiologic role in the pathogenesis of type 2 DM by promoting oxidative stress, systemic inflammation, and endothelial dysfunction. Lowering homocysteine levels by daily supplementation with folic acid and vitamins B_6 and B_{12} did not reduce the risk of developing type 2 DM among women at high risk for CVD.[36] In a meta-analysis of 5 clinical trials evaluating extended-release niacin for women with dyslipidemia, improvements were noted in terms of lower LDL-C and triglycerides.[28]

Homocysteine has been linked to fragility fractures, including hip fractures in older men and women.[37,38] Clearly, a need exists for long-term clinical trial data to determine the role of each B vitamin in skeletal health, and several clinical trials are ongoing to evaluate this.

In a meta-analysis of 14 trials evaluating B vitamins (B_6, B_{12}, and folic acid) and cognition, it was concluded that there was no evidence that any of these vitamins alone or in combination provided any benefit against cognitive decline in people with normal or impaired cognitive function.[39]

Vitamin C. Ascorbic acid, a water-soluble vitamin, is needed for collagen formation and tissue repair, as well as for metabolism of folic acid, iron, phenylalanine, tyrosine, norepinephrine, and histamine; use of carbohydrates; synthesis of lipids and proteins; immune function; hydroxylation of serotonin; and preservation of blood vessel integrity. Ascorbic acid enhances absorption of nonheme iron. It is absorbed from the jejunum.

Dietary sources include citrus fruits, green vegetables (peppers, broccoli, cabbage), tomatoes, and potatoes. Vitamin C supplements gradually lose potency with storage, and in foods, vitamin C is rapidly destroyed by exposure to air, by drying or salting, and by up to 50% through ordinary cooking.

The DRI of vitamin C for women aged 51 to 70 years is 75 mg. Requirements may be increased in acquired immunodeficiency syndrome, gastrectomy, ileal resection, surgery, and tuberculosis and in heavy smokers.

A severe deficiency in vitamin C can cause scurvy, a disease that results in extreme weakness, lethargy, easy bruising, and bleeding.

Toxicity can occur in patients with a history of oxalate-containing renal stones. High-dose ascorbic acid (but not sodium ascorbate) may decrease urine pH, causing renal tubular reabsorption of oxalate, with the possibility of precipitation of oxalate stones in the urinary tract. High doses may cause diarrhea. Withdrawal scurvy may occur after prolonged administration of 2 g to 3 g per day.

Most prospective studies showed no association between vitamin C and breast cancer risk; however, an inverse association was reported in a meta-analysis of 12 case-control studies.[40] In a population-based prospective cohort study, women aged 40 to 75 years at baseline were followed for 12 years, with a strong inverse association between plasma vitamin C level and a 62% reduction in DM risk.[41]

Vitamin C is important to overall health; dietary sources such as fruits and vegetables should be promoted to reach the DRI. The role of vitamin C in chronic diseases requires further study.

Vitamin D. Vitamin D is a sterol-like compound synthesized in nature by interaction between 7-dehydrocholesterol and ultraviolet light that, by a photochemical reaction, opens up the B ring of the steroid nucleus. Typically, this synthesis takes place in the skin of many animals, including humans. This compound—also called vitamin D_3 or cholecalciferol—is biologically inactive.

After cutaneous synthesis, cholecalciferol is absorbed into the bloodstream, where it is transported to the liver and rapidly hydroxylated at the 25 position to produce 25-hydroxycholecalciferol or 25-hydroxyvitamin D (25[OH]D), commonly considered to be inactive as well, although this issue is not completely resolved. The 25(OH)D is measurable in serum, and as such it serves as the functional indicator for vitamin D status and probably also as an important storage form of the vitamin in the body.[42]

The final step in the activation of the molecule is further hydroxylation at the 1 position of the A-ring to produce 1,25-dihydroxycholecalciferol, or calcitriol. Calcitriol is one of the most potent biologic molecules known, working at submicrogram levels. It has been recognized for some years that the calcitriol circulating in the blood is normally synthesized in the kidney in response to fibroblast growth factor 23, parathyroid hormone, and hypophosphatemia. Secreted calcitriol goes to the intestinal mucosa, where it induces the synthesis of the calcium transport apparatus in the mucosal cell, which mediates the active absorption of calcium from food into the bloodstream.

Another form of vitamin D is a similar compound, ergocalciferol, or vitamin D_2, which in experimental animals has an ability to prevent rickets in a way roughly similar to that of cholecalciferol. Ergocalciferol is produced synthetically by irradiation of a product of ergot mold.

Both forms of vitamin D (D_2 and D_3) are measured in international units (IU), with 1 μg of cholecalciferol being equivalent to 40 IU. These forms had been considered to be equipotent, but it is clear that vitamin D_3 is substantially more potent than vitamin D_2 by a factor of at least 4.[43]

Vitamin D is essential for the efficient intestinal absorption of calcium and thus for bone health. In women with a severe vitamin D deficiency, gross absorption of dietary calcium is no more than 10%, and net absorption may be zero or even negative. Calcium absorption, bone mineral density (BMD), and other bone health benefits plateau at a 25(OH)D level of 50 nmol/L (20 ng/mL).[44,45] However, some studies suggest that calcium absorption efficiency varies inversely with serum 25(OH)D up to levels of about 80 nmol/L (32 ng/mL), above which further increases in vitamin D status produce no further improvement in absorption efficiency.[46]

Similarly, in a population-based study of the National Health and Nutrition Examination Survey III data, BMD and lower-extremity neuromuscular function improved as vitamin D status improved up to levels above 80 nmol/L (32 ng/mL).[47,48] Such a small fraction of the population has values above 80 nmol/mL that it is not clear from the available data whether a plateau is reached; it is possible that even higher values for serum 25(OH)D may be needed to optimize bone and neuromuscular health.

Studies have found that vitamin D (≥600 IU/d for ages 1-70 y and 800 IU/d for ages older than 70 y) with supplemental calcium can reduce the rate of postmenopausal bone loss, especially in older women.[44] Results from the Women's Health Initiative found that participants taking calcium (1,000 mg/d) plus vitamin D (400 IU/d) had a small but significant 1% improvement in hip BMD.[49] Vitamin D supplementation also has been found to improve muscle strength and balance and to reduce the risk of falling.[50] Meta-analyses of RCTs in postmenopausal women (mean age, 71-85 y) show that vitamin D doses of 700 IU to 800 IU per day were associated with significant reductions in the risk of hip and nonvertebral fractures. No significant changes were found in outcomes for either of those fracture sites in trials that used less than 700 IU per day.[51]

It has become clear that the hydroxylation at the 1 position of the A-ring step occurs not solely in the kidney but in many other tissues as well and that the calcitriol synthesized in most of those tissues serves an autocrine function (ie, it acts and is degraded locally in the cells and tissues concerned).[52] It links extracellular stimuli to tissue-specific transcription of the genetic code for the synthesis for a variety of protein products. In the intestinal mucosa, one of the products concerned is a calcium transport protein, but in many other tissues where calcitriol binding occurs, the proteins concerned are related primarily to cell differentiation, cell proliferation, cell apoptosis, cell adhesion, and various aspects of the immune response.

In the past, most clinicians did not assess vitamin D nutritional status, which can be evaluated by measuring serum 25(OH)D. Some uncertainty remains with respect to the level of serum 25(OH)D that signifies the bottom end of the healthy range, but it is clear that earlier laboratory reference ranges are not coextensive with the healthy range. Some experts believe that the bottom end of that healthy range is at least as high as 75 nmol/L to 80 nmol/L (30-32 ng/mL), and some of the cancer and autoimmune studies suggest that the bottom end of the healthy range may be as high as 100 nmol/L to 125 nmol/L (40-50 ng/mL). However, many experts believe that there is a threshold at approximately 20 ng/mL (50 nmol/L), with minimal additional benefit above this level.[44,53] Measurement of calcitriol levels is not usually helpful for diagnostic purposes because calcitriol has a short half-life in the blood, and its level reflects effective calcium intake status rather than vitamin D status. Calcitriol will normally be high on a low calcium intake and normally low on a high calcium intake.

In 2011, the Institute of Medicine (IOM) set the tolerable upper intake level of vitamin D at 4,000 IU per day, which correlates with 25(OH)D levels of 125 nmol/L (50 ng/mL).[44] It is difficult to establish a true oral intake requirement, because much of the vitamin D that people use every day probably comes by way of cutaneous synthesis within their own bodies. This source varies by degree of skin exposure to the sun, the time of day at which such exposure occurs, the latitude at which one lives, the age of the person concerned, and skin pigmentation. Thus, dark-skinned city dwellers at mid-latitudes and above are at a disadvantage. In all studies published to date, those people have values for serum 25(OH)D substantially lower than those of light-skinned persons, and as a group are more commonly vitamin D deficient.

The IOM did not recommend increasing sun exposure to achieve adequate 25(OH)D levels and based the dietary guidelines on an assumption of minimal to no sun exposure. For the typical white person living in the Northeast United States, sunlight exposure of 5 to 15 minutes on the arms and legs between the hours of 10 AM and 3 PM 2 to 3 times a week has been proposed by some. Women with dark skin may require as much as 5 to 10 times longer skin exposure, because their darker skin pigment markedly reduces vitamin D production from sunlight. Moreover, solar radiation is classified as a carcinogen, so the recommendation to increase sun exposure to raise vitamin D levels is controversial and was not endorsed by the IOM. Wearing a sunscreen with a sun protection factor of 8 or more blocks the skin's ability to produce vitamin D by 95%.

The IOM's recommended dietary allowances of 600 IU per day of vitamin D for adults aged up to 70 years and 800 IU per day for those aged older than 70 years are public health guidelines for a generally healthy population (Table 2), and the IOM acknowledged that some people may have greater requirements.[45] The National Osteoporosis Foundation and the North American Menopause Society (NAMS) recommend 800 IU to 1,000 IU per day of vitamin D_3 for women aged 50 years and older.[18,54] Although doses as high as 10,000 IU per day are considered safe, long-term studies of safety at these high doses are lacking.

NONPRESCRIPTION OPTIONS

Table 2. Institute of Medicine Committee to Review Dietary Reference Intakes for Vitamin D and Calcium Recommended Dietary Allowances, by Life Stage

Life-stage group, age and sex	Vitamin D RDA, IU/d[a]	Vitamin D Serum 25(OH)D, ng/mL[b]	Vitamin D UL, IU/d[c]	Calcium RDA, mg/d[a]	Calcium UL, mg/d[c]
1-3 y M+F	600	20	2,500	700	2,500
4-8 y M+F	600	20	3,000	1,000	2,500
9-13 y M+F	600	20	4,000	1,300	3,000
14-18 y M+F	600	20	4,000	1,300	3,000
19-30 y M+F	600	20	4,000	1,000	2,500
31-50 y M+F	600	20	4,000	1,000	2,500
51-70 y M	600	20	4,000	1,000	2,000
51-70 y F	600	20	4,000	1,200	2,000
71+ y M+F	800	20	4,000	1,200	2,000
Pregnant or lactating F					
14-18 y	600	20	4,000	1,300	3,000
19-50 y	600	20	4,000	1,000	2,500
Infants					
0-6 mo M+F	400[d]	20	1,000	200[d]	1,000
6-12 mo M+F	400[d]	20	1,500	260[d]	1,500

Abbreviations: F, female; IU, international unit; M, male; RDA, recommended dietary allowance; UL, tolerable upper intake level above which there is risk of adverse events.
a. Intake that covers needs of ≥97.5% of population.
b. Levels corresponding to the RDA and covering the requirements of ≥97.5% of the population.
c. Not intended as a target intake (no consistent evidence of greater benefit at intake levels above the RDA).
d. Reflects adequate intake reference value rather than RDA, which has not been established for infants.
Adapted from Ross AC, et al.[45]

Currently, *Canada's Food Guide* agrees with the IOM's recommended dietary allowances of vitamin D for its citizens. It also recommends that all Canadians aged older than 2 years, including pregnant and lactating women, consume 500 mL (2 cups) of vitamin D-fortified milk or soy beverages every day.[55] Health Canada recommends that, in addition to following *Canada's Food Guide*, everyone aged older than 50 years should take a daily vitamin D supplement of 400 IU.

The actual requirement for additional oral intake will vary from person to person, although it will be similar within various age and ethnic groups. Although the optimal range for 25(OH)D levels continues to be debated, some experts recommend doses of vitamin D to ensure maintenance of a serum 25(OH)D level of 80 nmol (32 ng/mL) or higher. As a rough guide, the serum 25(OH)D level, under steady-state dosing, will rise by about 1 nmol/L per μg cholecalciferol per day. Thus, a person with a serum 25(OH)D value of 50 nmol/L (20 ng/mL) may need at least 30 μg of additional vitamin D$_3$ per day (1,200 IU) to reach a level of 80 nmol/L (32 ng/mL)—or, to use the units commonly reported in the United States, serum 25(OH)D will rise by about 1 ng/mL for every 100 IU per day of additional cholecalciferol.

Studies have shown that more than 60% of people—whether institutionalized or free living, using common vitamin D supplements or not—have serum 25(OH)D values less than 80 nmol/L (32 ng/mL).[56,57] Vitamin D insufficiency is highly prevalent among people aged older than 90 years.[58]

The IOM sets the current tolerable upper limit at 4,000 IU per day.[44] A 2007 study found no concerns at regular intakes below 40,000 IU per day, concluding that 10,000 IU per day is safe for essentially the entire adult population.[59] However, studies of the long-term safety of such high doses are lacking, and there are no reasons to use as much as 10,000 IU per day on a regular basis.

A major source of vitamin D is cutaneous synthesis. Curiously, although low latitudes are associated with a greater ultraviolet B irradiance, the prevalence of vitamin D insufficiency is no different in the southern tier of US states than in the northern, most likely because there is more sun avoidance in southern states.

A few food sources of vitamin D are available—primarily oily fish (eg, salmon). But only wild-caught fish, deriving their vitamin D from ingested phytoplankton, are good sources; farm-raised fish have far less vitamin D. Fish liver oil has long been the classic source of vitamin D, and years ago cod and halibut liver oils were used as mainstays in the prevention of rickets in children. Some mushrooms contain vitamin D. (Further information on vitamin D content in mushrooms and other foods can be found on the US Department of Agriculture Web site, http://ndb.nal.usda.gov/ndb/search/list.) For decades, milk has been fortified with a small amount of vitamin D (100 IU/8-oz serving), and some orange juices have been fortified to the same level. Small amounts of vitamin D have been added to certain ready-to-eat cereals. Other fortified foods are likely to be marketed soon.

Women aged older than 70 years who have little or no sun exposure and rely on diet alone for vitamin D intake are likely to have suboptimal 25(OH)D levels. Current daily requirements can usually be met with an oral multivitamin supplement (typically containing 400 IU vitamin D) plus dietary intake of fortified foods. Because vitamin D must be metabolized before it is biologically active, taking vitamin D at the same time as a calcium supplement is not necessary. However, many calcium supplements contain vitamin D, providing the convenience of obtaining both nutrients in a single-dose form.

The principal high-potency form of the vitamin available to clinicians was once 50,000 IU of vitamin D_2 as an oral prescription product. Now there are several OTC products containing 1,000 IU to 50,000 IU vitamin D_3 per dose, allowing consumers to obtain the vitamin D they need without a prescription.

With fortified foods and with supplements, reading labels is important. When vitamins D_2 and D_3 were thought to be equally potent, manufacturers were free to use either form of the vitamin in their products. Now consumers with vitamin D deficiency should generally seek out products with D_3.

Vitamin E. This fat-soluble vitamin, α-tocopherol, acts in conjunction with selenium as an antioxidant, protecting polyunsaturated fatty acids in various cell structures and protecting RBCs from hemolysis. Deficiency of this vitamin is rare.

Food sources include nuts, seeds, whole grains, vegetable oil, and wheat germ. The DRI of vitamin E for women aged 51 to 70 years is 15 mg (22.5 IU). High dietary intake of polyunsaturated fatty acids may increase this requirement. The National Institutes of Health recommends basing the DRI on the α-tocopherol form of vitamin E because it is the most active, usable form. The expression of vitamin E activity has been changed from IU to α-tocopherol equivalents, with 1.5 IU equal to 1 mg α-tocopherol equivalent.

Among healthy adults, no acute AEs have been noted with vitamin E use at doses of up to 1,500 IU per day, thus this is the tolerable upper limit for intake of vitamin E (1,500 IU or 1,000 mg per day). However, the Physicians' Health Study suggested an increased risk of hemorrhagic stroke at doses of 400 IU on alternate days.[60] Moreover, a meta-analysis of 19 trials among patients with chronic diseases found a significant deleterious relationship between high-dosage (defined as ≥400 IU/d) vitamin E and all-cause mortality, although the trials were often small.[61] A 2014 USPSTF statement has recommended against the use of vitamin E for cancer or CVD prevention.[2]

The digestive tract requires fat to absorb vitamin E, thus people with malabsorption syndromes are more likely to become deficient. People with Crohn disease or cystic fibrosis often have chronic diarrhea and may need to supplement their diet with vitamin E.

General guidelines caution that vitamin E doses higher than 400 IU per day are to be avoided in people taking warfarin and related anticoagulants because of its interference with platelet function, which can have an additive effect, decreasing blood clotting.

The Heart Outcomes Prevention Evaluation (HOPE) study examined vitamin E supplementation and cardiovascular events in high-risk patients.[62,63] This was based on the belief that oxidation of the LDL-C molecule is important in the development and progression of atherosclerosis; thus, antioxidants might be useful in the treatment of CVD. This double-blind study of secondary prevention followed more than 4,000 patients in each of the vitamin E and placebo groups for 4.5 years. Patients were aged 55 years or older and were at high risk for cardiovascular events from either CVD or DM. The study compared vitamin E 400 IU per day or placebo with either an angiotensin-converting enzyme inhibitor or placebo. The study demonstrated that vitamin E had no apparent benefit in patients at high risk for cardiac events.

Precautions when using over-the-counter anticoagulant therapies

- Use is contraindicated in patients with active bleeding (eg, abnormal uterine bleeding, peptic ulcer, intracranial bleeding) or a history of bleeding (hemostatic disorders), with drug-related hemostatic problems, and in those taking prescription anticoagulant medications (eg, warfarin or antiplatelet agents such as ticlopidine, clopidogrel, dipyridamole).
- Caution is advised when using more than one over-the-counter anticoagulant therapy, including aspirin (including low-dose aspirin for cardiovascular benefit), aspirin-containing products, nonsteroidal anti-inflammatory drugs, vitamin E, fish oil, dong quai, evening primrose oil, feverfew, garlic, ginger, and Ginkgo biloba).
- Use should be discontinued 7 to 10 days before dental or surgical procedures; use can usually be resumed after discharge.

In the HOPE extension trial, effects of long-term vitamin E supplementation on cardiovascular events and cancer were examined.[63] Study patients were aged 55 years and older and had a history of coronary artery disease or PAD, stroke, or DM, plus 1 other CVD risk factor. Patients were randomized to receive either 400 IU per day vitamin E or placebo. Median follow-up was 7 years. Results demonstrated no significant difference in the primary outcomes of MI, stroke, or cardiovascular death. Vitamin E had no effect on occurrence of cancer.

The Women's Health Study evaluated vitamin E taken long term in the primary prevention of CVD and cancer. The study randomized 39,876 women (aged >45 y) to receive 600 IU of natural-source vitamin E or placebo on alternate days, with a follow-up of 10 years.[64] Women with either factor V Leiden or the prothrombin mutation had a 49% hazard reduction in venous thrombosis associated with vitamin E treatment (relative hazard, 0.51; 95% CI, 0.30-0.87; P for trend=.014). Results demonstrated a nonsignificant 7% risk reduction for nonfatal MI, nonfatal stroke, or cardiovascular death. No difference was seen in total mortality. No significant difference between groups was noted regarding frequency of cancer. Supplementation with vitamin E reduced the risk of venous thromboembolism in women, and those with a previous history or genetic predisposition may particularly benefit.

A meta-analysis of 12 clinical trials with 167,025 participants concluded that vitamin E supplementation was not associated with a reduction in total mortality, cancer incidence, or cancer mortality.[65] Vitamin E supplementation does not seem to provide protection against cancer or CVD. Perhaps 600 IU vitamin E may protect women at high risk for venous thromboembolism from this event.

Vitamin K. Vitamin K is found as phylloquinone (vitamin K_1; sources include green leafy vegetables) and menaquinone (vitamin K_2; sources include meat, eggs, dairy, and natto). Although Vitamin K has been associated with reduced fracture risk in observational studies, many clinical trials have shown no benefit. Vitamin K_1 and vitamin K_2 may have different skeletal benefits. The relationship between vitamin K and skeletal health requires further study. Only food sources of vitamin K are recommended.

Vitamin K supplements are contraindicated in women taking warfarin. The DRI of vitamin K for women aged 51 to 70 years is 90 μg.

In a prospective cohort study, 24,340 participants aged 35 to 64 years were followed for cancer incidence and mortality in relation to dietary intake of vitamin K. The results suggest that dietary intake of menaquinones, which is highly determined by the consumption of cheese, is associated with a reduced risk of incident and fatal cancer.[66]

Minerals

Trace elements and metals in biologic fluids are essential nutrients for humans. They act as "biochemical triggers," some forming complexes with enzymes and helping in the binding of biologic ligands.

Calcium. Calcium, a divalent, cationic element, is the fifth most abundant element in the earth's crust, present in pearls and marble, ivory and antlers, and corals and bone. Calcium is also the most abundant mineral in the human body. An adult human body contains 1,000 g to 1,200 g of calcium, 99% of which is in bones and teeth. As an element, calcium can neither be synthesized nor degraded as it moves through the processes of cellular- and organ-level metabolism.

Calcium requirements for skeletal maintenance fluctuate throughout a woman's life. During the teen years, calcium requirements are high because of the demands of a rapidly growing skeleton. At the time of puberty, girls have been found to acquire more bone mineral content per lean body mass than boys.[67-69] This additional bone mineral content is presumed to be a source of calcium for reproductive purposes, such as creating an entire fetal skeleton, and it may correspond to the loss of bone mineral content that is seen at the time of menopause.

During a woman's reproductive years, less calcium is required for bone health as bone turnover stabilizes at a low level and peak adult bone mass is achieved and maintained. Calcium requirements remain stable until menopause, when the bone resorption rate increases because of the decrease in ovarian estrogen production. Calcium needs rise at that time because of decreased efficiency in the use of dietary calcium.[42] This is largely because of estrogen-related shifts in intestinal calcium absorption and renal conservation.

The amount of calcium needed is also affected by the decrease in intestinal absorption that occurs with age. Net calcium absorption averages about 10% of intake, with transient increases during adolescent growth spurts and pregnancy. By age 65 years, calcium absorption efficiency is typically 50% below adolescent peak absorption.[70]

One factor that may limit calcium absorption is a lack of vitamin D resulting from age-related declines in several functions, including ingestion, cutaneous synthesis of the parent vitamin, renal synthesis of the active form of the vitamin (1,25-dihydroxyvitamin D), and intestinal responsiveness. Dietary factors limiting calcium absorption include consumption of oxalic acid (found in spinach, rhubarb, and certain other green vegetables), large amounts of grains that contain phytates (eg, wheat bran, soy protein isolates), and possibly, tannins (found in tea). Evidence indicates that other dietary components, such as fat, phosphorus, magnesium, and caffeine, have negligible effects on calcium absorption at generally prevalent intake levels.

In RCTs, calcium plus vitamin D has been shown to reduce or halt bone loss in healthy postmenopausal women and in postmenopausal women with substantial bone loss or previous fracture, especially in the 5 or more years after menopause.[71] A review of more than 20 studies found that postmenopausal women receiving calcium supplementation had bone losses of 0.014% per year compared with 1.0% per year in untreated women.[72] In longer-term trials, the beneficial effects of calcium supplementation were sustained for up to 4 years.

Older studies found that in the presence of adequate vitamin D, calcium also reduced the incidence of spine, hip, and other fractures. Some other large trials did not show significant efficacy of daily oral calcium supplements in preventing fracture.[49,73,74] Studies of calcium and vitamin D and calcium alone found no efficacy in reducing fracture risk using prespecified intent-to-treat analysis.[49,73,75,76] However, in 2 studies, baseline calcium intake was already at or close to the response threshold, and calcium intake for the other studies was not reported. Additionally, treatment adherence was poor (35%-55%) in 2 studies, but when analysis was confined to treatment-adherent participants, significant reductions in fracture risk were found. A NAMS position statement on the role of calcium in perimenopausal and postmenopausal women reached the conclusion that primary analysis (intent-to-treat) of the effect of calcium intake on fractures did not show efficacy and that secondary evidence (patient compliance) revealed benefit.[77]

Calcium seems to potentiate the effect of exercise on BMD in postmenopausal women, primarily in those with daily calcium intake of more than 1,000 mg.[78]

Calcium, either alone or with vitamin D, is not as effective as pharmacotherapy with menopausal estrogen-alone therapy, estrogen-progestogen therapy, an estrogen agonist/antagonist, or a bisphosphonate. However, supplemental calcium substantially improves the efficacy of these agents in reducing menopause-related bone loss.[79] Because of the well-established need for adequate calcium intake, all key clinical trials with either an estrogen agonist/antagonist or a bisphosphonate have provided supplemental calcium to treatment and to placebo arms. Although it is likely that calcium potentiates the positive BMD effects of an estrogen agonist/antagonist and bisphosphonates as it does for estrogen-alone therapy and estrogen-progestogen therapy, this conclusion can only be surmised.

The importance of an adequate calcium intake for skeletal health is well established.[77] Calcium also has been associated with beneficial effects in several nonskeletal disorders, primarily colorectal cancer, hypertension, and obesity, although the extent of those effects has not been fully elucidated. Calcium supplements may slightly increase the risk of nephrolithiasis.[49]

Calcium nutritional status is very difficult to assess using usual laboratory tests. Serum calcium is maintained in the normal range in most cases, even in the presence of severe deficiency. Some combination of a history of low calcium intake, coupled with decreased bone mass for age, increased bone-remodeling indices, and high serum parathyroid hormone, will usually be characteristic of calcium deficiency; however, each of these associated changes can be produced by other causes. Because inadequate calcium intake is prevalent, and given the intake guidelines from the IOM, it is safe to assume that most patients need more calcium.[44,71]

Women with low 25(OH)D levels are unlikely to absorb calcium optimally. Given the fact that low serum vitamin D levels are linked to calcium deficiency, laboratory tests for vitamin D are being used more often in lieu of specific tests for calcium deficiency.

The IOM, the National Institutes of Health, and Osteoporosis Canada have all published calcium intake guidelines.[44] The National Osteoporosis Foundation has also updated its guidelines.[80] A woman's calcium requirement rises at menopause (or whenever estrogen is lost). This is because calcium absorption efficiency and renal conservation are to some extent estrogen dependent and deteriorate in the estrogen-deprived state.

Recommended intakes are probably sufficient for most people to maintain skeletal mass during the peak adult years and to minimize age-related bone loss during involution (Table 3).[44,77,80-82] These recommendations are based mainly on several clinical trials in which intakes of 1,500 mg to 2,500 mg per day, coupled with adequate vitamin D status and protein intake, reduced parathyroid hormone secretion to premenopausal normal values, stopped (or slowed) age-related bone loss, and reduced osteoporotic fractures by up to 55%. Intakes that would be optimal for other health or disease endpoints are less well studied, but such data as are available indicate an intake requirement at least as high as that for the protection of bone mass. The NAMS position statements on calcium and on osteoporosis concluded that the target calcium intake for most postmenopausal women is 1,200 mg per day.[18,77]

It is currently difficult to pin down the calcium-intake status of the population because of the rapidly changing environment with respect to food fortification and supplement use. From food sources alone, median calcium intakes for women aged 40 to 60 years are less than 600 mg per day and have been approximately stable at that level for many years, despite education and other campaigns to improve calcium intake. This leaves a substantial gap that ranges from 400 mg to 900 mg per day to be filled by fortified foods, supplements, or both. Specific populations of postmenopausal women at extra risk for inadequate calcium intake include women who are lactose intolerant, who follow a pure vegetarian diet (typically getting only 250 mg/d of calcium), or who have poor eating habits. The extent of inadequacy in the general population led the 2010 US Department of Agriculture to classify calcium as a shortfall nutrient in its dietary guidelines for Americans.[5]

It has been shown, moreover, that clinician attention to recommending an adequate calcium intake has dropped by nearly 50% since the introduction of bisphosphonate drugs for osteoporosis.[83] Because patients tend to find nutritional advice from their clinicians more credible than the comparable advice they get from all other sources, it is critically important that clinicians continue to emphasize the importance of adequate calcium intake.

Dietary sources are the preferred means of obtaining adequate calcium intake because there are other essential nutrients in high-calcium foods. For most US residents, dairy products (eg, milk, cheese, yogurt, ice cream) are the major contributors of dietary calcium, providing approximately 70% of the total calcium intake of postmenopausal women aged 60 years and older. An 8-oz serving of milk or yogurt or a 1-oz to 1.5-oz cube of hard cheese contains about 300 mg of calcium. All other (nondairy) foods combined contribute only 150 mg to 250 mg calcium to a typical adult diet. Hence, meeting current intake recommendations from commonly available foods generally requires consumption of approximately 3 servings of dairy food per day. Reduced-fat or low-fat products contain at least as much calcium per serving as high-fat dairy products, and they offer alternatives for women concerned about body weight and lipid profiles.

Because many people will choose not to achieve the recommended 3 dairy servings per day, food manufacturers have introduced a variety of calcium-fortified products, including fruit juices, breakfast cereals, and breads. These foods are not equally well engineered because the added calcium may exhibit reduced bioavailability or such poor physical properties so that the fortificant settles into the bottom of the carton (as with soy beverages). Thus, although calcium fortification of foods is a welcome improvement in the nutritional value of available foods, it still functions in a climate of "buyer beware," and the consumer would be well advised to choose brands that have demonstrated fortificant bioavailability.

The best way to understand the calcium content of a tablet supplement or a food item is to look at the label. A 100% daily calcium value is 1,000 mg, so if the label shows that the item contains 40% of the daily value, the amount of calcium is 400 mg.

An estimated 25% of the US population and 70% of the world's population exhibit some degree of "lactase nonpersistence" (ie, inability to metabolize lactose in dairy products), which in some people may produce diarrhea, bloating, and gas when dairy products are consumed (ie, lactose intolerance). Lactase nonpersistence is more common among people of East Asian, African, and South American descent. Other GI problems (eg, celiac disease, irritable bowel syndrome, Crohn disease, infection) or their treatment with intestinal antibiotics can cause temporary or permanent lactose intolerance. Many women with lactase nonpersistence can tolerate milk normally if they have never stopped drinking it since youth or if they increase intake gradually, thereby conditioning their intestinal flora to produce lactase. The National Medical Association has issued 2 consensus reports recommending 3 servings of dairy per day for all African Americans.[84,85] Those few who remain intolerant may substitute yogurt and lactase-treated milk. True milk intolerance or allergy is rare. Calcium supplements or calcium-fortified foods should be considered if dietary preferences or lactase nonpersistence restricts consumption of dairy foods.

Calcium supplements offer a convenient alternative to women unable to consume enough calcium from diet alone. Their use should be confined to what their name denotes, supplementing an already nearly adequate diet. Dependence on supplements for basal intake is not wise and probably not effective, because a low calcium intake is commonly a marker for a globally poor diet, and fixing only the calcium component is not an adequate response to a patient's need. Nevertheless, calcium supplements do play an important role, particularly as adjuvants in the treatment of existing disease such as osteoporosis.

As with food fortification, not all supplements are engineered equally. In the past, some calcium tablets did not disintegrate in the body to release the nutrient. Because calcium supplements (such as calcium-fortified foods) are not regulated as drugs, caution is advised. Brands that have demonstrated calcium bioavailability are the best choices. Calcium supplements vary in type of calcium salt (and hence calcium content), formulation, price, and to some extent, absorbability.

- The 2 most-often used calcium supplement types contain either calcium carbonate or calcium citrate, but a wide variety of calcium salts are found in calcium supplements, including calcium acetate, calcium citrate malate, calcium gluconate, calcium lactate, calcium lactogluconate, and calcium phosphate (the latter being a collective term that describes supplements consisting of either the monobasic, dibasic, or tribasic phosphate salt of calcium). Calcium is also available in bone meal (basically calcium phosphate) as well as in dolomite or oyster shell (both basically calcium carbonate) supplements. In the past, some of these have contained toxic contaminants, especially lead; however, analyses of the most commonly used brands did not reveal toxic levels of contaminants.

- Different calcium salts contain different percentages of calcium. Calcium carbonate provides the highest percentage (40%); thus 1,250 mg of calcium carbonate provides 500 mg of calcium. Calcium citrate (tetrahydrated form) contains 21% calcium; 2,385 mg of calcium citrate therefore provides 500 mg of calcium. All marketed calcium supplements list the actual calcium content, and this value needs to be taken into consideration when calculating daily intake.

- Various formulations of calcium supplements are available, including oral tablets, chewable tablets, dissolvable oral tablets, and liquids. Another formulation for patients

CHAPTER 7

with difficulty swallowing is an effervescent calcium supplement, typically calcium carbonate combined with materials such as citric acid that facilitate dissolving in water or orange juice.

- Absorbability is also a concern. Contrary to popular belief, calcium carbonate and calcium citrate are equally well absorbed if taken with meals, the normal way of assimilating any nutrient. Calcium citrate malate is highly bioavailable, as are supplements containing calcium that is chelated to an amino acid (eg, bisglycinocalcium), but these lesser-used supplements are typically more expensive than calcium carbonate. Studies comparing various commonly used calcium compounds found little differences in their bioavailability when supplements were taken with food. Calcium absorption is optimized if taken with meals and intake is spread out over the day, but contrary to previous advice, there is no practical limit to the amount that can be taken at one time. When taken without food, calcium citrate may be more bioavailable than calcium carbonate. Pharmaceutical formulation of the supplement (ie, the other ingredients in the tablet and how they are packed together) actually makes more of a difference in absorbability than does the chemical nature of the calcium salt. For example, 2 different calcium carbonate tablets may differ in absorbability by as much as 2-fold.[86]

The AE profile from recommended levels of calcium intake is insignificant, but the risk of nephrolithias was 17% higher with calcium/vitamin D supplements than with placebo.[49] Some women have difficulty swallowing a large tablet or have GI AEs. Tolerability can be addressed by getting most or all of a requirement from food or by switching the type of calcium or reducing the dose. Adverse GI events are often related to a woman's taking more calcium than required, not dividing doses, or perhaps confusing supplemental intake with recommended total daily intake.

There are no reported cases of calcium toxicity from food calcium sources, even in pastoral populations whose calcium intake may be in excess of 6,000 mg per day (almost entirely from dairy sources). All reported cases of calcium intoxication have come from the prolonged use of calcium supplement sources, principally calcium carbonate. Even from this source, intakes associated with toxicity have usually been above 4,500 mg per day, taken over prolonged periods. Intake of more than 2,500 mg per day (the upper limit for healthy adults set by the IOM) can increase the risk of hypercalcemia, which in extreme cases can lead to kidney damage. It is not necessary to measure urine calcium excretion before increasing calcium intake to recommended levels in women who have not had a renal calculus, but a woman diagnosed with renal calculi should not consume calcium supplements above the level recommended for her age (Table 3)[44,77,80-82] until the specific cause of the stone has been determined.

Table 3. Recommended Daily Calcium Intake in Perimenopausal and Postmenopausal Women

National Osteoporosis Foundation 2008	
Women aged 50 y and older	1,200 mg
NAMS 2006	
Women aged 50 y and older	1,200 mg
Osteoporosis Canada 2002	
Women aged 50 y and older	1,500 mg
Institute of Medicine 2011	
Aged 31-50 y	1,000 mg
Aged 51 y and older	1,200 mg
National Institutes of Health 1994	
Premenopausal women aged 25-50 y	1,000 mg
Postmenopausal women aged <65 y using ET	1,000 mg
Postmenopausal women not using ET	1,500 mg
All women aged 65 y and older	1,500 mg

Abbreviation: ET, estrogen therapy.
Committee to Review Dietary Reference Intakes for Vitamin D and Calcium, Food and Nutrition Board[44]; North American Menopause Society[77]; National Osteoporosis Foundation[80]; Brown JP, et al[81]; NIH Consensus conference.[82]

Chromium. Chromium helps to maintain normal blood glucose levels. No DRI of chromium for women aged 51 to 70 years has been established; the adequate intake established by the National Academy of Sciences for women aged 50 years and older is 20 μg per day.[17]

Food sources include cereals, meats, poultry, fish, and beer. Promotion of high doses of chromium supplements for weight loss has become popular, but valid trials of both safety and efficacy are lacking. The role of chromium supplements in patients with chromium deficiency or glucose intolerance has not been defined.

Iron. Iron serves numerous important functions in the body relating to the metabolism of oxygen, not the least of which is its role in hemoglobin transport of oxygen to tissues. Almost two-thirds of iron in the body is found in hemoglobin.

Excess iron results in cellular dysfunction, leading to toxicity and even death. Although early research linked high iron stores with increased rates of MI in men, later studies have not supported such an association.

A reduction in iron negatively affects the function of oxygen transport in RBCs. The World Health Organization considers iron deficiency the top nutritional disorder in the world.[87] As much as 80% of the world's population may be iron deficient, and 30% may have iron deficiency anemia. Iron deficiency severity ranges from iron depletion, which yields little physiologic damage, to iron deficiency anemia, which can affect the function of numerous organ systems.

The most common causes of iron deficiency anemia are GI bleeding or excess menstrual flow. During perimenopause, women experiencing prolonged or repeated heavy uterine bleeding may need additional iron if they develop iron deficiency anemia. After menopause, most women should not choose a multivitamin or mineral supplement containing iron because iron is no longer lost through menstrual bleeding. The DRI of elemental iron for menstruating women is 18 mg per day; after menopause, 8 mg per day is sufficient. Women who use multivitamins should be advised to use an appropriate formulation.

In addition to GI bleeding and excess menstrual flow, other conditions associated with a high risk of developing iron deficiency anemia include kidney failure (especially for those on dialysis); chronic infectious, inflammatory, or malignant disorders (eg, arthritis and cancer); and GI malabsorption diseases (eg, celiac disease and Crohn disease). Not all these conditions will respond to iron supplementation. Many persons (particularly menstruating women and vegetarians) who engage in regular, intense exercise have marginal or inadequate iron status requiring iron supplementation. Signs of iron deficiency anemia include fatigue and weakness, decreased work performance, difficulty maintaining body temperature, decreased immune function, and glossitis (inflamed tongue).

Iron is readily available in food (eg, organ meats, beef, turkey, clams, oysters, oatmeal, beans) and fortified foods (eg, breakfast cereals). When iron deficiency anemia is diagnosed, OTC or prescription oral iron supplements are often recommended. Prescription intravenous iron therapy may be called for in extreme cases of anemia or in persons unable to adequately absorb oral iron supplements. Total dietary iron intake in vegetarian diets may meet recommended levels; however, it is less available for absorption than in diets that include meat.

Supplemental iron is available in 2 forms: ferrous and ferric. Ferrous iron salts (ferrous fumarate, ferrous sulfate, and ferrous gluconate) are the best absorbed forms of iron supplements. *Elemental iron* is the amount of iron in a supplement that is available for absorption.

Magnesium. Magnesium is a divalent, cationic element, and like calcium, it is relatively abundant in the earth's crust. An adult human body contains between 25 g and 35 g magnesium, approximately one-half of which is in the skeleton. Like calcium, magnesium is a chemical element that can neither be synthesized nor degraded in the process of its use by living organisms.

Magnesium is a necessary cofactor for numerous cellular enzymes involved in intermediary and energy metabolism. In magnesium deficiency, global cellular functions are impaired, although there is no discrete disease syndrome that is characteristic of magnesium deficiency. Magnesium is said to function as a physiologic calcium-channel blocker, modulating the entry of calcium into the cytosol of various functioning tissues. When magnesium is deficient, cell calcium rises, with resultant hypertonia, muscle cramps, and elevated vascular tone.

Magnesium absorption from the diet is much more efficient than that of calcium, with net absorption usually in the range of 40% to 60% of ingested intake. Urinary magnesium can be reduced sharply with inadequate intake but may rise substantially in uncontrolled DM and with certain diuretics.

With severe magnesium deficiency, calcium homeostasis is seriously disrupted. The parathyroid glands cannot respond to hypocalcemia by secretion of parathyroid hormone, and the bone-resorptive apparatus is not able to respond to parathyroid hormone; therefore, hypocalcemia, refractory to any intervention other than magnesium repletion, ensues. Clinically recognizable magnesium deficiency occurs when there is excessive loss of body electrolytes through the intestine (eg, intestinal fistulas and various hypersecretory malabsorption syndromes), as well as during recovery from alcoholism. Milder degrees of deficiency, to the extent they occur, are presumably because of either inadequate dietary intake or to hypermagnesiuria induced, for example, by DM or certain diuretics. The full extent of the clinical expression of magnesium deficiency is uncertain but seems to include a higher risk of hypertensive CVD, excessive platelet aggregation and platelet-induced thrombosis, and at least in some persons, osteoporosis.

Magnesium is sometimes mentioned as a necessary supplement for the protection of bone health, for absorption of calcium, or both. However, in most trials focused on BMD or osteoporotic fracture, benefits of calcium were observed without magnesium supplements. Moreover, a study with calcium absorption as the endpoint found that adding 789 mg to 826 mg per day of magnesium, more than double the daily average magnesium intake (280 mg) for postmenopausal women, had no effect on calcium absorption.[88] There are, however, 2 lines of evidence suggesting that subclinical magnesium deficiency may complicate the osteoporotic disease process in certain patients.

Celiac disease is not simply a syndrome of malabsorption but of excess electrolyte loss through the intestine, and a nonnegligible fraction of patients with osteoporosis have silent celiac disease as a cause of or contributor to their osteoporosis.[88] These persons clearly need calcium supplementation, but available evidence suggests that they benefit from magnesium supplementation as well. Patients with osteoporosis, even though they lack overt intestinal symptoms and nevertheless have positive endomysial antibodies, would not be harmed by magnesium supplementation and might be helped.

A second line of evidence comes from the demonstration that many patients with vitamin D deficiency fail to show the expected parathyroid hormone response to their inefficient calcium absorption. These persons have presumptive magnesium deficiency by virtue of a positive magnesium tolerance test and response of parathyroid hormone to supplementation with magnesium citrate. The cause of the magnesium deficiency in these persons is unknown, and the ultimate significance of their silent magnesium deficiency remains unclear.[89]

The daily recommended intake for magnesium is 320 mg per day for women. The evidence supporting this recommendation is weak because there are no generally agreed-on indicators of optimal magnesium status. For the most part, this estimate is based on the amount of ingested magnesium needed to maintain zero magnesium balance, which, as with other nutrients, is a weak criterion.

Median magnesium intake in adult US women is approximately 230 mg per day, and roughly 60% to 70% of the US population regularly has an intake below the DRI.[42] This ostensible shortfall is about as large as the intake gap for calcium and vitamin D, but its clinical significance is much less clear. Until firmer evidence becomes available, it would seem both prudent and safe to attempt to improve magnesium intake status for most adults.

Magnesium is fairly widely distributed in a variety of foods, the richest sources being nuts, certain seeds, legumes, and various marine fish. Dairy foods are also good sources of magnesium, and in typical diets will often be the major source of magnesium. If a woman reaches the target figure for calcium (3 servings of dairy/d), she would automatically receive from that source alone roughly 40% of her recommended daily intake of magnesium.

Several popular calcium supplements combine calcium and magnesium. There is lore to the effect that magnesium must be present for calcium to be absorbed, which is the ostensible rationale for a combination supplement product. That statement is correct only for severe magnesium deficiency (as in malabsorption syndromes) and has been shown to be incorrect for typical adults. In controlled trials using isotopically labeled calcium sources, even a doubling of magnesium intake had no influence on calcium absorption efficiency. Moreover, all the trials establishing the efficacy of calcium in slowing age-related bone loss and reducing osteoporotic fracture risk were performed without supplementing magnesium intake.

In women with excessive magnesium loss, usually because of GI disease (eg, diarrhea, vomiting), magnesium supplementation would be appropriate.

There are no known cases of magnesium toxicity from food sources. Magnesium taken by mouth as various salts tends to have a cathartic effect, and one such preparation (magnesium citrate) has routinely been used as a means of cleaning out the GI tract before endoscopy or surgery. Anything that represents more than modest supplementation with magnesium salts is likely to elicit some degree of catharsis. The tolerable upper limit published by the IOM for magnesium applies only to supplemental sources and not to food sources.[90] That value has been set at 350 mg of supplemental magnesium per day.

Zinc. Found in almost every cell, zinc is an essential mineral that stimulates the activity of approximately 100 enzymes. Zinc is involved in nucleic acid and protein synthesis and degradation, is needed for DNA synthesis and wound healing, supports the immune system, and helps maintain the senses of taste and smell. The DRI of zinc for women aged 51 to 70 years zinc is 8 mg.

Zinc is found in a wide variety of foods such as oysters, red meat, poultry, beans, nuts, seafood, and dairy. Zinc absorption is greater from a diet high in animal protein than a diet rich in plant proteins. Vegetarians may need as much as 50% more zinc than nonvegetarians because of the lower absorption of zinc from plant foods.

Women who experience chronic diarrhea should be careful to add sources of zinc to their daily diet and may benefit from zinc supplementation. Anyone who has had GI surgery or digestive disorders that result in malabsorption, Crohn disease, or short-bowel syndrome are at greater risk of zinc deficiency and should be evaluated for a zinc supplement if diet alone fails to maintain normal zinc levels.

The effect of zinc treatments on the severity or duration of cold symptoms is controversial. A study of more than 100 employees of the Cleveland Clinic indicated that OTC zinc lozenges decreased the duration of colds by one-half, although no differences were seen in duration of fevers or level of muscle aches.[91]

Iron fortification programs for iron deficiency anemia may affect the absorption of zinc and other nutrients. Fortification of foods with iron does not significantly affect zinc absorption, but large amounts of iron supplements (>25 mg) may decrease zinc absorption. Taking iron supplements between meals will help decrease its effect on zinc.

Other minerals. For most people, some other additional vitamins or minerals will be present in a wholesome diet that includes 5 or more servings of fruits and vegetables per day. However, supplementation may be required.

Boron. Boron acts as a cofactor in magnesium metabolism and thus helps in bone regulation. There is no DRI for boron. Food sources are potatoes, legumes, milk, avocado, and peanuts. A daily multivitamin and mineral supplement containing 3 mg to 9 mg is adequate. Overdose can cause nausea, vomiting, and diarrhea.

Copper. Copper is a component of enzymes involved in iron metabolism. The DRI of copper for women aged 51 to 70 years is 900 µg daily. Food sources include organ meats, seafood, nuts, seeds, wheat bran, whole-grain products, and cocoa.

Manganese. Manganese is involved in bone formation as well as in enzymes in amino acid, cholesterol, and carbohydrate metabolism. Adequate intake is 1.8 mg daily.

Phosphorus. Phosphorus is an important mineral for bones, with too much or too little resulting in bone loss. One symptom of phosphorus deficiency is bone pain. Low phosphorus levels can result from poor eating habits, intestinal malabsorption, and excessive use of antacids that bind to phosphorus. Food sources include milk, yogurt, ice cream, cheese, peas, meat, eggs, some cereals, and breads. Soft drinks are an additional source. The DRI of phosphorus for women aged 50 years and older is 700 mg, with upper limits set at 4,000 mg per day for those aged 50 to 70 years and 3,000 mg per day for women aged older than 70 years.

Selenium. Selenium acts to defend against oxidative stress and the reduction and oxidation of vitamin C and other substances and in the regulation of thyroid hormone action. Food sources include organ meats, seafood, and plants (depending on soil content). The DRI of selenium for women aged 51 to 70 years is 55 µg. Overdose results in hair and nail brittleness and loss. The conclusion of a 2013 review was that the limited trial evidence that is available to date does not support the use of selenium supplements in the primary prevention of CVD.[92]

Other supplements

Currently popular nonbotanical dietary supplements in the United States and the natural health products in Canada do not have direct menopause-related symptom relief but are used for general health benefits by midlife women.

Coenzyme Q10

This fat-soluble, vitamin-like compound—also called CoQ10 or ubiquinone—is found in humans and other mammals. CoQ10 is a cofactor in energy-production reactions, particularly adenosine triphosphate, and functions as an antioxidant, protecting against free radical damage within mitochondria. It is found in all cells in the human body, with the highest concentrations in the heart, kidney, liver, and pancreas.

CoQ10, as oral tablets and capsules, is marketed in the United States and Canada as a dietary supplement and a natural health product, respectively; they are not regulated as drugs. As such, evidence for safety and efficacy is limited. Most information available is from anecdotal reports, case reports, and uncontrolled clinical studies.

Widely used throughout Europe and Asia, CoQ10 is claimed to be of benefit in CVD, including angina, congestive heart failure, and hypertension, as well as musculoskeletal disorders, DM, and obesity. However, study results are mixed.

- *Congestive heart failure.* CoQ10 supplementation is commonly used by patients with congestive heart failure in an attempt to replace levels lost in myocardial cells. The extent of CoQ10 deficiency correlates with the severity of heart failure. A 2013 meta-analysis of 13 trials showed significant improvement in the ejection fraction with the use of CoQ10 compared with controls when used for short-term (≤28 wk).[93] More clinical trials evaluating objective measures of cardiac performance as well as clinical outcomes in diverse populations over longer duration are needed. Encouraging results were seen in a trial of 443 elderly Swedish citizens with the use of combined selenium and CoQ10 supplementation. Over a follow-up of 5.2 years, a significant reduction in cardiovascular mortality occurred in the treatment arm compared with placebo.[94] The large, ongoing Q-Symbio trial will help provide further evidence when results are available.[95] CoQ10 has not been recommended as a therapy for heart failure by the American College of Cardiology or the American Heart Association.[96]

- *Hypertension.* CoQ10 has been shown to reduce blood pressure without significant AEs, and it appears effective as an adjunctive therapy for hypertension; however, at this time, it remains unclear whether CoQ10 should be used as an antihypertensive agent on its own.[97,98]

- *Statin-induced myopathies.* It has been proposed that CoQ10 depletion may be a contributing factor for statin-induced myopathies. Although statins have been shown to reduce serum CoQ10 levels by blocking the synthesis of mevalonic acid (a precursor of CoQ10), studies on the effects of CoQ10 supplementation on statin-induced myalgias have been inconsistent.[99-103]

- *Migraine.* CoQ10 may prevent migraines by improving oxidative phosphorylation in the mitochondria.[104] In a small RCT of 42 patients with migraine, CoQ10 was shown to be superior to placebo for attack frequency, headache days, and days with nausea at doses of 100 mg 3 times daily.[105] It can take up to 3 months to see benefit.[106]

- *Breast cancer.* Interest in the potential effect of CoQ10 in cancer began after lesser amounts were noted in the blood of patients with breast cancer. Studies of CoQ10 in patients with cancer are limited. A 2013 clinical trial found no improvement in treatment-induced fatigue in newly diagnosed patients with breast cancer using standard doses of CoQ10.[107] Caution is suggested because of its potential for interfering with the effectiveness of chemotherapy.[108]

Dosing. Dosing recommendations for CoQ10 range from 30 mg to 300 mg per day, depending on the indication. Doses higher than 100 mg should be taken in divided doses (2 or 3 times/d). Patients should be advised to take it with food.

Adverse events. CoQ10 is relatively safe, with a low incidence of AEs.[109] Adverse events of CoQ10 include nausea,

Chapter 7

epigastric pain, heartburn, headache, and fatigue. Use cautiously in liver disease because doses higher than 300 mg for extended periods may elevate liver enzymes.[110]

Interactions. CoQ10 may reduce the anticoagulant effects of warfarin. Because CoQ10 can lower blood pressure, caution should be taken when using in combination with antihypertensives or at the same time as herbal medications or supplements with additive hypotensive effects. Smoking has also been shown to decrease CoQ10 levels.[111]

Fish oil/Omega-3 and omega-6 fatty acids
Essential nutrients for humans include the parent fatty acids of the omega-3 and omega-6 families of polyunsaturated fatty acids.

Omega-3 fatty acids are polyunsaturated fats and include the 3 major dietary fatty acids: α-linolenic acid, eicosapentaenoic acid, and docosahexaenoic acid.[112] Fish oil is composed of eicosapentaenoic acid and docosahexaenoic acid, whereas α-linolenic acid is derived primarily from plant sources. The human body cannot produce omega-3 fatty acids, so they must be ingested in diet or taken as supplements.

These fatty acids are associated with cardiovascular and other health benefits; however, most of the cardiovascular and triglyceride-lowering benefits have been seen with fish oils (eicosapentaenoic acid and docosahexaenoic acid).[113] The body will convert α-linolenic acid into small amounts of eicosapentaenoic acid and docosahexaenoic acid; however, the conversion process may be inefficient, and nutritional sources must be relied on for an optimal level.

The most abundant sources of docosahexaenoic acid and eicosapentaenoic acid are fatty fish such as salmon, sardines, herring, mackerel, black cod, and bluefish. The α-linolenic acid is found in vegetable oils such as canola, soy, and especially flaxseed, as well as in dairy products and some red meat.

Dietary supplementation of omega-3 fatty acids has been suggested as useful in a variety of conditions. These include CVD, asthma, dementia and cognitive performance with aging, multiple sclerosis, Parkinson disease, premenstrual syndrome, rheumatoid arthritis, systemic lupus erythematosus, irritable bowel disease, renal disease, and various skin conditions. As with many supplements, the quality of studies varies. With the exception of effects on CVD and its risk factors, study results have been either insignificant or inconclusive.

- *Cardiovascular disease.* Omega-3 fatty acids from fish oils may have a number of reported benefits on CVD risk factors, including lowering triglyceride levels, improving blood pressure, preventing arrhythmias, and decreasing platelet aggregation.[112] When considering fish oil for treatment of dyslipidemia, it is important to note that it does not affect HDL-C. The greatest effect on lowering triglycerides has been in patients with very high baseline levels.[114] Prospective cohort studies have indicated a lower risk of fatal CHD in primary prevention from fish consumption once or twice per week.[115] Several prospective clinical trials have shown positive results with omega-3 fatty acids for the secondary prevention of cardiac events,[116-118] but later trials have failed to replicate these findings.[119,120] Several meta-analyses that have included these later trials have concluded that even though omega-3 fatty acid supplementation may protect against vascular events, there is no clear effect on cardiovascular death or major CVD events.[121-123]

- *Alzheimer disease.* Epidemiologic data have indicated that dietary use of omega-3 fatty acids, specifically docosahexaenoic acid, may be protective against Alzheimer disease. No controlled trials assessing docosahexaenoic acid on the treatment or prevention of Alzheimer disease have been completed at this time; however, several are ongoing.[124] A small trial showed improvement in memory function in 36 elderly patients with mild cognitive impairment with the use of fish oils over 12 months.[125] Larger clinical trials are required.

- *Depression.* Numerous studies have been published on the use of omega-3 fatty acids in depression with varying results.[126] Several meta-analyses have found a benefit of omega-3 fatty acids in treating depression and augmenting the effects of antidepressants[127,128]; however, a 2012 meta-analysis found the efficacy became nonsignificant with the inclusion of later published trials.[129]

Omega-6 fatty acids are polyunsaturated fatty acids and include linoleic acid, γ-linoleic acid, and arachidonic acid. Sources of linoleic acid include plant-based oils such as corn, safflower, soybean, and evening primrose seed. Omega-6 fatty acids may compete for common enzymatic processes with omega-3 fatty acids.[130] Most American diets provide at least 10 times more omega-6 than omega-3 fatty acids. It is not known whether a desirable ratio of omega-6 to omega-3 fatty acids exists or to what extent high intakes of omega-6 fatty acids interfere with any benefits of omega-3 fatty acid consumption.

Dosing. Fish oil capsules containing varying amounts of omega-3 and omega-6 fatty acids are available as OTC dietary supplements in the United States and natural health products in Canada. The US government has approved a prescription form of omega-3 fatty acids (omega-3 acid ethyl ester concentrate) with higher concentrates of docosahexaenoic acid and eicosapentaenoic acid than standard fish oil, as an adjunct to the diet for the treatment of very high triglycerides. The American Heart Association advises that treating hypertriglyceridemia should be done under a clinician's care.

Fish oils are well tolerated at doses of 4 g or less daily. Dosing recommendations vary from 1 g to 4 g per day, depending on the indication. Doses of 3 g to 4 g per day are required for triglyceride lowering. Standard fish oil contains 120 mg docosahexaenoic acid and 180 mg eicosapentaenoic acid in a 1-g capsule. Omega-3 fatty acid supplements containing varying docosahexaenoic acid and eicosapentaenoic acid concentrations are also available.

Adverse events. Fish oil supplements can produce heartburn, nausea, dyspepsia, loose stools, and bad breath, as well as a fishy aftertaste.

Fish oil supplements are generally derived from small pelagic fish or from formulations produced by algae; furthermore, mercury is tightly bound to fish proteins instead of fatty acid; therefore, fish oil supplements contain little to no mercury.[131,132]

Interactions. Supplements of fish oil greater than 3 g per day have the potential to slow blood clotting and potentially increase bleeding by decreasing platelet aggregation. Caution should be used when taking other herbal medications or drugs that have antiplatelet effects, as well as anticoagulants such as warfarin. Fish oils may also decrease blood pressure and may have additive effects with blood pressure medications.

Glucosamine and chondroitin
Glucosamine is an amino monosaccharide that is present in almost all human tissues, especially cartilaginous tissues. Chondroitin is a complex carbohydrate that helps cartilage retain water.

These agents have been promoted for pain relief, primarily in osteoarthritis. They are sometimes taken individually but primarily in combination and are used as alternatives or along with analgesics and nonsteroidal anti-inflammatory drugs (NSAIDs). In the United States and Canada, glucosamine and chondroitin are sold as dietary supplements and as natural health products, respectively; thus, they are not regulated as drugs.

Glucosamine is stabilized as 1 of 2 salts, glucosamine sulfate or glucosamine hydrochloride. The sulfate form has been the most studied, and it is unknown whether the hydrochloride salt is as effective. One study comparing the 2 salt forms demonstrated no significant differences with efficacy or AEs between the formulations.[133] Persons may respond differently to the 2 salts. Chondroitin is available as the sulfate salt.

Glucosamine sulfate (alone and with chondroitin sulfate) has been shown to be symptomatically effective in a number of studies and may have a structure-modifying effect on knee osteoarthritis. In animal studies, most of the oral dose is absorbed and incorporated into biologic structures, including the liver, kidneys, and articular cartilage. It is assumed that glucosamine sulfate supplementation facilitates the production and regeneration of cartilage.

Clinical studies have been conducted on glucosamine sulfate for osteoarthritis for more than 20 years, primarily in Europe, where it is available by prescription. Two systematic reviews, one a Cochrane review, have found clinical trial evidence supporting the safety and efficacy of glucosamine sulfate for relieving pain and improving function in patients with osteoarthritis.[134,135] The Cochrane review identified 25 RCTs evaluating oral glucosamine in osteoarthritis.[135] In several placebo-controlled trials, oral glucosamine sulfate was found to be superior to placebo in most but not all trials. In 5 trials comparing glucosamine sulfate and NSAIDs, glucosamine was superior in 2 of the trials and equivalent in 2 trials.

Chondroitin is used in an attempt to influence cartilage loss, with the assumption that because it is partially absorbed in the intestine, some of it may reach joints. Few studies have been done examining the effect on joint space; more have looked at pain relief. There has been some speculation that chondroitin has anti-inflammatory effects, but evidence is lacking. In vitro studies suggest that chondroitin may inhibit some of the cartilage-degrading enzymes. No large clinical trials have addressed the efficacy of chondroitin alone in the treatment of osteoarthritis. The results of a meta-analysis of available trials suggest the benefit of chondroitin on osteoarthritis symptoms may be minimal.[136]

The Glucosamine/Chondroitin Arthritis Intervention Trial, the first such large-scale, US multicenter clinical trial, examined the combination of glucosamine hydrochloride and chondroitin sulfate for relief of mild pain in knee osteoarthritis. In this 6-month study, these substances were compared separately or in combination with each other with celecoxib and with placebo. Glucosamine hydrochloride and chondroitin sulfate together or alone did not provide statistically significant pain relief; however, patients with moderate to severe pain had a significantly higher rate of response in the combination group compared with placebo.[137]

Several trials have assessed the structure-modifying effect of glucosamine sulfate and chondroitin sulfate using plain radiography to measure joint-space narrowing.[138-140] In 2 earlier trials, glucosamine had positive effects on the rate of progression of the disease on knee osteoarthritis,[138,139] as well as preventing total joint replacement.[141] Results from the Glucosamine/Chondroitin Arthritis Intervention Trial showed glucosamine (alone and with chondroitin) had no effect on overall progression of knee osteoarthritis at 2 years. However, a subset of patients with grade 2 osteoarthritis showed a trend toward improvement, although this was not statistically significant.[142] A meta-analysis of 6 RCTs showed that glucosamine sulfate may delay the radiologic progression of knee osteoarthritis over 2 to 3 years, and another meta-analysis of 10 trials found no effect of glucosamine sulfate supplementation on joint space narrowing.[143,144] The structure-modifying effect of glucosamine remains unclear.

Please see Chapter 4 for more information on arthritis.

Dosing. Nearly all trials used glucosamine at doses of 500 mg 3 times daily or 1,500 mg once a day. Chondroitin has been typically studied at a dose of 400 mg 3 times daily.

Adverse events. Glucosamine and chondroitin are considered to be safe, and no serious AEs have been reported. In a Cochrane review, the reported AEs for glucosamine were similar to placebo, although some studies noted GI complaints and sleepiness.[135]

Glucosamine used in supplements is obtained from chitin, extracted from marine exoskeletons. Thus, for women with shellfish allergies, this supplement should be used with caution, depending on the severity of the allergy.

Interactions. Concerns have been raised that these agents may interfere with glycemic control in women with type 2 DM because animal models have demonstrated such effects; however, animals may handle glucosamine differently than do humans. A trial of 35 patients with type 2 DM showed no changes in glycemic control from daily therapy with 1,500 mg glucosamine sulfate and 1,200 mg chondroitin sulfate.[145] Glucosamine alone or in combination with chondroitin may increase the anticoagulation effects of warfarin. Patients on warfarin should be advised to avoid glucosamine and chondroitin or have their INR closely monitored.[146]

Inferior oral supplements of glucosamine (alone and with chondroitin) may also contain a large quantity of sodium chloride or potassium chloride or both, unneeded but less-expensive "salts." These products should be avoided.

S-Adenosylmethionine

S-Adenosylmethionine (SAM-e) is a metabolite of folate that can be found in every living cell. Via enzymatic transmethylation, it plays a role in the formation, activation, or metabolism of neurotransmitters, hormones, proteins, and phospholipids. SAM-e is used as a mood enhancer and for joint and liver health. This chemical is available as an oral supplement, marketed as a dietary supplement in the United States and as natural health product in Canada. In some European countries, SAM-e is a prescription drug. SAM-e has been studied for treatment of depression and osteoarthritis and for prevention of liver disease.

- *Depression.* Several systematic reviews and meta-analyses have found SAM-e to be well tolerated and effective for the treatment of mild to moderate depression.[126,147] Many of the studies included in these analyses have used the intravenous or intramuscular forms of SAM-e. Compared with conventional antidepressant therapy, SAM-e has been found to be equivalent to tricyclic antidepressants; however, few studies have compared SAM-e to other antidepressants. SAM-e has not been well studied in severe depression, although preliminary data have suggested that SAM-e may be effective as adjunctive therapy to antidepressants, especially in those patients who were not responders to selective serotonin-reuptake inhibitors.[148] Dosage for depression is 800 mg to 1,600 mg per day.

- *Osteoarthritis.* A number of clinical trials have been completed assessing the use of SAM-e for pain relief in osteoarthritis.[149] In all trials, SAM-e was significantly more effective than placebo in decreasing the pain of osteoarthritis and equally effective as NSAIDs. A Cochrane systematic review found a small clinical effect with SAM-e in improving osteoarthritis pain and function; however, studies were not adequately sized and were too heterogeneous to make conclusions.[150] Dosage for osteoarthritis is 1,200 mg per day.

- *Liver disease.* Even though SAM-e has been studied in a range of chronic liver disease, the greatest interest has been with intrahepatic cholestasis; however, studies have been found to be inadequate to make comparisons with prescription therapies. A Cochrane review found no evidence to support the use of SAM-e for alcoholic liver disease.[151] Dosages used in studies for liver disorders is 200 mg to 400 mg per day.

Adverse events. Supplementation with SAM-e is well tolerated, with an AE profile that includes occasional GI upset, nausea, dry mouth, headache, dizziness, restlessness, and insomnia.[148] For study results and additional resources on supplements, see the Web site of the National Center for Complementary and Alternative Medicine (http://nccam.nih.gov/research/results).

Over-the-counter hormones

Three OTC hormone preparations require special mention: topical progesterone, dehydroepiandrosterone (DHEA), and melatonin. These steroid-containing products are not government regulated as drugs but rather as dietary supplements. Dietary supplements are not required to prove safety and efficacy before marketing.

Topical progesterone

Many brands of topical progesterone can be purchased without a prescription in the United States as lotion, gel, and cream preparations. Progesterone cannot be sold without a prescription in Canada. Progesterone is the progestogen secreted by the human ovary and hence is called *bioidentical* or *natural* to distinguish it from synthetic progestins. Although bioidentical to endogenous progesterone, the "natural" progesterone used for therapy is synthesized commercially by a chemical process using plants such as soybeans and wild yam.

Topical progesterone preparations vary widely in dosages, formulations, additional ingredients, and recommended application sites. In addition, the concentration of the OTC brands varies as well (eg, creams range from no active ingredient to ≥450 mg progesterone/oz compared with prescription custom-compounded progesterone cream that usually contains 400 mg-450 mg progesterone/oz). Furthermore, some products may not contain the progesterone amounts as claimed by the manufacturer.[152]

Women purchase millions of dollars of various OTC topical progesterone creams each year. Marketers claim progesterone cream balances the hyperestrogenic surges of perimenopause (so-called estrogen dominance) and thus relieves hot flashes and other menopause-related symptoms. Some marketers tout other benefits, including breast enlargement and protection against osteoporosis and breast cancer.

Although clinical experience is extensive, scientific evidence of efficacy for menopause-related symptoms is limited. In 3 clinical trials evaluating the use of topical progesterone cream for hot flashes, results were insufficient to support a claim of efficacy.[153-155] Nonetheless, some practitioners recommend using creams that contain more than 400 mg progesterone per ounce (either OTC or custom compounded 1.5%-3%) for perimenopausal women to achieve physiologic (not pharmacologic) levels of progesterone during the time of estrogen dominance. Daily doses vary from 10 mg to 40 mg of progesterone per day.[156] Progesterone cream can be applied to the palms, inner arms, chest, or inner thighs, although applying to palms seems inadvisable because transference to others, including infants and children, is theoretically possible.

Both anecdotal and limited clinical trial evidence suggest that absorption of OTC topical progesterone cream varies among formulations, as well as among women.[156,157] Studies have shown that progesterone in cream formulations can be absorbed through the skin; however, serum levels of progesterone are often low.[156,158,159] It has been proposed that RBCs may play a role in transporting progesterone directly to tissue, and therefore serum levels may not reflect tissue levels; however, this has not been studied adequately for any firm conclusions.[160]

The effects of transdermal progesterone on endometrial protection with estrogen use are unknown.[156] Longer-term studies have reported that transdermal progesterone may fail to attenuate the mitotic effects of estrogen on the endometrium.[161] Studies have also shown no improvement for endpoints of BMD or cardiovascular markers.[153,154] Topical progesterone cream should not be recommended to lower the risk for osteoporosis or CVD, nor should it be used to prevent estrogen-induced endometrial hyperplasia.[156]

Overall, the OTC progesterone cream is well tolerated, with headache and vaginal bleeding being the most commonly reported AEs in studies.[155] It is unclear whether they are safe for women with a history of a hormone-dependent neoplasm.

Over-the-counter topical creams made from the wild yam plant are marketed as containing a progesterone precursor (diosgenin) that can provide the health benefits attributed to progesterone cream. However, diosgenin cannot be converted into progesterone within the body. Some wild yam creams contain progesterone that has been added to the cream. But many wild yam creams contain only progesterone precursors and thus do not provide any absorbable progesterone. Data do not support any menopause-related health claims for wild yam creams.

Dehydroepiandrosterone

Dehydroepiandrosterone (DHEA) and its sulfoconjugate, dehydroepiandrosterone sulfate (DHEAS), are androgen prohormones. In women, endogenous DHEA is produced by the adrenal glands (90%) and the ovaries (10%). Almost all DHEA is converted to DHEAS, which degrades more slowly than does DHEA. Dehydroepiandrosterone levels peak in women at age 25. Levels decline steadily after age 30 until they become almost undetectable by age 70. A temporary increase in the rate of decline seems to be related to menopause. The fall in secretion of DHEA and DHEAS by the adrenal gland parallels the decline in formation of androgen and estrogen by steroidogenic enzymes in specific-target peripheral tissues.

As no specific receptor has yet been identified, DHEA and DHEAS serve as precursors to androgens such as testosterone and dihydrotestosterone, as well as estrogen, all of which have steroid receptors and are biologically active.[162]

Because DHEA production declines with advancing years, supplements containing DHEA are promoted by marketers as agents to ward off a variety of age-related symptoms. However, no relationship between decreasing DHEA levels and accelerated aging has been proven.

Most often, DHEA is sold as a single-ingredient oral supplement, although it is sometimes packaged with herbs or other ingredients. Although DHEA is a hormone, it is only regulated in the United States as a dietary supplement, not as a drug. In Canada, DHEA is classified as a controlled substance and requires a prescription.

Products vary widely in their amount of DHEA. An analysis of 16 DHEA supplements found that less than 50% of products contained the product specifications stated on the product label.[163]

Long-term oral DHEA treatment is innately suboptimal because oral DHEA must first undergo significant hepatic first-pass metabolism, the rate of which unpredictably accelerates over time. The dose of DHEA must thus be increased, resulting in an increase in AEs. Transdermal or vaginal DHEA offers more promise for future research. Oral administration is associated with increases in testosterone levels and, because of the first-pass effect, estradiol and estrone levels as well. With transdermal DHEA, only increases in testosterone levels are seen.

Although DHEA has been studied for a variety of conditions, including sexual function, depression, osteoporosis, aging, and general well-being, most trials have evaluated its use to treat adrenal insufficiency, for which it appears to be effective. Some trials have indicated a role for DHEA in improving physical and psychological well-being and energy, although not all studies have demonstrated a clear relationship between these endpoints and DHEA. It has been proposed that the behavioral improvements in postmenopausal women may be from the neuroendocrine effects of DHEAS on the secretion of pituitary endorphins, although in general, women with physiologic, age-related declines in DHEA secretion have shown little benefit from exogenous DHEA. A review of the literature concluded that the studies evaluating the role of DHEA in improving mood and well-being were inconclusive.[162]

- *Sexual function.* The effects of DHEA on sexual function have been explored. One review identified 8 trials investigating the effect of oral DHEA on sexual function in healthy postmenopausal women.[164] Only 3 of the studies found a positive effect on sexual function; however, these studies were limited with small sample size, inadequate study power, and short duration of use. Studies using longer duration and validated instruments found no improvement in sexual function. In contrast, intravaginal administration of DHEA has shown promise as an option for women with dyspareunia from urogenital atrophy. A trial of 218 postmenopausal women found improvements in vaginal atrophy and sexual function parameters with the use of vaginal DHEA cream daily over 12 weeks.[165,166]

- *Cognition.* A cross-sectional study of 295 women found that higher endogenous DHEAS levels were independently associated with better cognitive function.[167] But it is still unknown whether administering DHEA will have a positive effect on cognition.

- *Bone loss.* The value of DHEA in preventing bone loss is unclear. Increased spinal BMD, but not hip, was seen with 50 mg oral DHEA coadministered with calcium and vitamin D for 1 year in a small clinical trial of women aged 65 to 75 years (n=58).[168] Similarly, a 2-year trial of women aged older than 60 years taking 50 mg DHEA had small but inconsistent effects on BMD.[169] Other studies have found significant increases in hip BMD in elderly women with low baseline levels of DHEAS, but this effect has not been observed in all studies.[170-173] No fracture data are available.

- *Weight loss.* Dehydroepiandrosterone may have fat-reducing properties, although its role as an antiobesity drug is controversial. Some clinical data support the contention that DHEA supplementation improves lean body mass, waist circumference, and glucose tolerance.[174,175] In one study, DHEAS administration led to a better metabolic profile in obese postmenopausal women.[175]

Dose. The oral dose often used for low libido and adrenal insufficiency is 50 mg per day. At this dose, DHEA is converted to testosterone, whereas at higher doses (1,600 mg/d) DHEA will be converted to estrone and estradiol. The optimal vaginal dose that did not affect estrogen levels in studies was 0.5% (6.5 mg) DHEA daily.[166]

Adverse events. Dehydroepiandrosterone seems to be well tolerated in older women at doses of 50 mg or less. Few AEs have been reported at these doses, although in some women, androgenic AEs (eg, facial hair growth, acne) may occur. Nausea, vomiting, dermatitis, and jaundice have been noted with chronic use of low-dose DHEA. With higher doses, reported AEs include jaundice, elevated liver function tests, virilization, AEs on the breast, and depressed mood. A slight decrease in HDL-C is seen with oral DHEA, but the long-term risk of CVD or other long-term risks is unknown.

Dehydroepiandrosterone should be avoided in women of reproductive age who are thinking of becoming pregnant because there is a potential risk of virilization of the female fetus.[176] Dehydroepiandrosterone also is contraindicated in women who have hormone-dependent cancers. The National Institute on Aging recommends against taking DHEA supplements to reverse the effects of aging.[177]

Please see chapter 8 for more information about androgens.

Melatonin
Melatonin (N-acetyl-5-methoxytryptamine), an endogenous pineal gland hormone, regulates the "central clock" and the rest-activity cycles. It is produced from its precursor, tryptophan, with the process regulated by the suprachiasmatic nucleus of the hypothalamus, the site of the body's circadian clock. Endogenous melatonin levels are highest in childhood, drop significantly during puberty, and decline steadily thereafter throughout life.[178] From a circadian perspective, light suppresses melatonin secretion during the day to a level that is virtually unmeasurable. Melatonin blood levels begin to increase in the evening and peak between midnight and 3:00 AM, resulting in a direct sedative effect and drop in body temperature, thus promoting sleep.[179] In postmenopausal versus premenopausal women under consistent routine conditions, melatonin was shown to peak earlier in the night without differences in time of melatonin onset or amplitude.

The active urinary metabolite of melatonin, 6-sulfatoxymelatonin, is significantly lower in persons with insomnia, suggesting that melatonin suppression or deficit might be responsible for sleep difficulties, particularly in older adults. Low secretors of melatonin may have a greater response to melatonin supplementation.[180] Melatonin has been studied in a wide variety of special populations disposed to low melatonin levels, for example, in brain injury.[181]

Certain pharmacologic agents such as NSAIDS, benzodiazepines, and β-adrenergic receptor blockers can inhibit endogenous melatonin synthesis. Acute and chronic alcohol use, tryptophan deficiency, and caffeine are also associated with decreased melatonin function. Monoamine oxidase inhibitors, noradrenergic uptake inhibitors, selective serotonin-reuptake inhibitors, and neuroleptics enhance melatonin function.

Although melatonin is a hormone, it is regulated in the United States only as a dietary supplement and as a natural health product in Canada, not as a drug. Melatonin is available over the counter in most pharmacies and health food stores. However, the lack of regulation and its availability in small doses with increased vehicle-to-drug ratio increases the likelihood of misformulation and poor release of melatonin.

Melatonin has been widely used by women, but its effects on sleep and behavioral sedation are inconsistent in studies.

- *Circadian rhythm sleep disorders*. Melatonin supplementation may shift the circadian rhythm and has been proposed for circadian rhythm sleep disorders (ie, shift work) and to prevent or treat jet lag, particularly in those who have crossed several time zones.[182,183] Additionally, melatonin has been evaluated in conditions with circadian rhythm disturbances, such as in dementia.[184]

- *Insomnia*. Some studies have shown melatonin benefit in improving sleep latency and sleep duration, especially in older persons, although most studies have been small and of short duration. A meta-analysis of 19 trials concluded that melatonin had a modest but significant improvement in sleep latency, total sleep time, and sleep quality; however, this effect may be smaller than what has been shown for other sleep medications.[185] The dose range of melatonin in these studies varied from 0.3 mg to 5 mg, and duration of use ranged from 7 days to 128 days. A greater effect on sleep latency and total sleep time was seen in studies using higher doses and longer durations, but there was no effect on sleep quality with dose or duration. There are limited data that show that melatonin provides relief from menopause-related sleep disturbances or that melatonin retards aging. A meta-analysis of 9 studies demonstrated that melatonin was effective for delayed sleep-phase disorder.[186] Dose range was 0.3 mg to 5 mg, with 5 mg being the most commonly used. Duration was 10 days to 4 weeks, but dose and duration were not considered in this analysis.

- *Nocturnal blood pressure*. Studies have evaluated the effects of melatonin on nocturnal blood pressure, with inconsistent results. A 2011 meta-analysis showed that controlled-release melatonin may significantly reduce nocturnal blood pressure, but this same effect was not observed with immediate-release formulations.[187]

- *Benzodiazepine withdrawal*. Similar to benzodiazepines, melatonin augments γ-aminobutyric acid receptors and may be useful in weaning patients from long-term benzodiazepine use. In one study, discontinuation of benzodiazepine therapy in patients with insomnia was achieved using a 2-mg controlled-release melatonin formulation for 6 weeks, with good sleep quality preserved at 6 months.[188] In another study, melatonin improved sleep quality in patients undergoing benzodiazepine withdrawal.[189]

Dosing. The optimal dose of melatonin for long-term safety is not known. For sleep disorders, it has been used in doses varying from 0.5 mg to 5 mg daily, taken approximately 1.5 to 2 hours before going to bed. It is generally regarded as safe for short-term use (≤3 months).[190] Melatonin is available in 2 formulations: quick release and sustained release. Because melatonin has a short half-life of approximately 30 to 60 minutes, the quick release may be preferable for initiating sleep, whereas a sustained-release formulation is likely beneficial to sustain sleep. Studies using sustained-release formulations have had better outcomes on sleep parameters.[191,192]

Adverse events. The incidence of AEs with melatonin is very low and not much different than that of placebo.[183] Adverse events such as abdominal cramps, hangover effects, dizziness, fatigue, irritability, and impaired balance are associated with high doses (>3 mg/d) of melatonin. High doses also exacerbate depression; its use is best avoided in women with a history of mental illness.

Interactions. Melatonin should be used cautiously with other central nervous system depressants (sedatives, anxiolytics) because there may be an additive effect. Melatonin may impair the antihypertensive effect of the calcium channel blocker, nifedipine.[193] In addition, there have been case reports of melatonin decreasing prothrombin times in patients on warfarin.[183] Data regarding its use in postmenopausal women with DM are conflicting because there have been reports of increased insulin resistance with melatonin.[194]

References

1. US Food and Drug Administration. FDA issues dietary supplements final rule [press release]. FDA Web site. FDA Website. June 22, 2007. www.fda.gov/NewsEvents/Newsroom/PressAnnouncements/2007/ucm108938.htm. Updated April 10, 2013. Accessed April 29, 2014.
2. Moyer VA; US Preventive Services Task Force. Vitamin, mineral, and multivitamin supplements for the primary prevention of cardiovascular disease and cancer: US Preventive Services Task Force recommendation statement. *Ann Intern Med*. 2014;160(8):558-564.
3. Mente A, de Koning L, Shannon HS, Anand SS. A systematic review of the evidence supporting a causal link between dietary factors and coronary heart disease. *Arch Intern Med*. 2009;169(7):659-669.
4. Guenther PM, Casavale KO, Reedy J, et al. Update of the Healthy Eating Index: HEI-2010. *J Acad Nutr Diet*. 2013;113(4):569-580.
5. US Department of Agriculture, US Department of Health and Human Services. *Dietary Guidelines for Americans, 2010*. 7th ed. Washington, DC: US Government Printing Office; 2010.
6. Appel LJ, Moore TJ, Obarzanek E, et al. A clinical trial of the effects of dietary patterns on blood pressure. DASH Collaborative Research Group. *N Engl J Med*. 1997;336(16):1117-1124.
7. de Koning L, Chiuve SE, Fung TT, Willett WC, Rimm EB, Hu FB. Diet-quality scores and the risk of type 2 diabetes in men. *Diabetes Care*. 2011;34(5):1150-1156.

CHAPTER 7

8. Fung TT, Chiuve SE, McCullough ML, Rexrode KM, Logroscino G, Hu FB. Adherence to a DASH-style diet and risk of coronary heart disease and stroke in women. *Arch Intern Med.* 2008;168(7):713-720.
9. Fung TT, Hu FB, Wu K, Chiuve SE, Fuchs CS, Giovannucci E. The Mediterranean and Dietary Approaches to Stop Hypertension (DASH) diets and colorectal cancer. *Am J Clin Nutr.* 2010;92(6):1429-1435.
10. Dixon LB, Subar AF, Peters U, et al. Adherence to the USDA Food Guide, DASH Eating Plan, and Mediterranean dietary pattern reduces risk of colorectal adenoma. *J Nutr.* 2007;137(11):2443-2450.
11. Miller PE, Cross AJ, Subar AF, et al. Comparison of 4 established DASH diet indexes: examining associations of index scores and colorectal cancer. *Am J Clin Nutr.* 2013;98(3):794-803.
12. Salehi-Abargouei A, Maghsoudi Z, Shirani F, Azadbakht L. Effects of Dietary Approaches to Stop Hypertension (DASH)-style diet on fatal or nonfatal cardiovascular diseases—incidence: a systematic review and meta-analysis on observational prospective studies. *Nutrition.* 2013;29(4):611-618.
13. Bhupathiraju SN, Wedick NM, Pan A, et al. Quantity and variety in fruit and vegetable intake and risk of coronary heart disease. *Am J Clin Nutr.* 2013; 98(6):1514-1523.
14. Hartley L, Igbinedion E, Holmes J, et al. Increased consumption of fruit and vegetables for the primary prevention of cardiovascular diseases. *Cochrane Database Syst Rev.* 2013;6:CD009874.
15. Jansen RJ, Robinson DP, Stolzenberg-Solomon RZ, et al. Fruit and vegetable consumption is inversely associated with having pancreatic cancer. *Cancer Causes Control.* 2011;22(12):1613-1625.
16. Park SY, Ollberding NJ, Woolcott CG, Wilkens LR, Henderson BE, Kolonel LN. Fruit and vegetable intakes are associated with lower risk of bladder cancer among women in the Multiethnic Cohort Study. *J Nutr.* 2013;143(8):1283-1292.
17. National Academy of Sciences. Institute of Medicine. Food and Nutrition Board. *Dietary Reference Intakes (DRIs): Recommended Intakes for Individuals*. US Dept of Agriculture Web site. www.iom.edu/Activities/Nutrition/SummaryDRIs/~/media/Files/Activity%20Files/Nutrition/DRIs/5_Summary%20Table%20Tables%201-4.pdf. Modified December 9, 2013. Accessed April 29, 2014.
18. Management of osteoporosis in postmenopausal women: 2010 position statement of The North American Menopause Society. *Menopause.* 2010; 17(1):25-54.
19. Ye Y, Li J, Yuan Z. Effect of antioxidant vitamin supplementation on cardiovascular outcomes: a meta-analysis of randomized controlled trials. *PloS One.* 2013;8(2):e56803.
20. Thomson CA, Neuhouser ML, Shikany JM, et al. The role of antioxidants and vitamin A in ovarian cancer: results from the Women's Health Initiative. *Nutr Cancer.* 2008;60(6):710-719.
21. Xu X, Yu E, Liu L, et al. Dietary intake of vitamins A, C, and E and the risk of colorectal adenoma: a meta-analysis of observational studies. *Eur J Cancer Prev.* 2013;22(6):529-539.
22. Mathew MC, Ervin AM, Tao J, Davis RM. Antioxidant vitamin supplementation for preventing and slowing the progression of age-related cataract. *Cochrane Database Syst Rev.* 2012;6:CD004567.
23. Misotti AM, Gnagnarella P. Vitamin supplement consumption and breast cancer risk: a review. *Ecancermedicalscience.* 2013;7:365.
24. Kim J, Kim MK, Lee JK, et al. Intakes of vitamin A, C, and E, and beta-carotene are associated with risk of cervical cancer: a case-control study in Korea. *Nutr Cancer.* 2010;62(2):181-189.
25. Ghosh C, Baker JA, Moysich KB, et al. Dietary intakes of selected nutrients and food groups and risk of cervical cancer. *Nutr Cancer.* 2008;60(3):331-341.
26. Lane JS, Magno CP, Lane KT, Chan T, Hoyt DB, Greenfield S. Nutrition impacts the prevalence of peripheral arterial disease in the United States. *J Vasc Surg.* 2008;48(4):897-904.
27. Myung SK, Ju W, Cho B, et al; Korean Meta-Analysis Study Group. Efficacy of vitamin and antioxidant supplements in prevention of cardiovascular disease: systematic review and meta-analysis of randomised controlled trials. *BMJ.* 2013;346:f10.
28. Goldberg AC. A meta-analysis of randomized controlled studies on the effects of extended-release niacin in women. *Am J Cardiol.* 2004; 94(1):121-124.
29. Langan RC, Zawistoski KJ. Update on vitamin B12 deficiency. *Am Fam Physician.* 2011;83(12):1425-1430.
30. Larsson SC, Orsini N, Wolk A. Vitamin B6 and risk of colorectal cancer: a meta-analysis of prospective studies. *JAMA.* 2010;303(11):1077-1083.
31. Oaks BM, Dodd KW, Meinhold CL, Jiao L, Church TR, Stolzenberg-Solomon RZ. Folate intake, post-folic acid grain fortification, and pancreatic cancer risk in the Prostate, Lung, Colorectal, and Ovarian Cancer Screening Trial. *Am J Clin Nutr.* 2010;91(2):449-455.
32. Kabat GC, Miller AB, Jain M, Rohan TE. Dietary intake of selected B vitamins in relation to risk of major cancers in women. *Br J Cancer.* 2008;99(5):816-821.
33. Toole JF, Malinow MR, Chambless LE, et al. Lowering homocysteine in patients with ischemic stroke to prevent recurrent stroke, myocardial infarction, and death: the Vitamin Intervention for Stroke Prevention (VISP) randomized controlled trial. *JAMA.* 2004;291(5):565-575.
34. Albert CM, Cook NR, Gaziano JM, et al. Effect of folic acid and B vitamins on risk of cardiovascular events and total mortality among women at high risk for cardiovascular disease: a randomized trial. *JAMA.* 2008;299(17):2027-2036.
35. Martí-Carvajal AJ, Solà I, Lathyris D, Karakitsiou DE, Simancas-Racines D. Homocysteine-lowering interventions for preventing cardiovascular events. *Cochrane Database Syst Rev.* 2013;1:CD006612.
36. Song Y, Cook NR, Albert CM, Van Denburgh M, Manson JE. Effect of homocysteine-lowering treatment with folic acid and B vitamins on risk of type 2 diabetes in women: a randomized, controlled trial. *Diabetes.* 2009;58(8):1921-1928.
37. van Meurs JB, Dhonukshe-Rutten RA, Pluijm SM, et al. Homocysteine levels and the risk of osteoporotic fracture. *N Engl J Med.* 2004;350(20):2033-2041.
38. Gjesdal CG, Vollset SE, Ueland PM, et al. Plasma total homocysteine level and bone mineral density: the Hordaland Homocysteine Study. *Arch Intern Med.* 2006;166(1):88-94.
39. Balk EM, Raman G, Tatsioni A, Chung M, Lau J, Rosenberg IH. Vitamin B6, B12, and folic acid supplementation and cognitive function: a systematic review of randomized trials. *Arch Intern Med.* 2007;167(1):21-30.
40. Howe GR, Hirohata T, Hislop TJ, et al. Dietary factors and risk of breast cancer: combined analysis of 12 case-control studies. *J Natl Cancer Inst.* 1990;82(7):561-569.
41. Harding AH, Wareham NJ, Bingham SA, et al. Plasma vitamin C level, fruit and vegetable consumption, and the risk of new-onset type 2 diabetes mellitus: the European prospective investigation of cancer—Norfolk prospective study. *Arch Intern Med.* 2008;168(14):1493-1499.
42. Standing Committee on the Scientific Evaluation of Dietary Reference Intakes. Food and Nutrition Board Institute of Medicine. Vitamin D. In: *Dietary Reference Intakes: Calcium, Phosphorus, Magnesium, Vitamin D, and Fluoride*. Washington, DC: National Academy Press; 1997:250-287.
43. Armas LA, Hollis BW, Heaney RP. Vitamin D2 is much less effective than vitamin D3 in humans. *J Clin Endocrinol Metab.* 2004;89(11):5387-5391.
44. Committee to Review Dietary Reference Intakes for Vitamin D and Calcium, Food and Nutrition Board. Overview of vitamin D. In: Ross AC, Taylor CL, Yaktine AL, Del Valle HB, eds. *Dietary Reference Intakes for Calcium and Vitamin D*. Washington DC: National Academies Press; 2011:75-124.
45. Ross AC, Manson JE, Abrams SA, et al. The 2011 report on dietary reference intakes for calcium and vitamin D from the Institute of Medicine: what clinicians need to know. *J Clin Endocrinol Metab.* 2011;96(1):53-58.
46. Heaney RP, Dowell MS, Hale CA, Bendich A. Calcium absorption varies within the reference range for serum 25-hydroxyvitamin D. *J Am Coll Nutr.* 2003;22(2):142-146.
47. Bischoff-Ferrari HA, Dietrich T, Orav EJ, Dawson-Hughes B. Positive association between 25-hydroxy vitamin D levels and bone mineral density: a population-based study of younger and older adults. *Am J Med.* 2004; 116(9):634-639.
48. Bischoff-Ferrari HA, Dietrich T, Orav EJ, et al. Higher 25-hydroxyvitamin D concentrations are associated with better lower-extremity function in both active and inactive persons aged ≥60 y. *Am J Clin Nutr.* 2004;80(3):752-758.
49. Jackson RD, LaCroix AZ, Gass M, et al; Women's Health Initiative Investigators. Calcium plus vitamin D supplementation and the risk of fractures. *N Engl J Med.* 2006;354(7):669-683. Erratum in: *N Engl J Med.* 2006;354(10):1102.
50. Bischoff HA, Stähelin HB, Dick W, et al. Effects of vitamin D and calcium supplementation on falls: a randomized controlled trial. *J Bone Miner Res.* 2003;18(2):343-351.
51. Bischoff-Ferrari HA, Willett WC, Wong JB, Giovannucci E, Dietrich T, Dawson-Hughes B. Fracture prevention with vitamin D supplementation: a meta-analysis of randomized controlled trials. *JAMA.* 2005;293(18):2257-2264.

52. Holick MF. Sunlight and vitamin D for bone health and prevention of autoimmune diseases, cancers, and cardiovascular disease. *Am J Clin Nutr.* 2004;80(6 suppl):1678S-1688S.

53. Lips P. Which circulating level of 25-hydroxyvitamin D is appropriate? *J Steroid Biochem Mol Biol.* 2004;89-90(1-5):611-614.

54. National Osteoporosis Foundation. *Get the Facts on Calcium and Vitamin D.* National Osteoporosis Foundation Web site. www.nof.org/articles/952. Accessed April 29, 2014.

55. Health Canada. Food and Nutrition. Vitamin D and calcium: updated dietary reference intakes. Health Canada Web site. www.hc-sc.gc.ca/fn-an/nutrition/vitamin/vita-d-eng.php#a10. Updated March 22, 2012. Accessed April 29, 2014.

56. Looker AC, Dawson-Hughes B, Calvo MS, Gunter EW, Sahyoun NR. Serum 25-hydroxyvitamin D status of adolescents and adults in two seasonal subpopulations from NHANES III. *Bone.* 2002;30(5):771-777.

57. Lappe JM, Davies KM, Travers-Gustafson D, Heaney RP. Vitamin D status in a rural postmenopausal female population. *J Am Coll Nutr.* 2006;25(5):395-402.

58. Passeri G, Pini G, Troiano L, et al. Low vitamin D status, high bone turnover, and bone fractures in centenarians. *J Clin Endocrinol Metab.* 2003;88(11):5109-5115.

59. Hathcock JN, Shao A, Vieth R, Heaney RP. Risk assessment for vitamin D. *Am J Clin Nutr.* 2007;85(1):6-18.

60. Sesso HD, Buring JE, Christen WG, et al. Vitamins E and C in the prevention of cardiovascular disease in men: the Physicians' Health Study II randomized controlled trial. *JAMA.* 2008;300(18):2123-2133.

61. Miller ER 3rd, Pastor-Barriuso R, Dalal D, Riemersma RA, Appel LJ, Guallar E. Meta-analysis: high-dosage vitamin E supplementation may increase all-cause mortality. *Ann Intern Med.* 2005;142(1):37-46.

62. Lonn E, Bosch J, Yusuf S, et al; HOPE and HOPE-TOO Trial Investigators. Effects of long-term vitamin E supplementation on cardiovascular events and cancer: a randomized controlled trial. *JAMA.* 2005;293(11):1338-1347.

63. Lonn E, Yusuf S, Arnold MJ, et al; Heart Outcomes Prevention Evaluation (HOPE) 2 Investigators. Homocysteine lowering with folic acid and B vitamins in vascular disease. *N Engl J Med.* 2006;354(15):1567-1577. Erratum in: *N Engl J Med.* 2006;355(7):746.

64. Glynn RJ, Ridker PM, Goldhaber SZ, Zee RY, Buring JE. Effects of random allocation to vitamin E supplementation on the occurrence of venous thromboembolism: report from the Women's Health Study. *Circulation.* 2007;116(13):1497-1503.

65. Alkhenizan A, Hafez K. The role of vitamin E in the prevention of cancer: a meta-analysis of randomized controlled trials. *Ann Saudi Med.* 2007;27(6):409-414.

66. Nimptsch K, Rohrmann S, Kaaks R, Linseisen J. Dietary vitamin K intake in relation to cancer incidence and mortality: results from the Heidelberg cohort of the European Prospective Investigation into Cancer and Nutrition (EPIC-Heidelberg). *Am J Clin Nutr.* 2010;91(5):1348-1358.

67. Leonard MB, Elmi A, Mostoufi-Moab S, et al. Effects of sex, race, and puberty on cortical bone and the functional muscle bone unit in children, adolescents, and young adults. *J Clin Endocrinol Metab.* 2010;95(4):1681-1689.

68. Järvinen TL, Kannus P, Sievänen H. Estrogen and bone—a reproductive and locomotive perspective. *J Bone Miner Res.* 2003;18(11):1921-1931.

69. Ferretti JL, Capozza RF, Cointry GR, et al. Gender-related differences in the relationship between densitometric values of whole-body bone mineral content and lean body mass in humans between 2 and 87 years of age. *Bone.* 1998;22(6):683-690.

70. Heaney RP, Recker RR, Stegman MR, Moy AJ. Calcium absorption in women: relationships to calcium intake, estrogen status, and age. *J Bone Miner Res.* 1989;4(4):469-475.

71. US Department of Health and Human Services. *The Surgeon General's Report on Bone Health and Osteoporosis: What It Means to You.* Bethesda, MD: US Department of Health and Human Services, Office of the Surgeon General, 2012.

72. Nordin BE. Calcium and osteoporosis. *Nutrition.* 1997;13(7-8):664-686.

73. Grant AM, Avenell A, Campbell MK, et al; RECORD Trial Group. Oral vitamin D3 and calcium for secondary prevention of low-trauma fractures in elderly people (Randomised Evaluation of Calcium Or vitamin D, RECORD): a randomised placebo-controlled trial. *Lancet.* 2005;365(9471):1621-1628.

74. Porthouse J, Cockayne S, King C, et al. Randomised controlled trial of calcium and supplementation with cholecalciferol (vitamin D3) for prevention of fractures in primary care. *BMJ.* 2005;330(7498):1003-1009.

75. Prince RL, Devine A, Dhaliwal SS, Dick IM. Effects of calcium supplementation on clinical fracture and bone structure: results of a 5-year, double-blind, placebo-controlled trial in elderly women. *Arch Intern Med.* 2006;166(8):869-875.

76. Bischoff-Ferrari HA, Dawson-Hughes B, Baron JA, et al. Calcium intake and hip fracture risk in men and women: a meta-analysis of prospective cohort studies and randomized controlled trials. *Am J Clin Nutr.* 2007;86(6):1780-1790.

77. North American Menopause Society. The role of calcium in peri- and postmenopausal women: 2006 position statement of the North American Menopause Society. *Menopause.* 2006;13(6):862-877; quiz 878-880.

78. Specker BL. Evidence for an interaction between calcium intake and physical activity on changes in bone mineral density. *J Bone Miner Res.* 1996;11(10):1539-1544.

79. Nieves JW, Komar L, Cosman F, Lindsay R. Calcium potentiates the effect of estrogen and calcitonin on bone mass: review and analysis. *Am J Clin Nutr.* 1998;67(1):18-24.

80. National Osteoporosis Foundation. *Calcium Basics.* National Osteoporosis Foundation Web site. http://nof.org/files/nof/public/content/file/214/upload/67.pdf. August 2010. Accessed April 29, 2014.

81. Brown JP, Josse RG; Scientific Advisory Council of the Osteoporosis Society of Canada. 2002 clinical practice guidelines for the diagnosis and management of osteoporosis in Canada. *CMAJ.* 2002;167(10 suppl):S1-S34. Erratum in: *CMAJ.* 2003;168(5):544; *CMAJ.* 2003;168(4):400; *CMAJ.* 2003;168)6:676.

82. NIH Consensus conference. Optimal calcium intake. NIH Consensus Development Panel on Optimal Calcium Intake. *JAMA.* 1994;272(24):1942-1948.

83. Stafford RS, Drieling RL, Hersh AL. National trends in osteoporosis visits and osteoporosis treatment, 1988-2003. *Arch Intern Med.* 2004;164(14):1525-1530.

84. Wooten WJ, Price W. Consensus report of the National Medical Association. The role of dairy and dairy nutrients in the diet of African Americans. *J Natl Med Assoc.* 2004;96(12 suppl):5S-31S.

85. National Medical Association. Lactose intolerance and African Americans: implications for the consumption of appropriate intake levels of key nutrients. *J Natl Med Assoc.* 2009;101(10 suppl):5S-23S.

86. Rafferty K, Walters G, Heaney RP. Calcium fortificants: overview and strategies for improving calcium nutriture of the US population. *J Food Sci.* 2007;72(9):R152-R158.

87. DeMaeyer EM, Dallman P, Gurney JM, Hallberg L, Sood SK, Srikantia SG; World Health Organization. *Preventing and Controlling Iron Deficiency Anaemia Through Primary Health Care: A Guide for Health Administrators and Programme Managers.* Geneva: World Health Organization; 1989.

88. Ott SM, Tucci JR, Heaney RP, Marx SJ. Hypocalciuria and abnormalities in mineral and skeletal homeostasis in patients with celiac sprue without intestinal symptoms. *Endocrinol Metab.* 1997;4:201-206.

89. Sahota O, Mundey MK, San P, Godber IM, Hosking DJ. Vitamin D insufficiency and the blunted PTH response in established osteoporosis: the role of magnesium deficiency. *Osteoporos Int.* 2006;17(7):1013-1021. Erratum in: *Osteoporos Int.* 2006;17(12):1825-1826.

90. Institutes of Medicine of the National Academies. *Dietary Reference Intakes: The Essential Guide to Nutrient Requirements.* Washington, DC; National Academies Press; 2006. www.nal.usda.gov/fnic/DRI/Essential_Guide/DRIEssentialGuideNutReq.pdf. Accessed April 29, 2014.

91. Mossad SB, Macknin ML, Medendorp SV, Mason P. Zinc gluconate lozenges for treating the common cold. A randomized, double-blind, placebo-controlled study. *Ann Intern Med.* 1996;125(2):81-88.

92. Rees K, Hartley L, Flowers N, et al. 'Mediterranean' dietary pattern for the primary prevention of cardiovascular disease. *Cochrane Database Syst Rev.* 2013;8:CD009825.

93. Fotino AD, Thompson-Paul AM, Bazzano LA. Effect of coenzyme Q10 on heart failure: a meta-analysis. *Am J Clin Nutr.* 2013;97(2):268-275.

94. Alehagen U, Johansson P, Björnstedt M, Rosén A, Dahlström U. Cardiovascular mortality and N-terminal-proBNP reduced after combined selenium and coenzyme Q10 supplementation: a 5-year prospective randomized double-blind placebo-controlled trial among elderly Swedish citizens. *Int J Cardiol.* 2013;167(5):1860-1866.

95. Mortensen SA. Overview on coenzyme Q10 as adjunctive therapy in chronic heart failure. Rationale, design and end-points of "Q-symbio"—a multinational trial. *Biofactors.* 2003;18(1-4):79-89.

96. Yancy CW, Jessup M, Bozkurt B, et al. 2013 ACCF/AHA guideline for the management of heart failure: a report of the American College of Cardiology Foundation/American Heart Association Task Force on Practice Guidelines. *J Am Coll Cardiol*. 2013;62(16):e147-e239.

97. Hodgson JM, Watts GF, Playford DA, Burke V, Croft KD. Coenzyme Q10 improves blood pressure and glycaemic control: a controlled trial in subjects with type 2 diabetes. *Eur J Clin Nutr*. 2002;56(11):1137-1142.

98. Rosenfeldt FL, Haas SJ, Krum H, et al. Coenzyme Q10 in the treatment of hypertension: a meta-analysis of the clinical trials. *J Hum Hypertens*. 2007;21(4):297-306.

99. Bookstaver DA, Burkhalter NA, Hatzigeorgiou C. Effect of coenzyme Q10 supplementation on statin-induced myalgias. *Am J Cardiol*. 2012;110(4):526-529.

100. Young JM, Florkowski CM, Molyneux SL, et al. Effect of coenzyme Q(10) supplementation on simvastatin-induced myalgia. *Am J Cardiol*. 2007;100(9):1400-1403.

101. Schaars CF, Stalenhoef FH. Effects of ubiquinone (coenzyme Q10) on myopathy in statin users. *Curr Opin Lipidol*. 2008;19(6):553-557.

102. Lamperti C, Naini AB, Lucchini V, et al. Muscle coenzyme Q10 level in statin-related myopathy. *Arch Neurol*. 2005;62(11):1709-1712.

103. Marcoff L, Thompson PD. The role of coenzyme Q10 in statin-associated myopathy: a systematic review. *J Am Coll Cardiol*. 2007;49(23):2231-2237.

104. Rozen TD, Oshinsky ML, Gebeline CA, et al. Open label trial of coenzyme Q10 as a migraine preventive. *Cephalalgia*. 2002;22(2):137-141.

105. Sándor PS, Di Clemente L, Coppola G, et al. Efficacy of coenzyme Q10 in migraine prophylaxis: a randomized controlled trial. *Neurology*. 2005;64(4):713-715.

106. Pringsheim T, Davenport W, Mackie G, et al; Canadian Headache Society Prophylactic Guidelines Development Group. Canadian Headache Society guideline for migraine prophylaxis. *Can J Neurol Sci*. 2012;39(2 suppl 2):S1-S59.

107. Lesser GJ, Case D, Stark N, et al; Wake Forest University Community Clinical Oncology Program Research Base. A randomized, double-blind, placebo-controlled study of oral coenzyme Q10 to relieve self-reported treatment-related fatigue in newly diagnosed patients with breast cancer. *J Support Oncol*. 2013;11(1):31-42.

108. Dhanasekaran M, Ren J. The emerging role of coenzyme Q-10 in aging, neurodegeneration, cardiovascular disease, cancer and diabetes mellitus. *Curr Neurovasc Res*. 2005;2(5):447-459.

109. Hidaki T, Fujii K, Funahashi I, Fukutomi N, Hosoe K. Safety assessment of coenzyme Q10 (CoQ10). *BioFactors*. 2008;32(1-4):199-208.

110. Greenberg S, Frishman WH. Co-enzyme Q10: a new drug for cardiovascular disease. *J Clin Pharmacol*. 1990;30(7):596-608.

111. Elsayed NM, Bendich A. Dietary antioxidants: potential effects on oxidative products in cigarette smoke. *Nutr Res*. 2001;21(3):551-567.

112. Harris WS, Miller M, Tighe AP, Davidson MH, Schaefer EJ. Omega-3 fatty acids and coronary heart disease risk: clinical and mechanistic perspectives. *Atherosclerosis*. 2008;197(1):12-24.

113. Lee JH, O'Keefe JH, Lavie CJ, Marchioli R, Harris WS. Omega-3 fatty acids for cardioprotection. *Mayo Clin Proc*. 2008;83(3):324-332. Erratum in: *Mayo Clin Proc*. 2008;83(6):730.

114. McKenney JM, Sica D. Role of prescription omega-3 fatty acids in the treatment of hypertriglyceridemia. *Pharmacotherapy*. 2007;27(5):715-728.

115. Zheng J, Huang T, Yu Y, Hu X, Yang B, Li D. Fish consumption and CHD mortality: an updated meta-analysis of 17 cohorts. *Public Health Nutr*. 2012;15(4):725-737.

116. Burr ML Fehily AM, Gilbert JF, et al. Effects of changes in fat, fish, and fibre intakes on death and myocardial reinfarction: diet and reinfarction trial (DART). *Lancet*. 1989;2(8666):757-761.

117. Marchioli R, Barzi F, Bomba E, et al; GISSI-Prevenzione Investigators. Early protection against sudden death by n-3 polyunsaturated fatty acids after myocardial infarction: time-course analysis of the results of the Gruppo Italiano per lo Studio della Sopravvivenza nell'Infarto Miocardico (GISSI)-Prevenzione. *Circulation*. 2002;105(16):1897-1903.

118. Yokoyama M, Origasa H, Matsuzaki M, et al; Japan EPA Lipid Intervention Study (JELIS) Investigators. Effects of eicosapentaenoic acid on major coronary events in hypercholesterolaemic patients (JELIS): a randomised open-label, blinded endpoint analysis. *Lancet*. 2007;369(9567):1090-1098.

119. Kromhout D, Giltay EJ, Geleijnse JM; Alpha Omega Trial Group. n-3 fatty acids and cardiovascular events after myocardial infarction. *N Engl J Med*. 2010:363(21):2015-2026.

120. Galan P, Kesse-Guyot E, Czernichow S, Briancon S, Blacher J, Hercberg S; SU.FOL.OM3 Collaborative Group. Effects of B vitamins and omega 3 fatty acids on cardiovascular disease: a randomized placebo controlled trial. *BMJ*. 2010;341:c6273.

121. Kotwal S, Jun M, Sullivan D, Perkovic V, Neal B. Omega 3 fatty acids and cardiovascular outcomes: systematic review and meta-analysis. *Circ Cardiovasc Qual Outcomes*. 2012;5(6):808-818.

122. Kwak SM, Myung SK, Lee YJ, Seo HG; Korean Meta-analysis Study Group. Efficacy of omega-3 fatty acid supplements (eicosapentaenoic acid and docosahexaenoic acid) in the secondary prevention of cardiovascular disease: a meta-analysis of randomized, double blind, placebo-controlled trials. *Arch Intern Med*. 2012;172(9):686-694.

123. Rizos EC, Ntzani EE, Bika E, Kostapanos MS, Elisaf MS. Association between omega-3 fatty acid supplementation and risk of major cardiovascular disease events: a systematic review and meta-analysis. *JAMA*. 2012;308(10):1024-1033.

124. Cole GM, Ma QL, Frautschy SA. Omega-3 fatty acids and dementia. *Prostaglandins Leukot Essent Fatty Acids*. 2009;812-3):213-221.

125. Lee LK, Shahar S, Chin AV, Yusoff NA. Docosahexaenoic acid-concentrated fish oil supplementation in subjects with mild cognitive impairment (MCI): a 12-month randomised, double-blind, placebo-controlled trial. *Psychopharmacology (Berl)*. 2013;225(3):605-612.

126. Ravindran AV, Lam RW, Filtreau MJ, et al; Canadian Network for Mood and Anxiety Treatments (CANMAT). Canadian Network for Mood and Anxiety Treatments (CANMAT) clinical guidelines for the management of major depressive disorders in adults. V. Complementary and alternative medicine treatments. *J Affect Disord*. 2009;117(suppl 1):S54-S64.

127. Appleton KM, Hayward RC, Gunnell D, et al. Effects of n-3 long-chain polyunsaturated fatty acids on depressed mood: systematic review of published trials. *Am J Clin Nutr*. 2006;84(6):1308-1316.

128. Lin PY, Su KP. A meta-analytic review of double-blind, placebo controlled trials of antidepressant efficacy of omega-3 fatty acids. *J Clin Psychiatry*. 2007;68(7):1056-1061.

129. Bloch MH, Hannestad J. Omega-3 fatty acids for the treatment of depression: systematic review and meta-analysis. *Mol Psychiatry*. 2012;17(12):1272-1282.

130. Riediger ND, Othman RA, Suh M, Moghadasian MH. A systematic review of the roles of n-3 fatty acids in health and disease. *J Am Diet Assoc*. 2009;109(4):668-679.

131. Foran SE, Flood JG, Lewandrowski KB. Measurement of mercury levels in concentrated over-the-counter fish oil preparations: is fish oil healthier than fish? *Arch Pathol Lab Med*. 2003;127(12):1603-1605.

132. Mozaffarian D, Rimm EB. Fish intake, contaminants, and human health: evaluating the risks and the benefits. *JAMA*. 2006;296(15):1885-1899. Erratum in: *JAMA*. 2007;297(6):590.

133. Qui G, Weng XS, Zhang K, et al. A multicentral, randomized, controlled clinical trial of glucosamine hydrochloride/sulfate in the treatment of knee osteoarthritis [article in Chinese]. *Zhonghua Yi Xue Za Zhi*. 2005;85(43):3067-3070.

134. Poolsup N, Suthisisang C, Channark P, Kittikulsuth W. Glucosamine long-term treatment and the progression of knee osteoarthritis: systematic review of randomized controlled trials. *Ann Pharmacother*. 2005;39(6):1080-1087.

135. Towheed TE, Maxwell L, Anastassiades TP, et al. Glucosamine therapy for treating osteoarthritis. *Cochrane Database Syst Rev*. 2005;(2):CD002946.

136. Reichenbach S, Sterchi R, Scherer M, et al. Meta-analysis: chondroitin for osteoarthritis of the knee or hip. *Ann Intern Med*. 2007;146(8):580-590.

137. Clegg DO, Reda DJ, Harris CL, et al. Glucosamine, chondroitin sulfate, and the two in combination for painful knee osteoarthritis. *N Engl J Med*. 2006;354(1):795-808.

138. Pavelká K, Gatterová J, Olejarová M, Machacek S, Giacovelli G, Rovati LC. Glucosamine sulfate use and delay of progression of knee osteoarthritis: a 3-year, randomized, placebo-controlled, double-blind study. *Arch Intern Med*. 2002;162(18):2113-2123.

139. Reginster JY, Deroisy R, Rovati LC, et al. Long-term effects of glucosamine sulphate on osteoarthritis progression: a randomized, placebo controlled trial. *Lancet*. 2001;357(9252):251-256.

140. Rozendaal RM, Koes BW, van Osch G, et al. Effect of glucosamine on hip osteoarthritis: a randomized trial. *Ann Intern Med*. 2008;148(4):268-277.

141. Bruyere O, Pavelka K, Rovati LC, et al. Total joint replacement after glucosamine sulphate treatment in knee osteoarthritis: results of a mean 8-year observation of patients from two previous 3-year, randomised, controlled trials. *Osteoarthritis Cartilage*. 2008;16(2):254-260.

142. Sawitzke AD, Shi H, Finco MF, et al. The effect of glucosamine and/or chondroitin sulphate on the progression of knee osteoarthritis: a report from the Glucosamine/Chondroitin Arthritis Intervention Trial. *Arthritis Rheum.* 2008;58(10):3183-3191.

143. Lee YH, Woo JH, Choi SJ, Ji JD, Song GG. Effects of glucosamine or chondroitin sulfate on the osteoarthritis progression: a meta-analysis. *Rheumatol Int.* 2010;30(3):357-363.

144. Wandel S, Jüni P, Tendal B, et al. Effects of glucosamine, chondroitin, or placebo in patients with osteoarthritis of hip or knee: network meta-analysis. *BMJ.* 2010;341:c4675.

145. Marshall PD, Poddar S, Tweed EM, Brandes L. Clinical inquiries: do glucosamine and chondroitin worsen blood sugar control in diabetes? *J Fam Pract.* 2006;55(12):1091-1093.

146. Knudsen JF, Sokol GH. Potential glucosamine-warfarin interaction resulting in increased international normalized ratio: case report and review of the literature and MedWatch database. *Pharmacotherapy.* 2008;28(4):540-548.

147. Carpenter DJ. St John's wort and S-adenosyl methionine as "natural" alternatives to conventional antidepressants in the era of the suicidality boxed warning: what is the evidence for clinically relevant benefit? *Altern Med Rev.* 2011;16(1):17-39.

148. Papakostas GI. Evidence for S-Adenosyl-L-Methionine (SAM-e) for the treatment of major depressive disorder. *J Clin Psychiatry.* 2009; 70(suppl 5):18-22.

149. De Silva V, El-Metwally A, Ernst E, Lewith G, Macfarlane GJ; Arthritis Research UK Working Group on Complementary and Alternative Medicines. Evidence for the efficacy of complementary and alternative medicines in the management of osteoarthritis: a systematic review. *Rheumatology.* 2011; 50(5):911-920.

150. Rutjes AW, Nüesch E, Reichenbach S, Jüni P. S-Adenosylmethionine for osteoarthritis of the knee or hip. *Cochrane Database Syst Rev.* 2009;(4):CD007321.

151. Rambaldi A, Gluud C. S-adenosyl-L-methionine for alcoholic liver disease. *Cochrane Database Syst Rev.* 2006;(2):CD002235.

152. Cooper A, Spencer C, Whitehead MI, Ross D, Barnard GJ, Collins WP. Systemic absorption of progesterone from Progest cream in postmenopausal women. *Lancet.* 1998;351(9111):1255-1256.

153. Wren BG, Champion SM, Willetts K, Manga RZ, Eden JA. Transdermal progesterone and its effect on vasomotor symptoms, blood lipid levels, bone metabolic markers, moods, and quality of life for postmenopausal women. *Menopause.* 2003;10(1):13-18.

154. Leonetti HB, Longo S, Anasti JN. Transdermal progesterone cream for vasomotor symptoms and postmenopausal bone loss. *Obstet Gynecol.* 1999;94(2):225-228.

155. Whelan AM, Jurgens TM, Trinacty M. Bioidentical progesterone cream for menopause-related vasomotor symptoms: is it effective? *Ann Pharmacother.* 2013;47(1):112-116.

156. Elshafie MA, Ewies AA. Transdermal natural progesterone cream for postmenopausal women: inconsistent data and complex pharmacokinetics. *J Obstet Gynaecol.* 2007;27(7):655-659.

157. Hermann AC, Nafziger AN, Victory J, Kulawy R, Rocci ML Jr, Bertino JS Jr. Over-the-counter progesterone cream produces significant drug exposure compared to a food and drug administration-approved oral progesterone product. *J Clin Pharmacol.* 2005;45(6):614-619.

158. Wren BG, McFarland K, Edwards L, et al. Effect of sequential transdermal progesterone cream on endometrium, bleeding pattern, and plasma progesterone levels in postmenopausal women. *Climacteric.* 2000; 3(3):155-166.

159. Vashisht A, Wadsworth F, Carey A, Carey B, Studd J. A study to look at hormonal absorption of progesterone cream used in conjunction with transdermal estrogen. *Gynecol Endocrinol.* 2005;21(2):101-105.

160. Stanczyk FZ, Paulson RJ, Roy S. Percutaneous administration of progesterone: blood levels and endometrium protection. *Menopause.* 2005;12(2):232-237.

161. Vashisht A, Wadsworth F, Carey A, Carey B, Studd J. Bleeding profiles and effects on the endometrium for women using a novel combination of transdermal oestradiol and natural progesterone cream as part of a continuous combined hormonal replacement regime. *BJOG.* 2005;112(10):1402-1406.

162. Panjari M, Davis SR. DHEA therapy for women: effect on sexual function and wellbeing. *Hum Reprod Update.* 2007;13(3):239-248.

163. Parasrampuria J, Schwartz K, Petesch R. Quality control of dehydroepiandrosterone dietary supplement products. *JAMA.* 1998; 280(18):1565.

164. Davis S, Panjari M, Stanczyk FZ. DHEA replacement for postmenopausal women. *J Clin Endocrinol Metab.* 2011:96(6):1642-1653.

165. Labrie F, Archer D, Bouchard C, et al. Effect of intravaginal dehydroepiandrosterone (Prasterone) on libido and sexual dysfunction in postmenopausal women. *Menopause.* 2009;16(5):923-931.

166. Labrie F, Archer DF, Bouchard C, et al. Intravaginal dehydroepiandrosterone (prasterone), a highly efficient treatment of dyspareunia. *Climacteric.* 2011;14(2):282-288.

167. Davis SR, Shah SM, McKenzie DP, Davison SL, Bell RJ. Dehydroepiandrosterone sulfate levels are associated with more favorable cognitive function in women. *J Clin Endocrinol Metab.* 2008;93(3):801-808.

168. Weiss EP, Shah K, Fontana L, Lambert CP, Holloszy JO, Villareal DT. Dehydroepiandrosterone replacement therapy in older adults: 1- and 2-y effects on bone. *Am J Clin Nutr.* 2009;89(5):1459-1467.

169. Nair KS, Rizza RA, O'Brien P, et al. DHEA in elderly women and DHEA or testosterone in elderly men. *N Engl J Med.* 2006;355(16):1647-1659.

170. Jankowski CM, Gozansky WS, Kittelson JM, Van Pelt RE, Schwartz RS, Kohrt WM. Increases in bone mineral density in response to oral dehydroepiandrosterone replacement in older adults appear to be mediated by serum estrogens. *J Clin Endocrinol Metab.* 2008;93(12):4767-4773.

171. Jankowski CM, Gozansky WS, Schwartz RS, et al. Effects of dehydroepiandrosterone replacement therapy on bone mineral density in older adults: a randomized, controlled trial. *J Clin Endocrinol Metab.* 2006;91(8):2986-2993.

172. Morales AJ, Haubrich RH, Hwang JY, Asakura H, Yen SS. The effect of six months treatment with a 100 mg daily dose of dehydroepiandrosterone (DHEA) on circulating sex steroids, body composition and muscle strength in age-advanced men and women. *Clin Endocrinol (Oxf).* 1998;49(4):421-432.

173. Kenny AM, Boxer RS, Kleppinger A, Brindisi J, Feinn R, Burleson JA. Dehydroepiandrosterone combined with exercise improves muscle strength and physical function in frail older women. *J Am Geriatr Soc.* 2010;58(9): 1707-1714.

174. Villareal DT, Holloszy JO. Effect of DHEA on abdominal fat and insulin action in elderly women and men: a randomized controlled trial. *JAMA.* 2004;292(18):2243-2248.

175. Gómez-Santos C, Hernández-Morante JJ, Tébart FJ, Granero E, Garaulet M. Differential effect of oral dehydroepiandrosterone-sulphate on metabolic syndrome features in pre- and postmenopausal obese women. *Clin Endocrinol (Oxf).* 2011;77(4):548-554.

176. Dudley SD, Buster JE. Alternative therapy: dehydroepiandrosterone for menopausal hormone replacement. In: Lobo RA, ed. *Treatment of the Postmenopausal Woman: Basic and Clinical Aspects.* 3rd ed. San Diego, CA: Academic Press; 2007:821-828.

177. National Institute on Aging. *Can We Prevent Aging?* National Institutes of Health Web site. www.nia.nih.gov/sites/default/files/can_we_prevent_aging_0.pdf. Published July 2010. Updated February 2012. Accessed April 29, 2014.

178. Claustrat B, Brun J, Chazot G. The basic physiology and pathophysiology of melatonin. *Sleep Med Rev.* 2005;9(1):11-24.

179. Rohr UD, Herold J. Melatonin deficiencies in women. *Maturitas.* 2002; 41(suppl 1):S85-S104.

180. Van Someren EJ. Melatonin treatment efficacy: for whom and for what? *Sleep Med.* 2007;8(3):193-195.

181. Laakso ML, Lindblom N, Leinonen L, Kaski M. Endogenous melatonin predicts efficacy of exogenous melatonin in consolidation of fragmented wrist-activity rhythm of adult patients with developmental brain disorders: a double-blind, placebo-controlled, crossover study. *Sleep Med.* 2007; 8(3):222-239.

182. Bjortvatn B, Palleson S. A practical approach to circadian rhythm sleep disorders. *Sleep Med Rev.* 2009;13(1):47-60.

183. Herxheimer A, Petrie KJ. Melatonin for the prevention and treatment of jet lag. *Cochrane Database Sys Rev.* 2002;(2):CD001520.

184. de Jonghe A, Korevaar JC, van Munster BC, de Rooij SE. Effectiveness of melatonin treatment on circadian rhythm disturbances in dementia. Are there implications for delirium? A systematic review. *Int J Geriatr Psychiatry.* 2010;25(12):1201-1208.

185. Ferracioli-Oda E, Qawasmi A, Bloch MH. Met-analysis: melatonin for the treatment of primary sleep disorders. *PLoS One.* 2013;8(5):e63773.

186. van Geijlswijk IM, Korzilius HP, Smits MG. The use of exogenous melatonin in delayed sleep phase disorder: a meta-analysis. *Sleep.* 2010;33(12):1605-1614.

Chapter 7

187. Grossman E, Laudon M, Zisapel N. Effect of melatonin on nocturnal blood pressure: meta-analysis of randomized controlled trials. *Vasc Health Risk Manag*. 2011;7:577-584.
188. Garfinkel D, Zisapel N, Wainstein J, Laudon M. Facilitation of benzodiazepine discontinuation by melatonin: a new clinical approach. *Arch Intern Med*. 1999;159(20):2456-2460.
189. Peles E, Hetzroni T, Bar-Hamburger R, Adelson M, Schreiber S. Melatonin for perceived sleep disturbances associated with benzodiazepine withdrawal among patients in methadone maintenance treatment: a double-blind randomized clinical trial. *Addiction*. 2007;102(12):1947-1953.
190. Buscemi N, Vandermeer B, Hooton N, et al. Efficacy and safety of exogenous melatonin for secondary sleep disorders and sleep disorders accompanying sleep restriction: meta-analysis. *BMJ*. 2006;332(7538):385-393.
191. Luthringer R, Muzet M, Zisapel N, Staner L. The effect of prolonged-release melatonin on sleep measures and psychomotor performance in elderly patients with insomnia. *Int Clin Psychopharmacol*. 2009;24(5):239-249.
192. Wade A, Downie S. Prolonged-release melatonin for the treatment of insomnia in patients over 55 years. *Expert Opin Investig Drugs*. 2008;17(10):1567-1572.
193. Lusardi P, Piazza E, Fogari R. Cardiovascular effects of melatonin in hypertensive patients well controlled by nifedipine: a 24-hour study. *Br J Clin Pharmacol*. 2000;49(5):423-427.
194. Cagnacci A, Arangino S, Renzi A, et al. Influence of melatonin administration on glucose tolerance and insulin sensitivity of postmenopausal women. *Clin Endocrinol (Oxf)*. 2001;54(3):339-346.

Chapter 8

Prescription Therapies

Prescription hormone drugs—including contraceptives, menopausal hormone therapy (HT), estrogen agonists/antagonists, estrogen combined with an estrogen agonist/antagonist, selective serotonin-reuptake inhibitors, and androgens—are among the treatments considered for women during perimenopause and beyond. Almost all are government approved for the indications for which they are most commonly prescribed, whereas some are prescribed off label (ie, used for an indication other than the US Food and Drug Administration [FDA]-approved indication).

Women sometimes elect nonprescription, over-the-counter (OTC) hormones for menopause symptoms. Over-the-counter hormone treatments are classified in the United States as either *dietary supplements* (*natural health products* in Canada) or *drugs*, depending on their intended use. As dietary supplements or natural health products, they are approved and regulated differently than are prescription drugs.

Hormone drugs that are custom compounded for a patient on the basis of an individual prescription are not required to be approved by FDA before they are sold or marketed to patients, even though some active ingredients in these compounded prescription drug products meet the specifications of the *United States Pharmacopeia* (USP). Because pharmacy compounding of custom or individualized medications is part of the routine practice of a pharmacy, the regulation of such prescription medications is generally done by state medical or pharmacy boards, not the federal government, unless 1) the medications being compounded are an exact copy of a commercially available drug product (in which case the compounding pharmacy is acting as a manufacturer and thus subject to FDA jurisdiction), or 2) the compounded prescription drugs pose a substantial and significant risk to patient safety or public health (for example, the 2012 episode of multiple patient deaths from intrathecal injection of a compounded drug product made by a compounding pharmacy in Massachusetts).

Contraceptives

Despite a decline in fertility during perimenopause, pregnancy is still possible until menopause is reached. Perimenopausal women who wish to avoid pregnancy should be counseled regarding various birth control methods. However, this population has special characteristics that influence contraceptive choice. Women of older reproductive age may be experiencing perimenopausal symptoms that could be managed with contraceptives. However, these women may have concomitant medical conditions that would make certain contraceptive methods inappropriate. Women aged older than 40 years are also more likely to desire long-acting or permanent contraception. Women of older reproductive age have lower rates of contraceptive failure than do younger women because of lower fecundity, less frequent sexual intercourse, and higher compliance with contraceptive regimens.[1] Hormonal contraceptives—with and without estrogen—and intrauterine devices (IUDs) offer viable options for perimenopausal women.[2]

For any woman who desires long-term protection from pregnancy, long-acting, reversible contraceptive methods, which include the copper IUD, the 2 levonorgestrel-releasing intrauterine systems (LNG-IUS), and the etonogestrel subdermal implant, provide superior contraceptive effectiveness, high user satisfaction, and easy insertion in an office or clinic setting.[3] For women who have completed their childbearing, long-acting reversible contraceptive methods are convenient and are less expensive and invasive than surgical sterilization.

The Centers for Disease Control and Prevention (CDC) has issued evidence-based guidelines, making contraceptive provision and clinical decision making easier: the Selected Practice Recommendations and the Medical Eligibility Criteria for Contraceptive Use.[4] The Selected Practice Recommendations explain how to safely initiate contraceptive methods at any time during the menstrual cycle and when it is necessary to perform a pelvic examination before contraceptive initiation (ie, only before intrauterine contraception). The Medical Eligibility Criteria for Contraceptive Use categorizes contraceptive methods according to their safety when used for women with a variety of medical conditions. For each condition, eligibility for the use of each contraceptive method is categorized into 1 of 4 categories: 1) a condition for which there is no restriction for use, 2) a condition in which the advantages generally outweigh the theoretical or proven risks, 3) a condition in which the theoretical or proven risks usually outweigh the advantages, and 4) a condition that represents an unacceptable health risk if the method is used.

According to the Medical Eligibility Criteria for Contraceptive Use guidelines, there are no contraceptive methods that are contraindicated on the basis of age alone (Table 1).[4] However, there are some medical conditions more common in older women that may make some contraceptive methods inappropriate (Tables 2 and 3).[4] Clinical judgment will be required to balance the risks and benefits when a woman has multiple medical conditions. The availability of safe, effective methods, including intrauterine contraception and implants, suggests that use of estrogen-containing methods should increasingly be used with caution in older women with cardiovascular risk factors.

It is important for perimenopausal women to be aware that use of oral contraceptives (OCs) or any other hormonal or intrauterine contraceptive method does not reduce the risk of

What does government approval mean?

In the US prescription drug-approval process, a manufacturer sends the results of research information on a particular product along with a proposed health indication to FDA. FDA then considers the product's effectiveness, dosage, adverse effects, and possible long-term risks. If FDA approval is given, the product may then be offered on the US market for the specified health indication (or indications), accompanied by the FDA-approved product labeling (ie, prescribing information or package insert). All advertising and education to physicians and consumers from the manufacturer must comply with the prescribing information.

In general, FDA approval for a new prescription drug product requires at least 1 but more often 2 randomized, prospective, controlled trials that must meet or exceed pre-agreed on efficacy endpoints and in which, on balance, the anticipated benefits of the drug outweigh the risks. There is no set formulary for determining whether the benefits outweigh the risks for a new prescription drug, and the approval decision by FDA is made on a case-by-case basis. There is inevitably some variability in the standard for approval from division to division within the Center for Drug Evaluation and Research at FDA, or even within the same division, and in the case of relative scarcity of available therapeutics for certain indications FDA has the discretion to approve a new drug for an unmet or undermet important medical need, even if the efficacy endpoint may not be reached or if the safety concerns are significant.

FDA also has the power to allow for new drugs to be approved using agreed-on surrogate endpoints (eg, CD4 counts in patient with HIV) or to allow drugs to be marketed after only 1 randomized, prospective trial (accelerated approval) if there is commitment to perform a second, larger study postmarketing (also known as a phase 4 commitment by the company).

Once a drug is on the market, clinicians can legally prescribe it for off-label (unapproved) indications (eg, prescribing an oral contraceptive to treat hot flashes in perimenopausal women). This is a common medical practice that relies on additional published research and clinical experience documenting safety, efficacy, and dose.

Off-label use of prescription drugs is common in pediatric and adult oncology patient populations, for example. Off-label prescribing is part of the routine practice of medicine and as a rule is not regulated by FDA but rather by individual state medical boards. Although advertising and promotion of off-label uses of prescription drugs to consumers is not permitted, off-label promotion of such uses to physicians is permissible under a fairly narrowly defined set of circumstances.

A similar regulatory process exists in Canada. Before drug products are authorized for sale, a manufacturer must present substantive scientific evidence that is reviewed by Health Canada to assess safety, efficacy, and quality as required by the Food and Drugs Act and Regulations.

In certain US states and in Canada and with the patient's permission, a pharmacist can substitute a generic equivalent drug, if available, for the one that was prescribed. Some insurance companies provide better coverage for generics.

Clinicians can also legally write a prescription for a custom drug formulation that is mixed (compounded) by a pharmacist. Although the active ingredients are government approved, the formulation is not and typically has not been tested for bioavailability, effectiveness dose, or safety.

Over-the-counter products that are intended to be used as dietary supplements (or natural health products in Canada) are regulated differently than drugs, and the marketer is not required to prove efficacy, safety, or minimal effective dose.

Prescription Therapies

Table 1. US Medical Eligibility Criteria for Contraceptive-Use Categories on the Basis of Age

Method	Age range, y	Eligibility
Estrogen-containing contraception	≥40	Benefits outweigh risks
Progestin-only pill	≥40	No restriction
Progestin implant	≥40	No restriction
DMPA	≥40 to 45	No restriction
	>45	Benefits outweigh risks
Cu-IUD	≥40	No restriction
LNG-IUS	≥40	No restriction

Abbreviations: DMPA, depot medroxyprogesterone acetate; Cu-IUD, copper intrauterine device; LNG-IUS, levonorgestrel-releasing intrauterine system.
Centers for Disease Control and Prevention.[4]

sexually transmitted infections. Accordingly, women at risk should protect themselves through use of safer sex practices.

Intrauterine contraception

Intrauterine contraception offers perimenopausal women safe, highly effective, convenient, and long-term contraception. The intrauterine contraception method is the most widely used reversible contraceptive around the world, with 85 to 100 million users. In the United States and Canada, however, intrauterine contraception is used by less than 5% of users.[5] Intrauterine contraception may be a particularly desirable alternative for midlife women, including those considering surgical sterilization.

One intrauterine contraception method government approved for 5 years of contraception in the United States and Canada is the LNG-IUS. Irregular uterine bleeding and spotting are the most commonly reported adverse events (AEs). These nuisances subside as women develop either light cyclical menses or amenorrhea. A few women continue to have ongoing, unpredictable, light uterine bleeding or spotting.

Use of the LNG-IUS reduces menstrual blood loss.[6,7] For perimenopausal women considering surgery to treat heavy menstrual bleeding, the high endometrial progestin levels associated with this device reduce blood loss as effectively as endometrial ablation, thereby allowing many women to avoid surgery.[8] In 2009, the LNG-IUS was approved in the United States and Canada to treat heavy menstrual bleeding in women desiring to use intrauterine contraception. Use of this IUS is as effective as gonadotropin-releasing hormone agonists in the off-label treatment of pain associated with endometriosis.[9] A third, noncontraceptive use of the LNG-IUS is to prevent bleeding and endometrial hyperplasia in postmenopausal women using estrogen therapy (ET), which represents an off-label use in the United States and Canada.[10]

In 2013, a second, smaller LNG-IUS received US government approval for up to 3 years of use and provides highly effective contraception. Because of its smaller dimensions, this can be an appropriate choice for nulliparous as well as perimenopausal women desiring intrauterine contraception.[11] Because of its lower dose of LNG, it has a lower rate of amenorrhea.

A third intrauterine contraception method available in the United States is nonhormonal—the copper IUD, which is approved for 10 years of contraception but remains highly effective for at least 12 years.[12] Canada has approved 2 copper IUDs, each providing up to 5 years of contraception. The principal AEs associated with use of the copper IUD are increased cramping and menstrual flow. Accordingly, the copper IUD may not be an optimal choice for women who have problems with dysmenorrhea or heavy menstrual bleeding at baseline.

Insertion of an intrauterine contraceptive is an office-based procedure, but the procedure is different for each type. Although uterine perforation rarely occurs during insertion of modern intrauterine contraception, expulsion rates can be as high as 5% in the first months after insertion. Clinicians trained in insertion have the lowest rate of expulsions and uterine perforations.

Progestin-only contraceptives

Progestin-only contraceptives can be used by most perimenopausal women for whom contraceptive doses of estrogen are contraindicated (Table 3).[4] Progestin-only contraceptives provide a safer alternative for cigarette smokers aged older than 35 years, women with hypertension (controlled and uncontrolled), and those with a history of venous thromboembolism (VTE).[13] Contraindications include a history of hormone-dependent cancer and unexplained abnormal uterine bleeding.

Progestin-only contraceptives are available in several routes of delivery: IUS, subdermal implant, injection, and oral tablet. With the exception of the oral tablet, these methods also offer noncontraceptive advantages such as

Chapter 8

Table 2. US Medical Eligibility Criteria for Contraceptive-Use Categories for Estrogen-Containing Contraception According to Medical Condition

Condition	Category
Smoking age ≥35 y	
<15 cigarettes/d	Risks outweigh benefits
≥15 cigarettes/d	Unacceptable risk
Obesity	
BMI 30-34 kg/m²	Benefits outweigh risks
BMI ≥35 kg/m²	Benefits outweigh risks
Hypertension	
Controlled hypertension	Risks outweigh benefits
Elevated BP	
Systolic >140-159 mm Hg or diastolic >90-94 mm Hg	Risks outweigh benefits
Systolic ≥160 mm Hg or diastolic ≥ 95 mm Hg	Unacceptable risk
Vascular disease	Unacceptable risk
Diabetes	
No vascular disease	Benefits outweigh risks
Vascular disease or >20 y duration	Risks outweigh benefits or unacceptable risk (based on severity of condition)
Stroke	Unacceptable risk
Current or history of ischemic heart disease	Unacceptable risk
Multiple risk factors for cardiovascular disease (older age, smoking, obesity, DM, hypertension)	Risks outweigh benefits or unacceptable risk (based on severity of condition)

Abbreviations: BMI, body mass index; BP, blood pressure; DM, diabetes mellitus.
Centers for Disease Control and Prevention.[4]

decreased bleeding. Although bleeding or spotting is commonly irregular, the amount and the days of bleeding are decreased overall.

Implant progestin-only contraceptives. An etonogestrel subdermal contraceptive implant (available in the United States and approval pending in Canada) consists of 1 toothpick-sized polymer capsule implanted under the skin of the inner arm by a healthcare professional and offers highly effective contraception for up to 3 years. The implant is radio-opaque in order to be located by x-ray and packaged in a preloaded inserter designed to prevent too-deep insertion. Irregular bleeding, spotting, or amenorrhea commonly occurs throughout implant use.

Injectable progestin-only contraceptives. Medroxyprogesterone acetate (MPA) provides highly effective, long-term contraception when the hormone is administered suspended in an injectable solution ("depot"). Intramuscular depot MPA (DMPA) is available in the United States and Canada. The 150-mg dose is injected into either the buttock or upper arm every 3 months and does not need to be adjusted for body weight. Although DMPA contraception is reversible, return of fertility after cessation of therapy can be delayed 12 to 18 months. Some DMPA users report weight gain. Less common AEs include change in libido, depression, and nervousness. Some consumers call DMPA "the birth control shot." Epileptic seizures and menstrual migraines may be reduced when amenorrhea is achieved with DMPA.

A DMPA version containing 31% less progestin (104 mg) is available in the United States but not in Canada. The dose is injected subcutaneously into the anterior thigh or abdomen every 3 months, using a smaller needle than for intramuscular administration, which may cause less pain. This subcutaneous SMPA formulation is also US government approved for the treatment of endometriosis-related pain.

Initially, irregular bleeding or spotting is common with use of an injectable progestin-only contraceptive. After 4 or more injections, at least one-half of users will experience amenorrhea. Use of injectable progestin suppresses ovarian estradiol production, which can reversibly lower bone mineral density (BMD).[14] Labeling contains a boxed warning of the loss of BMD. Two case-control studies concluded that DMPA was associated with an increased risk of fracture,

Table 3. US Medical Eligibility Criteria for Contraceptive-Use Categories for Use of Progestin-Only Contraception, According to Medical Condition

Condition	POP	DMPA	Implant	LNG-IUS
Smoking age ≥35 y	No restriction	No restriction	No restriction	No restriction
Obesity	No restriction	No restriction	No restriction	No restriction
Hypertension				
Controlled hypertension	No restriction	Benefits outweigh risks	No restriction	No restriction
Elevated BP				
Systolic >140-159 mm Hg or diastolic >90-94 mm Hg	No restriction	Benefits outweigh risks	No restriction	No restriction
Systolic ≥160 mm Hg or diastolic ≥95 mm Hg	Benefits outweigh risks	Risks outweigh benefits	Benefits outweigh risks	Benefits outweigh risks
Vascular disease	Benefits outweigh risks	Risks outweigh benefits	Benefits outweigh risks	Benefits outweigh risks
Diabetes				
No vascular disease	Benefits outweigh risks	Benefits outweigh risks	Benefits outweigh risks	Benefits outweigh risks
Vascular disease or >20 y duration	Benefits outweigh risks	Risks outweigh benefits	Benefits outweigh risks	Benefits outweigh risks
Stroke	Benefits outweigh risks (I) Risks outweigh benefits (C)	Risks outweigh benefits	Benefits outweigh risks (I) Risks outweigh benefits (C)	Benefits outweigh risks
Current or history of ischemic heart disease	Benefits outweigh risks (I) Risks outweigh benefits (C)	Risks outweigh benefits	Benefits outweigh risks (I) Risks outweigh benefits (C)	Benefits outweigh risks (I) Risks outweigh benefits (C)
Multiple risk factors for cardiovascular disease (older age, smoking, obesity, DM, hypertension)	Benefits outweigh risks	Risks outweigh benefits	Benefits outweigh risks	Benefits outweigh risks

Abbreviations: BP, blood pressure; C, continuation; DM, diabetes mellitus; DMPA, depot medroxyprogesterone acetate; I, initiation; LNG-IUS, levonorgestrel-releasing intrauterine system; POP, progestin-only pill.
Centers for Disease Control and Prevention.[4]

with a 54% increase after prolonged use.[15] However, a retrospective cohort study found DMPA users to have an elevated fracture risk at baseline, a factor that was not controlled for in previous studies.[16]

Oral progestin-only contraceptives. A progestin-only OC formulated with 0.35 mg norethindrone provides effective contraception for perimenopausal women. This contraceptive needs to be taken at the same time every day for maximum efficacy; norethindrone's effect on cervical mucus diminishes after only 27 hours.[4] There are no hormone-free (inactive) pills. Unscheduled bleeding is common and can be decreased by taking the pills at the same time every day. Amenorrhea is less common than with other progestin-only contraceptives. Many consumers refer to this type of OC as "the mini-pill" or "POP" (progestin-only pill).

Combination (estrogen-progestin) contraceptives
Many oral and 2 nonoral combination contraceptives (ie, one containing estrogen and progestin) are available.

Labeling for all combination contraceptives in the United States and Canada contains a boxed warning that cigarette smoking increases the risk of serious cardiovascular AEs from hormonal contraceptive use, that this risk increases with age and with heavy smoking (≥15 cigarettes/d), and that this risk is quite marked in women aged older than 35 years. Estrogen-containing contraceptives are generally contraindicated in women aged older than 35 years who smoke.[4]

Obesity is a relative contraindication for combination contraceptives in perimenopausal women. Combination contraceptives increase the risk of VTE. Although the incidence of VTE is very low in reproductive-aged women, the risk increases with age and body mass index.[2,17] Although CDC guidance suggests that the benefits of combination contraceptives outweigh risks in women aged 35 years and older who are obese, the American College of Obstetricians and Gynecologists (ACOG) recommends using caution when prescribing estrogen-containing hormonal methods in such women.[17]

Combination contraceptives are safe, effective birth control options for midlife women who are healthy, lean, and do not smoke. Combination OCs also provide important noncontraceptive benefits for such women, including regulation of irregular uterine bleeding, reduction of vasomotor symptoms (VMS), decreased risk of ovarian and endometrial cancer, and maintenance of bone density (with a potential for decreased risk of postmenopausal osteoporotic fractures).[5] The incidence of cardiovascular events (VTE, myocardial infarction, stroke) is rare in combination OC users who are appropriate candidates for combination contraceptives, and long-term use does not seem to affect the risk of breast cancer. These observations likely apply for nonoral combination contraceptives as well.

Oral combination contraceptives. Oral contraceptives are the most commonly used combination contraceptive, and dozens are available in North America. Many consumers refer to an OC as "the pill."

When prescribing combination OCs for perimenopausal women, some clinicians feel that prescribing ultra-low-dose OCs is prudent. However, use of traditional 20-μg ethinyl estradiol OC formulations (21 active tablets followed by 7 hormone-free days) is associated with higher rates of unscheduled bleeding and spotting. Newer formulations with 25 μg ethinyl estradiol and a triphasic regimen of the progestins desogestrel or norgestimate—both available in the United States but not in Canada—seem to achieve the low rates of unscheduled bleeding and spotting characteristic of higher-dose OCs.[18] Accordingly, these 25-μg estrogen formulations may be a prudent choice for perimenopausal women. Some perimenopausal women may note the occurrence of bothersome VMS or other symptoms during the 7-day hormone-free interval. Use of continuous OC tablets or formulations with shorter or no hormone-free intervals often reduces such symptoms.

Newer OC formulations use shorter or no hormone-free intervals. Several OC formulations are based on a 24-4 regimen (24 active pills followed by 4 inactive pills) rather than the traditional 21-7 cycle and contain ultra-low doses.[18,19] These formulations may have a better bleeding profile despite their ultra-low doses of ethinyl estradiol, although studies are lacking in perimenopausal women. In addition, with the shorter hormone-free interval of 4 days compared to 7 days, ovarian follicular activity is better suppressed.[20,21] This enhanced follicular suppression has the potential to lead to increased efficacy as shown in one study.[22] Use of the newer, ultra-low-dose pills containing only 10 μg of estrogen (24 estrogen-progestin pills, 2 estrogen-only pills, and 2 placebo pills) in a 24/4-day regimen also is associated with enhanced ovarian follicular suppression.[23]

Drospirenone differs from other synthetic progestins in that it is derived from 17α-spironolactone. The ethinyl estradiol plus drospirenone OC has similar efficacy to other low-dose OCs and is government approved for the treatment of symptoms of premenstrual dysphoric disorder.[24,25] Drospirenone has antimineralocorticoid activity, including the potential for hyperkalemia in high-risk patients.[26] As a practical matter, however, this does not seem to have resulted in any clinically concerning cases of hyperkalemia.[27] Drospirenone has mild antimineralocorticoid effects, but there is no evidence for sustained weight loss because of a diuretic effect. Because of conflicting data and interpretation, there has been controversy over the possibility that the risk of VTE in women using drospirenone-containing OCs may be higher than in women using OCs formulated with other progestins.[28] In 2013, FDA revised the label of drospirenone-containing products to report that there may be an increased risk of VTE, stating: "Some epidemiologic studies reported as high as a three-fold increase in the risk of blood clots for drospirenone-containing products when compared to products containing LNG or some other progestins, whereas other epidemiological studies found no additional risk of blood clots with drospirenone-containing products."[29] A 2014 large (N>85,000) prospective study conducted in the United States and 6 European countries found that the risk of VTE associated with the 24/4 drospirenone OC formulation is similar to that of OCs formulated with other progestins.[30]

An OC containing estradiol valerate and dienogest has been US-government approved (not available in Canada) for contraception and the treatment of heavy menstrual bleeding.[31] Before the availability of this formulation, the estrogen component of all low-dose OCs available in the United States has been ethinyl estradiol. Ethinyl estradiol is a potent synthetic estrogen with similar metabolic effects (eg, liver protein production) regardless of the route of administration because of its long half-life and slow metabolism. In contrast, estradiol valerate is a synthetic hormone that is extensively metabolized to estradiol and valeric acid before reaching the systemic circulation.[32] Data from menopausal use have shown that transdermally and vaginally administered estradiol is not associated with an increased production of liver proteins and, therefore, has a lower risk for thrombosis.[33] A daily dose of 2 mg of estradiol valerate has biologic effects on the uterus, ovary, and hypothalamic-pituitary-ovarian axis similar to those of a 20-µg dose of ethinyl estradiol.[32] Whether the estradiol valerate and dienogest OC will be safer than those formulated with ethinyl estradiol with respect to thromboembolism risk is unknown.

Use of extended OC formulations results in withdrawal bleeding less often than monthly. Evidence has consistently shown these regimens are equivalent to traditional cyclic regimens in terms of contraceptive efficacy and safety, and patients on continuous regimens report fewer menstrual symptoms (eg, headaches, genital irritation, fatigue, bloating, withdrawal bleeding, and cramping).[34] Extended regimens include 84 active tablets and 7 inactive tablets.[35] Scheduled withdrawal bleeding occurs every 3 months.

Unscheduled bleeding is common with the use of extended OC. In women using formulations with 84 tablets that contain estrogen and progestin, the addition of 7 tablets with 10 µg ethinyl estradiol at the time of the 7 inactive tablets seems to reduce the occurrence of unscheduled bleeding as well as scheduled bleeding.[36] An extended OC regimen with an ascending dose of ethinyl estradiol during the 84 combination tablets followed with 7 tablets of 10 µg ethinyl estradiol appears to be associated with less unscheduled bleeding than earlier extended OC formulations.[37] Yet another strategy to reduce unscheduled bleeding persisting for more than 7 days in women using extended OCs is to discontinue active tablets for 3 days. In women needing contraception, this strategy should only be employed after at least 21 days of continuous active tablets.[38]

One combination OC is designed to be taken 365 days a year without a hormone-free interval. Consisting of 90 µg LNG and 20 µg ethinyl estradiol, this continuous-formulation OC provides a steady low dose of hormones. No scheduled withdrawal bleeding will occur. Persistent unscheduled bleeding, however, is common.[39] Common AEs of combination OCs include nausea and breast tenderness, which tend to resolve as OC use continues. Use of continuous combination OCs does not cause weight gain or headaches.

Nonoral combination contraceptives. Government-approved nonoral combination contraceptives include a vaginal ring and a weekly patch, both worn for 3 of 4 weeks. The ring releases ethinyl estradiol and etonogestrel, and the patch delivers ethinyl estradiol and norelgestromin.[40-42] Etonogestrel and norelgestromin are the biologically active metabolites of desogestrel and norgestimate, respectively, both of which are progestins used in commonly prescribed combination OCs.

As with combination OCs, use of either the ring or patch results in cyclical monthly withdrawal bleeding. Because these methods are longer acting, patient adherence (and therefore contraceptive efficacy) may be higher than with OCs. Although AEs and contraindications are in general similar to those for combination OCs, breast tenderness is more common with initial use of the patch.[43]

Labeling indicates that women using the patch are exposed to about 60% more estrogen than with a typical OC containing 35 µg ethinyl estradiol.[44] As a result, labeling for the patch contains a warning that its risk of VTE may be higher than with other combination contraceptives. One epidemiologic study found that VTE risk was similar to that of combination OCs, and another study found the risk was 2 times higher with the patch.[45] Because age is itself an independent risk factor for VTE, some experts believe that the ring and OCs are more appropriate choices for perimenopausal women than the patch. The possibly elevated risk of VTE (compared with OC use) contrasts with HT, in which the transdermal route of hormone administration may be associated with a lower risk of VTE compared with the oral route. Whereas the contraceptive patch releases a relatively high dose of ethinyl estradiol, transdermal estrogen formulations used in treating menopausal women release relatively low doses of estradiol.[46]

Emergency contraception

Emergency contraception refers to contraceptive measures that, if taken after sex, may prevent pregnancy. It may be appropriate in certain cases, such as after unprotected sexual intercourse, a condom failure, an IUD partially or totally expelled, or if one or more OC active pills have been missed, because other contraceptive methods are more reliable.[47] It is meant only for occasional use, when primary means of contraception fail. The emergency contraception pill is often referred to as "the morning-after pill," but this phrase is figurative inasmuch as these products are licensed for use 72 to 120 hours after sexual intercourse. It is also important to remember that the most effective form of emergency contraception is the copper IUD. It is more than 99% effective as emergency contraception.[48] When used as emergency contraception, the IUD may inhibit fertilization and implantation and then can remain in place as long-acting reversible contraceptive.

Because emergency contraception methods act before implantation of the embryo, they are medically and legally considered forms of contraception according to the International Federation of Gynecology and Obstetrics and the US government.[49] These pills are not to be confused with "the abortion pill" (RU486).

The progestin-only formulation, approved in the United States and in Canada for emergency contraception, uses LNG as two 0.7-mg tablets taken 12 hours apart or as a single 1.5-mg dose formulation. The original government labeling indicated that this reduces the risk of pregnancy by 89%. Labeling does not include this figure, but states that if it is taken within 72 hours after coitus, 7 of 8 women who would have become pregnant will not and that it works even better if taken within the first 24 hours after coitus. Persons of any age can now purchase this without a prescription in the United States. Otherwise, emergency contraception is available by prescription. In Canada, it is available without a prescription, except in Quebec.

Ulipristal acetate was approved in 2010 for emergency contraception in the United States. Ulipristal acetate is approved for use as soon as possible and up to 5 days after unprotected intercourse. It is available by prescription only. Ulipristal is a progesterone receptor modulator. It is more effective than progestin only when used within 24 hours or up to 5 days after unprotected sexual intercourse.[50] One meta-analysis showed that ulipristal acetate almost halved the risk of pregnancy compared with LNG in women who received emergency contraception within 120 hours after sexual intercourse. Furthermore, when emergency contraception was used within 24 hours of unprotected sex, the risk of pregnancy was reduced by almost two-thirds with ulipristal acetate compared with LNG. In addition, ulipristal acetate is more effective as emergency contraception than LNG in women who are obese.[51]

Emergency contraception is not effective in women who are already pregnant. Inadvertent ingestion of emergency contraception during pregnancy, however, is not known to be harmful to the woman or her fetus.

Concomitant administration of St. John's wort and some enzyme-inducing drugs (including certain anticonvulsants and the antibiotic rifampicin) may reduce plasma progestin levels and thus the effectiveness of low-dose hormonal contraceptives, including OCs and emergency contraception.[4] Switching to methods like intrauterine contraception and DMPA that are not affected by enzyme-inducing drugs or using condoms for added protection are options for women taking medications that may impair the efficacy of an OC. For effective emergency contraception, larger doses of progestins may be required in women using these concomitant medications.

Noncontraceptive benefits of hormonal contraceptives

Perimenopausal use of combined OCs for contraception has been associated with many noncontraceptive benefits (Table 4); these benefits may also apply to vaginal ring and transdermal estrogen-progestin contraceptives.[17]

Hormonal contraceptives (including extended-use combination OCs, injectable progestin, and the LNG-IUS) are often used to reduce the frequency and amount of menses or eliminate menstruation entirely. The use of OCs reduces risk of epithelial ovarian cancer in carriers of the BRCA mutation as well as in women at average risk for this malignancy.[52] Because use of OCs does not appear to increase breast cancer risk in mutation carriers, use of OCs represents a valuable approach to ovarian cancer chemoprophylaxis in BRCA mutation carriers.

Transition from hormonal contraception to hormone therapy

For those women who choose to use menopausal HT, the challenge is determining when to make the transition from the use of hormonal contraception to the lower-dose menopausal hormone formulations. Making the transition too soon may expose a perimenopausal woman to the risk of unintended pregnancy and result in irregular bleeding. However, once it can be assured that menopause has been reached, the transition to HT is advised so that hormone-

---

Table 4. Noncontraceptive Benefits of Combined Oral Contraceptives for Perimenopausal Women

- Restoration of regular menses
- Decreased dysmenorrhea
- Reduced heavy menstrual bleeding
- Reduced pain associated with endometriosis (continuous use of oral contraceptives)
- Suppression of vasomotor symptoms
- Enhanced bone mineral density and possible prevention of osteoporotic fractures
- Decreased need for biopsies for benign breast disease
- Prevention of epithelial ovarian and endometrial malignancies
- Improvements in acne that may flare up with perimenopause

related risks are minimized through use of lower-dose hormone formulations.

Historically, monitoring follicle-stimulating hormone levels (FSH) has been used to determine when menopause is reached. However, using FSH in combination contraceptive users to determine when menopause has occurred may not be accurate.[47] The CDC, ACOG, and the North American Menopause Society (NAMS) all recommend hormonal contraceptive use for a woman until she has reached an age at which she is statistically likely to be postmenopausal. In nonsmoking women, the median age of menopause is approximately 51 to 52 years—meaning that 50% of nonsmoking 51-year-old women have not reached menopause. About 90% of women will have reached menopause by age 55. Therefore, clinicians may continue contraception for women who are appropriate candidates until they are in their mid-50s. With this approach, women who choose to transition from hormonal contraception to HT can accomplish this without any hormone-free days.[2] Women who were not using hormonal contraceptives for contraception (ie, those using it for cycle control) and who have other means of contraception (tubal ligation or vasectomy) can discontinue medication for several months around age 51. Such women, along with their healthcare professionals, can then determine whether they wish to initiate estrogen-progestogen hormone therapy.

Estrogen therapy and estrogen-progestogen therapy

Estrogen has been the only pharmacologic therapy government approved in the United States and in Canada for treating menopause-related symptoms; however, in 2013, FDA approved 7.5 mg paroxetine, the first nonhormonal agent for use in treating VMS.[53,54] In addition, in 2013, FDA approved a product combining the estrogen agonist/antagonist bazedoxifene (BZA) with conjugated estrogen (CE) for use in treating VMS and preventing osteoporosis.

Terminology
Estrogen-containing drugs for menopause use historically were divided into 2 categories: estrogen therapy (ET) and combined estrogen-progestogen therapy (EPT).[55] The approval of BZA/CE has created a new category of estrogen-containing drugs for use by postmenopausal women.

- *Estrogen therapy* is unopposed estrogen prescribed for postmenopausal women who have had a hysterectomy.

- *Estrogen-progestogen therapy* is a combination of estrogen and progestogen (either progesterone or progestin, synthetic forms of progesterone). Although the available data suggest that the benefits of EPT are almost exclusively because of the estrogen, progestogen reduces the risk of endometrial adenocarcinoma in women with a uterus, a risk that is significantly increased in women using unopposed estrogen.

- *Hormone therapy* encompasses ET and EPT. FDA, however, refers to EPT as HT.

Previously, the terms *estrogen replacement therapy* and *hormone replacement therapy* were used. However, *replacement* is a misnomer, because postmenopausal estrogen levels are low in all women. That is the norm. It is not a deficiency state for which replacement is required. Women have high levels of estradiol and other hormones for a period of approximately 40 years for purposes of reproduction. Prepubertal and postmenopausal levels are low, suggesting those phases in a woman's life are not the optimal time for conception. Use of HT after menopause is considered therapeutic for menopausal symptoms, not replacement for a deficiency state. Although FDA uses *estrogen therapy* to describe unopposed ET and *hormone therapy* to describe EPT, NAMS differs from FDA in using *estrogen-progestogen therapy* for combined therapy and *hormone therapy* to describe all HT, both ET and EPT.

Marketers use various terms to describe HT, which can lead to misunderstanding, particularly by the public. For example, the term *natural* is sometimes used to refer to the product source (eg, a plant) or to the chemical structure (ie, bioidentical to human estrogens). Some women erroneously believe that products marketed as natural, plant-based, or bioidentical are safer or better than other classes of hormones. Other women erroneously believe that natural or bioidentical products are extracted from harvested crops instead of being produced in a laboratory. All hormones produced, including compounded hormones, must go through multiple chemical processes in the laboratory to be suitable for human use. Healthcare professionals should be aware of these beliefs and counsel women that the primary factor in determining usefulness of a hormone is not its origin or whether it is bioidentical; the primary clinical question when selecting ET or EPT is to determine an individual woman's risk-benefit ratio for treatment of specific menopause-related symptoms and/or for disease prevention, as well as the proven safety, efficacy, and quality-control aspects of the treatment.

Estrogen therapy
The term *estrogen* describes a variety of chemical compounds that have an affinity for estrogen-receptors (ERs)-α and -β (not included in this list are estrogen agonists/antagonists, which also have affinity for these receptors).[56]

Estrogen types. Estrogens can be divided into 6 main types:

Human estrogens. The estrogens produced in the human body are estrone (E1), 17β-estradiol (often called estradiol or E2), and estriol (E3). Estradiol is the most biologically active, whereas estrone is 50% to 70% less active, and estriol, a weak estrogen, is only 10% as active as estradiol. Estradiol, the principal estrogen secreted by the ovaries, is metabolized to estrone; estradiol and estrone can be metabolized to estriol, although exogenous estriol cannot be converted.

Chapter 8

Among the human estrogens, only 17β-estradiol is available in a government-approved, single-estrogen product.

Nonhuman estrogens. Nonhuman estrogens refer to conjugated estrogens (CE), a mixture of at least 10 estrogens obtained from natural sources (the urine of pregnant mares), occurring as the sodium salts of water-soluble estrogen sulfates. Conjugated estrogens contain the sulfate esters of the ring B saturated estrogens—estrone (about 45%), 17β-estradiol, and 17α-estradiol—and the ring B unsaturated estrogens—equilin (about 25%), 17β-dihydroequilin, 17α-dihydroequilin, equilenin, 17β-dyhydroequilenin, 17α-dihydroequilenin, and $\Delta^{8,9}$-estrone (ie, $\Delta^{8,9}$-dehydroestrone sulfate). The pharmacologic effects of CE are a result of the sum of activities of these estrogens.

Synthetic estrogens. The 2 types of these synthetic mixtures are esterified estrogens (which contain 75% to 85% sodium estrone sulfate) and synthetic conjugated estrogens (SCE). There are 2 designations of SCE: SCE-A (with a mixture of 9 of the estrogens found in CE) and SCE-B (including the estrogens found in synthetic SCE-A plus $\Delta^{8,9}$-dehydroestrone sulfate—the 10 estrogens found in CE).

Synthetic estrogen analogs with a steroid molecular structure. These compounds include ethinyl estradiol and estropipate (formerly called *piperazine estrone sulfate*).

Synthetic estrogen analogs without a steroid skeleton. These stilbesterol derivatives are not used for menopause-related therapy.

Plant-based estrogens without a steroid skeleton. Also known as *phytoestrogens*, these plant-based estrogens can have weak estrogenic as well as antiestrogenic properties, depending on the target tissue. These are not prescription products.

Clinical pharmacology. Endogenous estrogens exert effects on almost all cells in the body. They are largely responsible for the development and maintenance of the female reproductive system and secondary sex characteristics. By direct action, they cause growth and development of the uterus, fallopian tubes, and vagina. Along with other hormones, such as pituitary hormones and progesterone, they cause enlargement of the breasts through promotion of ductal growth, stromal development, and the accretion of fat. Estrogens are intricately involved with other hormones, especially progesterone, in the processes of the ovulatory menstrual cycle and pregnancy, and affect the release of pituitary gonadotropins. They also contribute to the shaping of the skeleton, changes in the epiphyses of the long bones that allow for the pubertal growth spurt and its termination, maintenance of tone and elasticity of urogenital structures, and pigmentation of the nipples and genitals.

Estrogens act by regulating the transcription of a number of genes. Estrogens diffuse through cell membranes, distribute themselves through the cell, and bind to ER-α or ER-β. Then the complex, together with proteins that assist in activating or inactivating the nuclear-specific DNA sequences or hormone-response elements, which enhance the transcription of adjacent genes, in turn leads to the observed effects. In women, ERs have been identified in all tissues, including the reproductive tract, breast, brain, bone, and skin. Recently, nongenomic actions of estrogen have been identified.

Estrogens occur naturally in several forms. The primary source of estrogen in normally cycling adult women is the ovarian follicle, which secretes 70 μg to 500 μg of estradiol daily, depending on the phase of the menstrual cycle. This is converted primarily to estrone, which circulates in roughly equal proportion to estradiol, and to small amounts of estriol. After menopause, most endogenous estrogen is produced by conversion of androstenedione (secreted by the adrenal cortex) to estrone by peripheral tissues. Thus, estrone and the sulfate-conjugated form, estrone sulfate, are the most abundant circulating endogenous estrogens in postmenopausal women. Although circulating estrogens exist in a dynamic equilibrium of metabolic interconversions, estradiol is the principal intracellular human estrogen and is substantially more potent than estrone or estriol at the receptor.

Circulating estrogens modulate the pituitary secretion of the gonadotropins, luteinizing hormone (LH), and FSH through a negative feedback mechanism. Estrogen therapy acts to reduce the elevated levels of these hormones in postmenopausal women.

Pharmacokinetics. Estrogens used in oral ET are well absorbed from the gastrointestinal (GI) tract after release from the drug formulation. Maximal plasma concentrations are attained 4 to 10 hours after oral administration. Estrogens are also well absorbed through the skin and mucous membranes. When applied transdermally or topically in high enough doses, absorption is usually sufficient to cause systemic effects. Although absorption of estrogen given vaginally can equal that of oral estrogen, the low-dose formulations designed to achieve only vaginal benefits result in minimal systemic absorption.

Although naturally occurring estrogens circulate in the blood largely bound to SHBG and albumin, only unbound estrogens enter target tissue cells. The half-life of the different estrogens in CE ranges from 10 to 25 hours; the half-life of estradiol is approximately 16 hours (oral) and 4 to 8 hours (transdermal). After removal of transdermal patches, serum estradiol levels decline in about 12 to 24 hours to preapplication levels.

When orally administered, naturally occurring estrogens and their esters are rapidly metabolized in both the gut and the liver before reaching the general circulation, which is called the *first-pass effect*. This significantly decreases the amount of estrogen (primarily estrone sulfate) available for circulation. In addition, the first pass through the liver affects other liver functions and is presumed to be one of the reasons various routes of administration affect lipid profiles differently. Synthetic estrogens are degraded very slowly in the liver and other tissues, which accounts for their high potency.

Systemic estrogens administered by nonoral routes are not subject to first-pass metabolism, but they do undergo significant hepatic uptake, metabolism, and enterohepatic recycling.

Timed-release transdermal and topical preparations cause less variability in blood levels than oral preparations at steady state and exhibit near zero-order pharmacokinetics. However, there may be substantial patient variability in blood levels.

Transdermal and topical administration produce therapeutic plasma levels of estradiol with lower circulating levels of estrone and estrone conjugates and require smaller total doses than oral therapy.

Estrogen products. Estrogens are available in many prescription preparations, including as single agents in oral preparations (Table 5); transdermal patch, gel, or topical emulsion preparations (Table 6); vaginal preparations (Table 7); and combination (EPT) preparations (Table 8). Clinicians should refer to product labeling before prescribing.

All government-approved estrogen-containing products that achieve systemic levels at recommended doses in the United States and in Canada are approved for the treatment of moderate to severe VMS). All local vaginal estrogen-containing therapies are approved for treating moderate to severe vaginal dryness and symptoms of vulvovaginal atrophy (VVA). Only one vaginal product (Femring) delivers systemic doses and thus is approved also for VMS. Two vaginal products (Premarin Vaginal Cream and Estring) are approved for treatment of pain with intercourse. One product (Estring) is also indicated for urinary urgency and dysuria. When prescribing solely to treat vaginal symptoms, vaginal preparations should be used. One oral estrogen (Enjuvia) is also approved for the treatment of pain with intercourse.

Some estrogen-containing systemic products have government approval for the prevention of postmenopausal osteoporosis, based primarily on studies demonstrating preservation of bone mineral density. Not all marketers of estrogen-containing products have funded the large, long-term trials necessary to prove efficacy. Previously, some estrogen-containing products were also approved for the treatment of postmenopausal osteoporosis, but this indication was withdrawn from all such products by the government because they had not conducted the required fracture trials using women with documented osteoporosis. However, NAMS supports the use of HT for osteoporosis prevention and the extended use of HT for women at high risk of fracture when alternate osteoporosis therapies are not appropriate or cause AEs, assuming the benefits of HT exceed the risks.[55]

These are the most common types of estrogen products used in prescription preparations:

Conjugated estrogens. Most clinical studies have used CE. As a result, more is known about their efficacy and safety than any other estrogen product. Although Premarin has

Table 5. Oral Estrogen Therapy Products for Postmenopausal Use in the United States and Canada

Composition	Product name	Dosage, mg/d
Conjugated estrogens	Premarin	0.3, 0.45,[a] 0.625, 0.9,[a] 1.25
Synthetic conjugated estrogens, A	Cenestin[a]	0.3. 0.45, 0.625, 0.9, 1.25
	C.E.S.[b]	0.3, 0.625, 0.9, 1.25
	PMS-Conjugated[b]	0.3, 0.625, 0.9, 1.25
Synthetic conjugated estrogens, B	Enjuvia[a]	0.3, 0.45, 0.625, 0.9, 1.25
Esterified estrogens	Menest[a]	0.3, 0.625, 1.25, 2.5
	Estragyn[b]	0.3, 0.625
17β-estradiol	Estrace, various generics	0.5, 1.0, 2.0
Estropipate	Ogen[a]	0.625 (0.75), 1.25 (1.5), 2.5 (3.0)
	Various generics[a]	0.625 (0.75), 1.5 (3.0), 5.0 (6.0)

Products not noted are available in the United States and in Canada.
a. Available in the United States but not Canada.
b. Available in Canada but not the United States.
Please visit the NAMS Web site at www.menopause.org *for updates to this information.*

Table 6. Transdermal Estrogen Therapy Products for Postmenopausal Use in the United States and Canada

Composition	Product name	Dosage, mg
17β-estradiol matrix patch	Alora[a]	0.025, 0.05, 0.075, 0.1 twice/wk
	Climara	0.025, 0.0375,[a] 0.05, 0.075, 0.1 once/wk
	Estradot[b]	0.025, 0.0375, 0.05, 0.075, 0.1 twice/wk
	Menostar[a]	0.014 once/wk (for osteoporosis therapy)
	Minivelle	0.0375, 0.05, 0.075, 0.1 twice/wk
	Oesclim[b]	0.025, 0.0375, 0.05, 0.075, 0.1 twice/wk
	Vivelle[a]	0.025, 0.0375, 0.05, 0.075, 0.1 twice/wk
	Vivelle-Dot[a]	0.025, 0.0375, 0.05, 0.075, 0.1 once or twice/wk
	Various generics	
17β-estradiol reservoir patch	Estraderm	0.025,[b] 0.05,[a] 0.1 twice/wk
17β-estradiol transdermal gel	Divigel	0.25, 0.5, 1/d
	EstroGel,[a] Estrogel[b]	0.75/d
	Elestrin[a]	0.52/d
17β-estradiol topical emulsion	Estrasorb[a]	0.05/d (2 packets)
17β-estradiol transdermal spray	Evamist[a]	0.021 mg per 90 μL spray/d (increase to 1.5 mg per 90 μL spray/d if needed)

Products not noted are available in the United States and in Canada.
a. Available in the United States but not Canada.
b. Available in Canada but not the United States.
Please visit the NAMS Web site at www.menopause.org for updates to this information.

been on the US market for more than 65 years, no generic equivalent has been government approved.

The standard CE oral dose has been 0.625 mg daily, based on bone protection studies.[57] Studies have shown that many women receive substantial benefit from lower doses (0.45 mg or 0.3 mg per day), although some women require higher doses for symptom relief and osteoporosis prevention.[58]

In a 10.7-year follow-up study after trial completion with ET-arm surviving participants, a decreased risk of breast cancer was seen in CE users compared with placebo, and more health benefits in general were seen in younger women.[59] However, findings from a 13-year follow-up from the Women's Health Initiative (WHI) do not support the use of ET for chronic disease prevention, even in younger women.[60]

Synthetic conjugated estrogens. Two types of synthetic SCE mixtures are available as oral tablets—SCE-A (with 9 estrogens) and SCE-B (with 10 estrogens). The SCE-A available in the United States is Cenestin (Congest, C.E.S., and PMS-Conjugated in Canada). The SCE-B is Enjuvia, available in the United States but not in Canada. The government does not view Cenestin or Enjuvia as generic equivalents to Premarin, although Enjuvia contains the primary 10 estrogens included in Premarin. In Canada, C.E.S. has been approved as a generic equivalent to Premarin since 1963, although at least 1 study shows that it is not bioequivalent.[61] No synthetic CE product is government approved for osteoporosis.

Estradiol. Initially, 17β-estradiol (or simply estradiol) could be administered only by injection because it was not absorbed from the GI tract. After micronization was developed, an oral product (Estrace) was marketed; various oral generics are also available. An oral EPT formulation approved in the United States (Activella) combines estradiol with norethindrone acetate. Subsequently, transdermal estradiol delivery systems were developed, including weekly and twice-weekly patches, gels (Divigel, Estrogel, Elestrin), a transdermal spray (Evamist), and a topical emulsion of estradiol hemihydrate (Estrasorb).[46] Transdermal EPT formulations combine estradiol with the progestins norethindrone acetate (Combipatch) or levonorgestrel (Climara Pro). Vaginal forms of estradiol are also available (Estrace Vaginal Cream, Estring Vaginal Ring), as well as the estradiol acetate vaginal ring (Femring) that exerts systemic effects and the estradiol hemihydrate vaginal tablet (Vagifem). Estradiol valerate is widely used in Europe, but it is available in the United States only in an injectable formulation not used for menopausal HT

Estradiol is the most widely used estrogen in Europe. It is the one estrogen available commercially in government-approved formulations that can be considered bioidentical.

PRESCRIPTION THERAPIES

As with lower doses of CE, numerous studies have used lower doses of oral and transdermal estradiol for the treatment of VMS and for the prevention of bone loss. Ultra-low-dose 0.25 mg oral micronized 17β-estradiol and 0.014 mg transdermal 17β-estradiol per day have also significantly increased spine and hip BMD compared with placebo.[62,63]

Ultra-low-dose 0.014 mg per day transdermal 17β-estradiol, a product approved for prevention of osteoporosis, has also been shown to be significantly more effective than placebo in reducing the frequency and severity of moderate and severe hot flashes, demonstrating that lower doses than were used in the past may be effective for many women.[64]

Esterified estrogens. Esterified estrogens (Menest in the United States; Neo-Estrone in Canada) are oral products of synthetic estrogen mixtures containing 75% to 85% sodium estrone sulfate. They are not indicated for osteoporosis.

Estropipate. Formerly called *piperazine estrone sulfate*, this is an oral form of estrone sulfate that has been solubi-

Table 7. Vaginal Estrogen Therapy Products for Postmenopausal Use in the United States and Canada

Composition	Product name	Dosage
Vaginal creams		
17β-estradiol[a]	Estrace Vaginal Cream[b]	Initial: 2-4 g/d for 1-2 wk Maintenance: 1g/1-3x/wk (0.1 mg active ingredient/g)
Conjugated estrogens[a]	Premarin Vaginal Cream	*For vaginal atrophy:* 0.5-2 g/d for 21 d then off 7 d[c] *For dyspareunia:* 0.5 g/d for 21 d then off 7 d, or twice/wk[c] (0.625 mg active ingredient/g)
Esterone	Estragyn Vaginal Cream[d]	2-4 g/d (1 mg active ingredient/g) adjusted to lowest amount that controls symptoms
Vaginal rings		
17β-estradiol	Estring	Device containing 2 mg releases 7.5 µg/d for 90 d (for vulvovaginal atrophy)
Estradiol acetate	Femring[b]	Device containing 12.4 mg or 24.8 mg estradiol acetate releases 0.05 mg/d or 0.10 mg/d estradiol for 90 days. Both doses release systemic levels for treatment of vulvovaginal atrophy and vasomotor symptoms (Progestogen recommended)
Vaginal tablet		
Estradiol hemihydrate	Vagifem	Initial: 1 tablet/d for 2 wk Maintenance: 1 tablet 2 x/wk (tablet containing 10 µg of estradiol hemihydrate equivalent to 10 µg of estradiol; for vaginal atrophy)

Products not noted are available in the United States and in Canada.
a. Higher doses of vaginal estrogen are systemic, meant to relieve hot flashes as well as vaginal atrophy; lower doses are intended for vaginal symptoms only even though a small amount does get absorbed.
b. Available in the United States but not Canada.
c. NAMS recommends using lowest effective dose, typically 0.5 g to 1 g per day, 2 to 3 times per week.
d. Available in Canada but not the United States.
Please visit the NAMS Web site at www.menopause.org for updates to this information.

Table 8. Combination Estrogen-Progestogen Therapy Products for Postmenopausal Use in the United States and Canada

Composition	Product name	Dosage/d
Oral continuous-cyclic regimen		
Conjugated estrogens (E) + medroxyprogesterone acetate (P)	Premphase[a]	0.625 mg E + 5.0 mg P (2 tablets: E and E + P) (E alone for days 1-14, followed by E + P on days 15-28)
Oral continuous-combined regimen		
Conjugated estrogens (E) + medroxyprogesterone acetate (P)	Prempro[a]	0.3 or 0.45 mg E + 1.5 mg P (1 tablet)
	Premplus[b]	0.625 mg E + 2.5 or 5.0 mg P (1 tablet)
Ethinyl estradiol (E) + norethindrone acetate (P)	Femhrt,[a] femHRT LO[b]	2.5 µg E + 0.5 mg P (1 tablet)
	Femhrt,[a] femHRT[b]	5 µg E + 1 mg P (1 tablet)
17β-estradiol (E) + norethindrone acetate (P)	Activella[a]	0.5 mg E + 0.1 mg P (1 tablet); 1 mg E + 0.5 mg P (1 tablet)
	Activelle LD[b]	0.5 mg E + 0.1 mg P (1 tablet)
	Activelle[b]	1 mg E + 0.5 mg P (1 tablet)
17β-estradiol (E) + drospirenone (P)	Angeliq	0.5 mg E + 0.25 mg P (1 tablet)[a] 1 mg E + 0.5 mg P (1 tablet)[a] 1 mg E + 1 mg P (1 tablet)[b]
Transdermal continuous-combined regimen		
17β-estradiol (E) + norethindrone acetate (P)	CombiPatch,[a] Estalis[b]	0.05 mg E + 0.14 mg P (9 cm² patch, twice/wk); 0.05 mg E + 0.25 mg P (16 cm² patch, twice/wk)
17β-estradiol (E) + levonorgestrel (P)	Climara Pro	0.045 mg E + 0.015 mg P (22 cm² patch, once/wk)

Products not noted are available in the United States and in Canada.
a. Available in the United States but not Canada.
b. Available in Canada but not the United States.
Please visit the NAMS Web site at www.menopause.org *for updates to this information.*

lized and stabilized by piperazine. It is marketed as Ogen in Canada but not in the United States and Ortho-Est in the United States but not in Canada, as well as in generic formulations. Ogen is approved for the prevention of postmenopausal osteoporosis.

Ethinyl estradiol. This synthetic steroid is widely used in combination contraceptives. It is also available in one oral EPT product (Femhrt in the United States, femHRT in Canada).

Sometimes an estrogen product is described as a *natural hormone*. The word *natural* is a marketing term used in many industries, including foods, in an attempt to convey that the product is safer than another product. Sometimes the term is used to describe an estrogen with a plant origin. There is no evidence that so-called natural estrogen products have greater efficacy or safety than other hormones.[55,65]

Measuring estrogen potency presents a challenge because estrogens vary in their dose equivalency and in their effects on various target tissues. Oral micronized estradiol 1.0 mg is equivalent to CE 0.625 mg with respect to effects on liver function, whereas 0.5 mg oral micronized estradiol produces changes in bone density equivalent to CE 0.625 mg

(Table 9). Very few head-to-head trials have compared different estrogens. Clinicians tend to view estrogen products as equivalent on a dose-for-dose basis, although data do not support this assumption; metabolic pathways and AEs can vary in general and from woman to woman. Like most medications, HT must always be tailored to the individual.

Routes of administration. For menopause-related therapy, estrogen can be administered orally, transdermally, topically, or vaginally. Intramuscular preparations are not recommended for menopause therapy because serum estrogen levels associated with injections rise to very high levels after administration.

Oral. Oral ET remains the most widely used formulation in North America. With all oral estrogen products, estrone will be the predominant estrogen in the circulation because of the first-pass uptake and metabolism in the GI tract and the liver.

The hepatic effect with oral ET results in greater stimulation of certain proteins compared with transdermal therapy, including lipoproteins such as high-density lipoprotein cholesterol (HDL-C). Oral estrogen is also associated with about a 25% increase in triglycerides, increasing the risk of pancreatitis in women who already have hypertriglyceridemia. Oral ET stimulates hepatic globulins, coagulation factors, and some inflammatory markers such as C-reactive protein and MMP-9, with possible implications for coronary heart disease (CHD).[66]

There also may be differences in glucose-insulin metabolism, but these data are less clear cut. Other important inflammatory markers, such as E-selectin, decrease with both modes of administration. The multicenter, case-control, Estrogen and Thromboembolism Risk trial suggested that oral ET but not transdermal ET is associated with an increase of VTE.[67,68] In a very large population-based study, participants receiving an estradiol transdermal system had a significantly lower incidence of VTE than participants receiving oral ET.[69] Oral HT but not low-dose transdermal HT increased the risk of stroke in one nested case-control observational study.[70]

The 4-year, multicenter Kronos Early Estrogen Prevention Study (KEEPS) of 727 healthy women within 3 years of menopause is the first and only randomized, placebo-controlled clinical trial that compared the differential effects of oral versus transdermal estrogen on various health outcomes. Stroke and VTE events were comparable across oral, transdermal, and placebo groups, although the study was not powered to identify differences in these clinical end points.[71]

Oral ET affects levels of endogenous sex hormones such as testosterone, SHBG, dehydroepiandrosterone (DHEA), and androstenedione. Exogenous oral estrogen increases SHBG, thereby decreasing free testosterone. Transdermal estradiol avoids the first-pass hepatic effect, so does not significantly affect levels of SHBG or free testosterone.

Table 9. Approximate Equivalent Estrogen Doses for Postmenopausal Use

Oral	
Conjugated estrogens	0.625 mg
Synthetic conjugated estrogens	0.625 mg
Esterified estrogens	0.625 mg
Estropipate (0.75 mg)	0.625 mg
Ethinyl estradiol	0.005 mg-0.015 mg
17β-estradiol	1.0 mg
Transdermal/Topical	
Estradiol patch	0.05 mg-0.1 mg
Estradiol gel	1.5 mg/2 metered doses
Vaginal	
Conjugated estrogens	0.3125 mg
17β-estradiol	0.5 mg

Transdermal/Topical. Estrogen delivered in these ways can be prescribed in lower doses than by oral administration because they are not dependent on GI absorption or subjected to first-pass hepatic metabolism. There is variation in absorption among transdermal and topical estrogens, depending on how the patches are applied and the carrier vehicle.

In contrast to oral ET, transdermal and topical administration of estrogen have the advantage of not increasing triglycerides but the disadvantage of not increasing HDL-C. Because of less liver exposure, transdermal and topical ET may have less of an AE on gallbladder disease and coagulation factors.

Transdermal patch ET is associated with relatively stable serum estradiol levels, unlike fluctuating serum levels found with oral estrogen. Thus, when stable estrogen levels are required, transdermal ET is a better choice than oral ET. These controlled-release methods of administration may also result in fewer migraines.

Estraderm was the first transdermal patch approved for use in the United States and Canada; it administered estradiol from a reservoir patch. Other transdermal patches are now available, each delivering estradiol from a matrix patch. Matrix patches are typically associated with less skin irritation than the older reservoir patches. Patch adhesives differ among product options. The spray, gel, and emulsion formulations have the advantage over patches in that they are less likely to cause skin irritation, but the gel and emulsion products have the disadvantage that skin-to-skin contact within 2 hours after application can lead to transfer of small amounts of estradiol. Also, sunscreen application shortly before applying transdermal and topical products may substantially increase estradiol exposure. When sunscreen is applied before the spray, there is no significant change in estradiol absorption or exposure. Use of sunscreen on the same area after application of transdermal estradiol has both increased and decreased estradiol absorption.

Vaginal. There are several different ways to deliver estrogen vaginally—creams, rings, and tablets (Table 7). Vaginal estrogen cream has been available for decades; the tablet and ring products are newer. Small amounts of estrogen administered locally are effective for treating vaginal atrophy. Labeling for vaginal estrogen products often includes the same warnings, contraindications, and AEs as labeling for systemic estrogen products, despite the fact that low-dose vaginal ET does not typically result in significant systemic estrogen levels.[72,73]

Except for the estradiol acetate vaginal ring (Femring), vaginal estrogens are not used for systemic effects (eg, hot flashes), although a 2005 Cochrane review found documentation of increases in serum estradiol levels from use of vaginal estrogen cream, tablets, and rings.[73] Estradiol levels were all in the postmenopausal range but varied according to the dose of the product. Women may notice breast tenderness when initiating therapy, suggesting low levels of systemic absorption; adjustments in dose may be needed. No significant differences among AEs were reported among the different methods of vaginal delivery.

Adding a progestogen to low-dose vaginal ET is not typically recommended. However, a progestogen is recommended with Femring or higher doses of other vaginal ET because of the increased risk of endometrial cancer.

A woman's individual needs and preferences should be the primary factors in determining the estrogen delivery route. In some women, medical factors may be the determinant (eg, vaginal administration to treat vaginal atrophy or transdermal administration for women with hypertriglyceridemia). Other factors include cost and insurance coverage.

Progestogen therapy

Progestogen therapy can be an option to treat hot flashes and other conditions of women at menopause and beyond, but its primary use in menopausal treatment is to reduce the risk of endometrial cancer associated with unopposed estrogen.[74]

Terminology. The term *progestogen* includes progesterone and the synthetic progestational compounds termed *progestins*, a wide range of hormones with the properties of the naturally occurring progesterone.

Progesterone. Progesterone is the steroid hormone produced by the ovary after ovulation and by the placenta during pregnancy. Exogenous progesterone is a compound identical to endogenous progesterone. It can be synthesized in the laboratory for therapeutic use, and it is available as progesterone in the *US Pharmacopeia* (ie, it meets the specifications of the USP). Relatively recent advances have allowed progesterone crystals to be micronized, resulting in improved oral absorption. Prometrium, also available in a generic formulation, is the only FDA-approved bioidentical progestogen. Before micronization, the rapid inactivation and poor bioavailability of orally administered progesterone led to the development in the 1950s of progestins.

Progestin. Progestins are synthetic products that have progesterone-like activity but are not identical to the progesterone produced in the human body. Progestins can be classified as those more closely resembling in chemical structure of either progesterone or testosterone (also called *19-nortestosterone derivatives*).

Progestins structurally related to progesterone are further classified into 2 groups:

- *Pregnane derivatives* (acetylated) MPA, megestrol acetate, cyproterone acetate, and chlormadinone acetate; and pregnane derivatives (nonacetylated) dydrogesterone and medrogestone

- *9-norpregnane derivatives* (acetylated) nomegestrol and nestorone; and 9-norpregnane derivatives (nonacetylated) demegestone, trimegestone, and promegestone

Progestins structurally related to testosterone are also further classified into 2 groups:

- *Ethinylated*, which include estranges, norethindrone (NET; also called norethisterone), norethindrone acetate (NETA), norethynodrel, lynestrenol, and ethynodiol diacetate, and 18-ethylgonanes LNG, norgestrel, desogestrel, gestodene, and norgestimate

- *Nonethinylated* dienogest and drospirenone

Progestins obtained from the plant-derived precursor diosgenin (found in the wild yam and soybean) should not be referred to as *natural* because they undergo multiple chemical reactions during synthesis in the laboratory. Wild yam added to a cream has no progesterone activity.

Mode of action. In the human, 2 progesterone receptor (PR) proteins, PR-α and PR-β, have been identified. Whether the available progestogen therapies preferentially bind to PR-α or PR-β is unclear. The primary actions of progestogens have been characterized in most detail in the uterus. In this target tissue, progestogens function primarily as antiestrogens, decreasing the number of nuclear ERs most likely through downregulation of ERs. In the endometrium, progestogens increase the activity of 17β-hydroxysteroid dehydrogenase, resulting in conversion of estradiol to estrone, a biologically weaker estrogen. These changes result in less estrogen-induced endometrial stimulation.

Progestogen products. A wide variety of progestogen types, modes of administration, and dosage regimens are available,

Prescription Therapies

Table 10. Progestogens Available in the United States and Canada

Composition	Product name	Dosage/d
Oral tablet: progestin		
Medroxyprogesterone acetate	Provera, various generics	2.5 mg, 5 mg, 10 mg
Norethindrone	Micronor,[a] Nor-QD,[a,b] various generics	0.35 mg
Norethindrone acetate	Aygestin,[a,b] various generics	5 mg
Megestrol acetate	Megace,[a] various generics	20 mg,[b] 40 mg, 40-mg suspension
Oral capsule: progesterone		
Micronized progesterone (in peanut oil)	Prometrium, generic	100 mg, 200 mg[b]
Intrauterine system: progestin		
Levonorgestrel	Mirena[a]	20 µg/d approximate release rate (52 mg for 5-y use)
	Skyla[a]	6 µg/d release rate (13.5 mg for 3-y use)
Vaginal gel: progesterone		
Progesterone	Crinone[a] 4%,[b] 8%	45- or 90-mg applicator
Vaginal insert: progesterone		
Micronized progesterone	Endometrin[a]	100-mg insert

a. Not approved by FDA for menopausal hormone therapy.
b. Available in the United States but not Canada.
Please visit the NAMS Web site at www.menopause.org *for updates to this information.*

each having distinct AEs as well as different actions on the endometrium and other organ systems (Table 10). Very few clinical trials have evaluated the relative potencies of progestogens.

All government-approved progestogen formulations will provide endometrial protection if the dose and duration are adequate. Combined EPT products are available. Although these are convenient, and many women prefer to take one pill or use one patch, they do reduce dosing flexibility. All combined EPT products in the United States and in Canada are government approved for postmenopausal use (Table 8) and include endometrial protection.

The progestogen product most structurally related to progesterone is Prometrium. Generally speaking, progestins structurally related to testosterone are more potent than those related to progesterone and MPA.

Government approval of progestogen products to oppose menopausal ET is relatively recent, although progestogens have been used off label for this indication for decades. The most commonly used progestogen formulation for endometrial protection among US women is the oral progestin MPA, either alone or in combination with CE. It is also the most widely studied progestogen for postmenopausal use. Other progestins are combined with other estrogens in several oral and transdermal EPT products.

Low doses of transdermal progestogens should have metabolic advantages over higher doses of oral therapy because they avoid the first-pass hepatic effect; however, data on this are limited.

Anecdotal data and results from the Postmenopausal Estrogen/Progestin Interventions (PEPI) trial suggest that women who experience AEs, especially mood changes, with a synthetic progestin sometimes respond more favorably to progesterone.[75] Before the late 1990s, North American women seeking progesterone products had to rely on custom-compounded formulations. Prometrium, an oral capsule containing micronized progesterone, was first approved in Canada, then by the US government. Prometrium should never be used by a woman allergic to peanuts because the active ingredient is suspended in peanut oil. In addition, a small percentage of women may experience extreme dizziness or drowsiness during initial therapy, so women should use caution when driving or operating machinery. Bedtime dosing is advised. Some women report improved sleep with use of this product.[76]

Micronized progesterone formulations (cream, lotion, gel, oral capsule, suppositories) are also available by prescription through custom-compounding pharmacies.

It is important to note that topical cream or gel preparations with progesterone, obtained either OTC or custom compounded from a prescription, may not exert sufficient activity to protect the endometrium from unopposed estrogen. These products should not be used for this purpose until optimum therapeutic doses for the various formulations are established.

Because vaginal administration at typical doses avoids systemic effects, vaginal progestogen is an attractive option. The vaginal bioadhesive gel containing 4% or 8% micronized progesterone provides sustained and controlled delivery of progesterone to the vaginal tissue. In a trial using cyclic administration of the gel in women with secondary amenorrhea, no hyperplasia was observed after 3 months.[77] A 100-mg progesterone vaginal insert has been approved for luteal phase support for assisted reproductive technology but not for EPT, but some practitioners use it off label for vaginal progestogen.

The use of a progestin-releasing IUS to protect the endometrium is appealing because it delivers the progestin in the highest concentration precisely where it is needed. Mirena, a progestogen-containing IUS available in the United States and Canada, is not government approved for endometrial protection, although there are small studies suggesting that it is effective. There is some systemic absorption of LNG with Mirena. Its relatively low dose (20 µg/d) and 5-year life span make it an attractive alternative for perimenopausal women. The 3-year Skyla is lower dose (6 µg/d), smaller, and might be easier to insert for a postmenopausal uterus, but there are no data on its endometrial protection.

Estrogen-progestogen therapy
Many regimens are used when prescribing EPT, and descriptive terminology is often inconsistent. The clinical goal of these EPT regimens is to provide uterine protection, maintain estrogen benefits, and minimize AEs (particularly uterine bleeding, which is annoying to many women and often reduces compliance), although there is no consensus on how to accomplish this goal. Regimens may be classified as continuous-cyclic sequential, continuous cyclic long-cycle, and continuous-combined (Table 11).

Continuous-cyclic (sequential) estrogen-progestogen therapy. In this regimen, estrogen is used every day with progestogen added cyclically for 12 to 14 days during each month. The combination oral EPT product Premphase uses a sequential regimen of estrogen for 14 days followed by estrogen and progestin for 14 days, similar to OCs. In a typical continuous-cyclic regimen, progestogen is started on the first or fifteenth day of the month. Starting the first day of the month makes it easier for some women to track their uterine bleeding because the cycle day corresponds with the day of the month.

If women are on standard doses of estrogen (0.625 mg/d CE or 1 mg/d of micronized estradiol), uterine bleeding occurs in about 80% of women when the progestogen is withdrawn, although it sometimes starts 1 or 2 days earlier, depending on the dose and type of progestogen used.

Table 11. Estrogen-Progestogen Therapy Regimens, Terminology

Regimen	Estrogen	Progestogen
Continuous-cyclic (sequential)	Daily	12-14 d/mo
Continuous-cyclic (sequential) long cycle	Daily	14 d q 2-6 mo
Continuous-combined	Daily	Daily

Continuous-cyclic (sequential) long-cycle estrogen progestogen therapy. To lessen the exposure to progestogen and the incidence of uterine bleeding, a modified continuous-cyclic EPT regimen of daily estrogen with cyclic progestogen (eg, 12 mg/d MPA for 14 d/mo) added every 2 to 6 months has been evaluated. Although this regimen reduces the number of withdrawal bleeding episodes, it has resulted in heavier and longer bleeding episodes. The effect on endometrial protection is undetermined. Two studies did not find evidence of endometrial hyperplasia after 1 year in women using estrogen at standard (0.625 mg/d CE) or one-half standard (0.3 mg/d CE) doses with MPA administered either quarterly or every 6 months.[78,79] However, the Scandinavian Long Cycle Study, which used 2 mg per day of 17β-estradiol (twice the standard dose) with a progestin administered quarterly, was stopped after 3 of 5 scheduled years because of an increased incidence of hyperplasia compared with a monthly progestogen regimen.[80]

Until more data are available, the continuous-cyclic (sequential) long-cycle regimen is not recommended as standard therapy when using standard doses of estrogen (0.625 mg/d CE or 1 mg/d micronized estradiol). If prescribed, endometrial monitoring is mandatory. Some clinicians use the high negative-predictive value of a thin, distinct endometrial echo on transvaginal ultrasound in women who wish to pursue such a regimen. Many clinicians are using this regimen with low or ultra-low-dose estrogens, but careful monitoring of the endometrium is advised.

Continuous-combined estrogen-progestogen therapy. These regimens were developed to address the withdrawal uterine bleeding, which is a major reason for discontinuing EPT. In this regimen, a woman uses estrogen and progestogen every day. Within several months, the endometrium can become atrophic, and amenorrhea results.

Rates of endometrial hyperplasia are low, generally less than 1% in women using continuous-combined EPT preparations, based on short-term studies (usually no longer than 1 y). Such studies are not considered long enough to assess endometrial cancer risk. The continuous-combined regimen has been the predominant regimen used in North America.

Clinical goal of estrogen-progestogen therapy. The clinical goal of progestogen in EPT is to provide endometrial protection while maintaining estrogen benefits and minimizing unwanted progestogen-induced effects, as well as minimizing progestogen exposure. Research is insufficient to recommend 1 regimen over another.[55]

For the postmenopausal woman using systemic ET, adding progestogen therapy to ET reduces the risk of endometrial cancer induced by ET to the level found in women not taking hormones. Data from the PEPI trial showed that women who used unopposed ET during the 3-year trial had a significantly increased risk of hyperplasia (34%), whereas those using EPT had a risk of only 1%.[81] A Cochrane review reports that the addition of oral progestin to ET, administered as either continuous-cyclic or continuous-combined, is associated with reduced rates of hyperplasia.[82] Cyclic progesterone added to ET also has been shown to inhibit the development of endometrial hyperplasia. In the PEPI trial, combining CE (0.625 mg/d) with progesterone (200 mg/d for 12 d/mo) over a 3-year follow-up did not produce an increase in endometrial hyperplasia compared with placebo. Progestogen does not eliminate endometrial cancer risk because there is a risk independent of hormone use.

It has been suggested that continuous-combined EPT may be less protective than continuous-cyclic EPT, because the endometrium is not shed on a regular basis and the continuous progestogen may completely downregulate PRs, rendering them ineffective. However, epidemiologic studies of continuous-combined EPT indicate no increased risk and may even suggest some added protection against endometrial cancer.[83] A cohort study in more than 200,000 women in Finland compared the risk of endometrial cancer in HT users for at least 6 months with that in the general population.[84] The use of continuous-combined EPT for at least 3 years was associated with a 76% reduction in endometrial cancer. The use of sequential EPT for at least 5 years was associated with varying degrees of increased risk, depending on the progestogen interval used.

Studies have provided data regarding the necessary dose and duration of the progestogen course to oppose the estrogen-induced risk of endometrial hyperplasia and adenocarcinoma (Table 12). A progestin-containing IUD and a progesterone vaginal gel offer other possible options for endometrial protection, although long-term efficacy data and FDA approval are lacking regarding endometrial cancer protection.[85]

Uterine bleeding with estrogen-progestogen therapy. Various regimens have been designed to decrease bleeding during use of HT. Two types of bleeding are commonly seen:

- Withdrawal uterine bleeding: Bleeding that results from progestogen cessation (or withdrawal)

- Breakthrough uterine bleeding: Irregular bleeding that may occur with regimens using continuous progestogen

Breakthrough uterine bleeding has been observed in 40% of women on a continuous-combined regimen during the first 3 to 6 months. The probability of achieving amenorrhea is greater if EPT is started 12 months or more after menopause; women who are recently postmenopausal exhibit more breakthrough bleeding. Because of this observation, some clinicians start with a cyclic regimen for 1 year and then switch to continuous combined EPT. Most (75%-89%) women who start with continuous-combined therapy become amenorrheic within 12 months. However, irregular bleeding may persist intermittently for months or years. Persistent breakthrough bleeding with continuous-combined EPT may necessitate switching to another regimen.

A study comparing 2 continuous-combined regimens—CE 0.625 mg plus MPA 2.5 mg per day and 17β-estradiol 1 mg plus NETA 0.5 mg per day—found that within 3 months, 71.4% of the estradiol-NETA users experienced amenorrhea compared with 40.0% of the CE-MPA users, but after 6 months, the differences were not statistically significant.[86] This study confirmed other findings that recently postmenopausal women (within 1-2 y of last menses) experienced more breakthrough bleeding than women more than 3 years postmenopausal. Treatment with one of the 19-nortestosterone derivatives (NET, NETA, LNG, norgestimate) or oral micronized progesterone tends to produce less breakthrough uterine bleeding during the first few months of use.

In women using EPT beyond 2 years, those using a continuous-combined regimen have a lower rate of breakthrough uterine bleeding and fewer endometrial biopsies than those using the cyclic regimen.

Extrauterine effects of progestogens. Progestogens exhibit effects on organ systems other than the endometrium. These effects vary depending on the progestogen type, dose, route of administration, and the EPT regimen.

On the basis of clinical trial data showing significantly increased risks, no EPT (or ET) regimen should be initiated for the primary or secondary prevention of cardiovascular disease (CVD).[87,88] However, some observational studies have shown that ET has beneficial effects on atherosclerosis, vasodilation, plasma lipids, arterial response to injury, and insulin sensitivity. Adding some progestogens may diminish these beneficial effects, but they generally do not eliminate them. All progestogens negate the beneficial effect of estrogen on blood flow. Selecting a metabolically neutral progestogen such as micronized progesterone or norgestimate for EPT is recommended to maintain higher plasma levels of HDL-C. In animal studies, progestins with a higher androgenic potency reduce more of the beneficial effects of estrogens on vasodilation; progesterone and 19-norpregnane derivatives have less of an AE profile. These beneficial endpoints do not outweigh the overall lack of CVD benefit reported in randomized, controlled trials (RCTs).

For women with type 2 diabetes mellitus (DM) who are using EPT to treat acute menopause symptoms, continuous-cyclic EPT regimens are recommended to minimize progestogen exposure; low-dose oral micronized progesterone

Chapter 8

Table 12. Minimum Progestogen Dosing Requirements for Endometrial Protection With Standard Estrogen Dosing

	Continuous-cyclic EPT (daily, 12-14 d/mo)	Continuous-combined EPT (daily)
Oral tablets		
Medroxyprogesterone acetate	5 mg	2.5 mg
Norethindrone	0.35 mg-0.7 mg	0.35 mg
Norethindrone acetate	2.5 mg	0.5 mg-1 mg
Micronized progesterone	200 mg	100 mg
Intrauterine system		
Levonorgestrel[a]	–	20 µg/d or 6 µg/d
Vaginal		
Progesterone gel[a]	45 mg	45 mg

Standard estrogen dosing is 0.625 mg conjugated estrogens, 1 mg oral estradiol, 0.05 mg patch, or the equivalent.
Abbreviation: EPT, estrogen-progestogen therapy.
a. Not FDA-approved for endometrial protection with estrogen therapy.

is also recommended. Transdermal ET may offer advantages over the oral route in that serum triglycerides and other thrombotic factors are not increased further in patients with DM.

Progestogen has limited effect on the bone-enhancing action of ET. Although adding 2.5 mg MPA or 1 mg NETA to ET slightly enhances estrogen's ability to prevent BMD loss in early postmenopausal women, estrogen alone is adequate to maintain BMD. Estrogen-progestogen therapy reduces spine and hip fractures, but the role of progestogen in this effect is not known. The decision to add progestogen to ET should not be based on its skeletal effect.

Breast cancer risk is not decreased when progestogen is added to ET, and data indicate an increased risk with standard doses.[89-91] Mammographic density is increased with progestogen use, although this effect will reverse with discontinuation. Breast discomfort and pain may increase with progestogen use.[92] It is not clear whether there is a class effect from progestogen or whether a certain type of progestogen can influence breast cancer risk. In a large case-control study from France, micronized progesterone was not associated with an elevated risk as opposed to combinations using MPA or NETA.[93] Another case-control study showed no increase in breast cancer with micronized progesterone compared with an increase with other progestogens and a higher risk with combined-continuous regimens versus sequential regimens. The study has significant limitations because of confounding by socioeconomic status and the usual healthy-user bias. The differential effects of progestogens on breast cancer require further confirmation.[94]

Some progestogens may negatively affect mood, particularly in women with a history of mood disorders. Data are inadequate to recommend specific progestogens or EPT regimens for minimal AEs. In general, the AEs of added progestogen are mild, although they may be severe in a small percentage of women.

These findings have resulted in the discussion of prescribing less progestogen or even unopposed ET for women with an intact uterus. However, there is insufficient evidence regarding endometrial safety to recommend long-cycle progestogen (ie, progestogen for 12-14 d/3-6 mo), and there is clear evidence of endometrial cancer risk with use of unopposed estrogen. Using lower doses of estrogen should decrease the risk of endometrial cancer and allow for lower doses of progestogen.[55]

In 2013, FDA approved a new medication called a *tissue-selective estrogen complex* (TSEC), which pairs bazedoxifene (BZA) 20 mg, a novel selective ER modulator, with CE 45 mg for the treatment of moderate to severe VMS and for the prevention of osteoporosis in postmenopausal women with a uterus.[95] Endometrial safety was comparable to placebo, with cumulative amenorrhea of more than 83%, similar to placebo. This will offer women another option instead of using EPT.[96,97]

Estrogen therapy and estrogen-progestogen therapy contraindications and warnings. The package insert list of ET and EPT contraindications is the same for all HT products, whether their effects are systemic or local (Table 13). Not all experts agree that low-dose vaginal ET is contraindicated in all these situations. If in doubt, refer to current product labeling before prescribing any hormone regimen.

Systemic and local ET and EPT products marketed in the United States have "class labeling," which includes a boxed warning (indicating that the warning is significant) that ET

Prescription

Table 13. Contraindications for Estrogen Therapy or Estrogen-Progestogen Therapy

- Undiagnosed abnormal genital bleeding
- Known, suspected, or history of breast cancer
- Known or suspected estrogen-dependent neoplasia
- Active or history of deep vein thrombosis, pulmonary embolism
- Active or history of arterial thromboembolic disease (eg, stroke, myocardial infarction)
- Liver dysfunction or disease
- Known or suspected pregnancy
- Known hypersensitivity to ET or EPT

Abbreviations: EPT, estrogen-progestogen therapy; ET, estrogen therapy.

increases the risk of endometrial cancer. Progestogen is advised when prescribing systemic ET for women with an intact uterus.

In the boxed warning of all systemic ET and EPT products (and some local ET products), the government requires the notation that the WHI found increased risks of stroke and deep vein thrombosis. The label further states that ET or EPT should not be used for the prevention of CVD or dementia. Also noted is that the WHI Memory Study, a substudy of the WHI, reported an increased risk of developing probable dementia in postmenopausal women aged 65 years or older during 5.2 years of treatment with oral CE (0.625 mg/d) alone and during 4 years of treatment with oral CE (0.625 mg/d) combined with MPA (2.5 mg/d) relative to placebo. It is unknown whether this finding applies to younger women.[98,99]

The labeling also states that other doses of CE and MPA and other combinations and dosage forms of ET and EPT were not studied in the WHI and that in the absence of comparable data, these risks should be assumed to be similar. Because of these risks, ET and EPT should be prescribed at the lowest effective doses and for the shortest duration consistent with treatment goals and risks for the individual woman. Close clinical surveillance of all women using ET or EPT is important and should include endometrial sampling when indicated. There is no evidence that the use of compounded ET or EPT formulations will result in a different risk profile than FDA-approved ET and EPT formulations of equivalent dose.

Although not in the boxed warning, labeling also warns of an increased risk of breast cancer with ET and EPT. Refer to labeling for additional warnings for various ET and EPT products before prescribing.

Estrogen therapy and estrogen-progestogen adverse events. A number of AEs are associated with ET and EPT (Table 14), although these vary depending on route of administration, type of progestogen, and dose (see labeling for specific products before prescribing). Although not life threatening, these AEs have a negative effect on quality of life (QOL) and often lead to discontinuation of therapy.

Women using EPT often experience uterine bleeding. Some women regard this EPT-induced bleeding as an unacceptable nuisance, although the bleeding often decreases or stops over time. Adjusting doses and evaluating for other causes of bleeding is indicated. In studies using ultra-low-dose EPT (0.30 mg-0.45 mg CE or equivalent), bleeding is a less common AE.

In some women, EPT causes fluid retention in the hands and feet or abdominal bloating with gaseous distention. A few women experience GI irritation and nausea from oral EPT administration. An analysis from the Nurses' Health Study showed that the risk of gastroesophageal reflux symptoms significantly increased with increasing dose and length of exposure to HT.[100] A prospective cohort study involving 31,494 postmenopausal women from the Swedish Mammography Cohort found that HT was associated with an increase in acute pancreatitis.[101]

Scientific evidence has found no association of HT or menopause with weight gain.[55]

The most common AE of transdermal-patch ET or EPT is skin irritation at the patch application site. This can sometimes be alleviated by rotating the patch, putting it on the buttock, and ensuring that the site is very clean. Using OTC hydrocortisone cream can help, as well as switching to a different ET or EPT patch that may have a different type of adhesive that will not be as irritating. Using talcum powder around the patch edge can prevent formation of dirt rings (dirt rings can be cleaned with mineral oil).

Table 14. Potential Adverse Events of Estrogen Therapy or Estrogen-Progestogen Therapy

- Uterine bleeding (starting or returning)
- Breast tenderness (sometimes enlargement)
- Nausea
- Abdominal bloating
- Fluid retention in extremities
- Changes in the shape of the cornea (sometimes leading to contact lens intolerance)
- Headache (including migraine)
- Dizziness
- Mood changes with EPT

Abbreviation: EPT, estrogen-progestogen therapy.

the vaginal estrogen ring is generally well tolerated, headache, abdominal pain, and vaginal pain, irritation, and erosion have been reported. If the ring falls out, it can be rinsed off and reinserted. The ring does not usually interfere with sexual intercourse, although it can be removed before intercourse if it is uncomfortable for either partner.

Estrogen vaginal creams are considered messy by some women. There are anecdotal reports of estrogen absorption by the male partner during sexual intercourse, leading to gynecomastia. Estrogen cream should not be used as a lubricant at the time of intercourse.

Estrogens are partly metabolized by CYP-450 3A4. Inducers of 3A4, such as St. John's wort, rifampin, or carbamazepine, may decrease estrogen concentrations and thus its effectiveness, whereas inhibitors such as itraconazole and clarithromycin may increase estrogen concentrations and its AEs.

A number of strategies exist for dealing with other AEs of ET and EPT (Table 15). Although there is limited scientific evidence to support these tips, clinical experience has determined that they are helpful in some women.

An important principle to keep in mind when prescribing HT, and especially when managing AEs, is that each woman is an individual with her own psychology and physiology. Each woman should be advised that it may take time to find the best regimen for her and that regular reevaluation with attempts to taper the dose are important. Sometimes it may take more than 1 or 2 products or regimens to find the appropriate one for an individual. A certain amount of the search is trial and error.

Women should be counseled not to expect immediate results. Clinical data suggest that relief of VMS with low-dose ET or EPT is not fully evident until 8 to 12 weeks of use. Setting realistic expectations about outcomes with scientific support will help prevent disappointment.

Timing of initiation. The WHI designers did not expect the timing of HT initiation to affect the results. That concept was not appreciated when the trial was planned. Post hoc analyses revealed that the timing of HT initiation in naturally menopausal women is important.[102] For example, the absolute risk of CHD was lower in the younger, recently postmenopausal women in the WHI than in the older group.

In the WHI, heart attack risk increased during the first year of EPT use in older women but not in younger women. Many experts believe that HT may have beneficial effects in women whose arteries are still healthy, regardless of age. However, a WHI report that included combined data from the RCT and the observational study did not find that CHD risks varied by the timing of HT initiation.[55,103]

The 13-year comprehensive analysis of the WHI reported that women aged 50 to 59 years in the ET-alone arm had significantly more favorable all-cause mortality and fewer myocardial infarctions. But the overall risks and benefits from both trials do not support the use of HT for chronic disease prevention.[60] KEEPS did not find a CHD benefit.[71]

Table 15. Coping Strategies for Estrogen Therapy or Estrogen-Progestogen Therapy Adverse Events

Adverse effect	Strategy
Fluid retention	Restrict salt; maintain adequate water intake; exercise; try a mild prescription diuretic.
Bloating	Switch to low-dose nonoral continuous estrogen; lower progestogen dose to a level that still protects the uterus; switch to another progestin or to micronized progesterone.
Breast tenderness	Lower estrogen dose; switch to another estrogen; restrict salt; switch to another progestin; cut down on caffeine and chocolate.
Headaches	Switch to nonoral continuous estrogen; lower dose of estrogen or progestogen or both; switch to a continuous-combined regimen; switch to progesterone or a 19-norpregnane derivative; ensure adequate water intake; restrict salt, caffeine, and alcohol.
Mood changes	Investigate preexisting depression or anxiety; lower progestogen dose; switch progestogen; switch from systemic progestin to the progestin intrauterine system; change to a continuous-combined EPT regimen; ensure adequate water intake; restrict salt, caffeine, and alcohol.
Nausea	Advise taking oral estrogen tablets with meals or before bed; switch to another oral estrogen; switch to nonoral estrogen; lower estrogen or progestogen dose.

Abbreviation: EPT, estrogen-progestogen therapy.

The ongoing Early Versus Late Intervention Trial With Estradiol (ELITE) being conducted by the National Institute on Aging is evaluating whether the timing of ET initiation reduces subclinical atherosclerosis progression and cognitive decline in 2 populations of women: those less than 1 year and those more than 10 years postmenopause. Future studies, with hypotheses guided by the results of previous trials of HT, have the potential to create a new paradigm for the primary prevention of CHD disease in women.[104] However, a comprehensive review of the timing hypothesis states that data are both supportive and not supportive of this hypothesis, but the finding of fewer AEs in younger women further supports the safety of HT for symptomatic women in the perimenopausal transition and early stages of menopause.[105]

On the basis of the evidence, NAMS is not recommending HT be used solely for coronary protection in women of any age. Initiation of HT in women aged 50 to 59 years or in those within 10 years of menopause to treat menopausal symptoms does not seem to increase the risk of CHD events.[55]

In reviewing the data on the effect of HT on stroke risk, ET and EPT seem to increase the risk of ischemic stroke in postmenopausal women, but clinical trial data are not consistent in this finding. For the women in the WHI, there were 8 additional strokes per 10,000 women per year in the EPT arm (oral CE plus MPA) and 12 additional strokes per 10,000 women per year in the ET arm (oral CE) compared with placebo. In the Nurses' Health Study, the absolute risk of stroke, however, was lower in women aged 50 to 59 years (1 additional stroke/10,000 women/y of ET) or within 5 years of menopause (3 additional strokes/10,000 women/y of EPT) than in older women more distant from menopause.[106] No studies indicate that HT is effective for reducing the risk of stroke in women with CVD or for prevention of a first stroke, and it may actually increase the rate of first strokes in women aged older than 60 years starting HT. Although stroke was not increased in the group of women aged 50 to 59 years in the combined analysis of the WHI, it almost doubled in the EPT group that was less than 10 years since menopause.

Premature menopause (age <40 y) and primary ovarian insufficiency are conditions associated with a lower risk of breast cancer and earlier onset of osteoporosis and CHD, but there are no conclusive data as to whether ET or EPT will affect morbidity or mortality from these conditions. The risk-benefit ratio for younger women who initiate therapy at an early age may be more favorable but is unknown. The data for women experiencing menopause at the median age (51.3 y) should not be extrapolated to these younger women. If there are no contraindications, NAMS recommends the use of HT or oral contraceptives until the median age of natural menopause in women with primary ovarian insufficiency or premature menopause, with annual reevaluation.[55]

Weighing benefits and risks. After the July 2002 announcement of the first WHI results with CE plus MPA in predominantly asymptomatic postmenopausal women (mean age, 63 y), use of all systemic HT for any indication declined significantly, no doubt because clinicians and their patients were concerned about the risks identified in this study and the fact that HT was not demonstrated to be the preventive therapy people were expecting. Since that time, different methods of analyzing these data and information from other trials have softened some of the concerns. In addition, lower-dose products are available that may offer similar benefits with fewer risks.

Leading healthcare organizations support the use of HT in appropriate situations.[107] Use of HT should be consistent with treatment goals, benefits, and risks for the individual woman, taking into account cause of menopause, time since menopause, symptoms, and domains (such as sexuality and sleep) that may have an effect on QOL and the underlying risk of CVD, stroke, VTE, DM, and other conditions.[55,107]

It may be helpful when reviewing risks with women considering HT to put them into perspective. Overall, these risks are rare (<1 event/1,000 women/y) and even rarer when initiated in women aged younger than 60 years or within 10 years of menopause. Understanding risk is crucial in counseling and educating women about the role of HT and individualizing therapy.

The effects of ET or EPT on risks of breast cancer, CHD, stroke, total CVD, and osteoporotic fracture in perimenopausal women with moderate to severe menopause symptoms have not been established in clinical trials. The findings from trials in different populations should, therefore, be extrapolated with caution. No HT regimen should be used for primary or secondary prevention of CVD or stroke, and HT should be avoided in women who have an elevated risk for stroke.

Lower-than-standard doses of HT should be considered (ie, daily doses of 0.3 mg oral CE or the equivalent). Different estrogens, progestogens, and routes of administration offer potential advantages for some women. In the absence of clinical trial data for each estrogen and progestogen, clinical trial results for 1 agent can be generalized to all agents within the same family. Custom-compounded HT products are not advised. Women being prescribed these products need to be informed of the potential risks and limited data available on efficacy, safety, and bioavailability.

There is strong evidence that ET and EPT reduce the risk of postmenopausal fracture with long-term treatment. In the WHI, daily 0.625 mg oral CE with or without 5 mg MPA was used; fracture protection with other HT or in lower doses still remains to be determined. For women who require drug therapy for prevention of osteoporosis (including women at high risk of fracture during the next 5-10 y), HT can be considered as an option. The risks and benefits of HT, as well as those of other government-approved therapies, must be weighed. No HT products have been approved by FDA for treatment of osteoporosis, only for prevention.

Extended use of the lowest effective dose of systemic HT is acceptable under the following circumstances, provided that the woman is well aware of the potential risks and benefits and that there is clinical supervision:

- In the woman for whom, in her opinion, the benefits of menopause symptom relief outweigh risks, preferably after an attempt to stop HT has failed.
- In women who are at high risk of osteoporotic fracture and also have moderate to severe menopause symptoms.
- For further prevention of bone loss in the woman with established reduction in bone mass when alternate therapies are not appropriate for that woman, or cause AEs, or when the outcomes of the extended use of alternate therapies are unknown.

When considering HT, various modes of administration are associated with different pros and cons (Table 16).

When a decision is made to discontinue systemic HT, there are scarce data to inform the choice of abrupt cessation versus tapering the dose. In a Swedish trial of 81 women, there was no difference in the number or severity of hot flashes, QOL, or resumption of HT over 3 months, regardless of mode of cessation.[108] There seems to be little difference in terms of return of menopause symptoms. Approximately 50% of women experience a recurrence of symptoms when therapy is discontinued, independent of age and duration of HT use.[109] The decision to continue HT should be individualized on the basis of severity of symptoms and risk-benefit ratio considerations, provided that the woman (in consultation with her healthcare professional) believes that continuation of therapy is warranted.

Low-dose vaginal ET is generally recommended for postmenopausal women whose only menopause-related symptom is vaginal atrophy. For symptomatic vaginal atrophy that does not respond to nonhormonal vaginal lubricants and moisturizers, low-dose vaginal ET is effective and well tolerated, and systemic absorption is limited. Progestogen is generally not indicated, but endometrial safety data do not extend beyond 1 year. Low-dose, local ET should be continued so long as distressing vaginal symptoms remain. For women treated for nonhormone-dependent cancer, management of vaginal atrophy is similar to that for women without a cancer history. For women with a history of hormone-dependent cancer, management recommendations depend on each woman's preference in consultation with her oncologist.[72]

Monitoring therapy. Clinical monitoring of women using HT includes ongoing evaluation for potential AEs. At least yearly return visits are recommended, during which time the woman and her clinician should review the decision to use HT, including a discussion of any new research findings. More frequent visits may be required, especially for women just starting HT or for those having bothersome AEs. Regular mammography is indicated. Endometrial surveillance is not required for women using systemic ET and adequate progestogen. Data are insufficient to recommend annual endometrial surveillance in asymptomatic women using low-dose vaginal ET for the treatment of vaginal atrophy. If a woman is at high risk for endometrial cancer, using a higher dose of vaginal ET, or is having symptoms (spotting, breakthrough bleeding), endometrial evaluation may be required. The clinical goal is to use the lowest effective HT dose for the shortest time consistent with treatment goals.

Bioidentical hormone therapy

The term *bioidentical hormone therapy* means different things to different people. To some scientists and healthcare professionals, bioidentical hormones are those that are chemically identical to the hormones produced by women (primarily in the ovaries) during their reproductive years. To others, the term *bioidentical* is used to refer to compounded HT that is not manufactured by a commercial pharmaceutical company but rather made for a particular patient by a compounding pharmacy. FDA has stated that the term *bioidentical hormone replacement therapy* is a marketing term not recognized by FDA.[110] NAMS uses the term *bioidentical hormones* to refer to all hormones that are chemically identical to those made in the human body.

A woman's body makes various estrogens (such as 17β-estradiol, estrone, and estriol) as well as progesterone, testosterone, and other hormones. Thus, bioidentical HT can mean a medication that provides 1 or more of these hormones as the active ingredient.[111]

Some well-tested, government-approved, brand-name prescription hormones meet the definition of bioidentical. Several government-approved drugs in the United States and Canada contain 17β-estradiol, and those that are not taken orally remain in the body as 17β-estradiol. These include pills, patches, topical gels, sprays, and a vaginal ring. There also are government-approved progesterone products, such as oral capsules, 4% and 8% vaginal gels, and a vaginal insert, that meet the definition of bioidentical.

Compounded hormone formulations

For decades, pharmacists have compounded various drug formulations for individual patients as prescribed by their clinicians. Compounding of HT allows individualized dosing and combinations of therapy, depending on the prescribing physician's and a woman's preference or tolerance. It also allows for different modes of administration of hormones, including subdermal implants, sublingual tablets, rectal suppositories, and nasal sprays. Products can be prepared without the binders, fillers, dyes, preservatives, or adhesives that are found in patented, commercially available products. To a large extent, compounding was intended for the patient whose needs were not being met by FDA-approved products.

Table 16. Pros and Cons of Hormone Therapy Routes of Administration

Oral estrogen

Pros

- Familiar, easy
- Beneficial effect on HDL-C, LDL-C, and total cholesterol
- Large amount of data
- Usually relatively low cost

Cons

- Risk of thrombosis, stroke
- Increase in triglycerides, C-reactive protein, SHBG, thyroid binding globulin, other hepatic proteins
- Decreased free testosterone secondary to increased SHBG

Transdermal or topical estrogen

Pros

- Avoids hepatic first-pass effect
- Less increase of triglycerides than oral ET
- Less effect on C-reactive protein than oral ET
- Fewer GI AEs than oral ET
- Perhaps less risk of venous thrombosis than with oral ET

Cons

- Patch-adhesive sensitivity/residue
- Patch is visible
- Usually relatively higher cost
- Gels, creams can possibly transfer to others

Vaginal (local) estrogen

Pros

- Vaginal benefit at lower dose
- Low-dose therapy typically avoids adverse systemic effects

Cons

- Increase in vaginal discharge
- Some may consider less convenient to use
- Lack of long-term uterine safety data for low-dose products

Progestogens

Pros

- Reduced risk of endometrial hyperplasia and cancer in women with a uterus using ET
- Progesterone dosed at night can decrease insomnia, improve sleep

Cons

- EPT associated with greater risk of breast cancer than ET
- Some progestogens reduce beneficial effect of oral estrogen on HDL-C
- Bloating
- Dysphoric effect for some women

Abbreviations: AEs, adverse events; ET, estrogen therapy; GI, gastrointestinal; HDL-C, high-density lipoprotein cholesterol; HT, hormone therapy; LDL-C, low-density lipoprotein cholesterol; SBHG, sex hormone-binding globulin.

In the wake of the Women's Health Initiative findings, however, compounding became much more popular as symptomatic women with concerns about patented HT frequently became targets for unproven bioidentical HT products. Women were led to believe that bioidentical HT products were safer and more effective than government-evaluated and government-approved medications, even though they have not been tested for effectiveness and safety. Bioidentical HT safety information is often not provided to women because there is no standard label or standard patient package insert, and information given to a patient by a compounding pharmacy or a prescribing physician may vary greatly. As a result, many women are unaware of potential risks and are often surprised to learn that the hormones are produced in a laboratory.

Some active ingredients meet the specifications of the USP. Standardization may be uncertain. Hormonal drugs that are compounded from a prescription are legal but have not gone through the rigorous testing that determines the safety and efficacy required for FDA approval. Often, third-party payers do not reimburse prescription costs for compounded formulations because they are viewed as experimental drugs.[55,65,112]

In 2008, FDA sent warning letters to 7 compounding pharmacies about the false claims that they had made about bioidentical HT, and the frequency of warning letters to compounding pharmacies for problems relating to problems with manufacturing and/or safety has increased markedly in 2012 and 2013.[113]

In testimony before the US Senate Committee on Health, Education, Labor, and Pensions, the executive director of the Center for Pharmaceutical Safety reported that even though some active ingredients of bioidentical HT meet the specifications of the USP, adoption of USP standards is optional. Compounding pharmacies are licensed by the state, but state regulations are minimally enforced and vary from state to state. As a result of a 2002 challenge to FDA authority over compounding industries' advertising and promotion (an authority granted by the 1997 FDA Modernization Act), virtually all FDA's authority to oversee the compounding industry was limited.[114]

Several organizations, including NAMS, FDA, ACOG, the Society of Obstetricians and Gynaecologists of Canada, the Endocrine Society, the American Medical Association, and the American Cancer Society, agree that compounded bioidentical HT products would be predicted to have the same risks and no greater benefits than their government-approved counterparts. Risks actually may be increased with bioidentical HT, as inadequate progesterone absorption has been reported to result in an increased risk of endometrial cancer. There is no evidence to support the health benefit or safety claims made by bioidentical HT promoters.

Transdermal creams and pills of many varieties are compounded. Some of the most widely used compounded estrogen products contained estriol, a weak estrogen having 5% to 10% of the effect of estradiol. Limited data show that oral estriol helps to relieve hot flashes. Estriol alone or in an oral mixture of 2 estrogens (either 80% estriol and 20% estradiol or 50% each) or 3 estrogens (usually 80% estriol, 10% estrone, and 10% estradiol) is often promoted as providing the benefits of government-approved estrogen products without increasing the risk of breast or endometrial cancer. Although estriol is a weak estrogen, it can still have a stimulatory effect on the breast and endometrium. Claims supporting estriol or any compounded formulation as safer than the government-approved formulations have not been substantiated by any well-designed clinical trials.

FDA banned the use of estriol by compounding pharmacies that did not obtain an investigational new drug application for its use.[115] FDA also states that there is no scientific evidence for using saliva testing to adjust hormones.[55] Women with an intact uterus using compounded estrogen should also use progestogen to counter estrogen's stimulatory effect on the endometrium.

Before an oral-capsule micronized progesterone product was marketed in the United States, oral micronized progesterone USP was a frequently prescribed compound. Compounded products are still used and may be especially appropriate for women with peanut allergies (oral-capsule micronized progesterone contains progesterone that is suspended in peanut oil). A 100-mg dose of micronized progesterone USP is equivalent to about 2.5 mg MPA.

Compounded topical preparations of progesterone are also available, although topical progesterone products have not been shown to achieve adequate serum levels to counter the stimulatory effect of ET on the uterus.

Compounded formulations should be used with caution and only with informed patient consent. There may be women for whom the positives outweigh the negatives, but for most women, government-approved hormone products will provide the appropriate therapy without assuming the risks and cost of compounded preparations. It is the stated position of the pharmacy industry that a compounded prescription drug product is not appropriate for a patient for whom there exists a commercially available prescription drug that matches the patient's medical need.

Selective estrogen-receptor modulators

Selective estrogen-receptor modulators (SERMs) are estrogen-like compounds that act as estrogen agonists or antagonists, depending on the SERM and the target tissue. In this way, they differ from endogenous human estrogen, which affects most estrogen receptors (ERs) in a stimulatory manner.

Because SERMs vary in their agonist/antagonist properties, they can be used to selectively target, prevent, and treat several diseases, including breast cancer and osteoporosis. The ideal SERM would provide agonist effects on the bone to prevent bone loss and on the brain to treat hot flashes while providing neutral or estrogen antagonist effects on the breast and endometrium to reduce cancer risks. To date, the ideal SERM has not been discovered. SERMs allow for individualization depending on the medical needs of the postmenopausal woman.

> **Compounded bioidentical hormone therapy**
> FDA has stated that compounding pharmacies have made claims about the safety and effectiveness of bioidentical hormone therapy unsupported by clinical trial data and thus considered to be false and misleading, but in the absence of recognized jurisdiction over compounding pharmacies it is unclear what effect, if any, FDA statements will have on either compounding pharmacy practices or their advertising and promotional claims about their products. Pharmacies may not compound drugs containing estriol without an investigational new drug authorization. FDA also states that there is no scientific basis for using saliva testing to adjust hormone levels, and the American Congress of Obstetricians and Gynecologists and the North American Menopause Society have supported this contention.

SERMs in clinical use are categorized on the basis of their chemical structures. Tamoxifen, toremifene, and ospemifene (a toremifene derivative) are triphenylethylenes; raloxifene is a benzothiophene; and bazedoxifene is an indole derivative.

SERMs available in the United States and Canada include tamoxifen, used for prevention and treatment of breast cancer; toremifene, used for treatment of breast cancer; raloxifene, approved for prevention and treatment of osteoporosis and prevention of invasive breast cancer; and ospemifene, approved for treatment of dyspareunia. Tibolone, a synthetic steroid, widely used around the world for several menopause-related indications, is not available in the United States or Canada. In 2013, FDA approved the first pairing of an estrogen product (CE) with a SERM (BZA).[116-118] SERMs used for treatment of menopause symptoms are ospemifene and the SERM BZA combined with CE.

Bazedoxifene and conjugated estrogens

In the large, phase 3, Selective Estrogen Menopause and Response to Therapy (SMART) trials in postmenopausal women with a uterus at risk for osteoporosis, BZA and CE were evaluated as an alternative to estrogen combined with a progestogen.[116-119] In SMART 1 and 2, BZA 20 mg paired with CE 0.45 mg and 0.625 mg reduced menopausal symptoms, including hot flashes, prevented bone loss in postmenopausal women, and had a favorable safety profile on the breast, endometrium, and ovary. Cardiovascular and VTE events were similar to placebo in trials up to 2 years. Secondary endpoints showed improvements in sleep, health-related QOL, and treatment satisfaction. Compared with CE combined with MPA, BZA and CE showed less breast tenderness ($P<.001$ for both doses) and higher rates of amenorrhea, with similar breast density changes from baseline compared with placebo.[120,121]

Minimal increases in endometrial thickness from baseline (<1 mm) that were asymptomatic and similar to placebo were seen in SMART 1. No increase in endometrial hyperplasia was seen in trials up to 2 years.[119] No cardiovascular AEs or VTEs were seen, but the SMART trials enrolled generally healthy postmenopausal women; thus, the lack of cardiovascular AEs and VTEs does not provide adequate risk determination. Two-fold risk of VTE has been seen with BZA alone; no additive effect on VTE was found when BZA was combined with either dose of CE.[116]

Ospemifene

Ospemifene was government approved in 2013 for treatment of moderate to severe dyspareunia, a symptom of menopausal vulvar and vaginal atrophy (VVA). Two phase 2 studies found that ospemifene had significant estrogenic effects on the vaginal epithelium.[122,123] The percentages of superficial and intermediate cells significantly increased, whereas percentages of parabasal cells significantly decreased with ospemifene compared with placebo.

Ospemifene was evaluated for the treatment of postmenopausal women with vaginal dryness and dyspareunia associated with VVA in two 12-week, phase 3 studies; 2 long-term safety extension studies; and a 52-week safety and efficacy study.[122,124,125] Improvements from baseline over placebo were found in vaginal pH and vaginal maturation index (percentage of superficial and parabasal cells) at weeks 12, 26, and 52 (all $P<.0001$), leading to approval for treatment of moderate to severe postmenopausal dyspareunia.

No trials have evaluated ospemifene's effects on breast density or breast cancer. Ospemifene has not been evaluated in a large RCT for its effects on bone density to determine whether it can prevent or treat osteoporosis, although there are promising preclinical data. Ospemifene has not been shown to cause any increased risk of endometrial proliferation per biopsy in trials up to 52 weeks. Although risks of thromboembolic stroke, hemorrhagic stroke, and VTE with ospemifene 60 mg in clinical trials have been similar to placebo in healthy postmenopausal women studied up to 52 weeks, concern remains about potential risk of VTE because of class effect. No exacerbation of hot flashes was seen in trials of women with VVA.

Tamoxifen

Tamoxifen, the first clinically significant SERM, is approved for treatment of node-negative breast cancer after surgery and radiation therapy. It also is used to reduce the risk of invasive cancer in patients with ductal carcinoma in situ who have been treated with surgery and radiation. It is used to reduce the risk of breast cancer in women who are at high risk and as palliative treatment for metastatic breast cancer. Two European trials showed a significant reduction in ER-positive breast cancer in women treated with tamoxifen.[126,127] Tamoxifen is associated with an increased risk for endometrial polyps, endometrial cancer, and thromboembolic events. Tamoxifen is not approved for prevention or treatment of osteoporosis but is a partial estrogen agonist in bone and has been shown to prevent bone loss in postmenopausal women at the spine and hip, with less increase in bone density than with ET.[128,129]

Raloxifene

Raloxifene 60 mg is government approved for the prevention and treatment of osteoporosis and for the reduction in risk of invasive breast cancer in women with osteoporosis and in women at high risk of breast cancer. Raloxifene has beneficial effects on BMD, decreasing bone turnover and reducing osteoporotic vertebral but not hip or nonvertebral fractures in the Multiple Outcomes of Raloxifene Evaluation (MORE) trial.[130,131]

Raloxifene carries an increased risk of VTE and stroke. The most commonly reported AEs are hot flashes (increased frequency or severity), leg cramps, peripheral edema, arthralgia, flu-like syndrome, and sweating.

CHAPTER 8

Assuming no contraindications, raloxifene is an attractive option for younger postmenopausal women with osteoporosis who by their younger age will be at higher risk for vertebral fracture than for hip fracture. They may receive both bone and breast benefits.

The Study of Tamoxifen and Raloxifene. In older women with osteopenia or osteoporosis, raloxifene therapy is associated with a significant reduction in the incidence of ER-positive breast cancer.[132,133] The Study of Tamoxifen and Raloxifene (STAR) revealed that raloxifene is equivalent to tamoxifen in reducing the incidence of invasive breast cancer in postmenopausal women at high risk for the disease.[134,135] In STAR, raloxifene was associated with fewer VTE events and pulmonary emboli than tamoxifen. Use of each of these agents should be discontinued before and during prolonged immobilization. Raloxifene should be used with caution in women with hepatic impairment. Concomitant use with systemic ET is not recommended. Tamoxifen is associated with an increased risk for endometrial polyps, endometrial cancer, and thromboembolic events; raloxifene was associated with a reduction in endometrial cancer.

Raloxifene also significantly reduced the incidence of ER-positive breast cancer in the Raloxifene Use for the Heart (RUTH) trial.[136] Raloxifene was associated with an increased risk of VTE (absolute risk increase, 1.2/1,000 woman-years) and fatal stroke (absolute risk increase, 0.7/1,000 woman-years). The rare risk of fatal stroke reported in RUTH was seen in women who had an increased risk of stroke at baseline (Framingham Stroke Risk Score Q13). Raloxifene did not reduce the risk of heart disease.

Selective serotonin-reuptake inhibitors and serotonin norepinephrine-reuptake inhibitors

The selective serotonin-reuptake inhibitor (SSRI) paroxetine 7.5 mg was approved for the treatment of moderate to severe VMS associated with menopause in 2013. Higher doses of paroxetine were originally approved in 1992 for treatment of psychiatric conditions that currently include depression, anxiety disorder, social anxiety disorder, panic disorder, obsessive compulsive disorder, and generalized and posttraumatic stress disorder.

The effectiveness of paroxetine 7.5 mg in reducing VMS was demonstrated in 2 similarly designed RCTs, one of 12 weeks' duration, and one of 24 weeks' duration.[54] Symptomatic women aged 40 years and older (N=1,184) were enrolled. In the pooled analysis, paroxetine significantly reduced VMS at weeks 4 and 12 as well as at week 24 in the 24-week study. Severity of VMS also was reduced. Treatment benefit was maintained throughout the duration of the 24-week study.

The most common AEs in the paroxetine trials were nausea, fatigue, and dizziness, all occurring at a rate below 4%.[54] Two serious AEs were reported in the paroxetine arm: 1 death from acute respiratory failure in the presence of hypertensive CVD and hypertension-mediated pulmonary edema and 1 suicide attempt by a participant 1 week after receiving clonazepam for new-onset anxiety. Neither was thought to be related to the study drug. There were no reports of discontinuation symptoms that are known to occur with higher doses of SSRIs.

Paroxetine 7.5 mg is the first nonhormonal medication to be US government approved for VMS. It provides a good alternative for women, especially those who cannot or choose not to use HT. Data are lacking for women with breast cancer taking tamoxifen. Paroxetine inhibits cytochrome P-450 CYP2D6 enzyme, which converts tamoxifen to endoxifen, a key metabolite in the pharmacologic activity of tamoxifen against breast cancer.[137] One cohort study of 2,430 women taking tamoxifen with variable amounts of time taking an SSRI found that the greater the percentage of time spent on an SSRI, the higher the mortality rate from breast cancer.[138] Because CYP2D6 is polymorphic and affected by many factors, results have been inconsistent.[137]

Other SSRIs and serotonin norepinephrine-reuptake inhibitors (SNRIs) have been found to decrease VMS in small studies, but none of the other products have sought government approval. Please see Chapter 3 for more information about the use of SSRIs and SNRIs in managing VMS.

Androgens

Although androgens are defined as hormones that promote the development and maintenance of male secondary sexual characteristics and structures, they are important for women as well. Androgens are the immediate precursors for estrogen biosynthesis. In addition, androgens affect sexual desire, muscle mass and strength, BMD, and distribution of adipose tissue and may influence energy and psychological well-being (Table 17).[139]

The major androgens in women, as in men, are testosterone and dihydrotestosterone. Androstenedione and dehydroepiandrosterone (DHEA) are considered preandrogens.

Androgens are synthesized primarily in the ovary and adrenal glands, although significant peripheral conversion occurs. About 66% of circulating testosterone is tightly bound to sex hormone-binding globulin (SHBG), with approximately 33% bound to albumin.[140] It is believed that only the free, or unbound, fraction is bioactive (approximately 1%-2% of the total circulating testosterone). Serum testosterone concentrations in women are approximately 10% of those in men.

Although production of ovarian and adrenal androgens decreases with age, there is no abrupt decline in these hormones with menopause. Surgical menopause is an exception, because testosterone levels decrease by approximately 50% after bilateral oophorectomy.[139] In addition to oophorectomy, a number of factors, including hypopituitarism, adrenal insufficiency (which may be primary or secondary to glucocorticosteroid use), chemotherapy, and pelvic irradiation, reduce androgen production in women. Drugs that increase SHBG concentrations (such as oral estrogen and thyroxine) decrease bioavailable testosterone.[141]

Potential benefits
Androgen therapy is receiving increasing attention for treating postmenopausal women with sexual dysfunction, despite the fact that androgen levels did not predict sexual function in several large observational studies.[142] Intramuscular depot testosterone and oral methyltestosterone have been used in the past, and each has been shown to improve sexual interest.[143,144] However, neither of these treatment modalities is recommended. Intramuscular testosterone formulations for men provide doses too high for women. Oral methyltestosterone lowers high-density lipoprotein cholesterol.

Several large RCTs have shown that testosterone administered via a transdermal patch significantly increases the frequency of satisfying sexual activity, sexual desire, arousal, and orgasm frequency in naturally and surgically menopausal women with and without concurrent ET who present with low sexual desire associated with distress.[145-148] This appears to be androgen mediated, because the effect is not blocked by concurrent use of an aromatase inhibitor.[149] In a large RCT of testosterone gel (LibiGel) in postmenopausal women with distressing low sexual desire, there was no significant improvement in any measure of sexual function, including libido or satisfying sexual events, compared with placebo, despite increasing circulating testosterone to levels to those seen with the testosterone patch (BioSante, unpublished data, December 2011).

Androgen therapy may play a role in the maintenance of BMD and body composition in women. In a 9-week randomized study of estrogen alone versus combined estrogen-methyltestosterone therapy, both treatments reduced urinary markers of bone resorption, but only combined estrogen-methyltestosterone therapy resulted in an increase in serum markers of bone formation.[150] Estradiol plus testosterone implants significantly increase lumbar spine and hip BMD compared with estradiol implants alone, and methyltestosterone plus estradiol increases lumbar spine BMD more than estradiol given alone.[151,152] In addition, women who received both estradiol and testosterone implants experienced an increase in fat-free mass and a reduced ratio of fat mass to fat-free mass.[151] Testosterone plus estrogen therapy significantly improves BMD density and lean mass in women with hypopituitism compared with ET.[153]

Despite widespread promotion of DHEA for the management of female sexual interest/arousal disorder, evidence supporting its use is lacking. Systematic reviews have shown no benefit of DHEA oral or transdermal therapy for postmenopausal women for sexual function, well-being, cognitive function, lipids, or carbohydrate metabolism.[154]

Dehydroepiandrosterone does have a small effect on BMD.[154] A systematic review and meta-analysis found no benefit of DHEA therapy in women with adrenal insufficiency for sexual well-being but did find a small effect on health-related QOL and depression.[155]

Androgen products
There are no government-approved androgen-containing prescription products for treating female sexual interest/arousal disorder in US or Canadian women, and androgen therapy for women remains controversial.[156] A testosterone patch (300 μg) was approved in Europe for use in surgically menopausal women with hypoactive sexual desire disorder on concurrent ET, but it was withdrawn from the market voluntarily in 2012. A 1% testosterone cream available in Australia for the treatment of women can be obtained in the same manner. An androgen-containing product that combined esterified estradiol with methyltestosterone, which was indicated for the treatment of moderate to severe VMS unresponsive to estrogen, used to be available in the United States, but production of that product was discontinued. Although no longer available, several "quasi-generic" esterified estradiol plus methyltestosterone products are available by prescription.

In Canada, prescription oral testosterone undecanoate approved for men is sometimes used off label in women. It is supplied in 40-mg tablets. The absorption of testosterone undecanoate is highly variable, and the 40-mg dose can result in male levels of testosterone in women. In the United States, prescription androgen-containing skin patches and gel products are formulated for men and are difficult to dose for women. These various formulations cannot be recommended for women.

Table 17. Conditions Associated With Diminished Testosterone Levels in Women

- *Aging.* Adrenal and ovarian androgen production declines gradually with aging
- *Bilateral oophorectomy.* Surgical removal of both ovaries decreases circulating levels of testosterone by 40% to 50%
- *Pituitary/Adrenal insufficiency.* Very low testosterone levels are seen with pituitary or adrenal insufficiency, as in Sheehan syndrome or Addison disease
- *Oral ET or OCPs.* Free testosterone levels are decreased because of increased concentrations of SHBG with oral ET use
- *Chronic illness.* Low androgen concentration also may occur in those with major medical problems, including anorexia nervosa, advanced cancer, and burn trauma

Abbreviations: ET, estrogen therapy; OCPs, oral contraceptive pills; SHGB, sex hormone-binding globulin.
Davison SL, et al.[139]

Testosterone administered by intramuscular injection or with subcutaneous pellets often results in supraphysiologic levels in women, with the highest levels occurring near the time of administration. The effect often lasts for 3 months, and the pellet is difficult to remove should there be a need for discontinuation.

Custom-compounded preparations of micronized testosterone USP are available as topical creams or ointments, although there are no definitive studies on absorption rates, and these preparations are not government approved. A popular product is custom-compounded topical 1% or 2% testosterone USP cream or ointment applied several times weekly directly to the vagina and clitoral area or any skin surface. Testosterone is well absorbed through the skin; supraphysiologic levels will be obtained if large amounts are applied. Anecdotal evidence supports use of this therapy for improving libido; however, no controlled studies have confirmed the safety or efficacy of topical testosterone for sexual dysfunction in women.

In Canada, DHEA is classified as a controlled substance and requires a prescription. In the United States, DHEA is available as an oral dietary supplement and may be purchased without a prescription. Although the typical dose for women is 25 mg to 50 mg per day, there is limited regulation of available products and great variability in the actual amount of hormone present in each tablet.

Prescription androgen products, including testosterone patches and gels appropriately dosed for women, are under investigation for use in postmenopausal women with female sexual interest/arousal disorder.

Monitoring therapy

Clinical monitoring of women using androgens includes a subjective assessment of sexual response and satisfaction. Women also should be evaluated for potential AEs, including hirsutism, acne, and clitoromegaly. Intermittent monitoring of lipids and liver function tests may be prudent. Regular mammography is indicated. Measuring the free-testosterone level or free-androgen index (total testosterone/SHBG) in women using topical testosterone therapies will not help with the assessment of efficacy, but it may be used as a safety measure, with the goal of keeping the value within the normal range for women of reproductive age. However, commercial laboratory measurements of testosterone levels in women are quite variable.

The cause of female sexual interest/arousal disorder is often multifactorial and may include psychological problems (depression, anxiety disorders), conflict within the relationship, fatigue, stress, lack of privacy, issues relating to physical or sexual abuse, medications, or physical problems that make sexual activity uncomfortable (endometriosis, atrophic vaginitis). It is very important to assess and treat other potential causes of female sexual interest/arousal disorder before considering a trial of androgen therapy. Sex therapy is an effective and safe intervention and generally should be advised before a trial of androgen therapy.[157]

Potential risks

The potential risks of androgen therapy for women are not well defined.[158] When recommending such therapy, clinicians should fully inform women of potential risks and monitor for AEs. These include acne, weight gain, excess facial and body hair, permanent lowering of the voice, clitoral enlargement, changes in emotion (eg, increased anger), and adverse changes in lipids and liver function tests. Such effects are unlikely if androgen levels are maintained within normal physiologic ranges for women. Estrogenic risks and AEs are also possible because androgens are converted to estrogens.

Whether androgen use in postmenopausal women will increase the risk of CVD or breast cancer is unknown.[159,160] A report from the Nurses' Health Study suggested an increased risk of breast cancer in users of testosterone therapies, although studies on long-term risks are limited.[161] In a 1-year study of a testosterone transdermal patch, there were 4 cases of breast cancer (including one detected 3 months after initiation of the study) among the 593 women randomized to active treatment and no cases of breast cancer among the 277 women randomized to placebo.[145] An RCT examining the risk of breast cancer and CVD with the use of a topical testosterone gel was discontinued when the testosterone gel was found to be no more effective than placebo, despite achieving testosterone levels equivalent to those obtained with the testosterone patch.

Limited research is available on the use of androgens in women not using concurrent ET, although 1 clinical trial of the testosterone patch in these women demonstrated similar safety and efficacy as was seen in prior studies of the testosterone patch in menopausal women with hypoactive sexual desire disorder using concurrent ET.[145] Because androgen does not protect the endometrium against estrogen-induced hyperplasia, a progestogen should be added to an estrogen-androgen regimen in women with a uterus.

References

1. Trussell J, Guthrie K. Choosing a contraceptive: Efficacy, safety, and personal considerations. In: Hatcher RA, Trussell J, Nelson AL, Cates W, Kowal D, Policar MS, eds. *Contraceptive Technology*. 20th rev ed. New York: Ardent Media; 2011:45-74.
2. Kaunitz AM. Clinical practice. Hormonal contraception in women of older reproductive age. *N Engl J Med*. 2008;358(12):1262-1270.
3. Peipert JF, Zhao Q, Allsworth JE, et al. Continuation and satisfaction of reversible contraception. *Obstet Gynecol*. 2011;117(5):1105-1113.
4. Centers for Disease Control and Prevention. US Medical Eligibility Criteria for Contraceptive Use, 2010. *MMWR Recomm Rep*. 2010;59(RR-4):1-86.
5. Allen RH, Cwiak CA, Kaunitz AM. Contraception in women over 40 years of age. *CMAJ*. 2013;185(7):565-573.
6. Hubacher D, Grimes DA. Noncontraceptive health benefits of intrauterine devices: a systematic review. *Obstet Gynecol Surv*. 2002;57(2):120-128.
7. Hurskainen R, Teperi J, Rissanen P, et al. Clinical outcomes and costs with the levonorgestrel-releasing intrauterine system or hysterectomy for treatment of menorrhagia: randomized trial 5-year follow-up. *JAMA*. 2004;291(12):1456-1463.

8. Kaunitz AM, Meredith S, Inki P, Kubba A, Sanchez-Ramos L. Levonorgestrel-releasing intrauterine system and endometrial ablation in heavy menstrual bleeding: a systematic review and meta-analysis. *Obstet Gynecol*. 2009;113(5):1104-1116.

9. Petta CA, Ferriani RQ, Abrao MS, et al. Randomized clinical trial of a levonorgestrel-releasing intrauterine system and a depot GnRH analogue for the treatment of chronic pelvic pain in women with endometriosis. *Hum Reprod*. 2005;20(7):1993-1998.

10. Raudaskoski T, Tapanainen J, Tomás E, et al. Intrauterine 10 microg and 20 microg levonorgestrel systems in postmenopausal women receiving oral oestrogen replacement therapy: clinical, endometrial and metabolic response. *Br J Obstet Gynaecol*. 2002;109(2):136-144.

11. Nelson A, Apter D, Hauck B, et al. Two low-dose levonorgestrel intrauterine contraceptive systems: a randomized controlled trial. *Obstet Gynecol*. 2013;122(6):1205-1213. Erratum in: *Obstet Gynecol*. 2014;123(5):1109.

12. Long-term reversible contraception: twelve years of experience with the TCu380A and TCu220C. *Contraception*. 1997;56(6):341-352.

13. Association of Reproductive Health Professionals. *A Quick Reference Guide for Clinicians: Choosing a Birth Control Method*. September 2011. www.arhp.org/uploadDocs/choosingqrg.pdf. Accessed July 15, 2014.

14. Kaunitz AM, Arias R, McClung M. Bone density recovery after depot medroxyprogesterone acetate use. *Contraception*. 2008;77(2):67-76.

15. Lopez LM, Chen M, Mullins S, Curtis KM, Helmerhorst FM. Steroidal contraceptives and bone fractures in women: evidence from observational studies. *Cochrane Database Syst Rev*. 2012;8:CD009849.

16. Lanza LL, McQuay LJ, Rothman KJ, et al. Use of depot medroxyprogesterone acetate contraception and incidence of bone fracture. *Obstet Gynecol*. 2013;121(3):593-600.

17. ACOG Committee on Practice Bulletins-Gynecology. ACOG practice bulletin. No. 73: use of hormonal contraception in women with coexisting medical conditions. *Obstet Gynecol*. 2006;107(6):1453-1472.

18. Bachmann G, Sulak PJ, Sampson-Landers C, Benda N, Marr J. Efficacy and safety of a low-dose 24-day combined oral contraceptive containing 20 micrograms ethinylestradiol and 3 mg drospirenone. *Contraception*. 2004;70(3):191-198.

19. Nakajima ST, Archer DF, Ellman H. Efficacy and safety of a new 24-day oral contraceptive regimen of norethindrone acetate 1 mg/ethinyl estradiol 20 micro g (Loestrin 24 Fe). *Contraception*. 2007;75(1):16-22.

20. Vandever MA, Kuehl TJ, Sulak PJ, et al. Evaluation of pituitary-ovarian axis suppression with three oral contraceptive regimens. *Contraception*. 2008;77(3):162-170.

21. Fels H, Steward R, Melamed A, Granat A, Stanczyk FZ, Mishell DR Jr. Comparison of serum and cervical mucus hormone levels during hormone-free interval of 24/4 vs. 21/7 combined oral contraceptives. *Contraception*. 2013; 87(6):732-737.

22. Dinger J, Minh TD, Buttmann N, Bardenheuer K. Effectiveness of oral contraceptive pills in a large US cohort comparing progestogen and regimen. *Obstet Gynecol*. 2011;117(1):33-40.

23. Archer DF, Nakajima ST, Sawyer AT, et al. Norethindrone acetate 1.0 milligram and ethinyl estradiol 10 micrograms as an ultra low-dose oral contraceptive. *Obstet Gynecol*. 2013;122(3):601-607.

24. Pearlstein TB, Bachmann GA, Zacur HA, Yonkers KA. Treatment of premenstrual dysphoric disorder with a new drospirenone-containing oral contraceptive formulation. *Contraception*. 2005;72(6):414-421.

25. Yonkers KA, Brown C, Pearlstein TB, Foegh M, Sampson-Landers C, Rapkin A. Efficacy of a new low-dose oral contraceptive with drospirenone in premenstrual dysphoric disorder. *Obstet Gynecol*. 2005; 106(3):492-501.

26. Rapkin AJ, Winer SA. Drospirenone: a novel progestin. *Expert Opin Pharmacother*. 2007;8(7):989-999.

27. Bird ST, Pepe SR, Etminan M, Liu X, Brophy JM, Delaney JA. The association between drospirenone and hyperkalemia: a comparative-safety study. *BMC Clin Pharmacol*. 2011;11:23.

28. Dinger J, Shapiro S. Combined oral contraceptives, venous thromboembolism, and the problem of interpreting large but incomplete datasets. *J Fam Plann Reprod Health Care*. 2012;38(1):2-6.

29. US Food and Drug Administration. FDA Drug Safety Communication: Updated information about the risk of blood clots in women taking birth control pills containing drospirenone. FDA Web site. www.fda.gov/Drugs/DrugSafety/ucm299305.htm?source=govdelivery. Updated February 15, 2013. Accessed May 1, 2014.

30. Dinger J, Bardenheuer K, Heinemann K. Cardiovascular and general safety of a 24-day regimen of drospirenone-containing combined oral contraceptives: final results from the International Active Surveillance Study of Women taking Oral Contraceptives. *Contraception*. 2014;89(4):253-263.

31. Jensen JT, Parke S, Mellinger U, Machlitt A, Fraser IS. Effective treatment of heavy menstrual bleeding with estradiol valerate and dienogest: a randomized controlled trial. *Obstet Gynecol*. 2011;117(4):777-787.

32. Jensen JT. Evaluation of a new estradiol oral contraceptive: estradiol valerate and dienogest. *Expert Opin Pharmacother*. 2010;11(7):1147-1157.

33. Scarabin PY, Oger E, Plu-Bureau G; Estrogen and THromboEmbolism Risk Study Group. Differential association of oral and transdermal oestrogen-replacement therapy with venous thromboembolism risk. *Lancet*. 2003;362(9382):428-432.

34. Edelman AB, Gallo MF, Jensen JT, Nichols MD, Schulz KF, Grimes DA. Continuous or extended cycle vs. cyclic use of combined oral contraceptives for contraception. *Cochrane Database Syst Rev*. 2005;(3):CD004695.

35. Anderson FD, Gibbons W, Portman D. Safety and efficacy of an extended-regimen oral contraceptive utilizing continuous low-dose ethinyl estradiol. *Contraception*. 2006;73(3):229-234.

36. Kaunitz AM, Portman DJ, Hait H, Reape KZ. Adding low-dose estrogen to the hormone-free interval: impact on bleeding patterns in users of a 91-day extended regimen oral contraceptive. *Contraception*. 2009;79(5):350-355.

37. Portman DJ, Kaunitz AM, Howard B, Weiss H, Hsieh J, Ricciotti N. Efficacy and safety of an ascending-dose, extended-regimen levonorgestrel/ethinyl estradiol combined oral contraceptive. *Contraception*. 2014;89(4):299-306.

38. Sulak PJ, Kuehl TJ, Coffee A, Willis S. Prospective analysis of occurrence and management of breakthrough bleeding during an extended oral contraceptive regimen. *Am J Obstet Gynecol*. 2006;195(4):935-941.

39. Archer DF, Jensen JT, Johnson JV, Borisute H, Grubb GS, Constantine GD. Evaluation of a continuous regimen of levonorgestrel/ethinyl estradiol: phase 3 study results. *Contraception*. 2006;74(6):439-445.

40. Roumen FJ, Apter D, Mulders TM, Dieben TO. Efficacy, tolerability and acceptability of a novel contraceptive vaginal ring releasing etonogestrel and ethinyl oestradiol. *Hum Reprod*. 2001;16(3):469-475.

41. Abrams LS, Skee D, Natarajan J, Wong FA. Pharmacokinetic overview of Ortho Evra/Evra. *Fertil Steril*. 2002;77(2 suppl 2):S3-S12.

42. Ahrendt HJ, Nisand I, Bastianelli C, et al. Efficacy, acceptability and tolerability of the combined contraceptive ring, NuvaRing, compared with an oral contraceptive containing 30 microg of ethinyl estradiol and 3 mg of drospirenone. *Contraception*. 2006;74(6):451-457.

43. Audet MC, Moreau M, Koltun WD, et al; ORTHO EVRA/EVRA 004 Study Group. Evaluation of contraceptive efficacy and cycle control of a transdermal contraceptive patch vs an oral contraceptive: a randomized clinical trial. *JAMA*. 2001;285(18):2347-2354.

44. Van den Heuvel MW, van Bragt AJ, Alnabawy A, Kaptein MC. Comparison of ethinylestradiol pharmacokinetics in three hormonal contraceptive formulations: the vaginal ring, the transdermal patch, and an oral contraceptive. *Contraception*. 2005;72(3):168-174.

45. Cole JA, Norman H, Doherty M, Walker AM. Venous thromboembolism, myocardial infarction, and stroke among transdermal contraceptive system users. *Obstet Gynecol*. 2007;109(2 pt 1):339-346.

46. Kaunitz AM. Transdermal and vaginal estradiol for the treatment of menopausal symptoms: the nuts and bolts. *Menopause*. 2012;19(6):602-603.

47. Division of Reproductive Health, National Center for Chronic Disease Prevention and Health Promotion, Centers for Disease Control and Prevention (CDC). US Selected Practice Recommendations for Contraceptive Use, 2013: adapted from the World Health Organization selected practice recommendations for contraceptive use, 2nd edition. *MMWR Recomm Rep*. 2013;62(RR-05):1-60.

48. Cleland K, Zhu H, Goldstuck N, Cheng L, Trussell J. The efficacy of intrauterine devices for emergency contraception: a systematic review of 35 years of experience. *Hum Reprod*. 2012;27(7):1994-2000.

49. Cleland K, Wood S. A tale of two label changes. *Contraception*. 2014;90(1):1-3.

50. Glasier AF, Cameron ST, Fine PM, et al. Ulipristal acetate versus levonorgestrel for emergency contraception: a randomised non-inferiority trial and meta-analysis. *Lancet*. 2010;375(9714):555-562.

51. Glasier A, Cameron ST, Blithe D, et al. Can we identify women at risk of pregnancy despite using emergency contraception? Data from randomized trials of ulipristal acetate and levonorgestrel. *Contraception*. 2011;84(4):363-367.

52. Cibula D, Zikan M, Dusek L, Majek O. Oral contraceptives and risk of ovarian and breast cancers in BRCA mutation carriers: a meta-analysis. *Expert Rev Anticancer Ther.* 2011;11(8):1197-1207.
53. Brisdelle [package insert]. Miami, FL: Noven; 2013.
54. Simon JA, Portman DJ, Kaunitz AM, et al. Low-dose paroxetine 7.5 mg for menopausal vasomotor symptoms: two randomized controlled trials. *Menopause.* 2013;20(10):1027-1035.
55. North American Menopause Society. The 2012 hormone therapy position statement of: The North American Menopause Society. *Menopause.* 2012;19(3):257-271.
56. Barnes BB, Levrant SG. Pharmacology of estrogens. In: Lobo RA, ed. *Treatment of the Postmenopausal Woman: Basic and Clinical Aspects.* 3rd ed. San Diego, CA: Academic Press; 2007:767-777.
57. Management of osteoporosis in postmenopausal women: 2010 position statement of The North American Menopause Society. *Menopause.* 2010;17(1):25-54.
58. Lindsay R, Gallagher JC, Kleerekoper M, Pickar JH. Effect of lower doses of conjugated equine estrogens with and without medroxyprogesterone acetate on bone in early postmenopausal women. *JAMA.* 2002;287(20):2668-2676.
59. LaCroix AZ, Chlebowski RT, Manson JE, et al; WHI Investigators. Health outcomes after stopping conjugated equine estrogens among postmenopausal women with prior hysterectomy: a randomized controlled trial. *JAMA.* 2011;305(13):1305-1314.
60. Manson JE, Chlebowski RT, Stefanick ML. et al. Menopausal hormone therapy and health outcomes during the intervention and extended poststopping phases of the Women's Health Initiative randomized trials. *JAMA.* 2013;310(13):1353-1368.
61. Bhavnani BR, Nisker JA, Martin J, Aletebi F, Watson L, Milne JK. Comparison of pharmacokinetics of a conjugated equine estrogen preparation (premarin) and a synthetic mixture of estrogens (C.E.S.) in postmenopausal women. *J Soc Gyncecol Investig.* 2000;7(3):175-183.
62. Prestwood KM, Kenny AM, Kleppinger A, Kulldorff M. Ultralow-dose micronized 17beta-estradiol and bone density and bone metabolism in older women: a randomized controlled trial. *JAMA.* 2003;290(8):1042-1048.
63. Ettinger B, Ensrud KE, Wallace R, et al. Effects of ultralow-dose transdermal estradiol on bone mineral density: a randomized clinical trial. *Obstet Gynecol.* 2004;104(3):443-451.
64. Bachmann GA, Schaefers M, Uddin A, Utian WH. Lowest effective transdermal 17beta-estradiol for relief of hot flushes in postmenopausal women: a randomized controlled trial. *Obstet Gynecol.* 2007;110(4):771-779.
65. Cirigliano M. Bioidentical hormone therapy: a review of the evidence. *J Womens Health.* 2007;16(5):600-631.
66. Shifren JL, Rifai N, Desindes S, McIlwain M, Doros G, Mazer NA. A comparison of the short-term effects of oral conjugated equine estrogens versus transdermal estradiol on C-reactive protein, other serum markers of inflammation, and other hepatic proteins in naturally menopausal women. *J Clin Endocrinol Metab.* 2008;93(5):1702-1710.
67. Canonico M, Oger E, Plu-Bureau G, et al; Estrogen and Thromboembolism Risk (ESTHER) Study Group. Hormone therapy and venous thromboembolism among postmenopausal women: impact of the route of estrogen administration and progestogens: the ESTHER Study. *Circulation.* 2007;115(7):840-845.
68. Canonico M, Fournier A, Carcaillon L, et al. Postmenopausal hormone therapy and risk of idiopathic venous thromboembolism: results from the E3N cohort study. *Arterioscler Thromb Vasc Biol.* 2010;30(2):340-345.
69. Laliberte F, Dea K, Duh MS, Kahler KH, Rolli M, Lefebvre P. Does the route of administration for estrogen hormone therapy impact the risk of venous thromboembolism? Estradiol transdermal system versus oral estrogen-only hormone therapy. *Menopause.* 2011;18(10):1052-1059.
70. Renoux C, Dell'aniello S, Garbe E, Suissa S. Transdermal and oral hormone replacement therapy and the risk of stroke: a nested case-control study. *BMJ.* 2010;340:c2519.
71. North American Menopause Society. KEEPS report. Presented at NAMS 23rd Annual Meeting; October 3-6, 2012; Orlando, Florida. www.menopause.org/annual-meetings/2012-meeting/keeps-report. Accessed July 15, 2014.
72. Management of symptomatic vulvovaginal atrophy: 2013 position statement of The North American Menopause Society. *Menopause.* 2013(9):888-902.
73. Suckling J, Lethaby A, Kennedy R. Local oestrogen for vaginal atrophy in postmenopausal women. *Cochrane Database Syst Rev.* 2006;(4):CD001500.
74. Stanczyk FZ. Structure-function relationships, pharmacokinetics, and potency of orally and parenterally administered progestogens. In: Lobo RA, ed. *Treatment of the Postmenopausal Woman: Basic and Clinical Aspects*, 3rd ed. San Diego, CA: Academic Press; 2007:779-798.
75. Effects of estrogen or estrogen/progestin regimens on heart disease risk factors in postmenopausal women. The Postmenopausal Estrogen/Progestin Interventions (PEPI) Trial. The Writing Group for the PEPI Trial. *JAMA.* 1995;273(3):199-208.
76. Montplaisir J, Lorrain J, Denesle R, Petit D. Sleep in menopause: differential effects of two forms of hormone replacement therapy. *Menopause.* 2001;8(1):10-16.
77. Warren MP, Biller BM, Shangold MM. A new clinical option for hormone replacement therapy in women with secondary amenorrhea: effects of cyclic administration of progesterone from the sustained-release vaginal gel Crinone (4% and 8%) on endometrial morphologic features and withdrawal bleeding. *Am J Obstet Gynecol.* 1999;180(1 pt 1):42-48.
78. Ettinger B, Selby J, Citron JT, Vangessel A, Ettinger VM, Hendrickson MR. Cyclic hormone replacement therapy using quarterly progestin. *Obstet Gynecol.* 1994;83(5 pt 1):693-700.
79. Ettinger B, Pressman A, Van Gessel A. Low-dosage esterified estrogen opposed by progestin at 6-month intervals. *Obstet Gynecol.* 2001;98(2):205-211.
80. Odmark IS, Bixo M, Englund D, Risberg B, Jonsson B, Olsson SE. Endometrial safety and bleeding pattern during a five-year treatment with long-cycle hormone therapy. *Menopause.* 2005;12(6):699-707.
81. Effects of hormone replacement therapy on endometrial histology in postmenopausal women. The Postmenopausal Estrogen/Progestin Interventions (PEPI) Trial. The Writing Group for the PEPI Trial. *JAMA.* 1996;275(5):370-375.
82. Furness S, Roberts H, Marjoribanks J, Lethaby A. Hormone replacement therapy in postmenopausal women and risk of endometrial hyperplasia. *Cochrane Database Syst Rev.* 2012;8:CD000402.
83. Doherty JA, Cushing-Haugen KL, Saltzman BS, et al. Long-term use of postmenopausal estrogen and progestin hormone therapies and the risk of endometrial cancer. *Am J Obstet Gynecol.* 2007;197(2):139.e1-139.e7.
84. Jaakkola S, Lyytinen H, Pukkala E, Ylikorkala O. Endometrial cancer in postmenopausal women using estradiol-progestin therapy. *Obstet Gynecol.* 2009;14(6):1197-1204.
85. Levine H, Watson N. Comparison of the pharmacokinetics of crinone 8% administered vaginally versus Prometrium administered orally in postmenopausal women(3). *Fertil Steril.* 2000;73(3):516-521.
86. Johnson JV, Davidson M, Archer D, Bachmann G. Postmenopausal uterine bleeding profiles with two forms of combined continuous hormone replacement therapy. *Menopause.* 2002;9(1):16-22.
87. Rossouw JE, Anderson GL, Prentice RL, et al; Writing Group for the Women's Health Initiative Investigators. Risks and benefits of estrogen plus progestin in healthy postmenopausal women: principal results from the Women's Health Initiative randomized controlled trial. *JAMA.* 2002;288(3):321-333.
88. Grady D, Herrington D, Bittner V, et al; HERS Research Group. Cardiovascular disease outcomes during 6.8 years of hormone therapy: Heart and Estrogen/progestin Replacement Study follow-up (HERS II). *JAMA.* 2002;288(1):49-57. Erratum in: *JAMA.* 2002;288(9):1064.
89. Lyytinen H, Pukkala E, Ylikorkala O. Breast cancer risk in postmenopausal women using estradiol-progestogen therapy. *Obstet Gynecol.* 2009;113(1):65-73.
90. Chlebowski RT, Anderson GL, Gass M, et al; WHI Investigators. Estrogen plus progestin and breast cancer incidence and mortality in postmenopausal women. *JAMA.* 2010;304(15):1684-1692.
91. Fournier A, Boutron-Ruault MC, Clavel-Chapelon F. Breast cancer and hormonal therapy in postmenopausal women. *N Engl J Med.* 2009; 360(22):2366.
92. Crandall CJ, Aragaki AK, Chlebowski RT, et al. New-onset breast tenderness after initiation of estrogen plus progestin therapy and breast cancer risk. *Arch Intern Med.* 2009;169(18):1684-1691.
93. Fournier A, Berrino F, Clavel-Chapelon F. Unequal risks for breast cancer associated with different hormone replacement therapies: results from the E3N cohort study. *Breast Cancer Res Treat.* 2008;107(1):103-111. Erratum in: *Breast Cancer Res Treat.* 2008;107(2):307-308.
94. Cordina-Duverger E, Truong T, Anger A, et al. Risk of breast cancer by type of menopausal hormonal therapy: a case control study among post-menopausal women in France. *PLoS One.* 2013;8(11):e78016.
95. US Food and Drug Administration. FDA approves Duavee to treat hot flashes and prevent osteoporosis [press release]. FDA Web site. www.fda.gov/drugs/newsevents/ucm370679.htm. Last update October 3, 2013. Accessed July 15, 2014.
96. Pinkerton JV, Komm BS, Mirkin S. Tissue selective estrogen complex combinations with bazedoxifene/conjugated estrogens as a model. *Climacteric.* 2013;16(6):618-628.

97. Archer DF, Pinkerton JV, Kagan R, et al. Gynecologic safety of bazedoxifene/conjugated estrogens: pooled analysis of phase 3 trials [abstract]. *Menopause*. 2012;19(12)1374. Abstract S-10.
98. Shumaker SA, Legault C, Rapp SR, et al; WHIMS Investigators. Estrogen plus progestin and the incidence of dementia and mild cognitive impairment in postmenopausal women: the Women's Health Initiative Memory Study: a randomized controlled trial. *JAMA*. 2003;289(20):2651-2662.
99. Shumaker SA, Legault C, Kuller L, et al; Women's Health Initiative Memory Study. Conjugated equine estrogens and incidence of probable dementia and mild cognitive impairment in postmenopausal women: Women's Health Initiative Memory Study. *JAMA*. 2004;291(24):2947-2985.
100. Jacobson BC, Moy B, Colditz GA, Fuchs CS. Postmenopausal hormone use and symptoms of gastroesophageal reflux. *Arch Intern Med*. 2008;168(16):1798-1804.
101. Oskarsson V, Orsini N, Sadr-Azodi O, Wolk A. Postmenopausal hormone replacement therapy and risk of acute pancreatitis: a prospective cohort study. *CMAJ*. 2014;186(5):338-344.
102. Rossouw JE, Prentice RL, Manson JE, et al. Postmenopausal hormone therapy and risk of cardiovascular disease by age and years since menopause. *JAMA*. 2007;297(13):1465-1477. Erratum in: *JAMA*. 2008;299(12):1426.
103. Prentice RL, Manson JE, Langer RD, et al. Benefits and risks of postmenopausal hormone therapy when it is initiated soon after menopause. *Am J Epidemiol*. 2009;170(1):12-23.
104. Hodis HN, Mack WJ. Postmenopausal hormone therapy in clinical perspective. *Menopause*. 2007;14(5):944-957.
105. Clarkson TB, Meléndez GC, Appt SE. Timing hypothesis for postmenopausal hormone therapy: its origin, current status, and future. *Menopause*. 2013;20(3):342-353.
106. Grodstein F, Manson JE, Stampfer MJ, Rexrode K. Postmenopausal hormone therapy and stroke: role of time since menopause and age at initiation of hormone therapy. *Arch Intern Med*. 2008;168(8):861-866.
107. Stuenkel CA, Gass ML, Manson JE, et al. A decade after the Women's Health Initiative—the experts do agree. *Menopause*. 2012;19(8):846-847.
108. Lindh-Astrand L, Bixo M, Hirschberg AL, Sundström-Poromaa I, Hammar M. A randomized controlled study of taper-down or abrupt discontinuation of hormone therapy in women treated for vasomotor symptoms. *Menopause*. 2010;17(1):72-79.
109. Ockene JK, Barad DH, Cochrane BB, et al. Symptom experience after discontinuing use of estrogen plus progestin. *JAMA*. 2005;294(2):183-193.
110. US Food and Drug Administration. *Bio-identicals: Sorting Myths From Facts*. January 9, 2008. www.fda.gov/downloads/ForConsumers/ConsumerUpdates/ucm049312.pdf. Updated April 8, 2008. Accessed July 15, 2014.
111. Simon JA, Patsner B, Allen LV Jr, et al. *Understanding the Controversy: Hormone Testing and Bioidentical Hormones*. Proceedings from the Postgraduate Course presented prior to the 17th Annual Meeting of The North American Menopause Society. Cleveland, OH: North American Menopause Society; 2006. www.menopause.org/docs/default-document-library/pg06monogrpahC2AF519C07F6.pdf?sfvrsn=2. Accessed July 15, 2014.
112. Rosenthal MS. The Wiley Protocol: an analysis of ethical issues. *Menopause*. 2008;15(5):1014-1022.
113. US Food and Drug Administration. FDA takes action against compounded menopause hormone therapy drugs [press release].FDA Web site. January 9, 2008. www.fda.gov/NewsEvents/Newsroom/PressAnnouncements/2008/ucm116832.htm. Updated April 16, 2013. Accessed July 15, 2014.
114. Federal and state role in pharmacy compounding and reconstitution: exploring the right mix to protect patients. Hearing before the U.S. Senate Committee on Health, Education, Labor, and Pensions. Pharmwatch Web site. October 23, 2003. www.pharmwatch.org/comp/sellers.shtml. Accessed July 15, 2014.
115. US Food and Drug Administration. Reminder again: obtaining an IND for estriol. The Law of Compounding Medications and Drugs Web site. June 27, 2013. www.lawofcompoundingmedications.com/2013/06/reminder-again-obtaining-ind-for-estriol.html. Accessed July 15, 2014.
116. Lobo RA, Pinkerton JV, Gass ML, et al. Evaluation of bazedoxifene/conjugated estrogens for the treatment of menopausal symptoms and effects on metabolic parameters and overall safety profile. *Fertil Steril*. 2009;92(3):1025-1038.
117. Lindsay R, Gallagher JC, Kagan R, Pickar JH, Constantine G. Efficacy of tissue-selective estrogen complex of bazedoxifene/conjugated estrogens for osteoporosis prevention in at-risk postmenopausal women. *Fertil Steril*. 2009;92(3):1045-1052.
118. Pinkerton JV, Utian WH, Constantine GD, Olivier S, Pickar JH. Relief of vasomotor symptoms with the tissue-selective estrogen complex containing bazedoxifene/conjugated estrogens: a randomized, controlled trial. *Menopause*. 2009;16(6):1116-1124.
119. Pickar JH, Yeh IT, Bachmann G, Speroff L. Endometrial effects of a tissue selective estrogen complex containing bazedoxifene/conjugated estrogens as a menopausal therapy. *Fertil Steril*. 2009;92(3):1018-1024.
120. Harvey JA, Pinkerton JV, Baracat EC, Shi H, Chines AA, Mirkin S. Breast density changes in a randomized controlled trial evaluating bazedoxifene/conjugated estrogens. *Menopause*. 2013;20(2):138-145.
121. Pinkerton JV, Harvey JA, Pan K, et al. Breast effects of bazedoxifene-conjugated estrogens: a randomized controlled trial. *Obstet Gynecol*. 2013;121(5):959-968.
122. Bachmann GA, Komi JO; Ospemifene Study Group. Ospemifene effectively treats vulvovaginal atrophy in postmenopausal women: results from a pivotal phase 3 study. *Menopause*. 2010;7(3):480-486.
123. McCall JL, DeGregorio MW. Pharmacologic evaluation of ospemifene. *Expert Opin Drug Metab Toxicol*. 2010;6(6):773-779.
124. Simon JA, Lin VH, Radovich C, Bachmann GA; Ospemifene Study Group. One-year long-term safety extension study of ospemifene for the treatment of vulvar and vaginal atrophy in postmenopausal women with a uterus. *Menopause*. 2013;20(4):418-427.
125. Portman DJ, Bachmann GA, Simon JA; Ospemifene Study Group. Ospemifene, a novel selective estrogen receptor modulator for treating dyspareunia associated with postmenopausal vulvar and vaginal atrophy. *Menopause*. 2013;20(6):623-630.
126. Cuzick J, Forbes JF, Sestak I, et al; International Breast Cancer Intervention Study I Investigators. Long-term results of tamoxifen prophylaxis for breast cancer–96-month follow-up of the IBIS-I trial. *J Natl Cancer Inst*. 2007;99(4):272-282.
127. Powles TJ, Ashley S, Tidy A, Smith IE, Dowsett M. Twenty-year follow-up of the Royal Marsden randomized, double-blinded tamoxifen breast cancer prevention trial. *J Natl Cancer Inst*. 2007;99(4):283-290.
128. Powles TJ, Hickish T, Kanis JA, Tidy A, Ashley S. Effect of tamoxifen on bone mineral density measured by dual-energy x-ray absorptiometry in healthy premenopausal and postmenopausal women. *J Clin Oncol*. 1996;14;(1):78-84.
129. Love RR, Mazess RB, Barden HS, et al. Effects of tamoxifen on bone mineral density in postmenopausal women with breast cancer. *N Engl J Med*. 1992;26(13):852-856.
130. Delmas PD, Bjarnason NH, Mitlak BH, et al. Effects of raloxifene on bone mineral density, serum cholesterol concentrations, and uterine endometrium in postmenopausal women. *N Engl J Med*. 1997;337(23):1641-1647.
131. Ettinger B, Black DM, Mitlack BH, et al. Reduction of vertebral fracture risk in postmenopausal women with osteoporosis treated with raloxifene: results from a 3-year randomized clinical trial. Multiple Outcomes of Raloxifene Evaluation (MORE) Investigators. *JAMA*. 1999;282(7):637-645. Erratum in: *JAMA*. 1999;282(22):2124.
132. Martino S, Cauley JA, Barrett-Connor E, et al; CORE Investigators. Continuing outcomes relevant to Evista: breast cancer incidence in postmenopausal osteoporotic women in a randomized trial of raloxifene. *J Natl Cancer Inst*. 2004;96(23):1751-1761.
133. Grady D, Ettinger B, Moscarelli E, et al; Multiple Outcomes of Raloxifene Evaluation Investigators. Safety and adverse effects associated with raloxifene: multiple outcomes of raloxifene evaluation. *Obstet Gynecol*. 2004;104(4):837-844.
134. Jordan VC. Optimising endocrine approaches for the chemoprevention of breast cancer beyond the Study of Tamoxifen and Raloxifene (STAR) trial. *Eur J Cancer*. 2006;42(17):2909-2913.
135. Vogel VG, Constantino JP, Wickerham DL, et al; National Surgical Adjuvant Breast and Bowel Project (NSABP). Effects of tamoxifen vs raloxifene on the risk of developing invasive breast cancers and other disease outcomes: the NSABP Study of Tamoxifen and Raloxifene (STAR) P-2 Trials. *JAMA*. 2006;295(23):2727-2741. Erratum in: *JAMA*. 2006;296(24):2926; *JAMA*. 2007;298(9):973.
136. Barrett-Connor E, Mosca L, Collins P, et al; Raloxifene Use for the Heart (RUTH) Trial Investigators. Effects of raloxifene on cardiovascular events and breast cancer in postmenopausal women. *N Engl J Med*. 2006;355(2):125-137.
137. Hertz DL, McLeod HL, Irvin WJ Jr. Tamoxifen and CYP2D6: a contradiction of data. *Oncologist*. 2012;17(5):620-630.

138. Kelly CM, Juurlink DN, Gomes T, et al. Selective serotonin reuptake inhibitors and breast cancer mortality in women receiving tamoxifen: a population based cohort study. *BMJ.* 2010;340:c693.
139. Davison SL, Bell R, Donath S, Montalto J, Davis SR. Androgen levels in adult females: changes with age, menopause, and oophorectomy. *J Clin Endocrinol Metab.* 2005;90(7):3847-3853.
140. Dunn JF, Nisula BC, Rodboard D. Transport of steroid hormones: binding of 21 endogenous steroids to both testosterone-binding globulin and corticosteroid-binding globulin in human plasma. *J Clin Endocrinol Metab.* 1981;53(1):58-68.
141. Shifren JL, Desindes S, McIlwain M, Doros G, Mazer N. A randomized, open label, crossover study comparing the effects of oral versus transdermal estrogen therapy on serum androgens, thyroid hormones, and adrenal hormones in naturally menopausal women. *Menopause.* 2007;14(6):985-994.
142. Davis SR, Davison SL, Donath S, Bell RJ. Circulating androgen levels and self-reported sexual function in women. *JAMA.* 2005;294(1):91-96.
143. Buster JE, Kingsberg SA, Aguirre O, et al. Testosterone patch for low sexual desire in surgically menopausal women: a randomized trial. *Obstet Gynecol.* 2005;105(5 pt 1):944-952.
144. Lobo RA, Rosen RC, Yang HM, Block B, Van Der Hoop RG. Comparative effects of oral esterified estrogens with and without methyltestosterone on endocrine profiles and dimensions of sexual function in postmenopausal women with hypoactive sexual desire. *Fertil Steril.* 2003;79(6):1341-1352.
145. Davis SR, Moreau M, Kroll R, et al; APHRODITE Study Team. Testosterone for low libido in postmenopausal women not taking estrogen. *N Engl J Med.* 2008;359(19):2005-2017.
146. Shifren JL, Davis SR, Moreau M, et al. Testosterone patch for the treatment of hypoactive sexual desire disorder in naturally menopausal women: results from the INTIMATE NM1 Study. *Menopause.* 2006;13(5):770-779. Erratum in: *Menopause.* 2007;14(1):157.
147. Simon J, Braunstein G, Nachtigall L, et al. Testosterone patch increases sexual activity and desire in surgically menopausal women with hypoactive sexual desire disorder. *J Clin Endocrinol Metab.* 2005;90(9):5226-5233.
148. Shifren JL, Braunstein GD, Simon JA, et al. Transdermal testosterone treatment in women with impaired sexual function after oophorectomy. *N Engl J Med.* 2000;343(10):682-688.
149. Davis SR, Goldstat R, Papalia MA, et al. Effects of aromatase inhibition on sexual function and well-being in postmenopausal women treated with testosterone: a randomized, placebo-controlled trial. *Menopause.* 2006;13(1):37-45.
150. Raisz LG, Wiita B, Artis A, et al. Comparison of the effects of estrogen alone and estrogen plus androgen on biochemical markers of bone formation and resorption in postmenopausal women. *J Clin Endocrinol Metab.* 1996;81(1):37-43.
151. Davis SR, McCloud P, Strauss BJ, Burger H. Testosterone enhances estradiol's effects on postmenopausal bone density and sexuality. *Maturitas.* 1995;21(3):227-236.
152. Watts NB, Notelovitz M, Timmons MC, Addison WA, Wiita B, Downey LJ. Comparison of oral estrogens and estrogens plus androgen on bone mineral density, menopausal symptoms, and lipid-lipoprotein profiles in surgical menopause. *Obstet Gynecol.* 1995;85(4):529-537. Erratum in: *Obstet Gynecol.* 1995;85(5 pt 1):668.
153. Miller KK, Biller BM, Beauregard C, et al. Effects of testosterone replacement in androgen-deficient women with hypopituitarism: a randomized, double-blind, placebo-controlled study. *J Clin Endocrinol Metab.* 2006;91(5):1683-1690.
154. Davis SR, Panjari M, Stanczyk FZ. Clinical review: DHEA replacement for postmenopausal women. *J Clin Endocrinol Metab.* 2011;96(6):1642-1653.
155. Alkatib AA, Cosma M, Elamin MB, et al. A systematic review and meta-analysis of randomized placebo-controlled trials of DHEA treatment effects on quality of life in women with adrenal insufficiency. *J Clin Endocrinol Metab.* 2009;94(10):3676-3681.
156. Wierman ME, Basson R, Davis SR, et al. Androgen therapy in women: an Endocrine Society Clinical Practice guideline. *J Clin Endocrinol Metab.* 2006;91(10):3697-3710.
157. Sarwer DB, Durlak JA. A field trial of the effectiveness of behavioral treatment for sexual dysfunctions. *J Sex Marital Ther.* 1997;23(2):87-97.
158. Braunstein GD. Safety of testosterone treatment in postmenopausal women. *Fertil Steril.* 2007;88(1):1-17.
159. Sutton-Tyrrell K, Wildman RP, Matthews KA, et al; SWAN Investigators. Sex-hormone-binding globulin and the free androgen index are related to cardiovascular risk factors in multiethnic premenopausal and perimenopausal women enrolled in the Study of Women Across the Nation (SWAN). *Circulation.* 2005;111(10):1242-1249.
160. Bell RJ, Davison SL, Papalia MA, McKenzie DP, Davis SR. Endogenous androgen levels and cardiovascular risk profile in women across the adult life span. *Menopause.* 2007;14(4):630-638.
161. Tamimi RM, Hankinson SE, Chen WY, Rosner B, Colditz GA. Combined estrogen and testosterone use and risk of breast cancer in postmenopausal women. *Arch Intern Med.* 2006;166(14):1483-1489.

APPENDIX

How to Evaluate Scientific Literature

As new studies are published, the evidence base increases for understanding the risks and benefits of treatment options. A basic understanding of the types of studies and the meaning of the analyses helps healthcare professionals to evaluate the evidence and implications for clinical practice. Readers in search of more sophisticated discussions are urged to consult current clinical epidemiology texts.

Study types

Two major types of studies are *experimental* and *observational*.[1,2] There are also meta-analyses, which pool the results of clinical trials or other types of studies.

In experimental studies, interventions and conditions are strictly defined and controlled by the investigators. In observational studies, investigators observe outcomes in relation to variables of interest. They do not assign participants to an exposure of interest.

Experimental studies

Types of experimental studies are randomized controlled trials (RCTs), crossover trials, and quasi-experimental studies.

- *Randomized, controlled trials* are considered the strongest for therapeutic interventions. In RCTs, a group of participants with similar characteristics is identified (eg, low bone density). Each participant is then randomly assigned (similar to a flip of a coin; neither the participants nor the investigator chooses) to an *intervention group* (or groups) or to a *control group*. Participants typically have an equal and unbiased (random) chance of being assigned to each treatment under study. Randomized, controlled trials have the best chance of avoiding selection bias if the randomization is adequate and the study size is large. This is because known and unknown characteristics should be the same in each group. The baseline characteristics of the 2 groups should be presented and statistically compared in an RCT's final report. The Women's Health Initiative is an example of an RCT.

Randomized, controlled trials are best suited to situations in which exposure to treatment is modifiable, a legitimate uncertainty exists regarding benefit or harm of treatment, and outcomes are reasonably common. However, inclusion and exclusion criteria may limit the extrapolation of the results to other groups (limiting whether the results can be generalized).

The *power* of a trial is the likelihood that it will determine the effect of the intervention. The number of participants is determined when the trial is designed, based on the likelihood of the measured outcome events and the anticipated magnitude of the intervention's effect. If events do not occur as often as predicted, the trial may not have adequate power to determine the effect of the intervention. The *Methods* section of the published trial results will describe how the investigator calculated the number of participants required and will quantify the range of effect the study can detect (eg, the study was powered to detect more than a 20% reduction in heart attacks). *Publication bias* favors small trials with positive outcomes. An international registry of clinical trials requires submission of the planned trial (including design, interventions, and prespecified outcomes) so that a full accounting of the status of trials that are not completed or are completed, regardless of their outcomes, can be assessed.

Depending on the intervention, participants and investigators may be purposefully *blinded* or *masked* (ie, they do not know which treatment a participant is receiving). This helps reduce some forms of bias and the effects of the participant's or investigator's expectations of intervention benefit.

Classically, RCTs are used to assess for *efficacy* of the treatment in an ideal controlled setting. More often, an RCT will assess *effectiveness* (not efficacy) by studying the intervention under more usual circumstances. This is because a study for efficacy may not reflect its actual effectiveness in a real-world, clinical practice setting. Both types of RCTs often use a relatively narrowly

APPENDIX

defined patient population. Even though an RCT is quite internally valid (ie, the study was done well), it may not be accurate to extrapolate (generalize) the results from one RCT to another patient population that was not studied in the trial.

Other important issues when evaluating the results of an RCT include checking to see whether all participants who started the trial were accounted for at trial conclusion and whether the groups were treated equally aside from the experimental intervention.

- *Crossover trials* allow participants to serve as their own controls. Participants are randomly assigned to one treatment arm and later switched to the other treatment arm. This crossover study methodology has often been used in trials to assess the efficacy of medications. The design is difficult to do well because of its potential for residual effects between interventions. Often there will be a *washout* period (time during which no treatment is given) between interventions.

- *Quasi-experimental studies* are of 2 general varieties. In one, 2 interventions are simultaneously compared in 2 groups of participants, but interventions are not randomized for any given participant (eg, 2 hospitals comparing 2 types of wound closure for the same type of surgery).

   Another common quasi-experimental study is when participants serve as their own controls, and the investigator controls the intervention. The intervention is neither randomized nor is there a control population to which the response can be compared. After baseline evaluation, the intervention is given, and the participants are reevaluated to observe any changes in characteristics because of the intervention.

Observational studies

Types of observational studies include purely *analytic* (or *descriptive*) studies. Analytic studies (including cohort studies, case-control studies, and cross-sectional studies) have a nonrandomized control group (eg, women who did not use hormone therapy [HT] for any number of reasons would be compared with women who elected to use HT). What is sampled first—risk factor, outcome, or risk factor and outcome simultaneously—determines which analytic study design is being used. Case reports and case series are not analytic because they do not have control comparisons. Observational studies can assess associations and correlations between exposures and outcomes, but they cannot confirm cause-and-effect relationships.

- *Cohort studies (or longitudinal studies)* begin with a defined group of participants (eg, persons of a certain age or those who work in a certain industry) called the *cohort*. These studies sample persons from the general population and determine whether they have exposures or risk factors of interest (eg, HT users vs nonusers). This cohort of persons is then followed over time to study a variety of outcomes. Data are collected in a similar manner on all participants from the beginning of the study (the baseline) and frequently at set intervals during follow-up. The Nurses' Health Study is one of the best-known prospective (occurring over time) cohort studies.

   These studies provide a clearer temporal sequence of exposures and outcomes than other analytic studies, are well suited for common exposures, and can study multiple exposures and outcomes. However, they can be time-consuming and expensive, they have the potential for many forms of bias, and participants may be lost during follow-up. When too many patients are lost, the validity of the study is compromised.

   Cohort studies may follow relevant events as they occur over time (prospective), but they may also be performed in a historical or a concurrent (cross-sectional) manner. Evidence from prospective cohort studies is considered stronger than the other forms of analytic studies because data on exposures are collected before the outcomes occur.

   The term *retrospective* is sometimes used when referring to a historical cohort study, but it can be confusing. If the data are easily accessible, the researcher can retrospectively evaluate a cohort that was followed in time, but the time was in the past moving forward (historical cohort), not progressing from current time onward (concurrent cohort). An example of a retrospective cohort is an occupational cohort with known exposure to a carcinogen or toxin in the remote past and whose participants have already accrued outcomes. In the Nurses' Health Study and the Framingham Study, information was gleaned in a concurrent and prospective fashion (in contrast to a historical cohort). All participants in each of these circumstances were followed longitudinally forward in some time frame.

- *Case-control studies* begin with an outcome or disease of interest (eg, myocardial infarction [MI], breast cancer) and then compare the characteristics or exposures of participants with the outcome *cases* to *controls* who do not have the outcome or disease of interest. Case-control studies are prone to many more forms of bias. A frequent one is *recall bias* (ie, participants cannot remember exposures or risk factors accurately).

   Matching participants for specific characteristics and defining strict eligibility criteria lessens but cannot eliminate the possibility that the results are *confounded*. For example, women who use HT are known to smoke less and lead generally healthier lifestyles. Hormone therapy users have less cardiovascular disease primarily because of better lifestyle habits rather than from any beneficial effect of HT use. Smoking or other lifestyle patterns can confound the results when observational studies analyze

HT use and health outcomes. Matching cases and controls for smoking status (or adjusting for this variable) helps reduce this confounding.

Despite these limitations, case-control studies have many advantages. Because they begin with an outcome of interest, they can be performed efficiently and at less cost than cohort studies. They are important in situations in which it would be unethical to assign participants to an exposure (eg, chemotherapy) or when an outcome is rare (eg, X-chromosome abnormalities associated with primary ovarian insufficiency).

- *Cross-sectional studies* are snapshots in time. Here, cases and controls are evaluated at the same time for risk factors or characteristics and outcomes of interest. Cross-sectional studies are very useful for determining prevalence, for planning for healthcare needs, and for generating hypotheses.

- *Case reports* and *case series* describe the experience of a single patient or series of patients. Such reports are useful in bringing new diseases or phenomena to the attention of the clinical and scientific community and for generating new hypotheses. However, lacking a control group, case reports or series without further study are only suggestive.

Many of these basic designs can be modified or combined, and many hybrid studies exist. An example is a case-control study within a cohort; this is a very useful study design and can provide many advantages, including cost efficiency.

Meta-analyses

Meta-analysis describes an analytic technique used to pool the results of clinical trials or other types of studies (not only RCTs). Often, a meta-analysis is performed on a group of studies that are too small to have statistical significance by themselves but that may show significance when pooled. Specific criteria (eg, eligibility criteria of participants, follow-up rates, data quality) are established to determine which studies will be included in the analysis. Inasmuch as any biases present in the contributing studies will be present in the meta-analysis, the outcome of a meta-analysis is only as good as the studies included.

In general, meta-analyses are difficult to perform. They are best performed based on the original data obtained from each investigator from each individual study. International guidelines provide checklists to understand the quality of a meta-analysis of clinical trials (eg, Consolidated Standards of Reporting Trials [CONSORT] guidelines).[3,4]

Analyzing study results

The bottom-line question when evaluating a study is: "What are the results?" The results of cohort studies and clinical trials are most frequently presented as a *relative risk* (RR)—the likely level of greater or lower risk (eg, for HT users vs nonusers). The RR can be determined because these study designs follow participants longitudinally, and risk (which is time-dependent) can be determined in each comparison group.

Rate/Risk

The term *rate* is the number of events per the number of participants per the time interval (eg, 44/10,000/y). Knowing the exact number of events over time is very useful, because this determines the risk.

The Council for International Organizations of Medical Sciences Task Force has provided nomenclature to guide the interpretation of risks[5]:

- Rare = Less than or equal to 10 in 10,000 per year
- Very rare = Less than or equal to 1 in 10,000 per year

Rare outcomes would not be of such great concern to an individual woman making a decision about treatment. However, it is important to recognize that common exposures that produce rare outcomes can still have profound public health effects.

Relative risk

The RR is a ratio—the rate of disease or the outcome of interest in a group exposed to a potential risk factor or treatment, or having a characteristic of interest, divided by the rate of disease of interest in an unexposed group (ie, those without the risk factor, treatment, or characteristic of interest). The RR should be used only for prospective studies.

Rate is used in both the numerator and the denominator. These are the numbers of events, per numbers of participants, per time interval (eg, 50/100,000/y). For example, if the annual rate of MI in women who smoke is 220 per 100,000, and the annual rate in women who do not smoke is 110 per 100,000, the RR associated with smoking is:

$$RR = \frac{220}{100,000/y} \div \frac{110}{100,000/y} = 2.00$$

This means that compared with nonsmoking women, the risk of MI for a woman who smokes is twice that of a woman who does not smoke in the study.

An RR less than 1.0 suggests that the factor decreases risk. For example, an RR of 0.50 means that there is a 50% less chance (or risk) of the outcome studied in those with the risk factor versus those without the risk factor of interest. An RR of 0.3 means a 70% lower relative risk.

An RR greater than 1.0 suggests that the factor increases risk. For example, an RR of 1.2 means there is a 20% increase in risk in the group with the risk factor versus the group without the risk factor. An RR of 2.0 means double the risk.

Odds ratio

The odds ratio (OR) is an estimate used in many analytic studies. It best approximates the RR when the outcome is rare.

APPENDIX

Confidence interval

The confidence interval (CI), usually cited with the RR or the OR, indicates with a certain degree of assurance the range within which lies the true magnitude of the measured effect. The CI has 2 components—the degree of certainty and the range (eg, 95% CI, 1.09-1.32). The point estimate (the RR or OR number) is the best mathematical estimate from the data. Understanding the upper and lower limits of the range is often clinically useful. If the CI is *wide*, the reader's confidence in the validity of the RR would be less than if the CI is *narrow* (ie, closer to the value of the RR).

Often, a 95% CI is used. A 95% CI gives the range of values that have a 95% probability of containing the true RR or OR. When a 95% CI does not contain the number 1.0 (eg, 0.40-0.80 or 1.12-1.37), the measured RR or OR is statistically significant by at least $P<.05$. The CI is more clinically useful than the P value because the CI helps the reader to understand the best estimate of the effect, and it provides the mathematical estimated limits, which are useful in determining the best-case and worse-case scenarios.

P value

This term is the probability of obtaining the observed RR or OR (or a more extreme value) by chance (random sampling) alone. A P value of .01 means that there is a 1% mathematical probability that the observed difference between 2 groups occurred by chance. By convention, P is generally deemed statistically significant if it is below 0.05. This means that if 20 outcomes are evaluated in a single study, 1 of these outcomes is likely to show a positive result just because of chance alone ($P=.05$, or 1/20). By the time $P=.001$, the likelihood is only 1 in 1,000 that the results occurred by chance—in other words, the finding is more likely to be real.

It is important to remember that a study can be statistically significant and not clinically significant. However, if it is not statistically significant, it cannot reach clinical significance, and the result could be clinically nonsignificant or inconclusive. An example is when the study is underpowered.

Absolute risk/Attributable risk

The effect of RR on a population and on an individual basis depends on *incidence* (ie, the number of new cases in a given period). This can be quantified by the absolute risk or attributable risk (AR), which is the difference between the incidence rates in the exposed and unexposed groups—in other words, the *risk difference*. The AR quantifies the effect of exposure, providing a measure of its public health effect. For example, for the calculation about the risk of MI in women who smoke, the AR is

$$AR = \frac{220}{100,000/y} - \frac{110}{100,000/y} = \frac{110}{100,000/y}$$

This means that for every 100,000 women who smoke, there would be 110 additional cases of MI per year.

Often, AR is more clinically useful than RR in explaining risk to patients. The US Food and Drug Administration requires that the absolute risk reduction be included on the product information sheet.

Number needed to treat

To communicate this risk difference to patients, the number needed to treat (NNT) can be useful. The NNT is merely the reciprocal of the AR (ie, 1 divided by the AR). For example, in a 1-year study, if the rate of an outcome was 20 per 1,000 in an untreated group and 10 per 1,000 in a treated group, the NNT is

$$NNT = \frac{1}{(20/1,000) - (10/1,000)} = \frac{1}{(10/1,000)} = \frac{1}{0.01} = 100$$

This means that for every 100 people treated, there would be 1 fewer negative outcome over the year.

References

1. Koepsell TD, Weiss NS. *Epidemiologic Methods: Studying the Occurrence of Illness.* New York: Oxford University Press; 2003.
2. Porta M. ed. *A Dictionary of Epidemiology.* 5th ed. New York: Oxford University Press; 2008.
3. Moher D, Schulz KF, Altman D; CONSORT Group (Consolidated Standards of Reporting Trials). The CONSORT statement: revised recommendations for improving the quality of reports of parallel-group randomized trials. *JAMA.* 2001;285(15):1987-1991.
4. Stroup DF, Berlin JA, Morton SC, et al. Meta-analysis of observational studies in epidemiology: a proposal for reporting. Meta-analysis of Observational Studies in Epidemiology (MOOSE) Group. *JAMA.* 2000;283(15):2008-2012.
5. World Health Organization. *Guidelines for Preparing Core Clinical-Safety Information on Drugs.* 2nd ed. Report of CIOMS Working Groups III and IV. Geneva: World Health Organization; 1999.

INDEX

Note: Page numbers in italics indicate that content may appear in a table or figure on that page.

5α-reductase, 32-34

A

abnormal uterine bleeding (AUB), 47-50, *48, 51*
   endometrial cancer diagnosis, 150
   estrogen-progestogen therapy, 273
   management of, 51-55, *53,* 152-153
   overview of, 47-48
   perimenopause and, *48*
   possible causes, *49, 50*
abuse, physical and sexual, 195-197, *197*
acne, 29, 31
actinic keratoses, 29, 163
acupuncture, 81, 134, 209-210, 221-222
Addison disease, 14, *283*
adenomyosis, 48, *49, 50*
adrenal glands
   adrenal physiology and menopause, 10-11
   androgen production, 5
   sexual function and, 74
adrenergic system, 10-11
adrenocorticotropic hormone (ACTH), 9, 10-11
aerobic activity, *26,* 198-199. *See also* exercise
aging
   adrenal physiology, 10-11
   androgen therapy, 282-284, *283*
   antimüllerian hormone (AMH) levels, 6
   cognitive changes, 85-87
   fertility, decline in, 45
   fracture risk and, 122, *123*
   hypothalamic-pituitary-ovarian (HPO) axis, 9-10
   quality of life, 1-2
   sexual function and, *75*
   STRAW+10 staging system, 3-9, *4, 5, 7*
AIDS and HIV, 92-93, *92, 93,* 95, *125,* 153-154, *154*
alcohol
   bone health, 123, *123*
   cancer risk, 141, 146, 150
   cardiovascular health and, 112
   clinical evaluation, 187-188
   recommended consumption, 25
   sleep disturbances and, 81
aldosterone blockade, 116
alendronate, 127-129, *128*
alopecia, 31-34
Alzheimer disease, 86-87, 244
amenorrhea, 6, *15, 48*. *See also* primary ovarian insufficiency
American Cancer Society (ACS), *141, 145, 154,* 157, *160,* 184, 189, 280
American College of Cardiology (ACC), 108-111, 113, 116, 119
   2013 ACC/AHA guidelines, 109, 111, 113, 119
American Congress of Obstetricians and Gynecologists (ACOG) recommendations
   abuse screening, 196
   clinical breast examination, 184
   compounded hormone products, 280
   genetic testing, 192
   hormonal contraceptives, 120, 260, 263
   HPV vaccine, 154
   hyperplasia, 148
   infertility, 45
   mammograms, 189
   migraine with aura, 85
   periodic pelvic examination, 184
   routine cervical cancer screening, 154, *155*
   transvaginal ultrasound, 193
American Heart Association (AHA)
   blood pressure, 114
   diet and lifestyle, 24-25, 110-112, 215
   risk assessment, 108, 109, 215
American Society for Colposcopy and Cervical Pathology, 96, 154, 189
anabolic agents, osteoporosis treatments, 131-132
anal incontinence, 73
androgenetic alopecia (AGA), 31-34
androgens
   acne and, 29
   adrenal physiology and menopause, 7-11
   androgen receptors, 12
   dehydroepiandrosterone (DHEA), 5, 86, 247-248, 282-284
   eye changes, midlife, 34-37
   hair growth, 31-34
   hearing loss and, 37
   hormone therapy, 282-284, *283*
   menstrual cycle and, 5
   sexual function and, *75, 76*
   skin health and, 31
androstenedione, *5,* 8, 9, 10
anemia, 54, 240-241
angina, 107. *See also* cardiovascular disease
angiotensin-converting enzyme (ACE) inhibitors, 114, 116
angiotensin II receptor blockers (ARBs), 114, 116
anovulatory uterine bleeding, 48-49, *50*
antiandrogens, 33
anticoagulant therapy, adverse interactions with, 221-222, 236, 244, 246
anticonvulsants, 49, 59, 64, 83, *84, 91, 125,* 262
antidepressants, 58-59, 83, 91-92
antimüllerian hormone (AMH), 3-9, *4, 5, 7,* 46, 190, 191
antioxidants, 30, 111-112, 229, 236
antiresorptive agents, 127-129, *128*
antiviral therapy, 94
antral follicle count (AFC), 3-9, *4, 5, 7,* 46
anxiety disorders
   androgen and, 12
   evaluation and management, 89-92, *91*
   hormones and, 88-89, *90*
   patient history, 183
   sexual function and, *75, 76,* 78
   sleep quality and, 80
   symptoms of, 87-88, *89*
appetite suppressants, 26-27
aromatase inhibitors (AIs), 54, 56, *68, 125,* 147, 210
arrhythmia, 60, 107, 219, 244. *See also* cardiovascular disease
arthralgia, 133-136
arthritis, *14,* 22, 133-136, 245-246
aspirin, 113, 116, 119, 161
asthma, 140-141
atherosclerosis. *See* cardiovascular disease
Atopobium, 21
atrophic vaginitis, 21, 284
auditory examination, 185-186
aura, migraine headache and, 83-85

293

autoimmune disorders
    dry eye syndrome and, 35
    heart disease risk, 109
    primary ovarian insufficiency and, 13, *14*
    rheumatoid arthritis, 134-135
Ayurveda, 207-208, 211

B
bacteria. *See also* sexually transmitted infections (STIs)
    bacterial vaginosis, 65, *65*, 93
    vulvovaginal changes, 21
bariatric surgery, 27
barrier birth control methods, 47
Bartholin gland cysts, 67
basal cell carcinoma, 163
bazedoxifene (BZA), 12, 58, 126, 130, *131*, 263, 274, 281
behavioral counseling, health promotion, 197-199, *198*, *200*
behavior therapy, sleep disturbances, 81
benzodiazepines, 81, *91*, 187, 248, 249
beta-blockers, 114, 116
beta-carotene, 112, 229-231, *230*
bimatoprost, 33
bioidentical hormones, 58, 278-280
biopsy, endometrial, 51, 53
birth control. *See* contraceptives
bisphosphonate therapy, 37-38, 126, 127-129, *128*
black cohosh, 57, 58, 208, 217-218
bladder, urinary
    cancer of, *141*
    estrogen receptors, 11-12
    genitourinary syndrome of menopause, 60-63, *61*, *62*, *63*, *64*
    urinary incontinence, 68-73, *69*, *70*, *72*, *73*
bleeding, vaginal. *See* abnormal uterine bleeding (AUB); menstrual cycle
blood glucose, 23, 114-120, *117*
blood pressure
    body weight and, 22
    cardiovascular disease and, 109-110
    coenzyme Q10, 243
    contraceptive use and, *259*, 260
    diabetes mellitus and, 119, 120
    hypertension, *110*
    management of, 114
    menopause and, 108
    metabolic syndrome, 109
blood vessels, estrogen receptors, 11-12. *See also* cardiovascular disease (CVD)
body changes, midlife
    body weight, 22-27, *25*, *26*, *28*
    ears, 37
    eyes, 34-37
    hair, 31-34
    skin, 27, 29-31
    teeth and oral cavity, 37-38, *38*
    vulvovaginal, 21-22
body mass index (BMI), 23, 183-184, *185*
body weight, 22-27, *25*, *26*, *28*
    cancer risk, *141*, 144, 146, 149-150, *150*
    cardiovascular health and, 108, 112-113
    clinical evaluation, 186
    contraceptive use and, *259*, 260
    dehydroepiandrosterone (DHEA), 248
    diabetes mellitus, 114-115, *117*
    fracture risk, 123, *123*
    hot flashes and, 56, *57*
    medications for weight loss, 25-27
    metabolic syndrome, 22-23, 108, 109, 115
    midlife change in, 22-27, *25*, *26*, *28*
    osteoarthritis and, 134

physical exam, 183-184, *185*
    sexual function and, *75*
    weight management, 23-25, *25*, *26*
bone health
    androgen therapy, 283
    antiepileptic drug therapy, 140
    body weight and, 23
    dehydroepiandrosterone (DHEA), 248
    estrogen receptors, 11-12
    evaluation of, 124-126, *125*, *127*, 188
    hormone therapy and, 274, 277-278
    isoflavones, effects of, 214
    magnesium and, 241
    osteoporosis, overview, 121-122, *121*
    osteoporosis, pharmacologic interventions, 126-132, *128*, *130*, *131*
    osteoporosis, risk factors, 122-124, *123*, *124*
    osteoporosis, secondary, 124, *125*, *127*
    primary ovarian insufficiency and, 15
    raloxifene, 12
    smoking and, 187
    tamoxifen, 281-282
    thyroid disorders and, 138
    tooth loss and, 37-38, *38*
    vitamin D, 233-234
bone mineral density (BMD), 15, 37, *121*, 122, *123*, 125-126, 130-131, 187, 214, 234, 258, *262*
botanical remedies, 216-221
    Chinese medicine, 210-211
    homeopathy, 208-209
    overview, 216-217
    safety concerns, 221-*222*, 227-229
    sleep disturbances, 82
    weight loss and, 24
BRCA1 and *BRCA2* genes, 141, 142, 147, 155, 157-158
breast cancer
    androgen therapy, 284
    body weight and, 22
    hormone therapy and, 274, 277
    incidence, 141-142, *141*
    pharmacologic interventions, 146-148
    risk factors, 142-144, *143*, *144*, 145-146
    screening for, 144-*145*, 188-189
    selective estrogen-receptor modulators (SERMs), 11-12, 146-148, 280-282
bupropion, 27, 78
burning mouth syndrome, 38

C
caffeine, 25, 71, 81, 84, 188
calcitonin, 126, *128*, 130-131
calcitriol, 233, 234
calcium
    bone health and, 122, 123, *125*
    epilepsy and, 140
    magnesium and, 241
    sources and benefits, 237-240, *240*
    vitamin D and, 233-234
California Teachers Study, 145-146, 162
Canadian Cancer Society, *141*, 142, 145
cancer. *See also* breast cancer
    abnormal uterine bleeding, 48, *49*, *50*, 51, 53
    androgen therapy, 284
    antioxidants and, 229-230
    body weight and, 22, 184
    bone health, secondary osteoporosis, 124, *125*
    B vitamins, effects of, 232
    cervical, 96, *141*, 153-*154*, *155*, 189, 230
    chemotherapy, effects of, 17, 124

294

colorectal, 158-161, *160*, 189, 230, 232
endometrial, 146, 148-153, *149, 150, 151*
hormone therapy and, 274, 277
human papillomavirus (HPV), 95-96, 153-154, *154, 155*
lesbian health, 195
lichen sclerosus and, 66
lung, 158
ovarian, 12, *141*, 154-158, 1*56*, 229
pancreatic, *141*, 161-162
progestogen therapy and, 270-278, *272, 274, 275, 276*
risk factors, general, *141*
selective estrogen-receptor modulators (SERMs), 11-12, 146-148, 280-282
skin, 29-30, 162-163
spironolactone use and, 33
thyroid, 139
Candida albicans, 65
cardiovascular disease (CVD)
aspirin use, 113
body weight and, 22, 112-113
B vitamins, effects of, 232-233
contraceptive use and, 260-261
depression and, 89
diabetes mellitus and, 114-115, 118, 120-121
diet and, 229-230, 236-237, 244
gallbladder disease and, 132-133
hormone therapy and, 16, 108, 115-116, 269, 273, *275, 276*, 277
hypertension and, *110*
lifestyle and, 110-111
migraine headache and stroke, 85
overview of, 107
pharmacologic interventions, 113-116, *114*
risk factors, 108-110
screening for, 189
SERMS and, 281, 282
sleep and, 79, 80
thyroid disorders and, 137, 138
treatment for, 116
cataracts, 35-36
celiac disease, 14, *15, 125*, 241
Centers for Disease Control and Prevention (CDC), 66, 93, 120, *141*, 196, 255, *257, 258, 259*
cervical cancer, 96, *141*, 153-154, *154, 155*, 189, 230
chemotherapy
androgen therapy, 282-284, *283*
bone health and, 124
effects of, 17
hearing loss and, 37
hot flashes, 56
induced menopause, 3
premature menopause, 12-17, *14, 15, 16*
Chinese medicine, 207-211, 221-222
chlamydia, 92-94, *92, 93*
chloasma, 30
cholesterol, blood levels
changes in menopause, 108
diet and, 112
dyslipidemia, 110, *111*
estrogen therapy and, 269
gallbladder disease, 132-133
management of, 113-*114*
screening tests, 109
cholesterol, dietary, 25, 108, 112
chondroitin, 245-246
chronic reaction vulvitis, 66
circadian rhythm, 9, 10, 248-249
classical lichen planus, 67
climacteric, defined, 3

clinical depression, 87, *88. See also* depression
clinical evaluation
auditory exam, 185-186
blood pressure, 184
dental/oral examination, 185
diagnostic and screening tests, 188-193
eye exam, 185
family history, 183
lesbian health issues, 194-196, *195*
medical history, 182-183
overview, 181, *182*
physical examination, 183-186, *185*
physical or sexual abuse, 195-197, *197*
primary ovarian insufficiency, *16*
quality-of-life evaluation tools, 201-202
rectal exam, 185
sexual history, 183
skin exam, 185
social and cultural aspects of care, 193-194
social history, 183
clitoris, 60-63, *61, 62, 63, 64*, 78, *79*
clomiphene citrate challenge, 45
clonidine, 60
cluster headache, 82, 83
coenzyme Q10, 84, 243-244
cognitive behavioral therapy, sleep disturbances, 81
cognitive function
changes in, 85-87
dehydroepiandrosterone (DHEA), 248
depression and, 89
estrogen receptors, 11-12
fish oil, omega-3, and -6 fatty acids, 244
hormone therapy and, 16
isoflavones, effects of, 214-215
collagen fibers, skin, 29, 30
colon, estrogen receptors, 11-12
colonoscopy, 159-160
colorectal cancer
antioxidants, effects of, 230
B vitamins, effects of, 232
incidence, *141*, 158
risk factors, 159, *160,* 161
screening for, 159-161, 189
complementary and alternative medicine (CAM)
Ayurveda, 211
Chinese medicine, 209-211
herbal therapies, 24, 82, 216-221
integrative medicine, 207-208
isoflavones, 212-216, *212, 213*
naturopathy and homeopathy, 207-*209*
safety concerns, 217, 221-*222,* 227-229
yoga, 211-212
compounded bioidentical hormone therapy, 278-280
condylomata acuminatum (genital wart), 67
conjugated estrogens, 12, 53, 58, 62, *63*, 115, *130, 131*, 263, 265-266, *265, 267, 268, 269*, 281
contact dermatitis, 67
Continuing Outcomes Relative to Evista (CORE) trial, 146-147
contraceptives
abnormal uterine bleeding, 51-54, *53*
acne and, 31
breast cancer and, 143
cervical cancer and, 153
diabetes mellitus and, 120
hot flashes, 58
options during perimenopause, 46-47
overview of, 255-263, *257, 258, 259, 262*
progesterone receptors, 12
smoking and oral contraceptives, 111

coronary heart disease (CHD), 107, *114*, 115, 184, 189, 215, 229. *See also* cardiovascular disease (CVD)
corpus luteum, 4-*5,* 48
corticosteroids, 35, *49,* 64, 66, 67, 90, 134, 135
counseling
    health promotion, 197-199, *198, 200*
    sex therapy, 77
    social and cultural aspects of care, 193-194
cultural aspects of care, 193-194
cyanocobalamin, 231, 232
cyproterone acetate, 31, 33, 270

D
danazol, 54
DASH (Dietary Approaches to Stop Hypertension), 198, 229
dehydroepiandrosterone (DHEA), 5, 10-11, 86, 247-248, 282-284
dehydroepiandrosterone sulfate (DHEAS), 5, *51,* 190, 247
dementia, 86-87
denosumab, 126, *128,* 131
dental care, 129, 185
depot medroxyprogesterone acetate (DMPA), 52, 58, *257,* 258, *259,* 260, 262
depression, 26, 27, *75, 76,* 78, 79, 87-92, *88, 90, 91,* 183, 189-190, 211, 244, 246
desmopressin, 52, 54
diabetes, type 1, *14, 15*
diabetes mellitus
    blood pressure and, 119
    body weight and, 22
    bone health, *125*
    cardiovascular disease and, 114-115, 118
    complications of, 118
    endometrial cancer risk, 148, 149, *150*
    hormone therapy and, 119-121, 273-274
    management of, 118-119
    overview of, 116-118, *117*
    screening for, 190
Diagnostic and Statistical Manual for Mental Disorders (DSM-5), 73, *74, 88,* 89, 90
diet. *See also* vitamins
    bone health, 122, 123
    cancer risk and, 146, 161, 162
    cardiovascular health and, 108, 111-112
    clinical evaluation, 186
    cognitive health and, 86
    colorectal cancer, 159
    fish, benefits of, 244-245
    health promotion counseling, 197-198, *198*
    lactose intolerance, 239
    mental health and, *91*
    sleep disturbances and, 81
    vitamin and mineral intake recommendations, 229-*230*
    weight management, 23-*25, 26*
Dietary Guidelines for Americans, 24, 198, 229
Dietary Reference Intakes (DRIs), 229-*230,* 233
Dietary Supplement Health and Education Act (DSHEA), 227-228
diethylstilbestrol, 96, 154, *155,* 182, 189
dihydrotestosterone (DHT), 5, 247, 282
docosahexaenoic acid, 244-245
dong quai, 218, 221, *222*
drugs. *See* pharmacology
dry eye syndrome, *14,* 35
ductal lavage, 144, 145
dyslipidemia, 3, 109, 110, 111, 113, 114, 119, 183, 233, 244
dysmenorrhea, *48,* 217-218
dyspareunia, 12, 13, 17, 21, 49, 60, 62, *63,* 66, 73, 75, *76-78,* 182, 185, 248, *267,* 281
dysphoria, 87, *88. See also* depression
dysthymia, 87, *88. See also* depression

E
early menopause, 3, 6-8, *7*
ears, 37, 185-186
embolism, 116, 260-261, 269, 281, 282. *See also* cardiovascular disease
emergency contraception, 261-262
endocrine system
    fertility assessments and, 6
    hypothalamic-pituitary-ovarian axis, 9
    menopause transition and, *7*-8
    postmenopause, 8-9
    primary ovarian insufficiency and, 13, *14*
endometrium
    abnormal uterine bleeding, 47-55, *49, 50, 51, 53,* 150, 152-153, 273
    endometrial ablation, 54
    endometrial adenocarcinoma, *49*
    endometrial biopsy, 51, 53, 193
    endometrial cancer, 146, 148-153, *149, 150, 151*
    endometrial hyperplasia, 7, *49*
    endometriosis, 12, 14, 155
    endometritis, *49,* 54
    evaluation of, *51*
    menstrual cycle, 4-6, *5*
    progestogen therapy, 270-278, *272, 274, 275, 276*
epilepsy, 139-140
erosive lichen planus, 66-67
erosive osteoarthritis, 133-134
escitalopram, 92
esterified estrogens, 267
estradiol
    asthma and, 140
    bone loss and, 122
    clinical evaluation, 190
    diabetes mellitus and, 117-118
    estrogen receptors, 11-12
    estrogen therapy, *265,* 266-270, *266, 267, 268, 269*
    menopause transition, 6-8, *7*
    menstrual cycle, 4-6, *5*
    ovarian reserve, evaluating, 45
    postmenopause, 8-9
    primary ovarian insufficiency, hormone therapy, 15-16
    STRAW+10 staging system, 3-9, *4, 5, 7*
estrogen
    abnormal uterine bleeding, 47-55
    alcohol use and, 187
    asthma and, 140
    body weight and, 22
    bone loss and, 122, 123
    breast cancer and, 142-143
    cardiovascular health and, 108, 115-116
    cervical cancer, 153
    clinical evaluation, 190-192, *191*
    cognitive changes and, 85-87
    colorectal cancer, 161
    contraceptives, overview of, 255-263, *257, 258, 259, 262*
    diabetes mellitus and, 119-121
    endometrial cancer and, 148-*150,* 152
    epilepsy and, 139
    estrogen-progestogen therapy, 263, 272-278, *272, 274, 275, 276*
    estrogen therapy, 10, 77, 263-270, *265, 266, 267, 268, 269, 279*
    gallbladder disease and, 133
    genitourinary syndrome of menopause, 60-63, *61, 62, 63, 64*
    hair growth and, 31-32
    hearing loss and, 37
    hot flashes, 57, 58
    hypothalamic-pituitary-ovarian axis, 9

hypothyroidism and, 137
menopause transition, 7-8
menstrual cycle and, 4-6, 5f
migraine headache and, 84-85
mood disturbances and, 89, *90*, 92
osteoporosis treatments, 126, 129-130, *130*, *131*
ovarian cancer and, 156
phytoestrogens (isoflavones), 212-216, *212*, *213*
postmenopause, 8-9
primary ovarian insufficiency and, 15
receptor (ER) activity, 11-12
selective estrogen-receptor modulators (SERMs), 11-12, 146-148, 280-282
sexual function and, 73-76, *75*
skin pigmentation and, 30
sleep disturbances, 81-82
vulvovaginal changes, midlife, 21-22
estrogen response elements (EREs), 11-12
estrone, *5*, 8-9, 11-12
estropipate, 267-268
eszopiclone, 59, 81, 92
ethinyl estradiol, 268-*269*
ethinyl estradiol plus drospirenone, 91
ethnicity
    breast cancer, 142
    cancer risk, 141
    diabetes rates, 117
    endometrial cancer, 148
    gallbladder disease, 132
    hormone levels and, 8
    hot flashes, 56
    osteoporosis rates, 121-122
    sleep disturbances, 79
    social and cultural aspects of care, 193-194
    vitamin D intake, 112
etidronate, 127-129, *128*
exercise, 23-24, *26*, *57*, 81, 86, *91*, 111-113, 123, 141, 145-146, 149-*150*, 198-199
expedited partner therapy, 93
extraurethral incontinence, 69-73, *69*, *70*, *72*, *73*
eyes
    antioxidants, effects of, 230
    eye exam, 185
    midlife changes in, 34-37
    vitamin A, 230-231

F
facial hair, 34
fallopian tubes, 47, 158
falls, risk and prevention, 123, *124*
familial adenomatous polyposis, 159, 160
fecal occult blood test, 159, 185
female pattern hair loss (FPHL), 31-34
Female Sexual Function Index, 76
fertility. *See also* primary ovarian insufficiency
    aging and, 45
    antimüllerian hormone (AMH), 6
    cancer and, 17
    fertility-enhancing options, 46
    ovarian reserve, evaluation of, 45-46
fibroids, 12, *49*, 51-54, *53*
fibromyalgia, 60, 64, 80, 136
FIGO (Féderation Internationale de Gynécologie et d'Obstétrique) staging system, 150-*151*
finasteride, 33
fluoxetine, 27, 59, 91
folate (folic acid), 112, 146, 161, 231, 232, 233
follicles, 4-9, *5*, *7*, 13

follicle-stimulating hormone (FSH)
    clinical evaluation, 190, 191-192
    hypothalamic-pituitary-ovarian axis, 9
    ovarian reserve, evaluating, 45-46
    primary ovarian insufficiency and, 14-15
    STRAW+10 staging system, 3-8, *4*, *5*, *7*
fractures, risk of, *121*, 122, *123*
fragile X syndrome, 14, 15
Framingham Heart Study, 36, 115, 123
Framingham Risk Score, 107-108, *109*, 110
FRAX, 122, *123*, 124, 126, 188

G
gabapentin, 59-60, 83, 140
gallbladder disease, 132-133
genes and genetics
    breast cancer, 142
    colorectal cancer, 159, 160-161
    endometrial cancer, *150*
    estrogen receptors, 11-12
    fracture risk, 122, *123*
    genetic testing, 192
    headaches, 82
    hot flashes and, 55-56
    ovarian cancer, *141*
    primary ovarian insufficiency, 13, *14*, 15
genital herpes, 92-93, *92*, *93*, 94
genital warts, 67, 92-93, *92*, *93*
genitourinary syndrome of menopause, 60-63, *61*, *62*, *63*, *64*
ginger, 221
Ginkgo biloba, 86, 218-219, 221
ginseng, 219, 221
glaucoma, 27, 33, 36, 185, 193
glucocorticoids, 10-11, 121, *123*, *125*, 126,140
goiter, 137, 138
gonadotropin and gonadotropin-releasing hormone (GnRH)
    abnormal uterine bleeding, 52, 53
    contraception, 257
    epilepsy, 139
    estrogen therapy, 264
    hot flashes, 79
    hypothalamic-pituitary-ovarian axis, 9, 11
    menstrual cycle, 6
    ovarian cancer, 155
    postmenopause, 8-9
    primary ovarian insufficiency, 13, 15
    vulvovaginal changes, 22
gonorrhea, 92-93, *92*, *93*, 94-95
gout, 135
Graves disease, 14, 137, 138
Greene Climacteric Scale, 182, 201, 202, 211

H
hair, 31-34
Hashimoto thyroiditis, 14, 136-138
headaches, 82-85, 243
health promotion, clinical evaluation, 197-199, *198*
hearing, 37, 185-186
heart health. *See* cardiovascular disease
hepatitis, 92-93, *92*, *93*, 95, 136
herbal supplements, 24, 82, 208-209, 210-211, 216-219, 220-*222*, 227-229
herpes, genital, 94
high-density lipoprotein cholesterol (HDL-C), 22, 108, *114*, 117, 181, 215, 231, 269, *279*, 283
hip fracture, 121-122. *See also* bone health
hirsutism, 31, 34
HIV (human immunodeficiency virus), 92-93, *92*, *93*, 95, *125*, 153, *154*

297

homeopathy
    integrative medicine, 207-208
    safety concerns, 221-222
    whole medical systems, 208-209
hormones. *See also* hormone therapy
    abnormal uterine bleeding, 49
    adrenal physiology and menopause, 10-11
    aging, STRAW+10 staging system, 3-9, 4, 5, 7
    bone loss and, 122, 123
    clinical evaluation, 190-192, 191
    cognition and, 85-87
    contraceptives, 47, 255-263, 257, 258, 259, 262
    depression and, 90-91
    diabetes, risk factors, 117-118
    dry eye syndrome, 35
    genitourinary syndrome of menopause, 60-63, 61, 62, 63, 64
    hair growth and, 31-32
    hypothalamic-pituitary-ovarian axis, 9-10
    melatonin, 82, 248-249
    menopause transition, 6-8, 7
    migraine headache and, 84
    mood disturbance and, 88-89, 90
    ovarian reserve, evaluating, 45-46
    over-the-counter hormones, 246-249
    postmenopause, 8-9
    premature menopause, 12-17, 14, 15, 16
    primary ovarian insufficiency and, 14-16
    seizures and, 139
    sexual function and, 73-76, 75
    skin physiology and, 29
    steroid hormones receptors, 11-12
hormone therapy
    abnormal uterine bleeding, 49, 51-54, 53
    administration routes, summary, 279
    androgen therapy, 282-284, 283
    asthma and, 140
    bioidentical hormone therapy, 278
    body weight and, 22
    breast cancer and, 142-144, 147-148
    cardiovascular health and, 108, 115-116
    cervical cancer, 153
    cognitive function and, 86
    colorectal cancer, 161
    compounded bioidentical hormone therapy, 278-280
    contraindications and warnings, 274-278, 275, 276
    cortisol levels and, 10
    depression and, 91-92
    diabetes mellitus and, 119-121, 120
    endometrial cancer and, 152
    epilepsy and, 139-140
    estrogen-progestogen therapy, 272-278, 272, 274, 275, 276
    estrogen therapy, 263-270, 265, 266, 267, 268, 269
    gallbladder disease and, 132-133
    genitourinary syndrome of menopause, 61-62
    hair loss, 32-33
    hearing loss and, 37
    hot flashes and, 58
    migraine headache and, 84-85
    natural hormone, defined, 268
    osteoporosis treatments, 129-132, 130, 131
    ovarian cancer and, 156
    overview of, 263
    progestogen therapy, 270-278, 271, 272, 274, 275, 276
    sexual function and, 77
    skin health and, 30
    sleep disturbances, 81-82
    transition from hormonal contraception, 262-263
hot flashes
    body weight and, 23
    cognitive changes and, 85
    cortisol levels and, 10
    epilepsy, patients with, 140
    homeopathic approaches, 208-209
    management of, 56-60, 57
    mood disturbances and, 89, 91
    overview of, 55-56
    palpitations, 107-108
    sleep and, 79-80, 81
    smoking and, 187
human chorionic gonadotropin (hCG), 9
human papillomavirus (HPV), 92-93, 95-96, 153-154, 155
hyperplasia, 48, 49, 50
hypertension. *See also* cardiovascular disease
    body weight and, 22
    cardiovascular disease and, 109-110
    cognitive function and, 86
    diabetes mellitus and, 120
    management of, 114
    metabolic syndrome, 109
    physical exam, 184
    treatment guidelines, 110
hyperthyroidism, 13, 14, 15, 125
hypertrophic lichen planus, 67
hypertrophic vulvitis, 66
hypothalamus
    amenorrhea, diagnosis of, 15
    hypothalamic-pituitary-ovarian axis, 9-10
    menopause transition, 8
    menstrual cycle and, 4-6, 5
hypothyroidism
    abnormal uterine bleeding, 49
    amenorrhea, 15
    overview, 136-138
    primary ovarian insufficiency, 13, 14
hysterectomy
    alternatives to, 54
    cognitive effects of, 86-87
    premature menopause, 13
    sexual function and, 77
    testosterone levels and, 9
hysteroscopy, 46, 54, 193

I
ibandronate, 127-129, 128
imaging
    abnormal uterine bleeding, 51
    breast cancer screening, 144-145, 189
    colorectal cancer screening, 159-160
    transvaginal ultrasonography, 193
incontinence, anal, 73
incontinence, urinary, 68-73, 69, 70, 72, 73
induced menopause, defined, 3
infection. *See also* sexually transmitted infections (STIs)
    abnormal uterine bleeding, 49, 50, 54
    Bartholin gland abscesses, 67
    urinary tract infection (UTI), 62-63, 64
    vulvovaginitis, 64-66, 65
infertility, 45-46. *See also* primary ovarian insufficiency
inflammatory arthritis, 134-135
inhibin A, 5, 9, 190, 191
inhibin B, 3-9, 4, 5, 7, 45, 190, 191
insomnia. *See* sleep
insulin, 114-118, 117
insulin-dependent diabetes, 116. *See also* diabetes mellitus
insulin resistance, 108, 109
integrative medicine, 207-208. *See also* complementary and alternative medicine (CAM)
intercourse, pain during, 21. *See also* dyspareunia, vulvovaginal health

International Federation of Gynecology and Obstetrics (FIGO), 48, *50*
interstitial cystitis, 72-73, *72, 73*
intimate partner violence, 195-*197*
intrauterine device (IUD), 47, 49, 52, 255, *257*
in vitro fertilization (IVF), 45-46
iron, 32, 54, 240-241
isoflavones, 58, 112, 212-216, *212, 213*

J
joint replacement, 134
juvenile diabetes, 116. *See also* diabetes mellitus

K
Kegel exercises, 70-71
keratin, 27
kidney disease
    bone health and, *125*
    diabetes mellitus and, 118, 120
    hypertension and, *110*
Kronos Early Estrogen Prevention Study (KEEPS), 86, 108, 115, 269, 276

L
labia majora/minora, 60-63, *61, 62, 63, 64*
Lactobacillus, 21
late menopause, 3, 6-8, *7*
late reproductive stage, STRAW, 6
leiomyoma, 48, *49, 50*
lesbian health issues, 194-196, *195*
letrozole, 147
leukemia, *49, 125*
lichen planus, 66-67
lichen sclerosus, 66
lifestyle modification, counseling on, 197-199, *198*
ligands, 11-12
lipomas, 163
liraglutide, 27
liver disease, *49, 125,* 218, 219, 246
lorazepam, 81
lorcaserin, 26
low-density lipoprotein cholesterol (LDL-C)
    cardiovascular disease and, 108, 110, *111*
    diet and, 112
    management of, 23, 113-*114*
    soy isoflavones, effects of, 112, 215
lubricants, vaginal, 61
lung cancer, *141*, 158
lungs, estrogen receptors, 11-12
luteal out-of-phase (LOOP) event, 7-8, *7*
luteal phase, 4-*5*
luteinizing hormone (LH)
    adrenal physiology and menopause, 10
    clinical evaluation, 190
    hypothalamic-pituitary-ovarian axis, 9
    menopause transition, *7*-8
    menstrual cycle, 4-6, *5*
    postmenopause, 8-9
    primary ovarian insufficiency and, 14-15
Lynch syndrome, 141, 155, *156*, 157-158, *159, 161*

M
macular degeneration, age-related, 36-37, 120
magnesium, 84, 123, 241-242
mammography, 144-*145*, 184, 189
manganese, 242
mastalgia, 7
medical history, patient exam, 182-183
medicine. *See* pharmacology

Mediterranean diet, 111-112, 229
medroxyprogesterone acetate (MPA), 52, *53*, 58, 119, *131*, 258, *259, 268, 271, 274*
melanoma, 29-30, *141*, 162-163
melatonin, 82, 248-249
memantine, 87
membrane-initiated estrogen signaling, 11
menopausal transition stage, STRAW, 2-3, *4*, 6-8, *7*
menopause. *See also* body changes, midlife
    adrenal physiology and, 10-11
    demographics, 1
    hypothalamic-pituitary-ovarian axis, 9-10
    ovarian aging and hormone production, 3-9, *4, 5, 7*
    overview of, 1
    premature, 12-17, *14, 15, 16*
    quality of life, 1-2
    steroid hormone receptors and, 11-12
    terminology, 2-3
menopause transition, defined, 2-3
menorrhagia, 7, *48*, 49, 52
menstrual cycle
    abnormal uterine bleeding, 47-55, *49, 50, 51, 53*
    epilepsy and, 139
    hypothalamic-pituitary-ovarian axis, 9-10
    menopause transition, 6-8, *7*
    migraine headache and, 84
    mood disturbances, 89, *90*, 91
    postmenopausal bleeding, 9
    premature menopause and, 14
    STRAW+10 staging system, 3-9, *4, 5, 7*
mental health. *See also* anxiety disorders; depression
    changes in, 87-92, *88, 89, 90, 91*
    clinical evaluation, 16, 189-190
    diet and, 244
    evaluation and management, 89-92, *91*
    psychological history, 183
    quality of life, 1-2, 201-202
    s-adenosylmethionine (SAM-e), 246
    sexual function and, *75*, 78
    sleep and, 79
metabolic syndrome, *14*, 22-23, 108, 109, 115
metformin therapy, 118-119
midlife body changes. *See* body changes, midlife
migraine, 7, 82, 83-85, 243
minerals, 32, 54, 84, 122, 123, *125*, 140, 229-*230*, 233-234, 236, 237-242, *240, 241*-243
mixed incontinence, 69-73, *69, 70, 72, 73*
moisturizers, vaginal, 60-*62*, 77, *78*, 278
mood disturbance, 88-89, *90*
moxibustion, 211
muscle-contraction headache, 82-83
myocardial infarction, 107. *See also* cardiovascular disease

N
naltrexone, 27
National Cancer Institute, 142, *143, 145*, 153
National Center for Complementary and Alternative Medicine (NCCAM), 207, 246
National Cholesterol Education Program Adult Treatment Panel (ATP III), 22-23, 109, 110, *111*
National Health and Nutrition Examination Survey (NHANES), 109, 121, 136, 184, 233-234
National Institutes of Health (NIH), 139-140, 236
National Intimate Partner and Sexual Violence Survey, 196
National Lipid Association, 113
National Osteoporosis Foundation (NOF), 121, 234, 238, *240*
naturopathy
    integrative medicine, 207-208
    safety concerns, 221-*222*

whole medical systems, 208-*209*
Neisseria gonorrhoeae, 94-95
nervous system
    burning mouth syndrome, 38
    diabetes mellitus, 118
    estrogen receptors, 11-12
    sacral neuromodulation stimulation (InterStim), 71
neurotransmitters, 12, 74, 85-87
niacin (vitamin B$_3$), 113, *114*, *230*, 231, 233
nicotine, sleep disturbances and, 81
night sweats, 55-60, *57*
nonsteroidal anti-inflammatory drugs (NSAIDs), 54, 84, 134, 135
norepinephrine, 10, 56, 58, 59, 74, 80, 282
Nurses' Health Study, 36, 108, 115, 132, 142, 146, 184, 187, 275, 277, 284, 290

O
obesity and overweight
    abnormal uterine bleeding, *49*
    body changes, midlife, 22-27, *25*, *26*, *28*
    breast cancer and, 144
    cancer risk and, *141*, 146
    cardiovascular health and, 108, 112-113
    clinical evaluation, 186
    contraceptive use and, *259*, 260
    dehydroepiandrosterone (DHEA), 248
    diabetes mellitus, 114-115, 117
    endometrial cancer risk, 149-*150*
    hormone levels and, 8, 9
    hot flashes and, 56, *57*
    medications for weight loss, 25-27
    metabolic syndrome, 109
    osteoarthritis and, 134
    physical exam, 183-184, *185*
    surgery for, 27
oligomenorrhea, 13, 14, *48*, *191*
omega-3 fatty acids, 58, 86, 111, 230, 244-245
omega-6 fatty acids, 244-245
oophorectomy
    adrenal physiology and, 11
    androgen therapy, 282-284, *283*
    bone health and, 124
    cognitive effects of, 86-87
    hot flashes, 56
    induced menopause, 3, 12-17, *14*, *15*, *16*
    testosterone levels and, 9
oral cavity
    midlife changes, 37-*38*
    tobacco use and, 187
oral contraceptives. *See* contraceptives
orlistat, 26
ospemifene, 12, 61, 62, *63*, 77, *78*, 185, 281
osteoarthritis, 22, 133-136, 245-246
osteoblasts, 122, 132
osteoclasts, 122, 127-129, *128*
osteoporosis. *See also* bone health
    antiepileptic drug therapy, 140
    body weight and, 23
    estrogen receptors, 11-12
    evaluation of, 124-126, *125*, *127*
    overview, 121-122, *121*
    pharmacologic interventions, 126-132, *128*, *130*, *131*
    primary ovarian insufficiency and, 15
    raloxifene, 12
    risk factors, 122-124, *123*, *124*
    secondary, causes of, 124, *125*, *127*
    thyroid disorders and, 138
    tooth loss and, 37-*38*
ovarian cancer, 12, *141*, 154-158, *156*, 229

ovaries
    aging and hormone production, 3-9, *4*, *5*, *7*
    androgen therapy, 282-284, *283*
    antral follicle count, 6
    clinical evaluation, 190, 192
    diabetes, risk factors, 117-118
    estrogen receptors, 11-12
    hirsutism, 34
    hypothalamic-pituitary-ovarian axis, 9-10
    menstrual cycle, 4-6, *5*
    ovarian cysts, *14*
    ovarian reserve, evaluation of, 45-46
    ovarian stromal hyperplasia, 9
    pelvic examination, 184-185
    polycystic ovary syndrome (PCOS), 12, *15*, 34, *49*
    premature menopause, 12-17, *14*, *15*, *16*
    progesterone receptors, 12
    sexual function and, 74
    spironolactone, 33
overactive bladder (OAB) syndrome, 71-73, *72*, *73*
overweight. *See* obesity and overweight
ovulation
    epilepsy and, 139
    menopause transition, 7-8, *7*
    menstrual cycle, 4-6, *5*
    ovulatory dysfunction, bleeding and, 48, *50*
    postmenopause, 9

P
Paget disease, *61*, 67, *127*
pain
    genitourinary syndrome of menopause, 60-63, *61*, *62*, *63*, *64*
    pelvic examination, 185
    urinary bladder, *72*
    vulvovaginal changes and, 21-22
PALM-COEIN classification, 48, *50*
palpitations, 107-108
pancreatic cancer, *141*, 161-162
pantothenic acid, 231
Pap (Papanicolaou) screening, 96, 153-*154*, *155*, 185
papulosquamous lichen planus, 67
parathyroid hormone, 126, *128*, 131-132, 233, 238, 241, 242
paroxetine, 58-59, 91, 263, 282
paroxysmal hemicrania, 82, 83
Partner Violence Screen, 196
pelvic examination, 184-185, 192
pelvic floor exercises, 70-71
pelvic inflammatory disease, 14, *49*
pelvic radiation therapy, 3, 17, 124
perimenopause. *See also* body changes, midlife
    abnormal uterine bleeding, 47-55, *49*, *50*, *51*, *53*
    birth control options, 46-47
    defined, 3
    epilepsy and, 139
    hot flashes, 55-60, *57*
    mood disturbances, 88-89, *90*
    sleep disturbances, 79-82
periodontal disease, 37-*38*
periovulatory phase, 4-5
peripheral vascular disease, 107. *See also* cardiovascular disease
pharmacology
    abnormal uterine bleeding, *49*, 51-54, *53*
    ACE inhibitors, 116
    acne medications, 31
    Alzheimer disease, 87
    androgen receptors, 12
    androgen therapy, 282-284, *283*
    angiotensin-converting enzyme (ACE) inhibitors, 116
    angiotensin II receptor blockers (ARBs), 116

anxiety, treatment for, 91-92
arthritis, osteoarthritis, 134
arthritis, rheumatoid, 135
aspirin, 113, 116, 119, 161
beta-blockers, 116
bioidentical hormone therapy, 278-280
blood pressure regulation, 114
bone health, osteoporosis interventions, 15, 37-38, 126-132, *128, 130, 131*
bone health, secondary osteoporosis, 124, *125*
cancer, breast, 146-148
contraceptives, 31, 47, 255-263, *257, 258, 259, 262*
counseling about medications, 200-201
depression, treatment for, 91-92
diabetes mellitus, 118-119
dry eye syndrome, 35
dyslipidemia, 110, *111,* 113-*114*
epilepsy, 139-140
estrogen receptor modulation, 12
estrogen therapy, 263-270, *265, 266, 267, 268, 269*
genitourinary syndrome of menopause, 61-62
glaucoma, 36
gout, 135
government regulation of, 256
hair loss, 32-33
headaches, 83, 84
hearing loss, 37
hirsutism, 34
hormone therapies, overview of, 255
hot flashes, 58-60
metformin therapy, 118-119
off-label use, defined, 256
ovarian cancer risk reduction, 157
overactive bladder syndrome, 72-73
prescription drug abuse, 188
primary ovarian insufficiency, hormone therapy, 15-16
progesterone receptors, 12
progestogen therapy, 270-278, *271, 272, 274, 275, 276*
selective estrogen-receptor modulators (SERMs), 11, 12, 58, 146, 147, 280-282
selective serotonin-reuptake inhibitors (SSRIs), 56, 58, 59, *75,* 78, 92, *125,* 220, 246, 255, 282
serotonin norepinephrine-reuptake inhibitors (SNRIs), 56, 58, 282
sexual function improvement, 77-78
sexually transmitted infections, 94, 95, 96
sleep disruption, treatment of, 81-82
statin therapy, 116, 119
urinary incontinence, *70,* 71
vaginal dryness, 77
weight loss, 25-27
phenytoin, 80, *91, 125,* 140
phosphorus, 243
photoaging, 29-30
physical abuse, 195-*197*
physical activity. *See* exercise
physical exam. *See* clinical evaluation
phytoestrogens, 11-12, 57, 58, 212-216, *212, 213,* 264
pituitary gland
    amenorrhea, diagnosis of, *15*
    hormone levels, evaluation of, 191-192
    hypothalamic-pituitary-ovarian axis, 9-10
    menopause transition, 8
    menstrual cycle and, 4-6, *5*
    plant sterols and stanols, 112
polycystic ovary syndrome (PCOS), 12, *15,* 34, 49, *50,* 117, 137, 149, *150,* 190
polyps, 48, *49, 50*
porphyria, *125*

Postmenopausal Estrogen/Progestin Interventions (PEPI), 22, 119, 132, 271, 273
Postmenopause. *See* body changes, midlife; menopause terminology
prediabetes, 116, *117. See also* diabetes mellitus
pregabalin, 60,136
pregnancy. *See also* fertility
    cardiovascular disease risk factors, 109
    fertility-enhancing options, 46
    menopause transition, 7-8
    ovarian reserve, evaluating, 45-46
premature menopause, 3, 12-17, *14, 15, 16*
premature ovarian failure, 3, 12-17, *14, 15, 16*
premenopause, 2
premenstrual dysphoric disorder (PMDD), 89, *90,* 91, 183
premenstrual syndrome (PMS), 89, *90,* 183, 217-218, 220-221
primary ovarian insufficiency, 3, 12-17, *14, 15, 16*
primordial follicle, 4-6, *5*
progesterone
    abnormal uterine bleeding, 52-54, *53*
    asthma and, 140
    body weight and, 22
    breast cancer and, 142-143
    cancer and, 152, 153, 156
    cardiovascular health and, 108, 115-116
    clinical evaluation, 190-192, *191*
    cognitive changes and, 85-87
    colorectal cancer, 161
    diabetes mellitus and, 117-121
    epilepsy and, 139
    hot flashes, 58
    hypothalamic-pituitary-ovarian axis, 9
    menopause transition, 8
    menstrual cycle and, 4-6, *5*
    primary ovarian insufficiency and, 15-16
    progestogen therapy, 270-278, *271, 272, 274, 275, 276, 279*
    receptor activity, 11-12
    sexual function and, 76
    sleep disturbances, 81-82
    topical progesterone, OTC, 246-247
progestin, 37, 58, 257-261
progestogen therapy, 270-278, *271, 272, 274, 275, 276, 279*
prolactin, 14, *16, 51,* 157, 190, *191*
pseudogout, 135-136
psoriasis, vulvar, 67
psychogenic headache, 82-83
pyridoxine (vitamin B$_6$), 231, 232

Q
quality of life, 1-2, 201-202
quigong, 211

R
race
    breast cancer, 142
    cancer risk, 141
    diabetes rates, 117
    endometrial cancer, 148
    gallbladder disease, 132
    hormone levels and, 8
    hot flashes, 56
    osteoporosis rates, 121-122
    sleep disturbances, 79
    social and cultural aspects of care, 193-194
    vitamin D intake, 112
radiation therapy, 12-17, *14, 15, 16,* 124
radioactive iodine therapy, 137, 138
raloxifene, 10, 12, 30, 126, *128,* 129, 146-147, 148, 281-282
ramelteon, 81

301

RANK ligand inhibitor, 126, *128,* 131
receptors, steroid hormones, 11-12, 33
rectal cancer, 158-161, *160,* 189
rectal exam, 185
red clover, 208, 212, 214
relaxation techniques, *57,* 81
reproductive aging, STRAW+10 staging system, 3-9, *4, 5, 7*
retina, 36-37
retinol, 230-231
retinopathy, 118, 120
rheumatoid arthritis, *14, 125,* 134-135
rhythm method, 47
riboflavin, 84, 231, 233
risedronate, 127-129, *128*

S
sacral neuromodulation stimulation (InterStim), 71
s-adenosylmethionine (SAM-e), 246
sclerostin antibody inhibitors, 132
screening tests, overview, 188-193. *See also* specific disease names
seborrheic dermatitis, 67, 163
seborrheic keratoses, 29
sedatives, 81-82
seizures, 139-140
selective estrogen-receptor modulators (SERMs), 11-12, 146-148, 280-282
selective progesterone-receptor modulators, 12
selective serotonin-reuptake inhibitors (SSRIs), 56, 58, 59, 75, 78, 92, *125,* 220, 246, 255, 282
    bone health effects, *125*
    depression treatment, 91-92
    hot flashes, 58-59, 282
    sexual function and, 78
selenium, 236, 243
serotonin, *26,* 81, 84, 85, 91
    black cohosh, 217
    migraine headache and, 84
    sexual function and, 74
    St. John's wort, 220
serotonin norepinephrine-reuptake inhibitors (SNRIs), 56, 58-59, 282
serotonin syndrome, 26
serrated polyp, 161
sex hormone-binding globulin (SHBG), 8, 32, 74, 78, 269, *279,* 282
sex therapy, 77
sexual abuse, 195-*197*
sexual health
    androgen therapy, 283, 284
    dehydroepiandrosterone (DHEA), 248
    genitourinary syndrome of menopause, 60-63, *61, 62, 63, 64*
    premature menopause and, 16-17
    sexual function, changes in, 73-78, *74, 75, 76, 77, 78, 79*
    sexual history, patient exam, 183
    vulvovaginal changes, midlife, 21-22
sexually transmitted infections (STIs)
    bacterial vaginosis, 93
    chlamydia, 93-94
    genital herpes, 94
    gonorrhea, 94-95
    hepatitis B and C, 95
    HIV, 95
    human papillomavirus (HPV), 95-96
    lesbian health, 195
    risk of and screening for, 92-93, *92, 93,* 192
    syphilis, 96
    trichomoniasis, 96
    vulvovaginitis, 64-66, *65*

short-lasting unilateral neuralgiform headache, 83
sigmoidoscopy, 159, 160, 189
sildenafil, 78
Sjögren syndrome, 14, 35, *61*
skin
    cancer, 29-30, *141,* 162-163
    changes in midlife, 27, 29-31
    dryness (xerosis), 30-31
    physical exam, 185
sleep
    disturbances in, 79-82
    melatonin, 248-249
    mood disturbances, 89, 91, 92
    weight gain and, 22
sleep apnea/hypopnea syndrome, 80
smoking, effects of
    adrenal function, 10
    bone health, *123*
    cardiovascular disease, 108, 111
    clinical evaluation, 187
    endometrial cancer, 150
    hearing loss and, 37
    hot flashes, *57*
    lung cancer, 158
    pancreatic cancer, 161-162
    skin health, 29, 30
smoking cessation, counseling on, 199
social history, patient exam, 183
soy, 58, 86, 112, 208, 212-216, *212, 213*
spironolactone, 31, 33
squamous cell hyperplasia, 66
Stages of Reproductive Workshop (STRAW), 2-9, *4, 5, 7,* 48, 191
statin therapy, 110, *111,* 112, 119
sterilization, 47
St. John's wort, 217, 220
strength training, *26,* 198-199
stress, *75,* 80, 88, *89,* 186-187
stress headaches, 82-83
stress incontinence, *69*-73, *70, 72, 73*
stroke. *See also* cardiovascular disease
    hormone therapy and, 108, 115-116, 269, 277
    migraine headaches and, 85
    risk of, 87
    SERMS and, 281
    vitamin E intake and, 236
strontium ranelate, 132
Study of Women Across the Nation (SWAN), 2, 8, 10, 117, 136, 186, 194
subclinical hyperthyroidism, 138
subclinical hypothyroidism, 137-138
substance abuse, 187-188
suicide, 26, 27, 88, 89, 282
sulphur, 209
sunscreen, 29-30
supplements, dietary
    antioxidants, 112
    calcium, 140, 239-240
    coenzyme Q10, 243-244
    cognitive health and, 86
    fish oil, omega-3 and -6 fatty acids, 244-245
    ginkgo biloba, 218-219
    ginseng, 219
    glucosamine and chondroitin, 245-246
    herbal therapies, overview, 216-217
    for hot flashes, 58
    iron, 54, 241
    isoflavones, 112
    kava, 219
    licorice, 219

magnesium, 242
over-the-counter hormones, 246-249
regulation of, 227-229
s-adenosylmethionine (SAM-e), 246
safety concerns, 221-*222*
sage, 220
vitamin D, 112, 123, 140
weight management, 24
surgery
    abnormal uterine bleeding, 54-55
    ovarian cancer risk reduction, 157-158
    urinary incontinence, 71
    weight loss procedures, 27
symptoms. *See also* body changes, midlife; clinical evaluation
    cognitive changes, 85-87
    estrogen-receptor modulation and, 12
    fertility, decline in, 45-47
    genitourinary syndrome of menopause, 60-63, *61, 62, 63, 64*
    headache, 82-85
    induced menopause, 14
    medical history, 182
    Menopausal Symptom List, 202
    psychological health, 87-92, *88, 89, 90, 91*
    sexual function, 73-78, *74, 75, 76, 77, 78, 79*
    sexually transmitted infections, 92-96, *92, 93*
    sleep disturbances, 79-82
    urinary incontinence and overactive bladder, 68-73, *69, 70, 72, 73*
    uterine bleeding, 47-55, *48, 49, 50, 51, 53*
    vasomotor (hot flashes), 55-60, *57*
    vulvar and vaginal issues, 63-68, *65, 68*
synthetic estrogen, 265-266, *265*
syphilis, 92-93, *92, 93,* 96

T
tamoxifen, 12, 36, *49,* 59, 146, 148, 156, 281-282
teeth
    bisphosphonate therapy and, 129
    midlife changes, 37-*38*
    physical exam, 185
telogen effluvium, 31-34
tension-type headache (TTH), 82-83
teriparatide, 126, *128,* 131-132
terminology of menopause, 2-3
testosterone
    aging and levels of hormone, 8
    androgen therapy, 282-284, *283*
    breast cancer and, 142-143
    clinical evaluation, 190
    cognitive changes and, 85-87
    hair growth and, 32
    menstrual cycle, 5
    postmenopause, 9
    receptor activity, 11-12
    sexual function and, 73-74, *75,* 76
thiamin (vitamin B$_2$), 231
thrombosis, 107, 108, 116, 237, 260, 269. *See also* cardiovascular disease
thyroid gland
    abnormal uterine bleeding and, *49*
    amenorrhea, diagnosis of, *15*
    cancer of, *141*
    clinical evaluation, 192
    hyperthyroidism, 138
    hypothyroidism, 136-138
    primary ovarian insufficiency and, 13, *14*
    thyroid disease, overview, 136
    thyroid nodules, 138-139
thyroiditis, 138

thyroid-stimulating hormone (TSH), 9, *16, 51, 127,* 136, 190, *191*
thyroxine, 32, *125,* 136, 192, 283
tibolone, 37, 131, 211, 216, 281
tissue-selective estrogen complexes (TSECs), 12, 58, 274
tobacco. *See* smoking, effects of
topical estrogen, 269-270, *269*
topiramate, 26-27, 140
tranexamic acid, 54
transdermal estrogen, 265-*266,* 269-270, *269*
transient ischemic attack (TIA). *See* cardiovascular disease (CVD)
transition, menopause, 2-3. *See also* body changes, midlife
transvaginal ultrasonography, *51,* 193
Treponema pallidum, 96
trichomoniasis, 64, 65, *92,* 96, 195
Trichomonas vaginitis, 65
trigeminal autonomic cephalgias, 82, 83
triglycerides
    body weight, 22-23
    cardiovascular disease, 108, 109, 110
    estrogen therapy and, 269
    management of, 113-*114*
triptan medications, 84
T-score, bone density, 15, *121,* 126
tubal ligation, 47
Turner syndrome, 13, 15, 37
Type 1 diabetes, 116, *125*
Type 2 diabetes, 116, *125,* 148, 149, *150. See also* diabetes mellitus

U
ulipristal acetate, 12, 262
ultrasonography
    abnormal uterine bleeding, *51*
    breast cancer screening, 145, 189
ultraviolet (UV) radiation, 27, 29-30
underweight, 23, *123,* 186
urethra, genitourinary syndrome of menopause, 60-63, *61, 62, 63, 64*
urethral diverticulum, *72-73*
urethral syndrome, *72-73*
urethritis, *72-73*
urgency incontinence, 69-73, *69, 70, 72, 73*
urinalysis, 192-193
urinary bladder
    cancer of, *141*
    estrogen receptors, 11-12
    genitourinary syndrome of menopause, 60-63, *61, 62, 63, 64*
urinary incontinence, 68-73, *69, 70, 72, 73*
urinary tract infection (UTI), 62-63, *64,* 218
US Preventive Services Task Force (USPSTF), 24, 37, 184, 189, 196, 236
uterine artery embolization, 13, *14*
uterine fibroids (leiomyoma)
    abnormal uterine bleeding, *49*
    estradiol and, 7
    management of, 51-54, *53*
    primary ovarian insufficiency and, 14
    progesterone receptors, 12
uterus
    abnormal uterine bleeding, 47-55, *49, 50, 51, 53,* 150, 152-153, 273
    clinical evaluation, 193
    endometrial cancer, 148-153, *149, 150, 151*
    estrogen receptors, 11-12
    medical history, 182
    menstrual cycle, 4-6, *5*
    pelvic examination, 184-185
    progesterone receptors, 12
    soy isoflavones, effects of, 216

V

vaccines, HPV, 154
vaginal atrophy, 14, 16, 21, 52, 60, *62*, *63*, 66, 68, 71, 77, *78*, 150, 185, 193, 248, *267*, 270, 278, 281
vaginal estrogen therapy, *269*, 270, 278
vaginal health. *See* vulvovaginal health
vaginal maturation index (VMI), 21
vaginal progestogen therapy, 272
valerian, 82, 220
valproate, 140
valvular heart disease. *See* cardiovascular disease (CVD)
vascular dementia, 87
vascular morbidity, diabetes and, 120-121
vasomotor symptoms
    acupuncture, 210
    black cohosh, 217-218
    body weight and, 23
    Chinese herbal therapy, 210-211
    cognitive changes and, 85
    cortisol levels and, 10
    epilepsy, patients with, 140
    homeopathic approaches, 208-*209*
    management of, 56-60, *57*
    mood disturbances and, 89, 91
    overview of, 55-56
    palpitations, 107-108
    postmenopause, 8
    sage, 220
    sleep and, 79-80, 81
    smoking and, 187
    soy isoflavones, 213-214
    St. John's wort, 220
venous thromboembolism (VTE), 116, 260-261, 281, 282
very-low-density lipoproteins (VLDLs), 108
violence, 195-*197*
viruses. *See also* sexually transmitted infections (STIs)
    HIV (human immunodeficiency virus), 92-93, *92*, *93*, 95, *125*, 153, *154*
    human papillomavirus (HPV), 92-93, *92*, *93*, 95-96, 153-*154*, *155*
    parvovirus B19, 136
vision
    antioxidants, effects of, 230
    aura, migraine headaches and, 83-85
    diabetes mellitus and, 118, 120
    eye exam, 185
    midlife eye changes, 34-37
    vitamin A, 230-231
vitamins
    B vitamins, 112, 231-233
    cardiovascular health and, 112
    cognitive health and, 86
    dietary intake recommendations, 229-*230*
    regulation of, 227-229
    toxicity, 231, 233
    vitamin A, 30, *125*, 229-230, *230*-231
    vitamin C, 229-*230*, 233
    vitamin D, 30, 32, 38, 112, 122, 123, 140, 146, 159, 162, 233-236, *235*
    vitamin E, 58, 229-*230*, 236-237
    vitamin K, 237
vitex, 220-221
vitreous, changes in, 36-37
vulvovaginal health
    androgen receptors, 12
    bacterial vaginosis, 93
    cancer, 96, *141*
    clinical evaluation, 67-*68*, 184-185, 193
    dermatoses, 66-67
    estrogen-receptors and, 12
    estrogen therapy, 265, *267*
    genitourinary syndrome of menopause, 60-63, *61*, *62*, *63*, *64*
    isoflavones, effects of, 214
    medical history, 182
    menopause, changes in, 21-22
    sexual function and, 73, 77
    vaginal dryness, 14
    vestibulodynia, 63-64
    vulvar disorders, causes of, *61*, 66
    vulvar masses, 67
    vulvar psoriasis, 67
    vulvar vestibulitis, 63-64
    vulvodynia, 63-64
    vulvovaginitis, 64-66, *65*

W

Waist circumference, 22, *28*, 112-117, 181, 183, 248
waist-to-hip ratio, 183-184
water intake, 31
weight, body. *See* body weight
Women Abuse Screening Tool, 196
Women's Health Initiative (WHI)
    cardiovascular disease, 108
    diabetes, 119-120
    gallbladder disease, 133
    hormone therapy, 276
    Memory Study, 86
    weight management, 22
    WHI Dietary Modification trial, 23, 161
    WHI Sight Exam Study, 36
Women's Health Study, 35, 113, 237
Women's Isoflavone Soy Health (WISH) study, 215-216
World Health Organization (WHO), 122, 143

X-Z

X chromosome disorders, *14*
xerosis, 30-31
yeast vaginitis, *65*
yoga, 77, 81, *91*, 211-212
zaleplon, 81
zinc, 32, 242
zoledronic acid, 127-129, *128*
zolpidem, 81
zona fasciculata, 10
zona glomerulosa, 10
zona reticularis, 10
Z-score, bone density, 15, *121*

CONTINUING MEDICAL EDUCATION (CME) ACTIVITY

Self-Assessment Examination

To claim CME credit, please read and study the entire *Clinician's Guide*, complete the examination, and submit the answer sheet and post-test evaluation to the North American Menopause Society (NAMS) by the expiration date of **October 15, 2017**. Physicians (MDs, DOs, and international equivalents) will receive 26.0 *AMA PRA Category 1 Credits*™. Other learners will be issued a certificate of participation. This activity includes 11.5 hours of pharmacotherapeutics education, which will be noted on the certificate of participation. CME credit and certificates of participation will be issued to those who achieve a passing grade of 70%.

Chapter 1. Menopause

1. Women have experienced menopause
    a. For thousands of years
    b. Only in recent history

2. The average age of menopause in the Western world is
    a. 48 years
    b. 52 years
    c. 55 years

3. In a woman with a uterus, menopause is defined as
    a. 1 year after the final menstrual period
    b. The final menstrual period
    c. The onset of vasomotor symptoms

4. Which of these is the least appropriate treatment in young women with primary ovarian insufficiency?
    a. Hormone therapy with a 100-μg transdermal estradiol patch and a cyclical progestogen
    b. A bisphosphonate to prevent bone loss
    c. Oral contraceptives

5. Premenopausal women undergoing cancer chemotherapy or radiation therapy
    a. Will become infertile permanently
    b. May be able to have fertility preserved

Chapter 2. Midlife Body Changes

6. At menopause, the decrease in estrogen will have several effects on the vagina. Which of these is *not* correct?
    a. The pH of the vagina is between 3.5 and 4.5, and there is an increase in mature superficial cells in the vaginal epithelium
    b. The pH of the vagina moves to an alkaline state, and lactobacilli are replaced by other flora
    c. Vaginal atrophy may occur and is characterized by vaginal walls that are thin, smooth, pale, and dry

7. In the United States, 73% of women aged 60 years and older are overweight. Which statement best describes weight changes during and after menopause?
    a. Both hormone therapy and menopause are strongly and directly associated with weight gain
    b. Menopause is associated with increased fat in the abdominal region and decreased lean body mass, independent of age
    c. The change in distribution of fat from subcutaneous stores to visceral abdominal fat may have beneficial metabolic effects

8. Which of these is *true* regarding the effect of sun exposure and sunscreen?
    a. Only ultraviolet B radiation is considered to be carcinogenic, and there is no suspected link between ultraviolet A radiation and melanoma
    b. The National Institutes of Health states that with typical use, sunscreens will significantly retard vitamin D production
    c. Sunscreen must have a sun protection factor (SPF) of 15 or higher to claim reduction in skin cancer

9. Which statement best describes the effect of hormone therapy (HT) on skin?
    a. Systemic HT has been shown to limit the loss of skin collagen, maintain skin thickness, and improve elasticity
    b. Systemic HT reduces the effect of genetic aging and damage from sun exposure
    c. Systemic HT reduces the risk of skin cancer but increases skin pigmentation (eg, chloasma)

10. Female pattern hair loss and telogen effluvium are the most common causes of hair loss in postmenopausal women. Work up of the patient with hair loss should *not* include
    a. A detailed history including clinical history; family history; hair loss history, including duration; pattern and percentage of loss; history of skin conditions; dietary and hair-care history
    b. A superficial skin biopsy of the scalp that includes several intact follicles
    c. Laboratory studies, including a complete blood count, comprehensive metabolic panel, thyroid function tests, and iron, ferritin, and zinc levels

11. Dry eye syndrome is one of the most common ocular complaints in menopausal patients. Which of these best describes the symptoms and initial treatment?
    a. Decreased tearing and increased intraocular pressure. Treat initially with systemic steroids.
    b. Dryness, scratchiness, and burning. Treat initially with ocular lubricants such as drops, gels, or ointments.
    c. Decreased visual acuity and excessive tearing. Treat initially with high-dose, oral estrogen.

12. The recommended approach to evaluating hearing loss in postmenopausal patients is to
    a. Use a self-assessment questionnaire, because they are inexpensive and 70% to 80% accurate
    b. Order audiometric testing on all patients aged older than 65 years
    c. Wait to hear complaints from the patient

13. Which of these statements is *false*?
    a. The rate of systemic bone loss is a predictor of tooth loss
    b. Fluctuations in sex hormones have been implicated in gingival inflammation
    c. Postmenopausal women are less susceptible to dental caries

Chapter 3. Clinical Issues
14. When assessing the etiology of sexual complaints, one should
    a. Assess biological factors initially and then proceed to psychological considerations if needed
    b. Assess biological and psychological factors to develop a differential diagnosis
    c. Assess psychological, sociocultural, interpersonal, and biological factors

15. Choose the *correct* statement.
    a. Most women do not have spontaneous desire
    b. Desire is composed of drive; belief, values, and expectations; and motivational components
    c. Low desire correlates well with serum dehydroepiandrosterone (DHEA) levels

16. Choose the *incorrect* statement.
    a. Only 3% of US women initiate a discussion of sexual problems with their healthcare providers
    b. Many patients think their doctors will dismiss their sexual concerns
    c. Women without sexual partners do not need counseling about sexual function

Chapter 4. Disease Risk
17. The American College of Cardiology/American Heart Association 2013 risk calculator assesses major risk factors for cardiovascular disease. Which important risk factor is not included when using this Web-based tool?
    a. Smoking
    b. Sex
    c. Family history

18. Oral estrogen with or without an oral progestogen increases risk for which of these conditions?
    a. Colon cancer
    b. Breast cancer
    c. Stroke

19. Your 59-year-old patient tripped and fell in the parking lot. The fall resulted in a vertebral fracture. You order a dual-energy x-ray absorptiometry (DXA) bone mineral density test. It shows that her bone density T-score is +0.9 at the femoral neck and +0.3 at the lumbar spine. Which of these diagnoses should be assigned?
    a. Normal
    b. Low bone density (osteopenia)
    c. Osteoporosis

20. After hip fracture, what proportion of women will require long-term care?
    a. 5%
    b. 10%
    c. 25%

21. Your 63-year-old patient has a T-score of −1.1 at the femoral neck and +0.9 at the lumbar spine. What is the most appropriate next step?
    a. Suggest treatment now because her T-score at the femoral neck is in the low bone density range
    b. Initiate therapy only if her 10-year predicted risk is ≥3% for hip fracture or ≥20% for major osteoporotic fracture
    c. Suggest that she increase her calcium and vitamin D and recheck bone density in 1 year

22. Which of these statements regarding osteoporosis medications is *true*?
    a. Bisphosphonates are associated with atypical femoral fractures
    b. Dental surgery is contraindicated in patients taking bisphosphonate therapy
    c. Teriparatide has been shown to reduce the risk of hip fractures
    d. Raloxifene reduces the risk of hip fractures

Chapter 5 Clinical Evaluation and Counseling

23. The most appropriate statement about history-taking is
    a. Given time constraints, it is best to review only menopausal symptoms and chief complaint
    b. Review problem list and chief complaint and proceed to physical exam
    c. Include review of symptoms and gynecologic, obstetric, serious illness, surgical, medication, sexual, psychologic, social, and family history

24. Which statement describes the best approach to managing modifiable risk factors?
    a. Discuss only the health risk factors the patient is interested in addressing
    b. Take a complete inventory of risk factors and health habits, educating the patient about the consequences of identified behaviors and providing support and tools to improve their lifestyle
    c. Because the patient who is overweight or obese may be uncomfortable discussing weight, let her other providers discuss it

25. Which statement about screening for common conditions is *false*?
    a. All postmenopausal women, regardless of age, should be screened for osteoporosis with dual-energy x-ray absorptiometry (DXA)
    b. Women aged older than 65 years with adequate negative cervical screening and no cervical intraepithelial neoplasia 2 or greater within the last 20 years need no further cervical cytology screening
    c. Screening for breast cancer-susceptibility genes requires availability of adequate resources to support the patient with positive results

26. Which statement is *most correct* about counseling?
    a. Topics that may be uncomfortable for the patient to discuss should be avoided
    b. When counseling, the clinician should use direct and nonjudgmental language that is culturally appropriate
    c. Same-sex couples are less likely to be affected by substance abuse and intimate partner violence and don't need to be screened for either

27. Quality of life (QOL) has become increasingly valued as a therapeutic outcome. Which statement about assessment is *incorrect* when describing QOL evaluation in the menopausal patient?
    a. Menopause-specific QOL scales (eg, Greene Climacteric Scale) may be categorized into 3 factors: vasomotor, somatic, and psychological
    b. The effect of hormone therapy on general quality of life (GQOL) is well documented and strongly associated with therapeutic effect
    c. Some QOL scales include mobility, self-care, usual activities, pain/discomfort, and anxiety/depression

Chapter 6. Complementary and Alternative Medicine

28. A postmenopausal woman aged 53 years is interested in starting black cohosh to help with mild vasomotor symptoms; however, she is concerned about its potential risks. Which one of these statements about black cohosh is *true*?
    a. Black cohosh causes heavy uterine bleeding so should be avoided in women who have fibroids or a clotting disorder
    b. Several case reports of kidney failure with black cohosh have been reported, so it should be avoided in women who have poor renal function
    c. Gastrointestinal adverse effects may occur with the first use of black cohosh

29. Which one of these statements about isoflavones is *true*?
    a. Isoflavones have a greater affinity for the estrogen-receptor (ER)-α than for the ER-β
    b. Evidence that isoflavones prevent bone loss in postmenopausal women is lacking
    c. Soy isoflavones in high doses consistently decrease breast cancer risk in postmenopausal women

30. Which one of these herbal therapies should be avoided if a woman is on an anticoagulant such as warfarin?
    a. Dong quai
    b. Vitex
    c. Licorice

Chapter 7. Nonprescription Options

31. Which statement is *true* regarding the DSHEA (Dietary Supplement Health Education Act of 1994)?
    a. Under the DSHEA, FDA is responsible for determining whether claims made about a dietary supplement are substantiated by adequate evidence
    b. Dietary-supplement marketers can make health claims for *natural conditions* (eg, hot flashes, age-related memory loss) without providing documentation for efficacy and safety
    c. FDA, not the manufacturer, is responsible for ensuring that package labels on dietary supplements are truthful and not misleading and that all ingredients and dose information is listed

32. 2011 Institute of Medicine (IOM) recommendations for dietary intake of vitamin D include
    a. 600 IU per day for adults aged 70 years and younger
    b. 800 IU per day for adults aged older than 70 years
    c. Setting tolerable upper limit of intake at 4,000 IU per day
    d. a and b only
    e. a, b, and c

33. Which of these statements regarding calcium supplementation in postmenopausal women is *false*?
    a. For women aged 40 to 60 years, median calcium intake from food sources alone is less than 600 mg per day
    b. Calcium intake is optimized if supplements are taken in 1 single dose without food
    c. Adverse events from recommended levels of calcium supplementation include nephrolithiasis

Chapter 8. Prescription Therapies

34. Which of these noncontraceptive uses of levonorgestrel-releasing intrauterine systems (LNG-IUS) in the United States is an approved FDA indication?
    a. To prevent bleeding and endometrial hyperplasia in postmenopausal women using estrogen therapy
    b. To treat heavy menstrual bleeding in women desiring to use intrauterine contraception
    c. To relieve pain associated with endometriosis

35. FDA has revised the label of these progestin-containing products to report that there may be a 3-fold increase in the risk of venous thromboembolism:
    a. Levonorgestrel-containing products
    b. Norgestimate-containing products
    c. Drospirenone-containing products

36. Compounded hormone therapy has been proven safe and has few risks.
    a. True
    b. False

37. Which of these are noncontraceptive benefits of combination oral contraceptives for perimenopausal women?
    a. Regulation of irregular menses
    b. Reduction of vasomotor symptoms
    c. Decreased risk of ovarian and endometrial cancer
    d. All of the above

38. What percentage of women reach menopause by age 55?
    a. 70%
    b. 80%
    c. 90%

39. Which of these statements is *false*?
    a. Estradiol is the most potent human estrogen
    b. Estriol reduces breast cancer
    c. Estrone is the most abundant circulating estrogen in postmenopausal women

40. The low-dose estradiol vaginal ring (Estring) is FDA approved for
    a. Vaginal atrophy/Genitourinary syndrome of menopause
    b. Dyspareunia from vaginal atrophy
    c. Urinary urgency and dysuria from vaginal atrophy
    d. All of the above

MENOPAUSE PRACTICE: A CLINICIAN'S GUIDE, 5th edition
CME ANSWER SHEET

Please circle the letter corresponding with the correct answer.

1.	a.	b.		11.	a.	b.	c.	21.	a.	b.	c.	31.	a.	b.	c.	
2.	a.	b.	c.	12.	a.	b.	c.	22.	a.	b.	c.	d.	32.	a.	b.	c.	d.	e.
3.	a.	b.	c.	13.	a.	b.	c.	23.	a.	b.	c.	33.	a.	b.	c.	
4.	a.	b.	c.	14.	a.	b.	c.	24.	a.	b.	c.	34.	a.	b.	c.	
5.	a.	b.		15.	a.	b.	c.	25.	a.	b.	c.	35.	a.	b.	c.	
6.	a.	b.	c.	16.	a.	b.	c.	26.	a.	b.	c.	36.	a.	b.		
7.	a.	b.	c.	17.	a.	b.	c.	27.	a.	b.	c.	37.	a.	b.	c.	d.
8.	a.	b.	c.	18.	a.	b.	c.	28.	a.	b.	c.	38.	a.	b.	c.	
9.	a.	b.	c.	19.	a.	b.	c.	29.	a.	b.	c.	39.	a.	b.	c.	
10.	a.	b.	c.	20.	a.	b.	c.	30.	a.	b.	c.	40.	a.	b.	c.	d.

Post-Test Evaluation

After completing this activity, do you feel prepared to
___ Initiate discussion with patients on menopause and healthy aging, including the effect on quality of life and sexuality?
___ Perform appropriate clinical assessments to diagnose conditions of menopause and aging, assess health risks, and identify any contraindications to medications?
___ Discuss a full range of management options with patients, based on their health risks, goals, and preferences?
___ Collaborate with other healthcare professionals to offer effective, individualized therapy for menopause symptoms and conditions?
___ Instruct and encourage patients to achieve a healthy lifestyle?

Do you face any barriers to achieving these objectives in your menopause practice? (Choose all that apply.)
___ Time   ___ Organizational/Institutional   ___ Financial   ___ Patient education/Compliance
___ Other (please explain) _____

What is your profession?
___ Physician (medical doctor or surgeon)   ___ Medical Resident   ___ Nurse   ___ Nurse Midwife
___ Nurse Practitioner   ___ Physician Assistant   ___ Pharmacist   ___ Researcher-Nonphysician
___ Dietitian or Nutritionist   ___ Mental Health Professional (nonphysician)   ___ Media/Publishing/Writing
___ Product Industry (eg, pharma)   ___ Other learner

To Apply for CME Credit

Learners may return this completed answer sheet and post-test evaluation form to NAMS by mail or fax or by emailing a scanned copy by the activity's expiration date of **October 15, 2017**, to

The North American Menopause Society
5900 Landerbrook Drive, Suite 390
Mayfield Heights, OH 44124
Fax: 440-442-2660
Email: nams@menopause.org

Keep a copy for your file. Each participant will receive a confidential report of the results along with the correct answer to each question. A certificate of credit will be sent to those who successfully complete the examination.

Name (please print) _____

Address _____

City _____

State/Province _____   **Zip/Country Code** _____   **Country** _____

Telephone _____   **Fax** _____   **Email** _____